D1201527

Atlas of CLINICAL SLEEP MEDICINE

Meir H. Kryger, MD, FRCPC
Clinical Professor of Medicine
University of Connecticut
Director of Research and Education
Gaylord Hospital Sleep Medicine
Wallingford, Connecticut

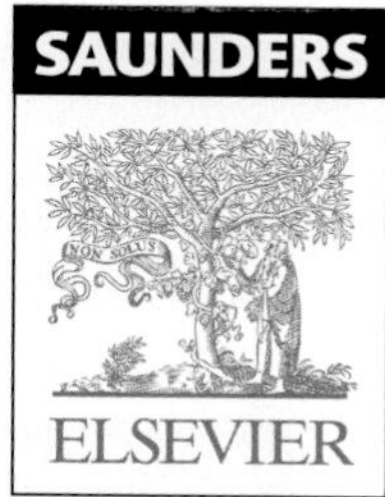

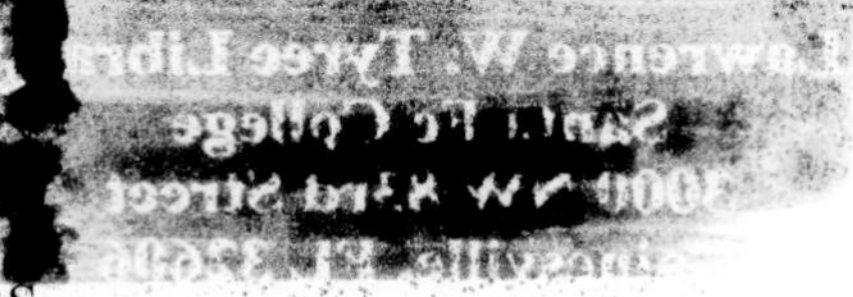

SAUNDERS
ELSEVIER

1600 John F. Kennedy Blvd.
Ste 1800
Philadelphia, PA 19103-2899

ATLAS OF CLINICAL SLEEP MEDICINE

ISBN 978-1-4160-4711-7

NOTICE

Knowledge and best practice in this field are constantly changing. As new research and experience broaden our knowledge, changes in practice, treatment and drug therapy may become necessary or appropriate. Readers are advised to check the most current information provided (i) on procedures featured or (ii) by the manufacturer of each product to be administered, to verify the recommended dose or formula, the method and duration of administration, and contraindications. It is the responsibility of the practitioner, relying on his or her own experience and knowledge of the patient, to make diagnoses, to determine dosages and the best treatment for each individual patient, and to take all appropriate safety precautions. To the fullest extent of the law, neither the Publisher nor the Editors assumes any liability for any injury and/or damage to persons or property arising out of or related to any use of the material contained in this book.

The Publisher

Library of Congress Cataloging-in-Publication Data
Atlas of clinical sleep medicine / [edited by] Meir Kryger.
p. ; cm.
Includes bibliographical references.
ISBN 978-1-4160-4711-7
1. Sleep disorders—Atlases. I. Kryger, Meir H.
[DNLM: 1. Sleep Disorders—diagnosis—Atlases. 2. Sleep—physiology—Atlases.
WM 17 A8812 2010]
RC547.A835 2010
616.8′498—dc22 2009002027

Acquisitions Editor: Dolores Meloni
Developmental Editor: Julia Bartz
Project Manager: Bryan Hayward
Design Direction: Steven Stave

Printed in China

Last digit is the print number: 9 8 7 6 5 4 3 2 1

This book is dedicated to
Barbara Rosenblum Kryger,
my wife, lifelong partner, and friend, who has been my muse, my inspiration, and my support

Contributors

Negar Ahmadi, MSc
Youthdale Child and Adolescent Sleep Centre, Toronto Western Hospital
Toronto, ON, Canada
Chapter 16

Todd Arnedt, PhD
Clinical Assistant Professor of Psychiatry and Neurology, University of Michigan Medical Center
Ann Arbor, MI
Chapter 7

Alon Y. Avidan, MD, MPH
Neurology Residency Program Director, Medical Director, UCLA Neurology Clinic
Associate Director, Sleep Disorders Center, Department of Neurology,
University of California–Los Angeles
Los Angeles, CA
Chapters 4, 10

Gregory Belenky, MD
Research Professor, Sleep and Performance Research Center and Program in Neuroscience, Washington State University
Spokane, WA
Chapter 3.3

Stewart Bohnet
Department of Veterinary and Comparative Anatomy, Pharmacology and Physiology,
Washington State University
Pullman, WA
Chapter 3.5

Frances Boquiren, BA
Student and Research Assistant, University of Toronto
Editorial Assistant, Department of Psychiatry, Toronto Western Hospital
Toronto, ON, Canada
Chapter 1

Victoria Boquiren, BSc
Ontario College of Art and Design
Toronto, ON, Canada
Chapter 1

Michel A. Cramer Bornemann, MD
Assistant Professor, Department of Neurology, University of Minnesota Medical School
Co-director, Minnesota Regional Sleep Disorders Center, Hennepin County Medical Center
Minneapolis, MN
Chapter 12

Orfeu Buxton, PhD
Instructor in Medicine, Division of Sleep Medicine, Harvard Medical School
Associate Neuroscientist, Brigham and Women's Hospital
Boston, MA
Chapters 3.1, 3.2

Ronald D. Chervin, MD, MS
Professor of Neurology, Michael S. Aldrich Collegiate Professor of Sleep Medicine
Director, University of Michigan Sleep Disorders Center, University of Michigan Medical School, University of Michigan Health System
Ann Arbor, MI
Chapter 7

Danny Eckert, PhD
Postdoctoral Fellow, Division of Sleep Medicine, Brigham and Women's Hospital
Boston, MA
Chapter 3.6

Carlo Franzini, MD
Professor of Physiology, Department of Human and General Physiology, Università di Bologna
Bologna, Italy
Chapter 3.8

Patrick M. Fuller, PhD
Instructor in Neurology, Harvard Medical School, Beth Israel Deaconess Medical Center
Boston, MA
Chapter 3.1

Charles F. P. George, MD, FRCPC, FCCP
Professor of Medicine, University of Western Ontario
Medical Director, Sleep Medicine Clinic, London Health Sciences Centre
London, ON, Canada
Chapters 14.4, 14.5

Ronald M. Harper, PhD
Distinguished Professor of Neurobiology, David Geffen School of Medicine at UCLA
Los Angeles, CA
Chapter 3.7

Don Hayes, Jr., MD
Assistant Professor, Division of Pediatrics and Internal Medicine
Medical Director, University of Kentucky Healthcare Children's Sleep Program
Associate Medical Director, University of Kentucky Healthcare Sleep Disorders Center, University of Kentucky College of Medicine
Lexington, KY
Chapter 11.2

Max Hirshkowitz, PhD
Associate (tenured) Professor, Baylor College of Medicine, Department of Medicine and Menninger Department of Psychiatry
Clinical Director, Sleep Disorders and Research Center, Michael E. DeBakey Veterans Affairs Medical Center
Houston, TX
Chapters 17, 18

Shahrokh Javaheri, MD
Professor Emeritus, University of Cincinnati
Medical Director, Sleepcare Diagnostics, VA Medical Center and Sleepcare Diagnostics
Cincinnati, OH
Chapter 13

Levente Kapás, MD
Associate Professor, WWAMI Medical Education Program, Washington State University
Spokane, WA
Chapter 3.9

James M. Krueger, PhD
Regents Professor, Sleep and Performance Research Center and Program in Neuroscience, Department of Veterinary and Comparative Anatomy, Pharmacology and Physiology, Washington State University
Pullman, WA
Chapters 3.3, 3.5, 3.9

Meir H. Kryger, MD, FRCPC
Clinical Professor of Medicine, University of Connecticut
Director of Research and Education, Gaylord Hospital Sleep Medicine
Wallingford, CT
Chapters 2, 9, 11.1, 11.3, 14.1, 14.2, 18, 19, 20

Carol A. Landis, DNSc
Professor, Department of Biobehavioral Nursing and Health Systems, University of Washington
Seattle, WA
Chapter 15.4

Kathryn A. Lee, RN, PhD
Professor, University of California, San Francisco
San Francisco, CA
Chapters 15.1, 15.3

Rachel Leproult, PhD
Department of Medicine, University of Chicago
Chicago, IL
Chapter 3.10

Victor Leyva-Grado, DMV, PhD
Department of Veterinary and Comparative Anatomy, Pharmacology and Physiology, Washington State University
Pullman, WA
Chapter 3.5

Mark W. Mahowald, MD
Professor, Department of Neurology, University of Minnesota Medical School
Director, Minnesota Regional Sleep Disorders Center, Hennepin County Medical Center
Minneapolis, MN
Chapter 12

Atul Malhotra, PhD
Medical Director, Brigham Sleep Disorders Research Program, Brigham and Women's Hospital
Boston, MA
Chapter 3.6

Wallace B. Mendelson, MD
Professor of Psychiatry and Clinical Pharmacology (retired), University of Chicago
Chicago, IL
Chapter 5

Tore A. Nielsen, PhD
Professor, Department of Psychiatry, Université de Montréal
Director, Dream and Nightmare Laboratory, Hôspital du Sacré-Coeur de Montréal
Montréal, QC, Canada
Chapter 6

William C. Orr, PhD
President and CEO, Lynn Health Science Institute
Clinical Professor of Medicine, Oklahoma University Health Sciences Center
Oklahoma City, OK
Chapter 14.3

Pier Luigi Parmeggiani, MD
Professor Emeritus, Department of Human and General Physiology, Università di Bologna
Bologna, Italy
Chapter 3.4

Barbara Phillips, MD, MSPH
Professor, Division of Pulmonary, Critical Care, and Sleep Medicine, University of Kentucky College of Medicine
Director, Sleep Center, University of Kentucky Healthcare Good Samaritan Hospital
Lexington, KY
Chapter 11.2

David M. Rector, PhD
Associate Professor, Department of Veterinary and Comparative Anatomy, Pharmacology and Physiology, Washington State University
Pullman, WA
Chapter 3.3

Kathryn J. Reid, PhD
Department of Neurology, Northwestern University Feinberg School of Medicine
Evanston, IL
Chapters 3.2, 8

Dominic Roca, MD
Director, Connecticut Center for Sleep Medicine
Pulmonary Intensivist, Stamford Hospital
Stamford, CT
Chapter 3.6

Thomas Roth, PhD
Sleep Disorders and Research Center, Henry Ford Hospital
Detroit, MI
Chapter 9

Philip Saleh, MSc
Youthdale Child and Adolescent Sleep Centre, Toronto Western Hospital
Toronto, ON, Canada
Chapter 16

Carlos H. Schenck, MD
Professor, Department of Psychiatry, University of Minnesota Medical School
Staff Psychiatrist, Minnesota Regional Sleep Disorders Center, Hennepin County Medical Center
Minneapolis, MN
Chapter 12

Colin M. Shapiro, BSc (Hons), MBB Ch, PhD, MRC Psych, FRPC(C)
Professor of Psychiatry, University of Toronto
Director of Neuropsychiatry, Youthdale Child and Adolescent Sleep Centre, Toronto Western Hospital
Toronto, ON, Canada
Chapters 1, 16

Amir Sharafkhaneh, MD, PhD
Assistant Professor, Baylor College of Medicine
Medical Director, Sleep Disorders Center, Michael E. DeBakey Veterans Affairs Medical Center
Houston, TX
Chapter 17

Deena Sherman, BA
Toronto, ON, Canada
Chapter 1

Karine Spiegel, PhD
INSERM / UCBL–U628, Physiologie intégrée du système d'éveil Département de Médecine Expérimentale, Faculté de Médecine, Université Claude Bernard
Lyon, France
Chapter 3.10

Leslie Swanson, PhD
Postdoctoral Fellow, University of Michigan Medical Center
Ann Arbor, MI
Chapter 7

Éva Szentirmai, MD
Assistant Professor, WWAMI Medical Education Program, Washington State University
Seattle, WA
Chapter 3.9

Eve Van Cauter, PhD
Professor, Department of Medicine, The University of Chicago
Chicago, IL
Chapter 3.10

Hans P. A. Van Dongen, PhD
Research Professor, Sleep and Performance Research Center, Washington State University
Spokane, WA
Chapter 3.3

Richard L. Verrier, PhD
Associate Professor of Medicine, Harvard Medical School, Cardiology Division, Beth Israel Deaconess Medical Center
Boston MA
Chapter 3.7

Susie Yim Yeh, MD
Pulmonary Intensivist, Division of Sleep Medicine, Brigham and Women's Hospital
Boston, MA
Chapter 3.6

Kin M. Yuen, MD, MS
Medical Director, Bay Sleep Clinic
Adjunct Clinical Instructor, Stanford University
Menlo Park, CA
Chapter 15.2

Phyllis C. Zee, MD, PhD
Department of Neurology, Northwestern University
Feinberg School of Medicine
Evanston, IL
Chapters 3.1, 3.2, 8

Michael Zupancic, MD
Pacific Sleep Medicine Services
San Diego, CA
Chapter 7

Foreword

During the Renaissance, scientists were often also artists. They had the mental agility to move back and forth between the sciences and the arts with ease and, more important, to integrate them. This led to each one influencing the other. Science affected the way art was created, and science was depicted in creative artistic formats. With the evolution of art into new forms that did not have much to do with science and the separate specialization of science, these two important human endeavors drifted far apart. If one searches the history of sleep, until the 1950s, it was encountered more frequently in the world of art than in the world of science. Artists depicted nightmares and night terrors, and authors described, with amazing accuracy, individuals who had various sleep disorders ranging from insomnia to sleep apnea. The description by Charles Dickens of Joe the fat boy in *The Pickwick Papers* describes the signs and symptoms of obstructive sleep apnea syndrome with uncanny accuracy.

In the 1950s, Drs. Aserinsky, Dement, and Kleitman ushered in the modern era of sleep research with their discovery of rapid eye movement (REM) sleep and the association of REM sleep and dreaming. This discovery promised to help gain insight into the nature of the mind–body connection. For the first time, scientists had a mental event, the dream, and a clear physiological correlate, REM sleep. Also, the nightly occurrence of REM sleep and its associated visual hallucinations was thought to provide insights into the nature of mental disorders that are characterized by waking hallucinations. While neither of these hopes came to fruition, this new discipline shed light on a third of our existence that was virtually unexplored. By analogy to geology, it was as though an additional third of the world's land mass was discovered. Questions arose such as: What do the brain and body do in sleep? What is the biologic basis of the dreams and nightmare we all experience, and what is their significance? Why do some people have difficulty sleeping whereas others cannot even stay awake during the day? With the observation that the control of many physiologic processes differed as a function of state (wake, REM, and NREM), the field of sleep medicine was born. Clearly one can have normal physiologic function while awake and serious pathophysiology while asleep.

Interestingly, as sleep medicine became a new discipline, artists were still fascinated with this mysterious third of existence. Thus, sleep medicine evolved in a parallel course with the depiction of sleep and dreams by authors and artists. The aim of this book is to meld the science of sleep with the arts. Previous Atlases have depicted polysomnograms associated with various aspects of sleep physiology and sleep disorders. Several other edited books have provided the reader with a broad understanding of sleep and its disorders. In fact, Dr. Kryger has written and edited several of these texts. Here the goal is more integrative: it is to give the reader an intellectual as well as sensory appreciation of the science of sleep and the practice of sleep disorders medicine. Not only is this book different in its approach, the content is also broader. Along with an in-depth presentation of sleep physiology and pathophysiology, there are chapters on the history of sleep as well as the depiction of sleep in the arts. This book aims not only to inform how to take a history from a sleep disorder patient, but also to educate what other individuals with this sleep disorder look like, what the patient's sleep study looks and sounds like, and how a patient's disorder is depicted in the arts. Thus, one will not only gain a familiarity with the disorder, but also a comfort in knowing all aspects of the patient's care management.

This book explains why sleep studies are run all night rather than sampling sleep for a few hours, what types of sleep studies are needed for which patients, and why highly prevalent sleep disorders went unnoticed by the medical community for decades. This book attempts to define the aspects of sleep that are essential to maximize an individual's productivity and health.

For non-sleep clinicians, this book will not only make them comfortable with the science of sleep, but it will give them a sense of what it is like to enter a sleep laboratory, what types of information can be gained from a sleep study, and, most important, what their patient will experience when a referral for a sleep study is made. For the sleep researcher/sleep clinician, this book will provide in-depth coverage of the sleep field with topics ranging from sleep history to basic sleep neurophysiology to the identification, diagnosis, and management of sleep medicine. For all of us, this book will not only stimulate our intellect but also our senses.

Thomas Roth
Detroit, Michigan, 2009

Preface

Our understanding of sleep and sleep disorders is fairly recent. Rapid eye movement (REM) sleep was first described in the same year as Watson and Crick published their important findings on the structure of DNA. Most people consider the discovery of REM the beginning of sleep science and sleep medicine. Up to that time, sleep was seldom mentioned by scientists but had been a topic for philosophers, such as Aristotle; playwrights, such as Shakespeare; novelists, such as Charles Dickens; and many visual artists, such as Vincent van Gogh. The visual artists did not simply portray sleep as a restful phase, but at times recorded the danger that sleep might bring.

In this book we are trying something new. We are trying to add to the knowledge about sleep by not simply focusing on words to transmit that knowledge, but also to use still and moving images and sounds to enhance the understanding of the science of sleep. I began by asking myself, "How would a great scientist and artist have tackled this job?" I immediately thought about Leonardo da Vinci and wondered how he would do such a project. I believe that he would have combined words with engaging visual imagery and whatever else was available in the scientific and communication universe of his day.

This book is substantially different than any book I've worked on before. Sleep medicine is a multidisciplinary field that is so much more than just sleep recordings—it is a perfect specialty in which to use multimedia for learning. Having grown up in medical school with Netter's brilliant atlases, my goal was to produce a volume in the spirit of Netter while including more types of content (images, videos, sleep recordings) than is possible with a conventional book. Putting together this book was like working on a painting—a giant mural. We had ideas about the information we wanted to convey, and we pondered how to use multimedia to present the knowledge, with a book being the anchor. I would like to thank the authors for the brilliant job they have done in capturing sleep medicine in a visual form.

I have always believed that knowledge of a medical field is not simply mastering the clinical facts but also understanding the interaction of history, the arts, and the scientific base that lead to the clinical facts. The anatomic drawings of Leonardo da Vinci remind us of the potential beauty of learning about science.

This is not the editor's first attempt at having at creating a multimedia platform for sleep disorders. Many years ago, I put together *Journey into Sleep*, a program that was CD-based that could link to Internet sites. The publishing world was convinced, as was I, that the physical book printed on paper was dead. We were all wrong. About a decade ago, it became apparent that CDs and DVDs as primary sources of content were doomed because the Internet was so much more convenient and that is where people expect to find certain types of content. However, physical books survived and have flourished. This book and its multimedia content were made possible by a flurry of recent technological changes: high-speed Internet, inexpensive mass storage, high-resolution graphics cards and computer displays, digital photography, and sleep data acquisition systems. There are many photographs in the Atlas. Acquiring the images required a high-resolution camera that could fit into a pocket. Patients were delighted that their images would be used for teaching and they gave permission to include them.

Previously, sleep medicine atlases displayed data originally collected on paper, which resulted in images that could be changed with great difficulty, and they could not emphasize certain teaching points easily. The examples in this book represent what is actually seen in the modern sleep disorders center, warts and all, using various data acquisition systems. The traces shown are real, and the montages used are those that enhance understanding and clarity.

By using digital data acquisition and analysis systems, we are able to emphasize the important teaching points much more easily than when paper was used. We are able to change the time base, compress the data, and split the screen so that the neurophysiologic variables can be shown optimally while the cardiorespiratory variables can be shown optimally as well using a different time base. It is as easy to see 8 hours on the screen as 30 seconds.

A clinician in sleep medicine uses information from several sources to establish a diagnosis and to determine optimal treatment. These sources include interviews with the patient, examination of the patient, evaluation of tests, and integration of this data with a knowledge base that includes understanding of the relevant pathophysiology. In a clinical learning setting, the mentor will transmit information to the trainee about each of these phases in the clinical interaction. In this book, we are attempting to emulate all parts of the process. We learn a great deal from what a patient tells us in his or her own words and from observing and evaluating the data. I hope that what is presented is helpful to the clinician and ultimately the patient. It is the patient who will benefit the most, and it is from the patient we learn the most.

We use the scoring rules recently published and explain them and show the reader not simply how to score but how to understand. We chose not to be constrained by the recommended epoch length and rules but to build from them and use the tools provided by modern systems to display the data as a clinician might in order to understand the signals coming from an ill patient.

The purpose of the book is to produce an atlas that would be useful for anyone wanting to learn about sleep. We hope that this work pleases the reader. We know it is not perfect, and as careful as we tried to be, we realize that readers will probably find errors. It is our hope that readers will provide us the feedback to help guide us as this book evolves.

Technical Details

All of the images and videos of patients, and sleep traces were obtained digitally in working sleep disorder centers.

Most of the photos and patient interviews were taken with small digital cameras that could fit into a pocket. The photos were usually captured using 5 or 8 megapixels. The patient video interviews were also taken with the same digital camera with a screen size of 640 by 480 pixels at 29 frames per second. The videos of sleeping patients were taken from data captured during the sleep recording. The images are in black and white (there is no "color" when using an infrared light source in the dark) and were compressed to the MPEG 4 format during acquisition. Most of the videos shown are totally unedited. When editing was necessary, Adobe Premier Elements, Quicktime, or Microsoft Moviemaker was used.

Almost all the sleep recordings were captured using a screen resolution of 1600 x 1200 pixels. The data were stored in the highest resolution without compression, if possible. These are working polysomnographic traces and they may not be the perfect configuration as described in scoring manuals, but they represent what is actually seen in the sleep disorders center. It is the editor's hope that the reader will learn how to best interpret and understand what is seen. That is the purpose of this atlas. The digitized images were then processed by artists at Elsevier to supply a uniform look and feel so that the overall appearance of the records had some visual consistency.

These photos and records span many years; thus, there is some variability in the resolution just as there is variability in the resolution of data acquisition systems. The screenshots obtained represent the spectrum of the most widely used data acquisition systems including Compumedics, Grass, Nihon Kohden, and Respironics.

Meir Kryger
Hamden, Connecticut
December, 2008

The Polysomnogram Recordings

The polysomnograms in the Atlas were generated from various data acquisition systems and represent the style of image obtained using the most commonly used modern systems and at times from older systems. Most often are shown the display and montage that someone interpreting the record might use. Frequently that would involve splitting the display into two windows: an upper window that displays the channels used for the recording and staging of sleep (most often a 30-second epoch) and a lower window that displays the channels used to best document movements and sleep breathing disorders (the epoch length usually varying from 30 seconds up to 10 minutes, depending on the abnormality being observed). The polysomnograms from the Atlas and other sources can also be viewed on the book's website in a size more closely approximating what might be seen on one's computer display.

Below are examples of the styles used when two windows are shown. The blue arrows point toward where the length of the epoch of the window is indicated.

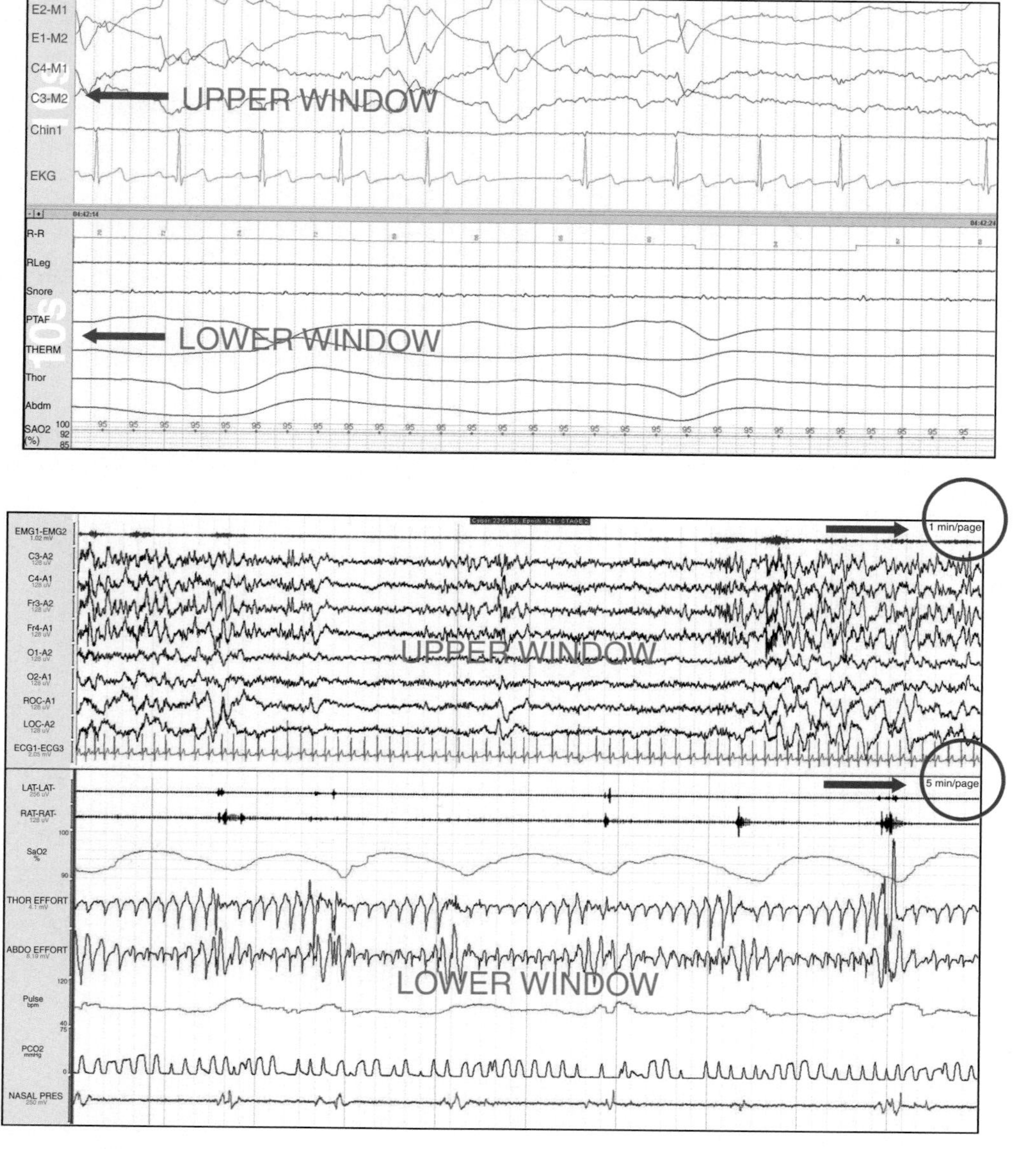

Acknowledgments

There are hundreds of people involved in the production of a book. These range from authors, to their editorial assistant secretaries, to the staff at Elsevier. It is not possible to name all the people that have played an important role in such a book. I thank them all.

I would like to thank the staff at Elsevier. I proposed a type of book that had not been produced before—a volume using still images and videos to teach about sleep. Elsevier encouraged the project from the very beginning. There were many technical and editorial challenges. I would like to thank Dolores Meloni, my editor at Elsevier, for her unwavering support. I would like to thank Julia Bartz, the developmental editor, who displayed never-ending calm and patience at every step. I would like to thank the design staff for the beautiful work they have done. I would like to thank the technical staff for having developed innovative methods to deal with the technical challenges at every step of the way.

I would like to thank the authors who have done a magnificent job in visually presenting information that normally would be described in words. It was not an easy task for them, and I thank them for their achievements.

I also want to thank Tom Roth and Bill Dement, who have always been an inspiration to me. The sleep field will never forget their important contributions to the health and safety of people around the world.

I would like to thank my family for understanding that I was trying to create something new.

Contents

Online Contents

CHAPTER 1

SLEEP IN ART AND LITERATURE

Colin M. Shapiro, Frances Boquiren, Victoria Boquiren, and Deena Sherman

It appears that every man's insomnia is as different from his neighbour's as are their daytime hopes and aspirations.

—F. Scott Fitzgerald

Anyone with the most rudimentary knowledge of sleep appreciates that there is light, medium, deep, and dreaming sleep (see Fig. 1-1).

The significance of these various levels and types of sleep has become much more appreciated over the last half-century. In the realm of the depiction of sleep and art there are a number of themes that repeatedly emerge. One is clearly the intense fascination with dreams and dream imagery. A second is religious themes, a third is the parallel between sleep and death, and for sleep researchers there is the depiction of sleeping individuals where a spot diagnosis might be attempted. Other themes include the issue of reward, abandonment of conscious control, and a depiction of innocence and serenity associated with sleep and the erotic.

The subject of sleep is revisited in art time and time again. Why do artists return to this inactive, common, basic human function? Certainly, a sleeping Venus is not as exciting as a dramatization of a bombing on a Spanish town or as uplifting as a starry night. The appeal of sleep lies in the fact that, although it is common, it is extremely complex. A sleeping woman takes on the posture of death but is very much alive. She is conscious but not cognizant. She lies physically in reality but her thoughts run in fantasy. Sleep delights, frightens, regenerates, and may even lead to fatigue. It can overpower like a heavy, irrepressible fog or elude us like the sweet thrills of happiness.

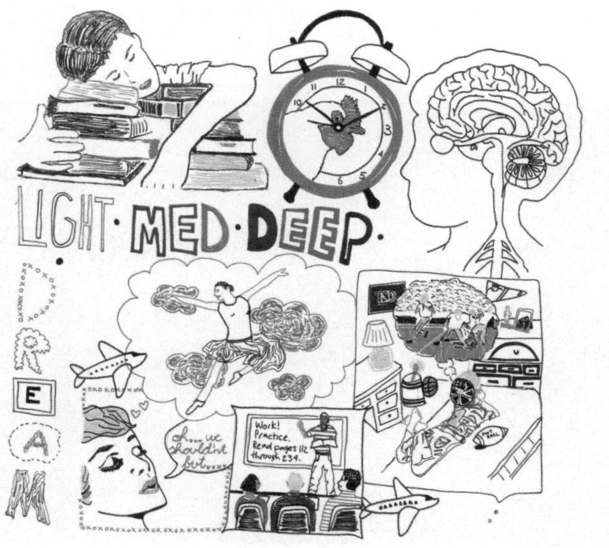

Figure 1-1.
Mahla Shapiro, *Light to Deep and Dreaming Sleep*, 2008.

Furthermore, although sleep is a basic human function, it is a unique experience for everybody. Thus, just as every man's sleeplessness differs from his neighbor's, so does his sleep. Sleep is a necessity and every person does it (or hopes to), but the actual experience cannot be shared. When one goes to sleep, he falls alone, and when he enters dreamland, he walks by himself. Here lies the appeal for artists. This inactive state contains so many connotations, evokes a large array of emotions, and holds an abundance of internal activity. How does one execute through painting one's experiences and thoughts on sleep? Artists encounter a great barrier to overcome in trying to convey a multifaceted action whose origins lie in inaction. It is extremely difficult for an artist to separate one sleeping figure who may represent strength in sleep from another that symbolizes vulnerability.

This chapter explores the various devices and methods artists use to articulate their explorations and understandings of sleep. Furthermore, it investigates the different themes and ideas that artists have had about this mysterious human experience.

Mythology

One way artists explore sleep is through mythology. Artists take advantage of the viewer's knowledge of and familiarity with the characters, stories, and settings of myth. This allows the artist to convey his or her definition of sleep by immersing it in these visual mythic cues. This is accomplished once the viewer recognizes these cues because it forces the viewer to ask herself, What are the implications of sleep in the context of the story?

An example of this is Sandro Botticelli's *Mars and Venus* (Fig. 1-2). In this painting, the fully clothed Venus sits at the left, upright and alert, whereas the sleeping Mars on the right lies languidly, incapacitated, exposed, and vulnerable. Venus appears to be in control while Mars is reduced to being a plaything for the baby satyrs. Thus, this painting likens the state of sleep to weakness. It is a powerful force that can overtake the god of war. Sleep is undesirable because it is capable of lowering the defenses of someone

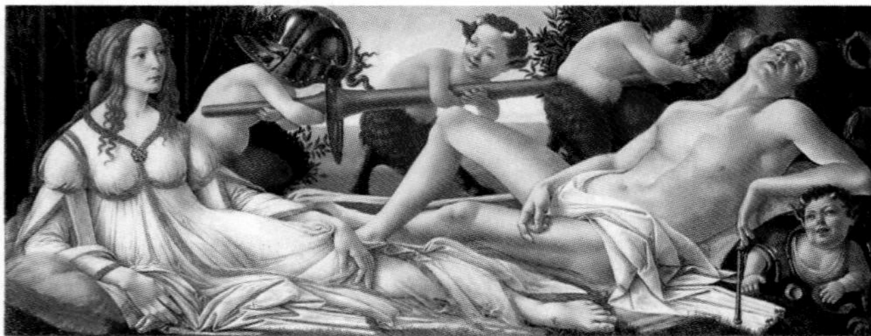

Figure 1-2.
Sandro Botticelli, *Mars and Venus*, ca. 1483. National Gallery of London.

as formidable as the god of war. The god of war becomes subject to humiliation. Furthermore, he has become prey to the outside world. This power of sleep is often not appreciated by patients, even those who suffer from sleep disorders, who may need to be reminded, for example, that sleep deprivation is used as a technique of torture. In other words, sleep is so highly necessary that "take those sleeping pills" may be the simplistic mantra.

Lorenzo Lotto's *Sleeping Apollo* (Fig. 1-3) portrays sleep in a manner similar to that of Botticelli's *Mars and Venus*. Once again, the sexes are divided; the naked female Muses are on the left and the slumbering Apollo sits on the right. Fame, who flies above Apollo, is ready to desert him and join the other Muses. The Muses have taken advantage of the sleeping Apollo to abandon their clothes and arts to frolic about.

Like Mars, Apollo is unaware of the activities of the waking world. The effects of sleep in both paintings produce a comic reaction. However, the way Mars and Apollo are portrayed in their sleep produces two decidedly different comic reactions. The sprawled, exposed sleeping Mars, with his own lance held by the baby satyrs, pointing at him, is an object to be ridiculed. The portrayal of sleeping Apollo is less negative. He sits more upright with what appears to be an instrument in his hand. He is depicted more like the dozing professor whose students have gone off to play.

Thus, sleep takes on a different meaning. The undignified position of Mars, the god of war, compounded with the connotations of strength, power, and chaos, portrays sleep as a weakening force that places one in a compromising position. On the other hand, in *Sleeping Apollo*, sleep appears not to take away strength or might, but reason. This is reinforced by the fact that Apollo is linked to reason and foresight. Sleep has removed him of rationality and made him completely oblivious to what has happened. This is further symbolized by the abandoning of the books and instruments of the Muses in front of him. Also, Apollo sits in the dark, enclosed by the trees; he is alone in the secluded realm of sleep and completely segregated from the outside world. Lack of rationality in sleep has become a key issue in the realm of forensic aspects of sleep, with recent media emphasis on the condition of sexsomnia and the consternation over the lack of mens rea in the sleeping state.

Giorgione's *Sleeping Venus* (Fig. 1-4), instead of two figures, has one, the female figure, who is sleeping. As in the other two paintings, Venus lies in a pastoral setting; but unlike in *Mars and Venus*, she is alone, and she is the one who is sleeping and nude. The curves of her body emulate the undulating hills. She has her left hand covering her genitals. This is an extremely erotic picture.

Sleep has taken on a different meaning here. Venus has become not someone to laugh at, like Mars or Apollo. Her strength or power or reason has not been taken away from her because of sleep. Rather, sexuality—which Venus is associated with—has become enhanced by sleep. According to Maria Ruvoldt, the conscious placement of her hand over her genitals refers to her procreative powers. Also, she has her right arm up to expose her armpit. This gesture is commonly associated with seduction in certain periods in Western art. Moreover, since the curves of her body imitate the landscape, there is a direct connection between her and nature, thus further associating her with fecundity.

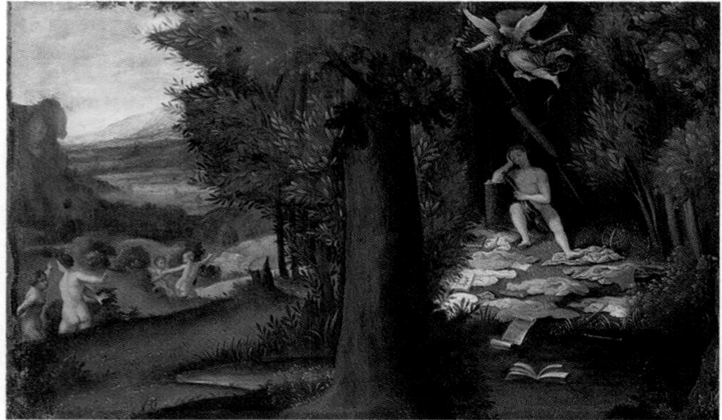

Figure 1-3.
Lorenzo Lotto, *Sleeping Apollo*, ca. 1530. Szepmuveseti Museum, Budapest.

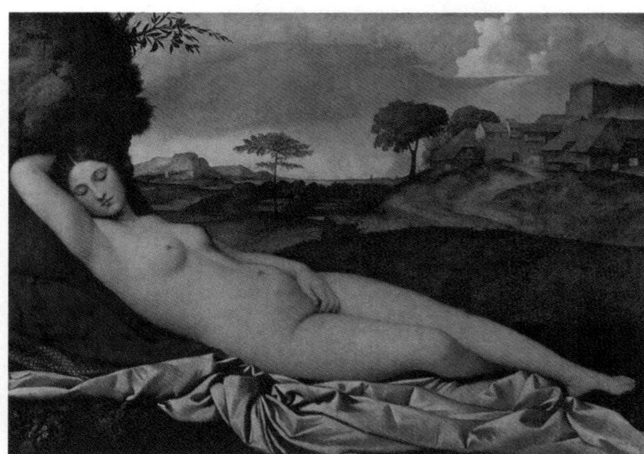

Figure 1-4.
Giorgione, *Sleeping Venus*, ca. 1508. Gemäldegalerie Alte Meister, Dresden, Germany.

Religion

Instead of mythology, Pierre Bonnard turns to the Bible in his representation of sleep. In his oil painting *Earthly Paradise* (Fig. 1-5), he depicts a slumbering Eve and an alert Adam. Bonnard utilizes the same pictorial language in his rendering of Eve: the exposed armpit and her rounded form alluding to nature. Her rendering and sleeping posture make her look thanatotic.

Although the pairing of the two biblical characters reminds us of Botticelli's *Mars and Venus*, they are not similar to the two mythical characters. By using the same visual language as Giorgione, Bonnard allows the female sleeper to be the empowered, natural being, as opposed to Botticelli's weakened male protagonist. One could argue, as the Art Institute of Chicago does, that "the male, seen as essentially intellectual, is able to transcend the earthly." However, one can interpret this as Eve being given more power because she was given more attention in terms of her physiognomy, rather than the awakened Adam. She is foreshortened and is positioned closest to the viewer. Furthermore, her color is in great contrast to the rest of the painting so that she becomes a focal point and detail is given to her face. On the other hand, Adam is rendered in shadow and only his profile is shown. Although he is standing—which could insinuate evolution—he is colored like the rest, to the point where he looks like a tree, or is simian-like.

In works such as Piero della Francesca's *Dream of Constantine* (Fig. 1-6), sleep is depicted as the state in which the divine communicates with humans. This is a common occurrence in mythology and religious stories. Well-known instances are the Bible's Jacob and his dream of the ladder that reached heaven, or the Egyptian Pharaoh's prophetic dreams that would be interpreted by Joseph. Whatever the story, it is necessary that the protagonist enter the state of sleep in order to hear God speak to him. In this early Renaissance painting, Constantine is shown reposed in a tent and is flanked by his sentinels. There is—or what appears to be—an angel swooping from the left-hand corner as if to deliver a divine message from God. This image depicts the moment, Laurie Schneider Adams tells us, when Constantine's dream "revealed the power of the Cross, and led to his legal sanction of Christianity." As opposed to Botticelli's *Mars and Venus* and Giorgione's *Sleeping Venus*, Constantine is neither emasculated nor empowered with sexual prowess. Sleep is depicted as a state wherein only the divine becomes revealed and the sleeper can realize higher states of consciousness. This is further exemplified by the contrast between Constantine and his guards. The leader is composed and peaceful in his rest as though receptive to a divine message. (This may be thought of as a foreshadowing of current research that links sleep in a critical way with the consolidation of memory.) The soldiers, on the other hand, appear languid and unaware of the angel that is delivering the message. The artist utilizes both this event and sleep as a way to demonstrate the former and to explore the latter. It is interesting to note that the title and content of the painting force the viewer to ask herself whether or not she is witnessing an event that is occurring in reality, or are we privy to the actual dream

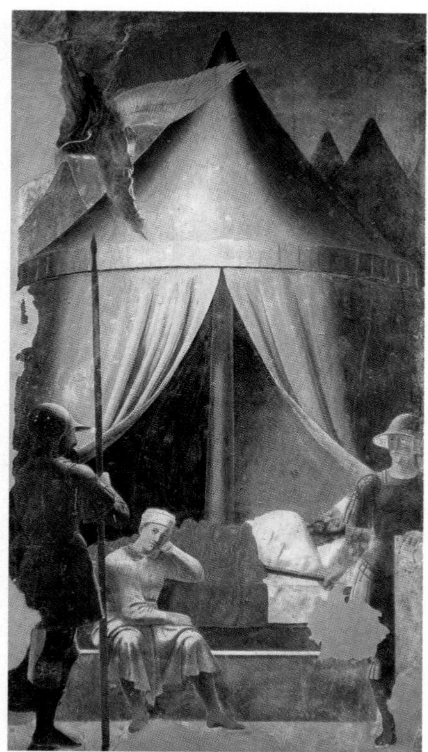

Figure 1-6.
Piero della Francesca, *Dream of Constantine*, ca. 1452. San Francesco, Arezzo, Italy.

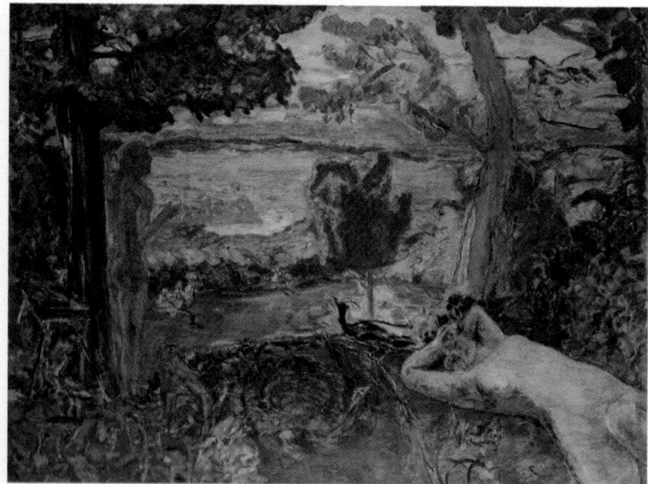

Figure 1-5.
Pierre Bonnard, *Earthly Paradise*, 1916–1920. The Art Institute of Chicago. (Used with permission. (C) 2008 Artists Rights Society [ARS], New York/ADAGP, Paris.)

of Constantine? Are we the awake sleepers who are also in Constantine's higher state and are witnessing the delivery of this divine message?

Sleep as Rest

John Keats equated sleep with rest.

WHAT is more gentle than a wind in summer?
What is more soothing than the pretty hummer
That stays one moment in an open flower,
And buzzes cheerily from bower to bower?
What is more tranquil than a musk-rose blowing
In a green island, far from all men's knowing?
More healthful than the leafiness of dales?
More secret than a nest of nightingales?
More serene than Cordelia's countenance?
More full of visions than a high romance?
What, but thee Sleep? Soft closer of our eyes!
Low murmurer of tender lullabies!
Light hoverer around our happy pillows!
Wreather of poppy buds, and weeping willows!
Silent entangler of a beauty's tresses!
Most happy listener! when the morning blesses
Thee for enlivening all the cheerful eyes
That glance so brightly at the new sun-rise.

From *Sleep and Poetry*

Although it may seem that only the mythical, powerful, and divine are depicted sleeping, there have been many examples of those in other social strata sleeping. Jan Steen's *The Dissolute Household* (ca. 1668) (Fig. 1-7) represents what modern times would term a "dysfunctional family." This family setting is the picture-perfect example of indulgence of many types: gambling, gluttony, and prostitution. All order is lost in this household where cards and oysters are strewn on the floor. The eye is immediately drawn to the woman at the table in restful sleep. Vernon Hyde Minor states that she is the wife of the man who is philandering with the prostitute. It is as though all the bawdiness has worn out the wife. This echoes the themes in Botticelli's *Mars* and Lotto's *Apollo*. Like Mars and Apollo, the weakened state of sleep/sleepiness/tiredness/fatigue (overlapping but distinct states) has made the wife vulnerable enough to become both the fool and the cuckold. Amidst all the indulgence and disorder, a monkey in the upper right corner plays with the clock and essentially "stops time." It is as though this morally challenged family is perpetually caught in this state of depravity. It insinuates that the only course of escape is to move into another state of being—sleep.

That sleep is a wondrous healing state of escape and rest and comfort for all is a common artistic theme, depicted in Laurent Delvaux and Peter Scheemakers' *Cleopatra* (Fig. 1-8). Jean-François Millet produced *Noonday Rest* in 1866 (Fig. 1-9). In 1875 John Singer Sargent emulated (see the signature) this image in *Noon* (Fig. 1-10). Van

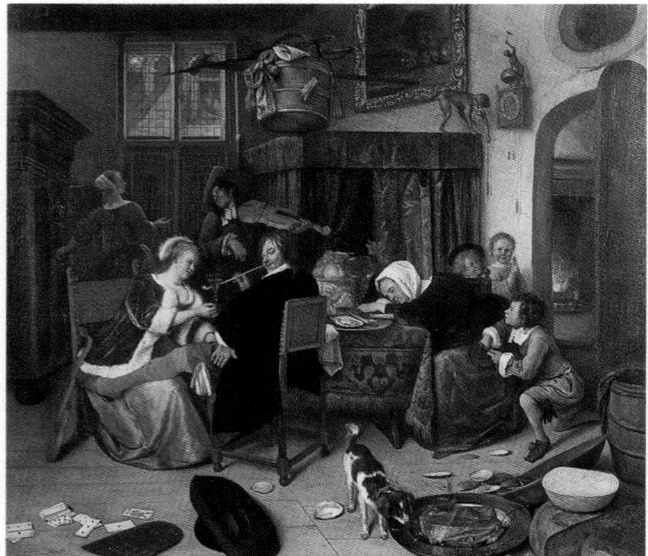

Figure 1-7.
Jan Steen, *The Dissolute Household*, ca. 1668. Wellington Museum, London.

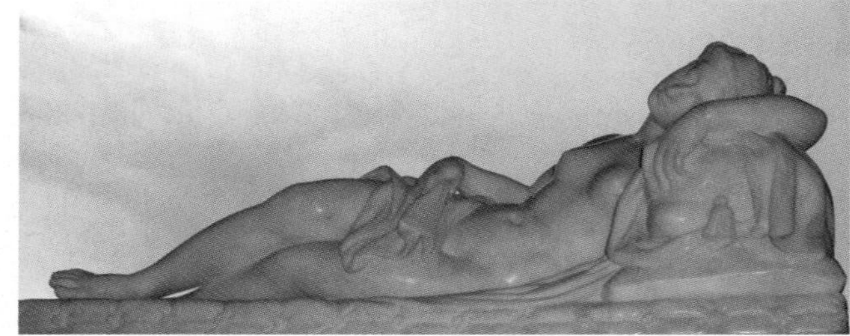

Figure 1-8.
Laurent Delvaux and Peter Scheemakers, *Cleopatra*, ca. 1723. Yale Center for British Art, New Haven, Conn.

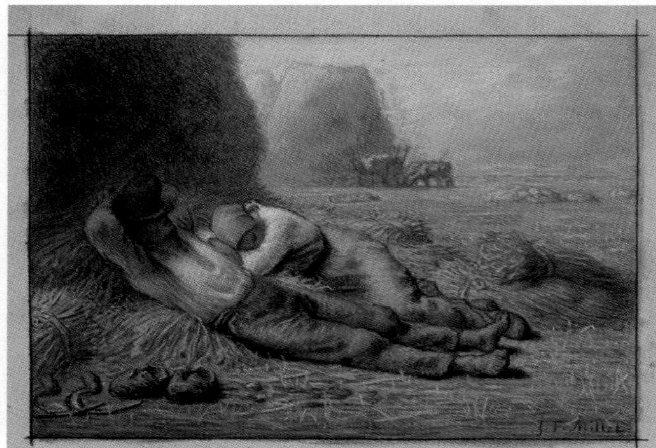

Figure 1-9.
Jean-François Millet, *Noonday Rest*, 1866. Museum of Fine Arts, Boston.

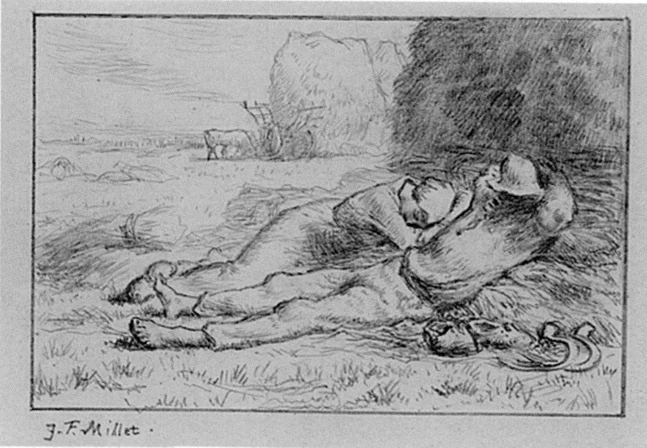

Figure 1-10.
John Singer Sargent, *Noon (after Jean-François Millet)*, ca. 1875. Metropolitan Museum of Art, New York.

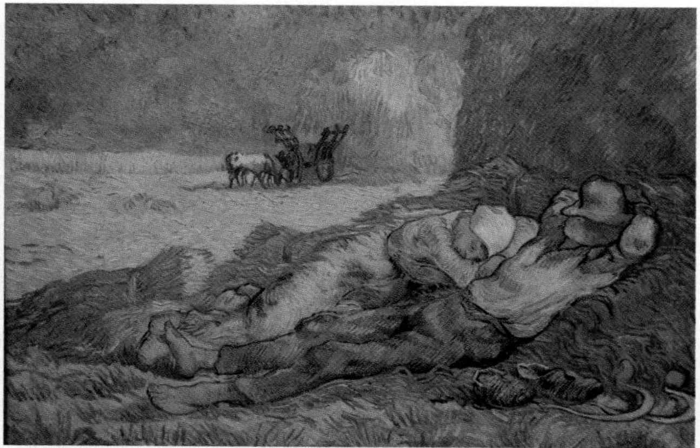

Figure 1-11.
Vincent Van Gogh, *Noon: Rest from Work* (after Jean-François Millet), 1890. Musée d'Orsay, Paris.

Gogh in turn emulated the same theme in *Noon: Rest From Work* in 1890 (Fig. 1-11). The luxury of sleep and rest is the image in *Repose* (ca. 1911) of this wealthy woman painted by John Singer Sargent (Fig. 1-12A).

In *The Cradle* (1872), Berthe Morisot portrays how complex something like sleep can be for the artist. The infant is peacefully asleep. The mother is calm, relaxed, and grateful—but vigilant as she watches over her baby (Fig. 1-12B).

In all of these examples a clear contrast is established: sleep and awake, unaware and alert, empowered and weakened. By depicting opposites side by side, artists enabled viewers to define these conscious states by what they were not. This is an extremely effective way to explore sleep beyond the physical signs but difficult from an epistemological perspective or psychological perspective. The alert poses of Botticelli's Venus and of Bonnard's Adam set against Mars and Eve, respectively, remind us of what sleep is not: a state of awareness and strength. For Lotto's Apollo, Steen's sleeping Wife, and even Giorgione's Venus, sleep is not being part of the active world. In Giorgione's *Sleeping Venus*, one could say that the landscape with the village painted in the right is Venus' antithesis. It is a reminder that while Venus is asleep, life in the town must and does continue. And lastly, for Piero della Francesca's Constantine, sleep is a demarcation between the blessed and the ignorant.

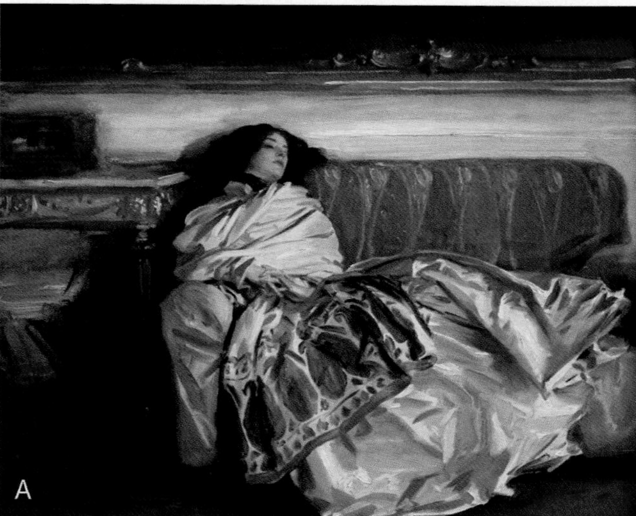

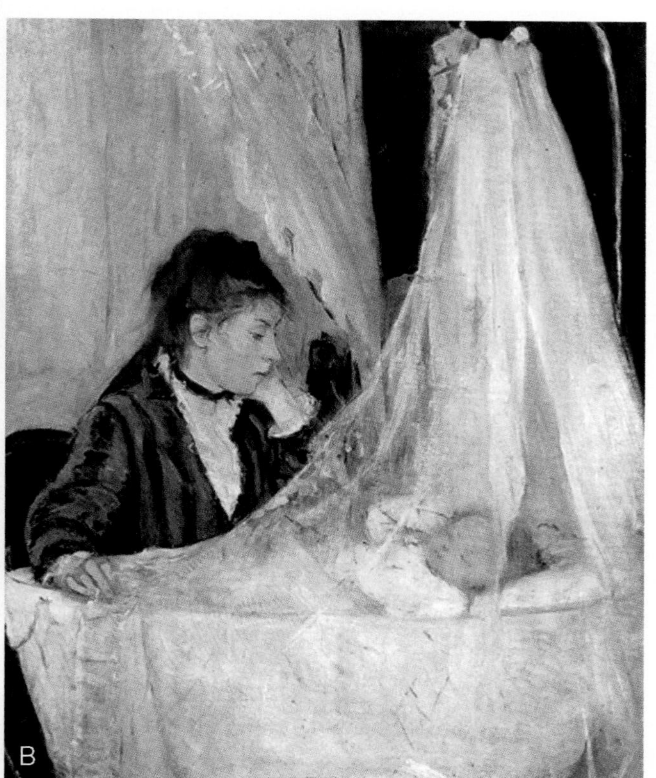

Figure 1-12.
A, John Singer Sargent, *Repose (Nonchaloire)*, 1911. B, Berthe Morisot, *Le berceau (The Cradle)*, 1872. Musée d'Orsay, Paris. National Gallery of Art, Washington, D.C.

Dreams, Danger, and Death

The painting of dreams is an excellent way for artists to explore sleep. Not only does it allow them to share their unique experiences and to move sleep from the external to the internal, it also is a way to combine elements that would not normally share the same space.

Francisco Goya, in *The Sleep of Reason Brings Monsters* (ca. 1799) (Fig. 1-13), clearly shows that dreams can be disturbing with invasion of the dreams by monsters. Henry Fuseli in *The Nightmare* (ca. 1781) shows a woman probably in a state of sleep paralysis (Fig. 1-14). She has visions of a devil-like creature on her abdomen and a horse's head peering at her from the left, but she cannot move.

Another example of dreaming is Henri Rousseau's *The Dream* (1910) (Fig. 1-15). In Rousseau's *The Dream*, there is a nude female lounging on a Victorian couch in the middle of a jungle. There are many hidden animals, but there is one in the center that draws the viewer's attention. It is an indefinable creature, which appears to be both human and animal, playing an instrument. The sky is light to indicate day; however, the moon is full and clearly visible. All these elements would not normally be together, yet the subject of dreaming allows them to be so. The juxtaposition of these things, combined with the realism in which they are rendered, evokes the feelings of eeriness and perplexity so often associated with dreams. There is a parody of the sleeping gypsy by Rousseau with the lion's belly enlarged and little remains of the gypsy's clothing. This was termed "The eaten gypsy" and reminds one that sleep may be restorative and positive but there is a lurking danger of sleep as well.

As we have seen, artists throughout time have actualized sleep through myth, religion, class, and dreams. Another recurring theme is death. That sleep may be a reversible form of death, and death a form of sleep, has always fascinated writers and artists, and even in the 19th century sleep and death were equated by some physicians.

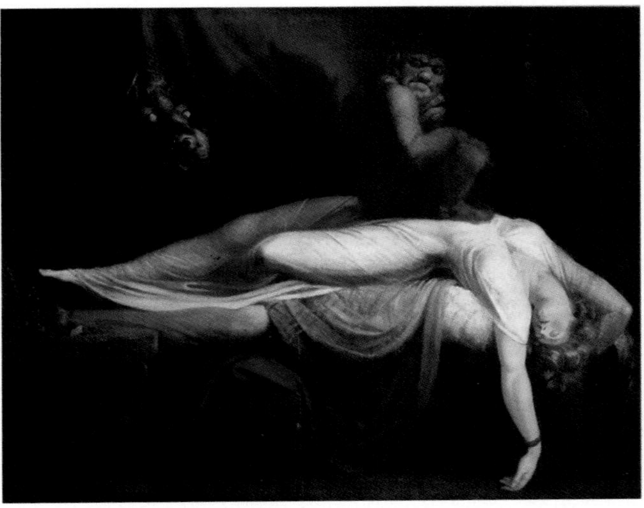

Figure 1-14.
Henry Fuseli, *The Nightmare*, 1781. Detroit Institute of the Arts, Detroit.

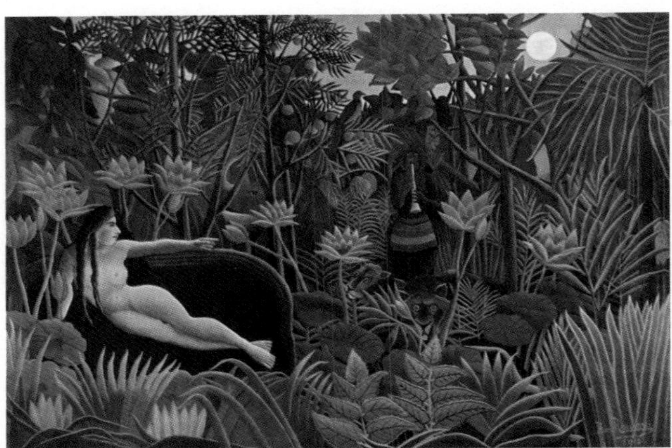

Figure 1-15.
Henri Rousseau, *The Dream*, 1910. Museum of Modern Art, New York.

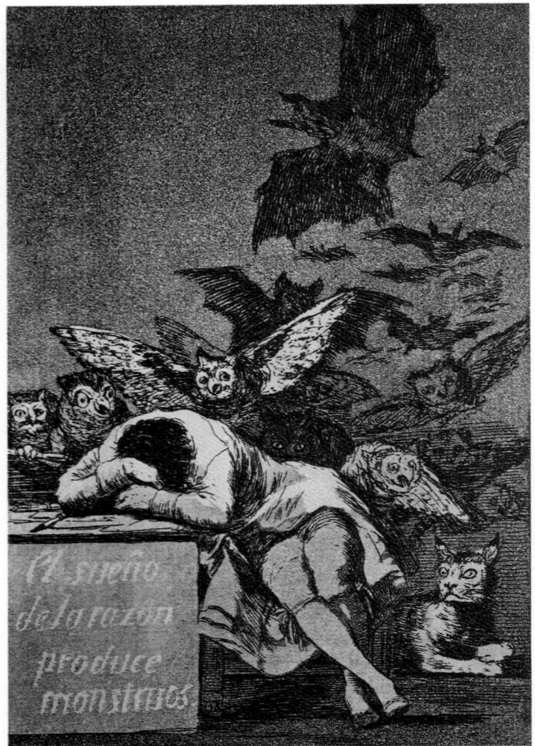

Figure 1-13.
Francisco José de Goya, *The Sleep of Reason Produces Monsters*, #43, 1799. From Los Caprichos.

William Shakespeare equated sleep with death.

To be, or not to be: that is the question. Whether 'tis nobler in the mind to suffer The slings and arrows of outrageous fortune, Or to take arms against a sea of troubles. And by opposing end them? To die: to sleep: No more; and by a sleep to say we end The heartache and the thousand natural shocks That flesh is heir to, — 'tis a consummation Devoutly to be wish'd. To die, to sleep; To sleep: perchance to dream: ay, there's the rub: For in that sleep of death what dreams may come?

From *Hamlet*, act 3, scene 1.

Sleep that knits up the ravell'd sleave of care,
The death of each day's life, sore labour's bath,
Balm of hurt minds, great nature's second course,
Chief nourisher in life's feast.

From *Macbeth*, act 2, scene 2.

Religion has, as noted above, contributed to views about sleep in general and artistic portraits in particular. For example, a bed made of arrows is not generally counted among the beds one would be happy to rest on. The bed of arrows, as shown in Figure 1-16, belongs to Bhishma, a hero of the Hindus.

According to historical record, Bhishma's bed of arrows was also his deathbed in a war that is said to have occurred around 6000 B.C. This emphasizes the perceived link of sleep and death.

Bhishma's body was so covered with arrows shot at him that when he lay down, the arrows made a bed. Only his head was not supported by arrows. So Bhishma asked Arjun, another war hero, to create a pillow of arrows for him. This Arjun did by putting the arrows into the ground for Bhishma's head. An interesting aspect of Bhishma's death is that he could control the exact time of his death.

The states of waking, dreaming, and deep sleep are associated with the syllable *aum* that Hindus chant when they meditate. When the sounds a-u-m that make up *aum* are chanted, it is believed that one goes through all of the three states. Meditation is a means of connecting with one's innermost self and is an integral part of Hinduism.

A more modern linking of sleep and death is shown by the painter John William Waterhouse in *Sleep and His Half-brother Death* (1874). As one moves from foreground to background, one clearly goes from life to death. There is no mistaking which of the brothers is alive even though both have similar postures (Fig. 1-17).

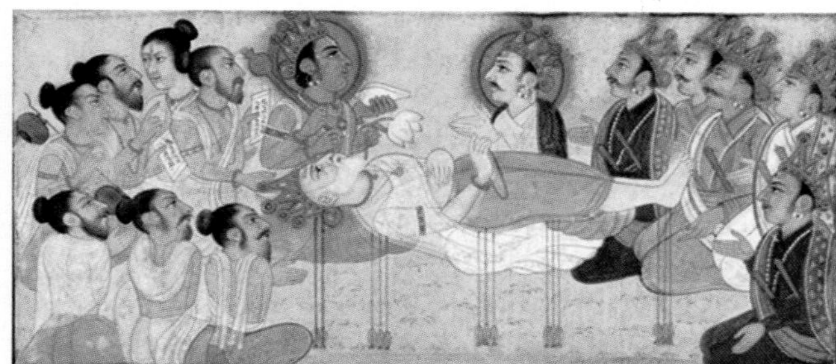

Figure 1-16.
The Death of Bhisma from *Mahabharata*, ca. 18th century. Smithsonian Institute, Washington, D.C.

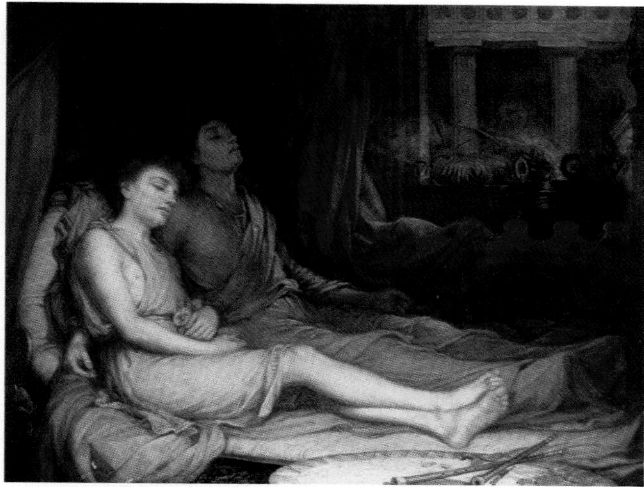

Figure 1-17.
John William Waterhouse, *Sleep and his Half-brother Death*, 1874. Private collection.

As understanding of sleep through science, philosophy, literature, and art changes throughout time, so will the visual renderings related to sleep and dreams. While one might at first glance think that the more we understand about sleep the less we will be fascinated and that there will be a commensurate decline in the involvement of all artists in the subject of sleep and dreams, this does not seem to be the case at all. Current artists seem to be engrossed by the subject, just as modern song writers and poets have continued the compositions of librettists of opera and classical poets (who often wrote about sleep and dreams). Whatever the case, we will continue to dream.

SELECTED READINGS

Adams LS: Art across Time, vol 2. Boston, McGraw-Hill, 1999, pp. 523, 582, 862.

Arnason HH: History of Modern Art. New York, Harry N. Abrams, 1998.

The Art Institute of Chicago: Master Paintings in The Art Institute of Chicago. Chicago: The Art Institute of Chicago, 1999, p. 121.

Minor VH: Baroque & Rococo: Art & Culture. Englewood Cliffs, N.J., Prentice Hall, 1999, p. 261.

Ruvoldt M: The Italian Renaissance Imagery of Inspiration: Metaphors of Sex, Sleep and Dreams. Cambridge, England, Cambridge University Press, 2004, pp. 40, 94.

Shapiro CM: Who Needs to Sleep Anyway? How Animals Sleep. Windsor, Ontario, Canada, Black Moss Press, 1996.

Shapiro CM, Trajanovic NN, Fedoroff JP: Sexsomnia—A new parasomnia? Can J Psychiatry 48(5):311–317, 2003.

Shapiro CM, Vaccarino K: Sleep in art. In Shapiro CM (ed): Sleep Solutions Manual. Pointe Claire, Quebec, Canada, Kommunicom Publications, 1995, pp. 223–246.

CHAPTER 2

HISTORY OF SLEEP MEDICINE AND PHYSIOLOGY

Meir Kryger

Although the field of medicine is fairly recent, historical, literary, and scientific descriptions have added to our knowledge. Obviously sleep disorders are not new, and it is appropriate to begin a historical timeline of sleep medicine and physiology with Hippocrates, the father of medicine.

Timeline

400 B.C. Hippocrates wrote, "I have known many persons in sleep groaning and crying out, some in a state of suffocation, some jumping up and fleeing out of doors, and deprived of their reason until they awaken, and afterward becoming well and rational as before, although they be pale and weak; and this will happen not once but frequently" (Fig. 2-1).

360 B.C. Dionysius, the tyrant of Heraclea (Fig. 2-2). Historical documents describe Dionysius as immensely obese and record that he died "choking on his own fat." His physicians may have used the first treatment of apnea, that is, sticking needles through the skin to arouse him from sleep.

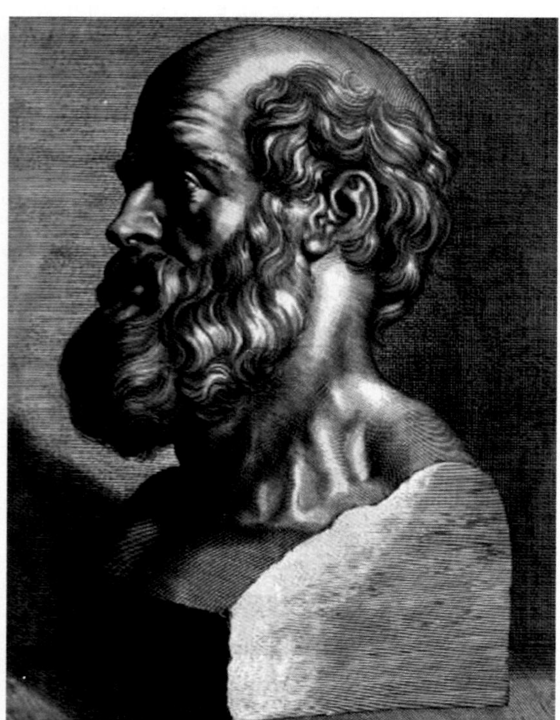

Figure 2-1.
Hippocrates, etching by Peter Paul Rubens.

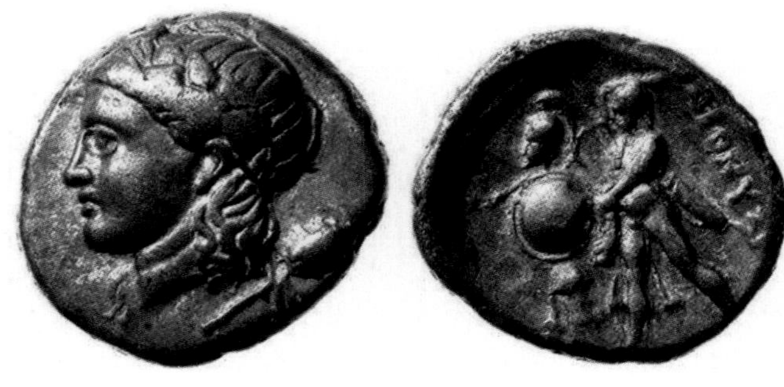

Figure 2-2.
Coin of Dionysius, which did not show him as obese.

Now up to a certain point under the flesh, completely callous as it was by fat, the needle caused no sensation; but if the needle went through so as to touch the region which was free of fat, then he would be thoroughly aroused.

—*Athenaeus,* The Deipnosophists.
translated by C. B. Gulick

350 B.C. Aristotle (Fig. 2-3) wrote about sleep and waking, whether they are a function of the body or the soul, and the significance of dreams. He observed that all creatures sleep.

Accordingly, almost all other animals are clearly observed to partake in sleep, whether they are aquatic, aerial, or terrestrial, since fishes of all kinds, and mollusks, as well as all others which have eyes, have been seen sleeping. "Hard-eyed" creatures and insects manifestly assume the posture of sleep; but the sleep of all such creatures is of brief duration, so that often it might well baffle ones observation to decide whether they sleep or not.

—*Aristotle,* On Sleep and Sleeplessness,
translated by J. I. Beare

1603 Shakespeare describes sleepwalking in *Macbeth*, act 5, scene 1. "**GENTLEWOMAN.** Since his Majesty went into the field, have seen her rise from her bed, throw her nightgown upon her, unlock her closet, take forth paper, fold it, write upon't, read it, afterwards seal it, and again return to bed; yet all this while in a most fast sleep" (Fig. 2-4). Falstaff, who appears in three Shakespeare

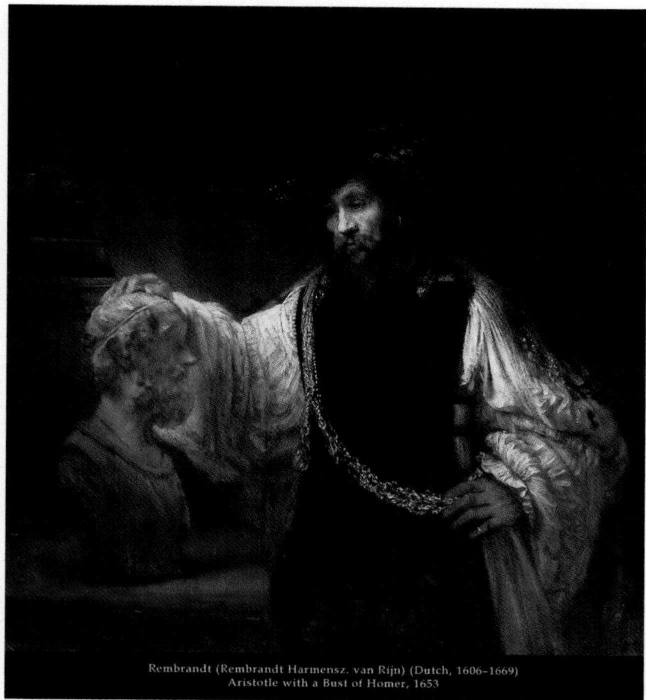

Figure 2-3.
Aristotle with a Bust of Homer, by Rembrandt van Rijin, 1653. Metropolitan Museum of Art.

plays, was obese, snored, and fell asleep at inappropriate times. These are symptoms of sleep apnea.

1605 Miguel de Cervantes Saavedra (Fig. 2-5), in his novel *The Ingenious Hidalgo Don Quixote of La Mancha*, probably described REM (rapid eye movement) sleep behavior disorder in Part 1, chapter 35:

> *[A]nd in his right hand he held his unsheathed sword, with which he was slashing about on all sides, uttering exclamations as if he were actually fighting some giant: and the best of it was his eyes were not open, for he was fast asleep, and dreaming that he was doing battle with the giant.*

1672 Sir Thomas Willis (of the circle of Willis) describes the features of restless legs syndrome (RLS). The condition will not receive a name until 1945 (Fig. 2-6).

1729 The first report of circadian rhythm was that of Jean-Jacques d'Ortous De Mairan, who set up an ingenious experiment using a mimosa plant that opened up its leaves at a certain time when it was sunny. He put the plant into a box so that there was no exposure to light, and the plant's leaves still opened at the same time. This plant was able to keep track of time (Fig. 2-7).

1816 William Wadd, Surgeon Extraordinaire to the King of England, writes a monograph entitled "Cursory Remarks on Corpulence; or Obesity considered as a Disease" in which he described sleepiness in obesity. One of his cases "became at length so lethargic, that he fell asleep in the act of eating, even in company."

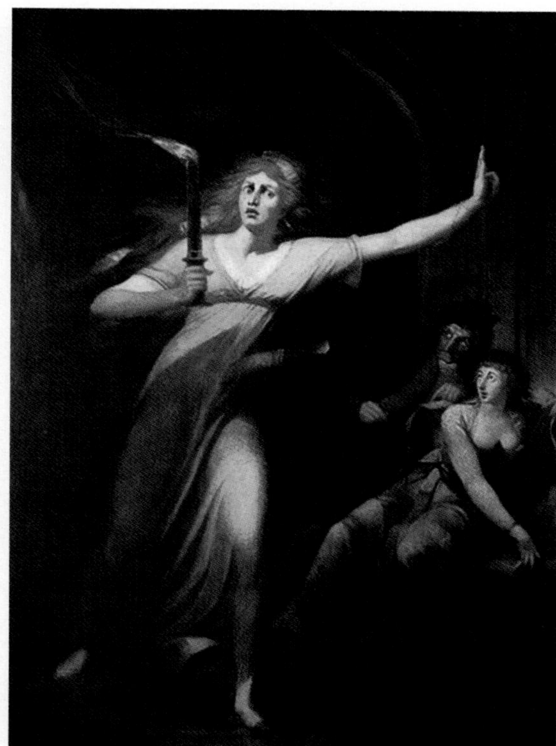

Figure 2-4.
Lady Macbeth Sleepwalking by Henry Fuseli, 1784. Louvre Museum.

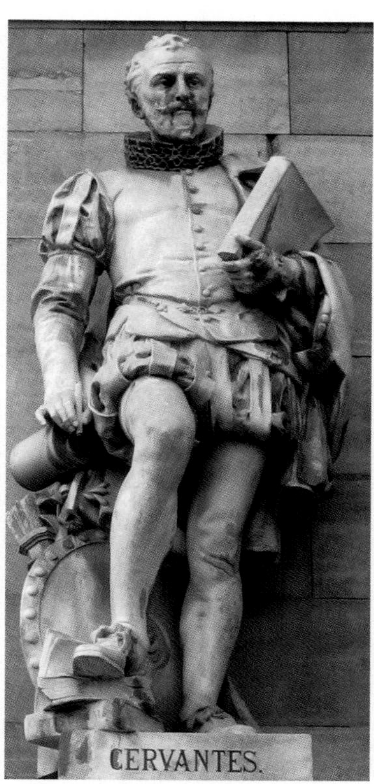

Figure 2-5.
Miguel de Cervantes described REM behavior disorder.

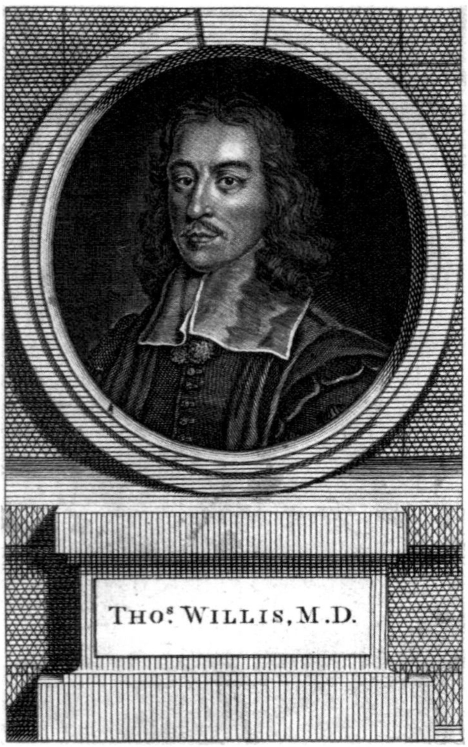

Figure 2-6.
Sir Thomas Willis.

1818 John Cheyne describes the breathing pattern named after him in "A case of Apoplexy in Which the Fleshy part of the Heart was converted into Fat." "For several days his breathing was irregular; it would entirely cease for a quarter of a minute, then it would become perceptible, though very low, then by degrees it became heaving and quick, and then it would gradually cease again: this revolution in the state of his breathing occupied about a minute, during which there were about thirty acts of respiration."

1832 Just after the discovery in 1831 by Samuel Guthrie of chloroform (which was later used as an anesthetic agent), Justus von Liebig discovered chloral hydrate, perhaps the first widely used and abused hypnotic agent.

1836 Charles Dickens (Fig. 2-8) publishes *The Posthumous Papers of the Pickwick Club*. In this book he describes Joe, the fat boy whose symptoms of snoring and sleepiness form the basis of the first article to describe the Pickwickian syndrome, published in 1956. "And on the box sat a fat and red-faced boy in a state of somnolency" (Fig. 2-9).

1862 Dr. Caffé in France is the first to describe a condition of hallucinations associated with sleepiness. It was incorrectly considered a form of epilepsy.

1864 Adolf von Baeyer discovers barbituric acid, the parent compound of the barbiturates.

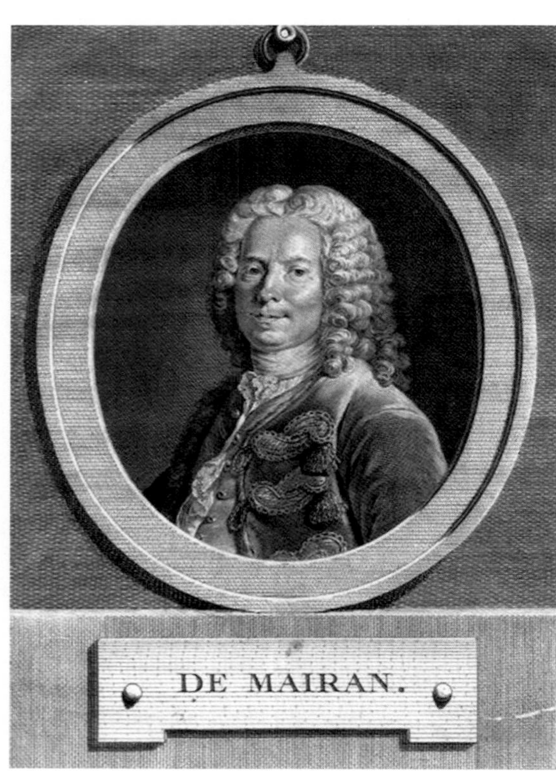

Figure 2-7.
Jean-Jacques d'Ortous de Mairan.

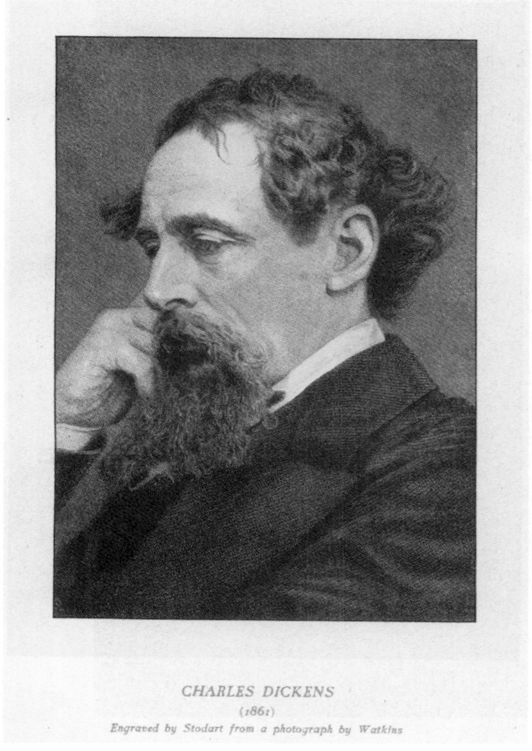

Figure 2-8.
Charles Dickens. (Courtesy M. H. Kryger.)

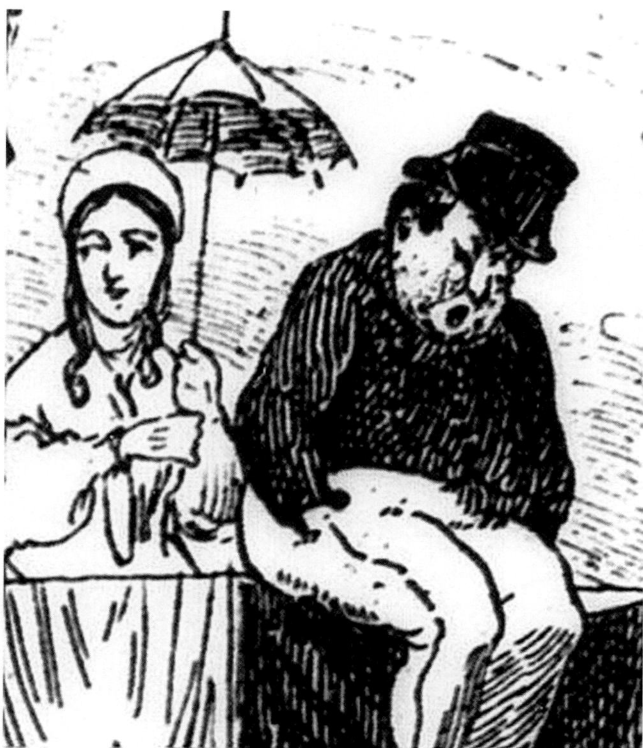

Figure 2-9.
Joe, the fat boy, "in a state of somnolency," *The Posthumous Papers of the Pickwick Club*. (Courtesy M. H. Kryger.)

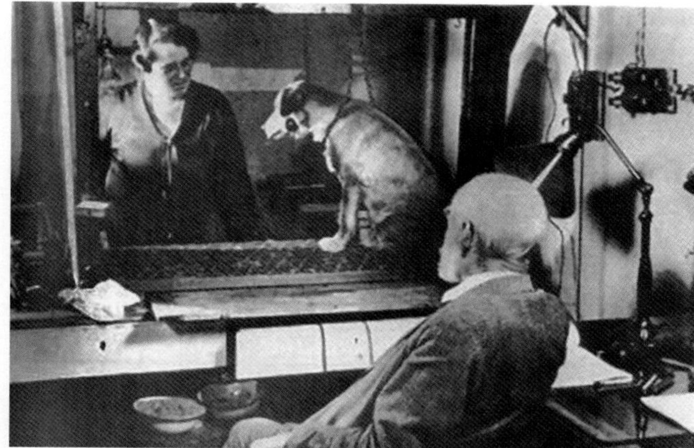

Figure 2-10.
Ivan Pavlov described conditional reflexes.

1869 William Hammond publishes *Sleep and its Derangements.* He uses the phrase "persistent wakefulness" to describe what would be called insomnia today. He also describes sleep state misperception, blaming the condition on increased blood flow to the brain.

1877 Karl Westphall is the first to describe sudden bouts of sleeping associated with loss of motor tone.

1880 Jean Baptist Edourd Gélineau is the first to use the term *narcolepsy* to describe a disease with irresistible sleep.

1890s Ivan Pavlov begins experiments on salivation in dogs in response to food and stimuli. His experiments led to his description of the existence of conditioned reflexes, a concept important in the psychological treatment of insomnia (Fig. 2-10).

1895 Nathaniel Kleitman, the first and most famous sleep researcher, is born.

1898 William Wells makes the association of nasal obstruction and daytime sleepiness: "[T]he stupid-looking lazy child who frequently suffers some headaches at school, breathes through his mouth instead of his nose, snorts, and is restless at night, and wakes up with a dry mouth in the morning, is well worthy of the selected solicitous attention of the school medical officer."

1902 Leopold Löwenfeld makes the statement that narcolepsy is associated with cataplexy.

1902 Emil Fischer and Joseph von Mering synthesize barbital, marketed in 1904 by the Bayer Company as Veronal. This became the first widely used barbiturate hypnotic.

1918 William Osler, in *Principles and Practice of Medicine*, describes sleeplessness and mental symptoms including drowsiness in congestive heart failure (Fig. 2-11).

1929 Hans Berger is the first to record an electroencephalogram.

1934 Luman Daniels points out that in narcolepsy there is sleepiness, cataplexy, hypnagogic hallucinations, and sleep paralysis.

1934 In a brilliant series of papers describing the clinical features of heart failure, W. R. Harrison describes the clinical consequences of Cheyne Stokes breathing in heart failure. He describes sleep onset and sleep maintenance insomnia, as well as paroxysmal nocturnal dyspnea, and

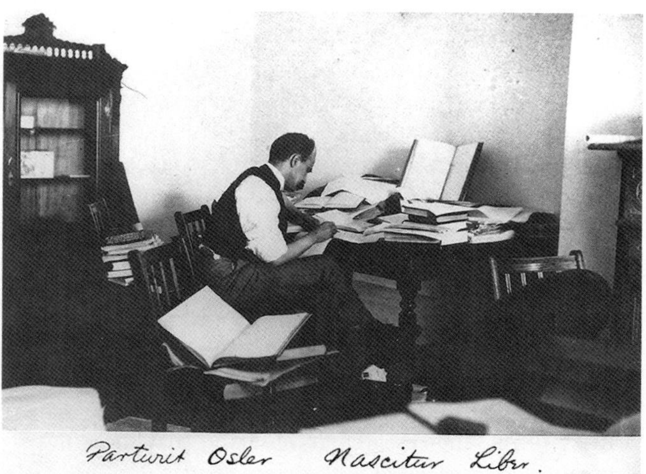

Figure 2-11.
Sir William Osler described drowsiness in heart failure.

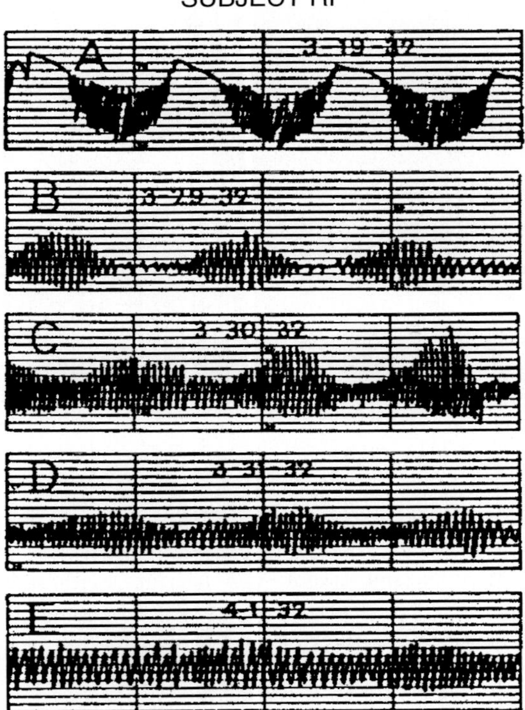

Figure 2-12.
Harrison shows in 1934 that CSR in heart failure improves with treatment.

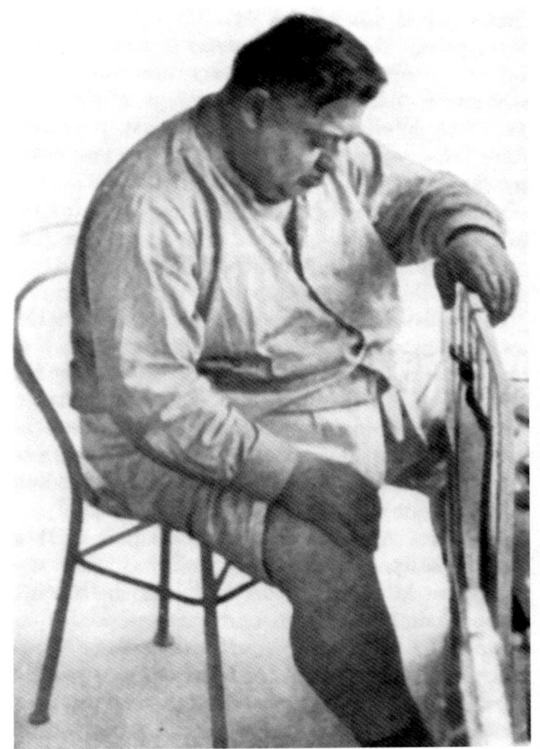

Figure 2-13.
Photo from article by Annie Spitz in 1937.

shows how the periodic breathing pattern improves with treatment of the heart failure (Fig. 2-12).

1935 Alfred Loomis describes the electroencephalogram findings of what was eventually called "nonrapid eye movement" (NREM) sleep.

1937 Annie Spitz describes three cases of what is clearly obstructive sleep apnea in patients who have right heart failure, Cheyne Stokes respiration, snoring, and sleepiness. Figure 2-13 is the first known published photograph of a sleep apnea patient.

1939 Nathaniel Kleitman publishes *Sleep and Wakefulness.* In his brilliant career he trained many of the pioneer researchers in sleep medicine (Fig. 2-14).

1949 Giuseppe Moruzzi and Horace Magoun describe the reticular activating system and the neurologic basis for wakefulness and arousal.

1945 Karl-Axel Ekbom introduces the term *restless legs syndrome* and describes the condition.

1953 Nathaniel Kleitman, at the University of Chicago, assigns a graduate student, Eugene Aserinski, to use eye muscle movements as a measure of the depth of sleep. The method used, electro-oculography, documented REM sleep. The researchers observed that these movements were associated with dream recall.

1956 Sydney Burwell and others describe the Pickwickian syndrome. The article, which focused on respiratory

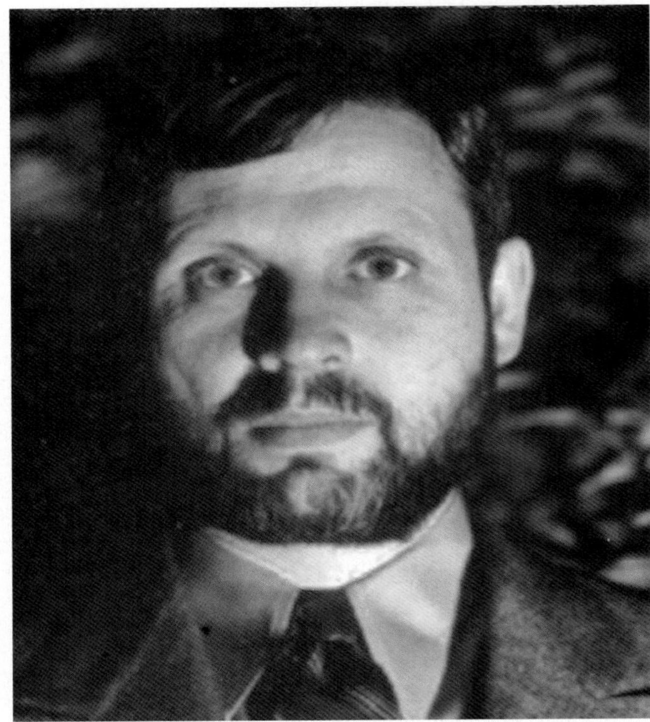

Figure 2-14.
Nathaniel Kleitman. (Courtesy W. C. Dement.)

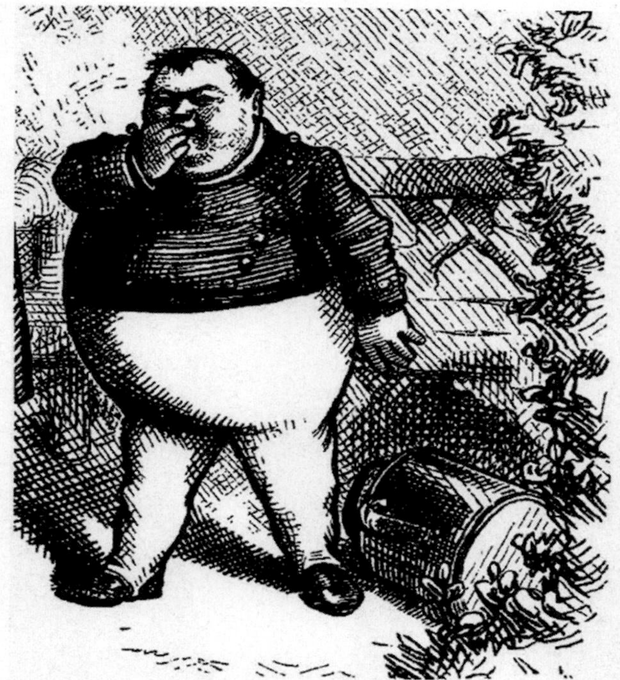

Figure 2-15.
Joe, the fat boy from article by Burwell. The illustration used by Burwell was not from the original illustrations of the novel.

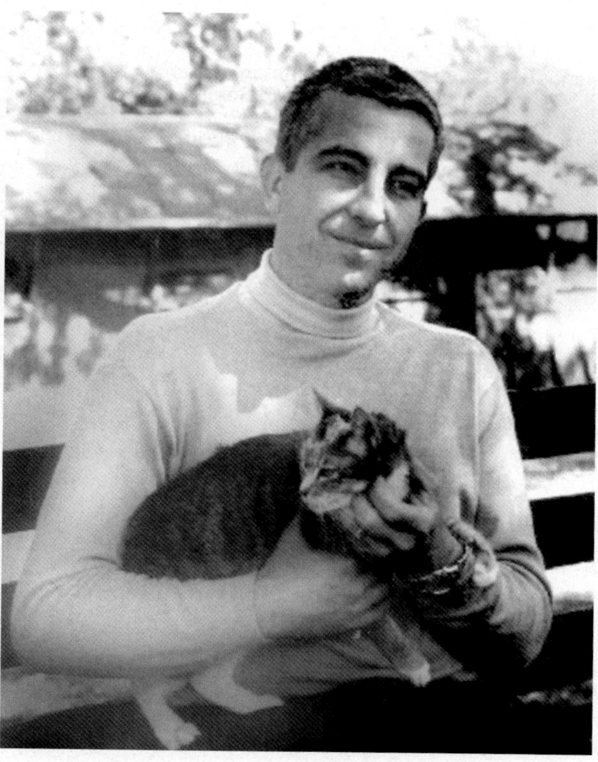

Figure 2-16.
William C. Dement at the beginning of his career, 1957.

failure, did not adequately explain the excessive daytime sleepiness that was the presenting complaint (Fig. 2-15).

1956 Leo Sternbach discovers the benzodiazepine RO6-690, which led to the approval of librium in 1960. Benzodiazepines replaced the barbiturates as hypnotics.

1957 William C. Dement describes REM sleep in the cat (Fig. 2-16).

1959 Michel Jouvet describes REM sleep atonia in cats. Within several years Allan Rechtschaffen, Dement, and Jouvet were to head research programs exploring the basic science of sleep (Fig. 2-17).

1960 Allan Rechtschaffen explores the psychophysiology of dreams.

1960 Gerry Vogel describes sleep-onset REMs in narcolepsy.

1961 The precursor of the Sleep Research Society is formed, and later becomes the Association for the Psychophysiological Study of Sleep (APSS). Ultimately the sleep scientists formed the Sleep Research Society.

1963 Richard Wurtman's group reports that melatonin synthesis in the pineal gland is controlled by light.

1964 The Association for the Psychophysiological Study of Sleep is founded. The APSS became the precursor for the Association of Sleep Disorders Centers (1975), the American Sleep Disorders Association (1987), and, ultimately, the American Academy of Sleep Medicine (1999).

1964–1968 Case reports from three centers in Europe (Carl Jung in Weisbaden in 1965; Henri Gastaut in Marseilles in 1965; Elio Lugaresi in Bologna in 1968) describe what we now know to be the sleep apnea syndrome (they called the cases Pickwick syndrome).

1967 Lawrence Monroe reports physiologic findings between good and poor sleepers. His description is a precursor of the concept of a hyperarousal state.

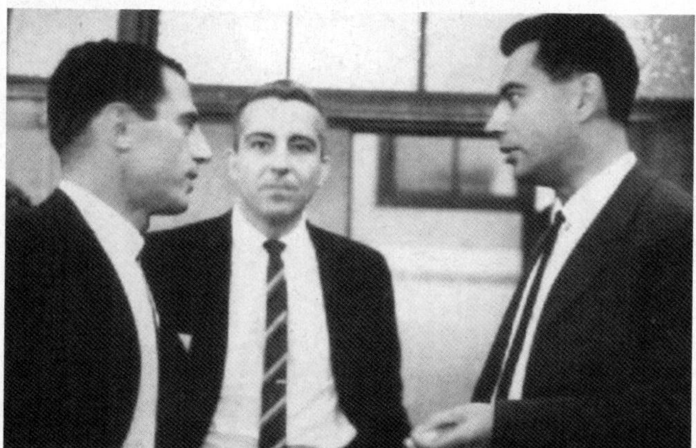

Figure 2-17.
Allan Rechtschaffen *(left)*, William C. Dement *(middle)*, and Michel Jouvet *(right)*, 1963. (Courtesy W. C. Dement.)

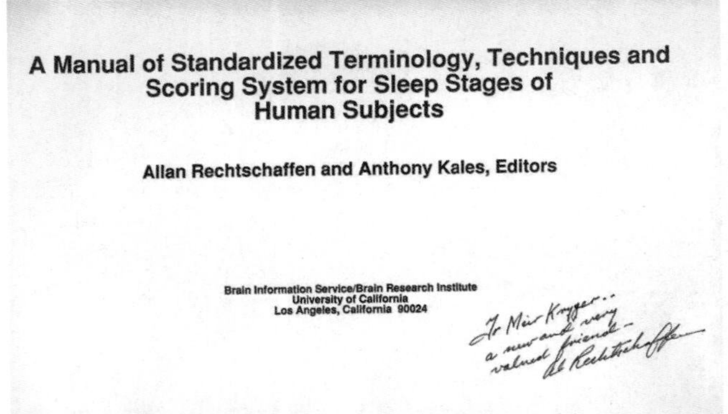
A Manual of Standardized Terminology, Techniques and Scoring System for Sleep Stages of Human Subjects

Allan Rechtschaffen and Anthony Kales, Editors

Brain Information Service/Brain Research Institute
University of California
Los Angeles, California 90024

Figure 2-18.
Rechtscahaffen and Kales sleep scoring manual. (Courtesy M. H. Kryger.)

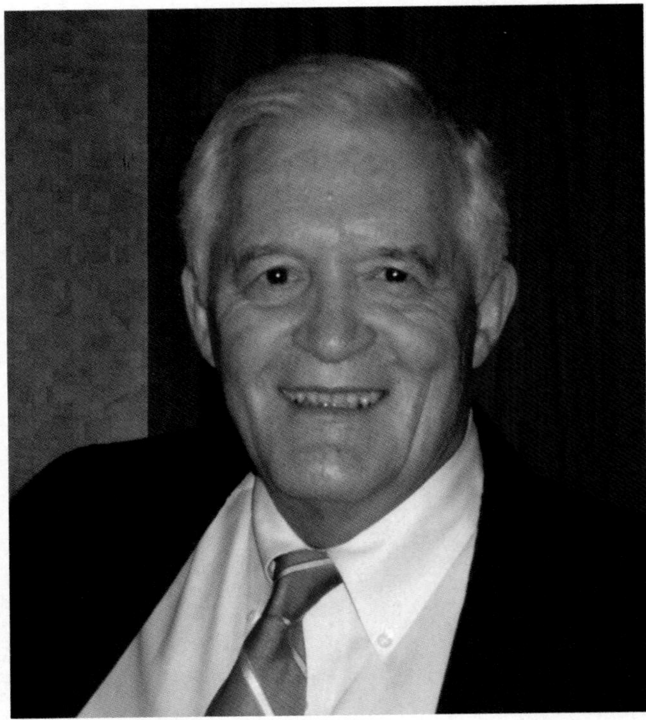

Figure 2-20.
Robert Moore.

1969 Allan Rechtschaffen and Anthony Kales produce a sleep scoring manual. It formed the basis of sleep staging for most research for the next 40 years (Fig. 2-18).

1970 William Dement founds the world's first sleep disorders center at Stanford University (Fig. 2-19).

1971 Ron Konopka and Seymour Benzer discover a mutant fly with a single gene mutation that could lengthen, shorten, or induce circadian arrhythmia, depending on the location of mutation in the gene.

1972 Robert Moore shows that destruction of the suprachiasmatic nucleus (SCN) results in loss of a circadian adrenal corticosterone rhythm, thus establishing the importance of the SCN in circadian physiology. Simultaneously, Frederick Stephan and Irving Zucker showed that ablation of the SCN abolishes behavioral rhythms (Fig. 2-20).

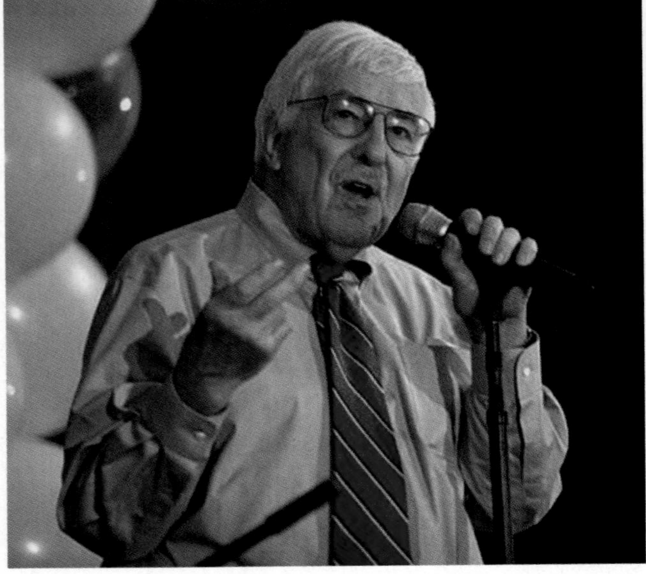

Figure 2-19.
William C. Dement, 2008.

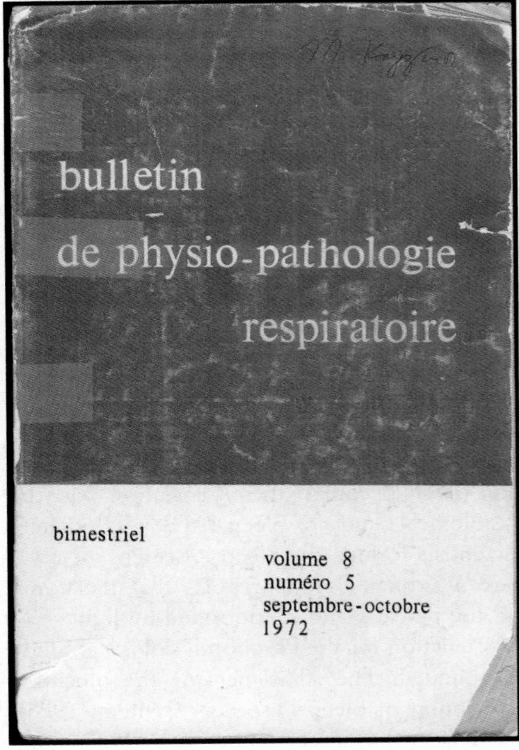

Figure 2-21.
The first major sleep apnea symposium was in Rimini.

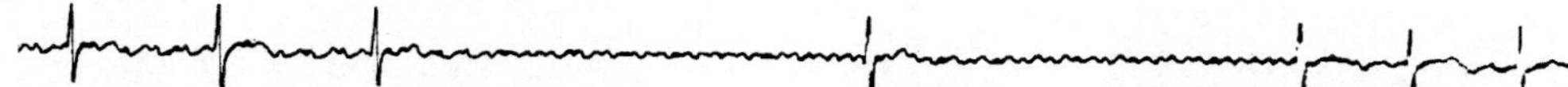

Figure 2-22.
Meir Kryger describes asystole in sleep apnea. A tracheostomy normalized the cardiac rhythm.

1972 The Rimini Symposium on Hypersomnia and Periodic Breathing, held in Italy, is the first major conference in which sleep apnea is the main focus. At this time the term *sleep apnea* had not yet been coined (Fig. 2-21).

1974 Meir Kryger describes one of the first cases of sleep apnea in North America, and documents that control breathing was normal, hypercapnea was not present, and upper airway resistance changed with position. Kryger showed that significant cardiac arrhythmias, such as bradycardia and asystole, are reversed by tracheostomy (Fig. 2-22).

1974 Hewlett-Packard introduces the first fiberoptic-based ear oximeter.

1976 The American Sleep Disorders Association is established. The name is later changed to American Academy of Medicine.

1976 Fred Turek and Michael Menaker establish that treatment with melatonin can alter the circadian clock of sparrows, laying the foundation for the use of melatonin and melatonin agonists as chronobiotic drugs today (Fig. 2-23).

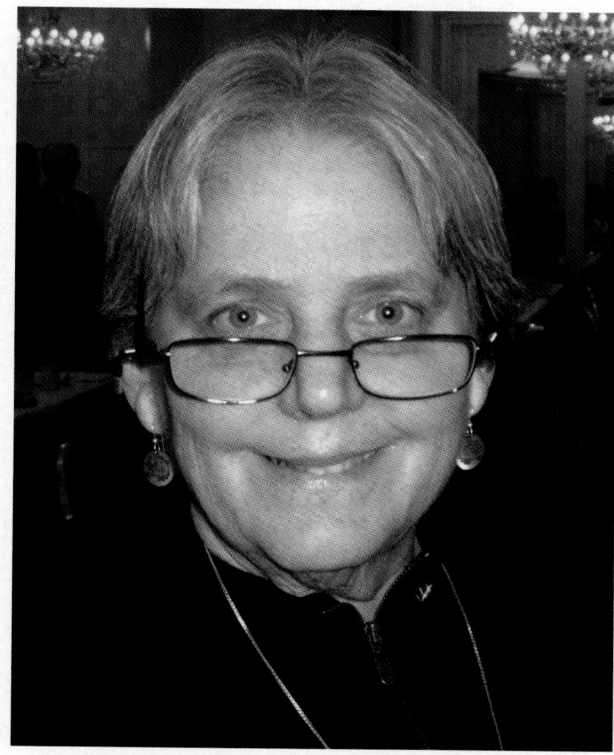

Figure 2-24.
Mary Carskadon.

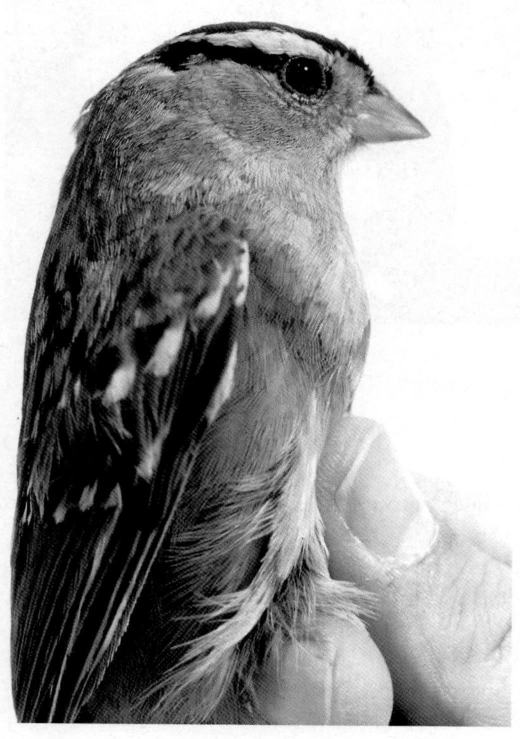

Figure 2-23.
Sparrow from experiments of Turek and Menaker.

1976 Mary Carskadon and colleagues report a large difference between subjective and objective measures of sleep in insomniacs, and showed that arousals increase with age (Fig. 2-24).

1976 *Sleep Apnea Syndrome* is published. This contains the papers presented at the first American symposium on the disorder (Fig. 2-25). The term *sleep apnea* was first introduced by Christian Guilleminault's team in 1975.

1976 Charles Czeisler describes 24-hour cortisol secretory patterns in humans (Fig. 2-26).

1978 The first issue of the journal *Sleep* is published. Christian Guilleminault is the editor (Fig. 2-27).

1981 Colin Sullivan describes the use of nasal CPAP (continuous positive airway pressure) in an article in *The Lancet.* This revolutionized the treatment of sleep apnea, which up to that time was treated surgically, usually with tracheostomy. Other advancements were made by David Rapoport and Mark Sanders (Fig. 2-28).

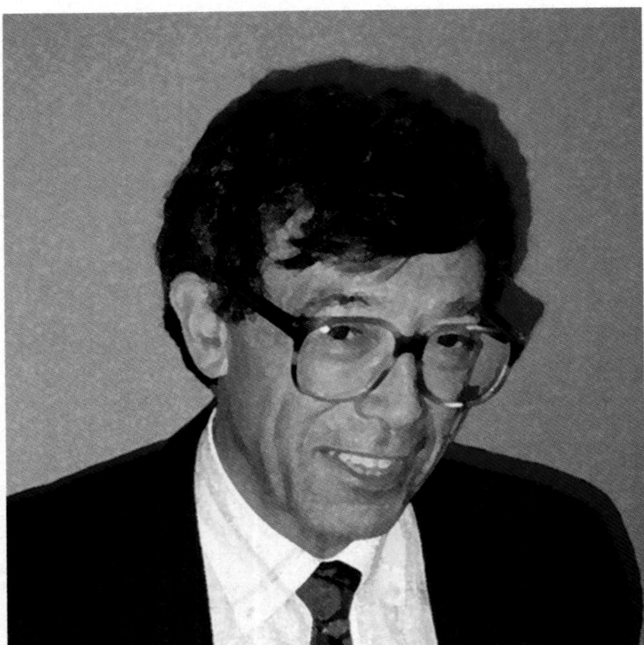

Figure 2-25.
Christian Guilleminault.

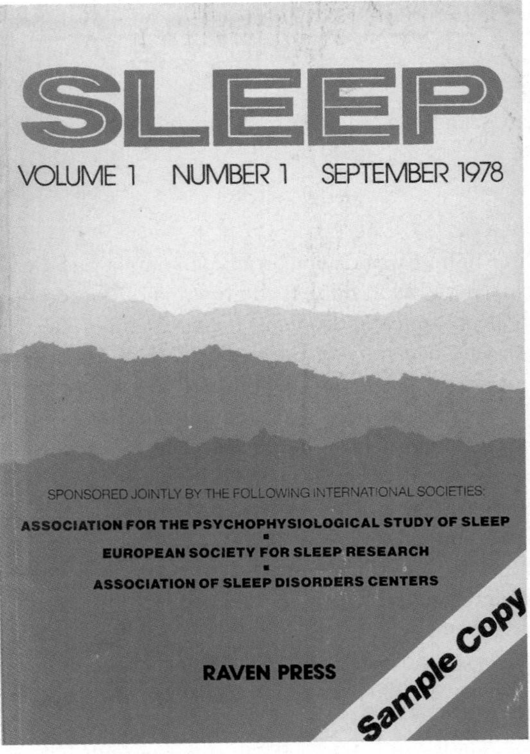

Figure 2-27.
First issue of *Sleep*.

1981 Thomas Roth's team reported on the many diseases associated with insomnia. Their report was the precursor for the concept of comorbid insomnia (Fig. 2-29).

1982 The National Institutes of Health holds the first consensus symposium conference on insomnia.

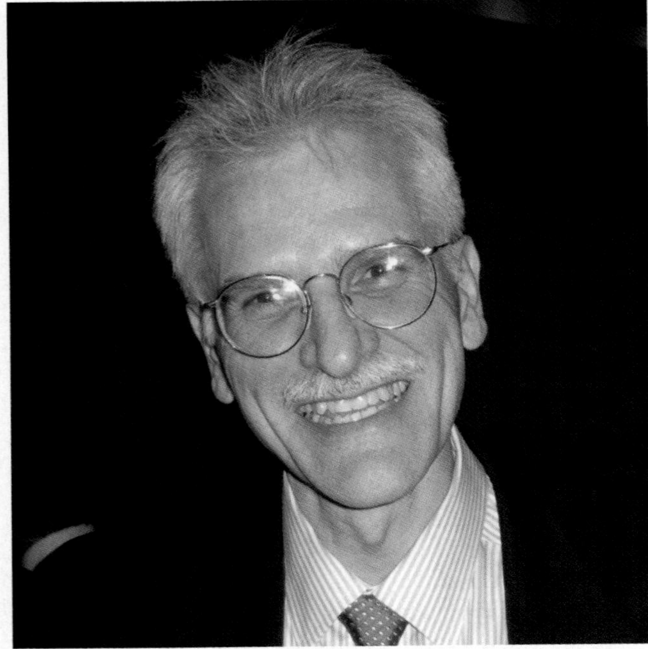

Figure 2-26.
Charles Czeisler.

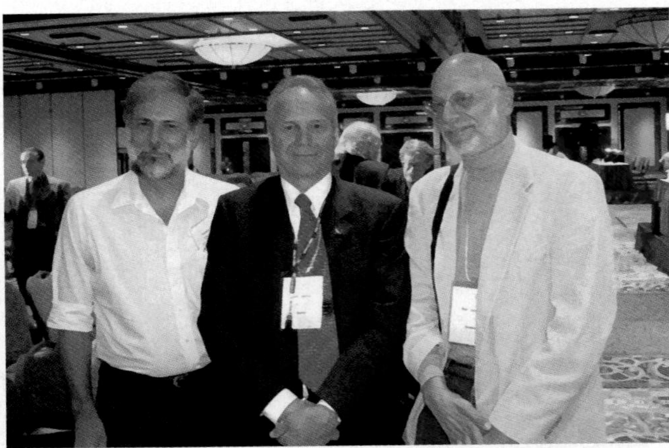

Figure 2-28.
Colin Sullivan *(center)*, David Rapoport *(left)*, and Mark Sanders *(right)*.

1986 The sleep group in Minnesota, led by Carlos Schenck (Fig. 2-30) and Mark Mahowald (Fig. 2-31), describes REM sleep behavior disorder, a condition in which people are not paralyzed during their dreams, but react physically to dream content.

1986 Sonia Arbilla and Salomon Langer describe zolpidem, the first nonbenzodiazepine with preferential affinity for a BZ1 receptor subtype.

1989 Jiang He and colleagues, as well as Christian Guilleminault and colleagues, show that untreated

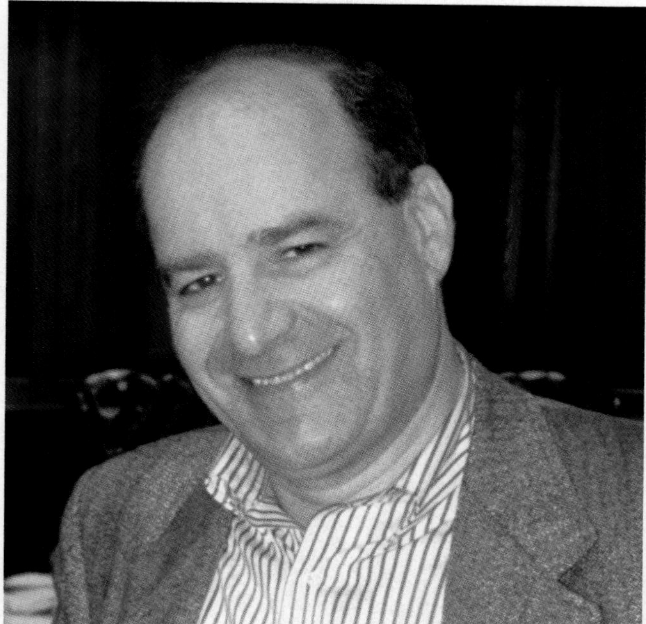

Figure 2-29.
Thomas Roth.

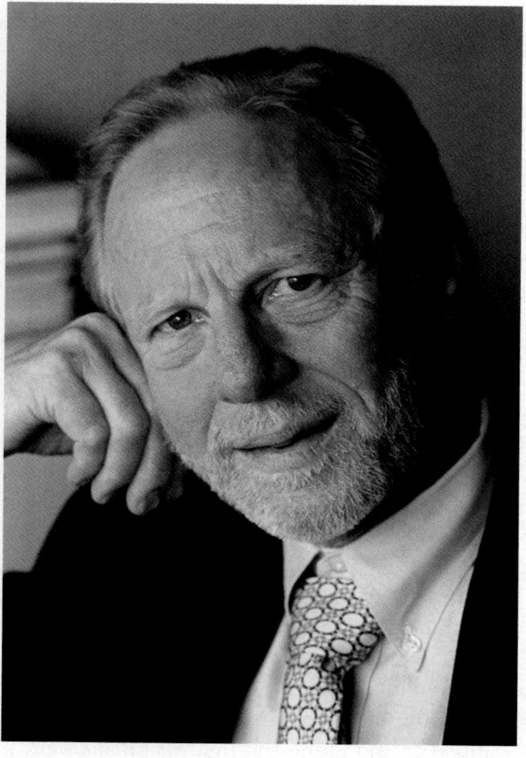

Figure 2-31.
Mark Mahowald.

patients with sleep apnea have a high mortality. This was shown to be particularly true for patients under 50 years of age.

1989 Meir Kryger, Tom Roth, and William Dement edit the first comprehensive sleep medicine textbook (Fig. 2-32).

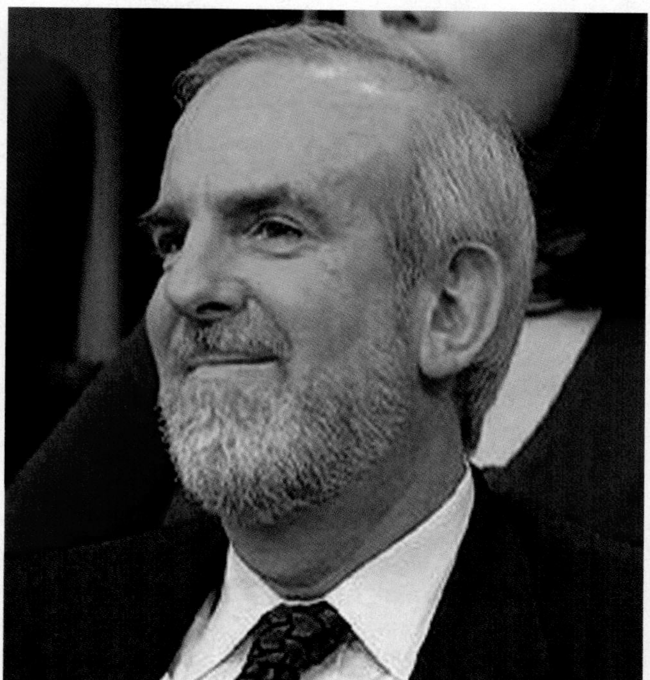

Figure 2-30.
Carlos Schenck.

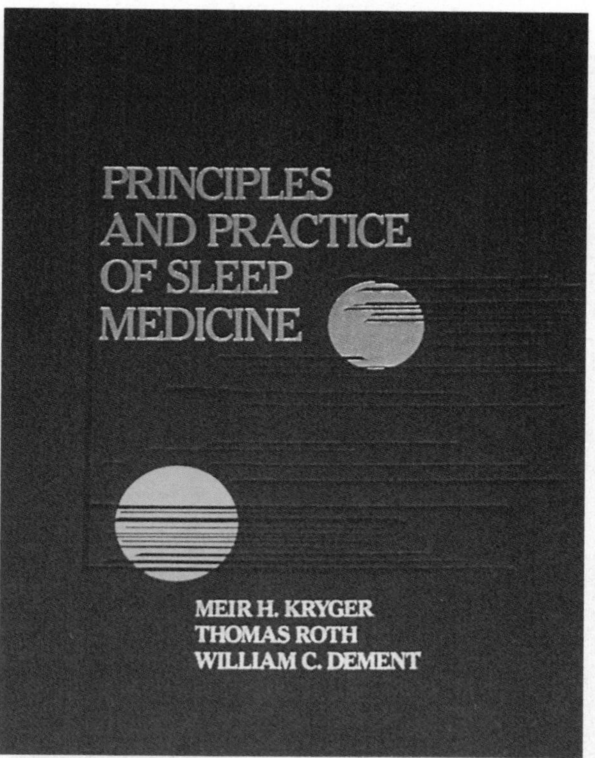

Figure 2-32.
Principles and Practice of Sleep Medicine, first edition.

1990 Michael Thorpy spearheads the creation of the first International Classification of Sleep Disorders (Fig. 2-33).

1990 The National Sleep Foundation is established in the United States.

1993 U.S. legislation establishes the Center for Sleep Disorders Research at the National Institutes of Health.

1993 Terry Young, in the first community-based epidemiologic study on sleep apnea, shows for the first time that sleep apnea is found to be extremely common among males. And for the first time the high prevalence among females was shown. Up to that time, it was thought that sleep apnea was rare among females.

1995 Nathaniel Kleitman gives a lecture at age 100 at the APSS (Fig. 2-34).

1997 Modafinil is shown to be effective as a stimulant. Ultimately it was found to be an efficacious treatment in narcolepsy, and later in other clinical conditions of excessive sleepiness.

1997 In 1994 the first circadian mutant mammal was produced by Martha Vitaterna, Lawrence Pinto, Fred Turek, Joseph Takahashi, and colleagues, by inducing mutations using a chemical mutagen and then screening animals for abnormal circadian phenotype. In 1997, Takahashi, Pinto, and Turek discover and clone the first mammalian circadian clock gene, called *Clock*. Soon many circadian genes were found to be similar in flies, mice, and humans, demonstrating the conservation of function over a prolonged period of evolutionary time. Figure 2-35 shows

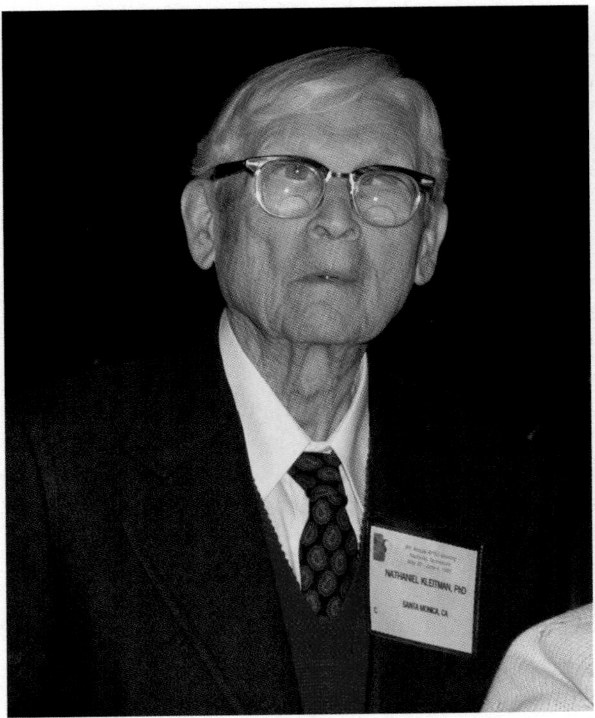

Figure 2-34.
Nathaniel Kleitman, age 100. (Courtesy M. H. Kryger.)

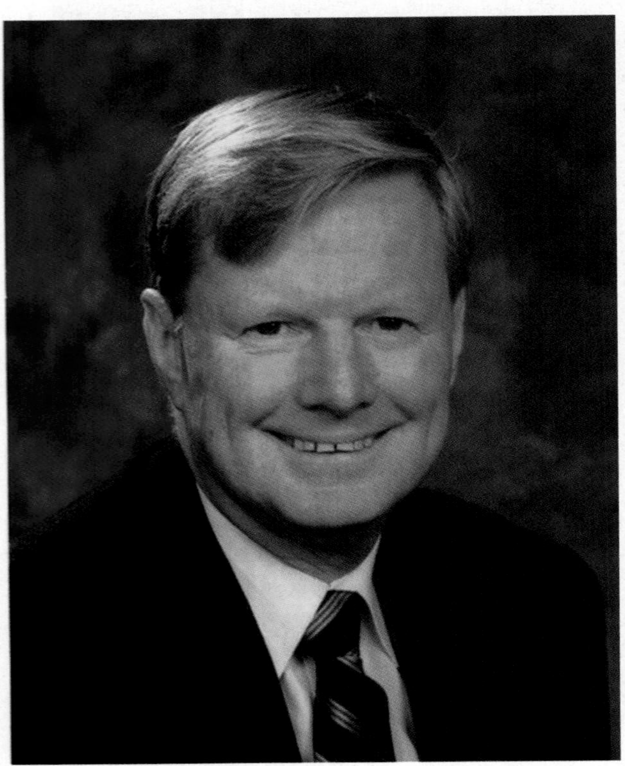

Figure 2-33.
Michael Thorpy.

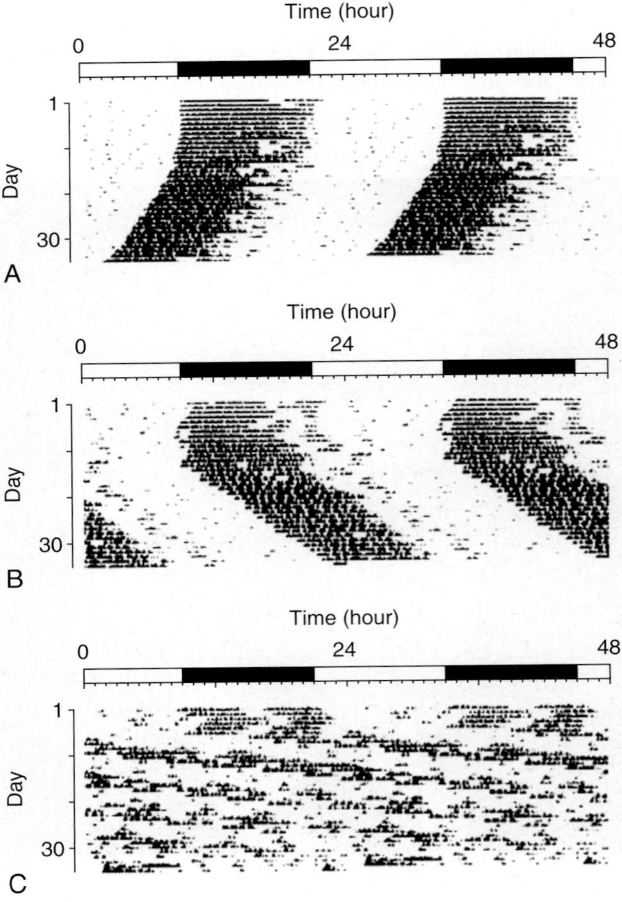

Figure 2-35.
Activity–rest plots in wild-type and two mutant animals.

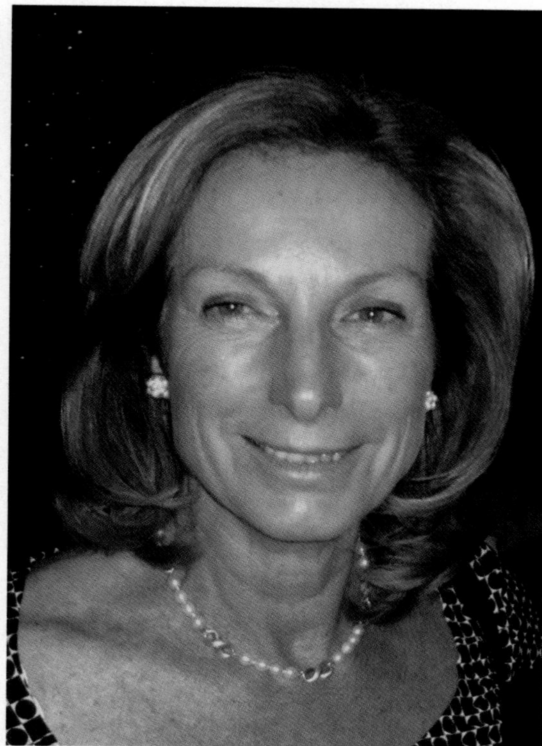

Figure 2-36.
Eve Van Cauter.

the circadian phenotype in wild-type, heterozygous, and homozygous mutant animals.

1999 Eve Van Cauter demonstrates that sleep restriction can induce, in otherwise healthy people, physiologic and endocrine changes indicative of early signs of insulin resistance. This led to a flood of epidemiologic, clinical, and animal studies for investigating the relationship between chronic partial sleep loss and obesity, diabetes, and cardiovascular disease (Fig. 2-36).

1999 Following a 10-year search, Emmanuel Mignot's group found that familial narcolepsy in dogs was due to mutations in the hypocretin receptor-2 (Fig. 2-37). Shortly after, Mashashi Yanagisawa's group independently found that hypocretin knockout mice also had narcolepsy.

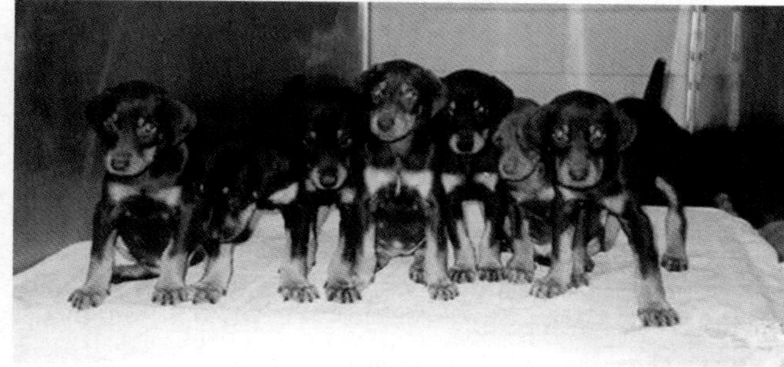

Figure 2-37.
Narcoleptic puppies.

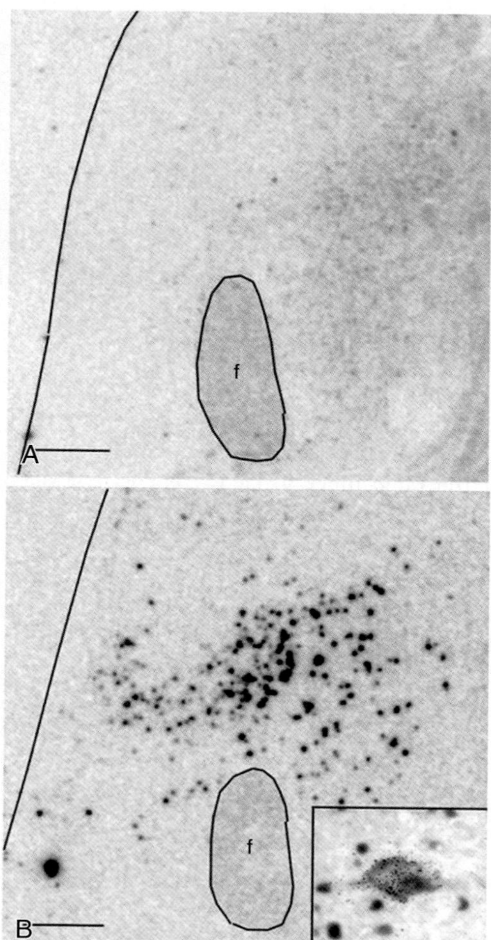

Figure 2-38.
A, narcolepsy. B, normal hypocretin gene expression in brain. (Courtesy E. Mignot.)

This was followed by the discovery at Stanford University, confirmed by Jerome Siegel's group at UCLA, that most cases of human narcolepsy, with cataplexy and HLA-DQB1*0602 positive, are associated with a loss of hypocretin peptide in the cerebrospinal fluid and the brain (Fig. 2-38).

2005 NIH holds a second consensus conference on management of insomnia.

2007 Juliane Winkelman found through a genome-wide association that single nucleotide polymorphisms with the BTBD9, MEIS1, and MAP2K5/LBXCOR1 region are associated with RLS. Hreinn Stefansson, David Rye, and colleagues also found independently that the BTBD9 polymorphism was associated with PLMs (and to a lesser extent RLS) and low ferritin levels.

2008 The Centers for Disease Control and Prevention (CDC) establish sleep as one of its areas of interest, thereby placing the topic onto the public health agenda.

CHAPTER 3 THE BIOLOGY OF SLEEP

3.1 Sleep Mechanisms

Patrick M. Fuller, Phyllis C. Zee, and Orfeu Buxton

Sleep Is Controlled by the Nervous System

Although it is generally believed that when asleep, the entire brain is "asleep," research suggests that sleep may also be a localized process and that the whole brain is not "asleep" at the same time. What is clear is that sleep is an active process whose timing and length are controlled by structures in the nervous system (Fig. 3.1-1).

Arousal Systems

For many years, the nature of the circuitry subserving the wake/arousal- and sleep-promoting brain regions remained elusive. The concept evolved that sleep control involved centers and processes that cause arousal and those that promote sleep (Figs. 3.1-2, 3.1-3).

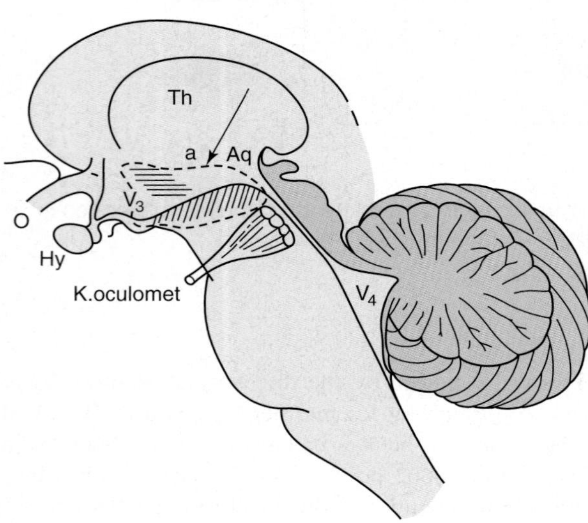

Figure 3.1-1.
An active role for the brain in sleep-wake behavior was first indicated in 1916 when Baron Constantine von Economo performed a postmortem brain analysis on victims of a viral encephalitis that profoundly affected sleep-wake regulation (i.e., encephalitis lethargica, or von Economo's sleeping sickness). As seen here in the original drawing taken from von Economo's clinico-anatomic studies, lesions at the junction of the midbrain and posterior hypothalamus *(diagonal hatching)* produced hypersomnolence. By contrast, lesions of the basal forebrain and anterior hypothalamus *(horizontal hatching)* produced profound insomnia. Von Economo also observed that lesions between these two sites *(arrow)*, which included the lateral hypothalamic area, caused narcolepsy. (From Von Economo C: Sleep as a problem of localization. J Nerv Ment Dis 71:249–259, 1930.)

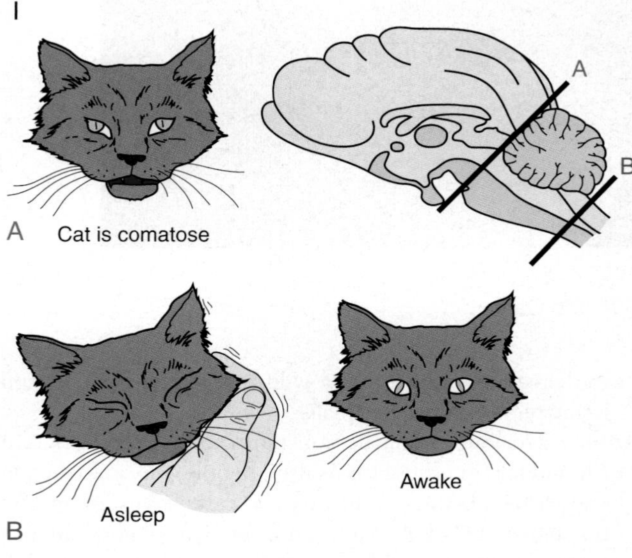

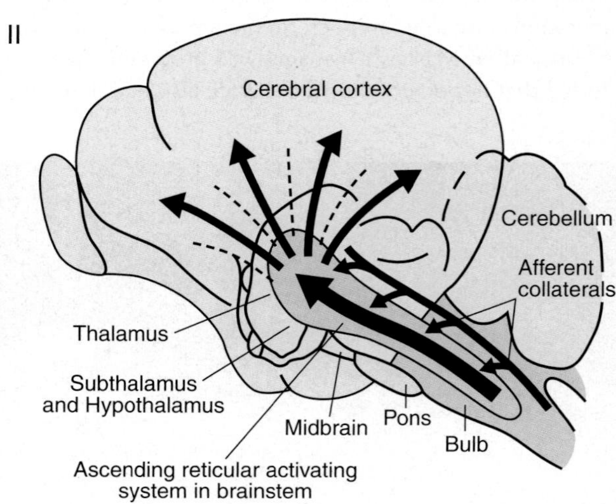

Figure 3.1-2.
See opposite page for legend

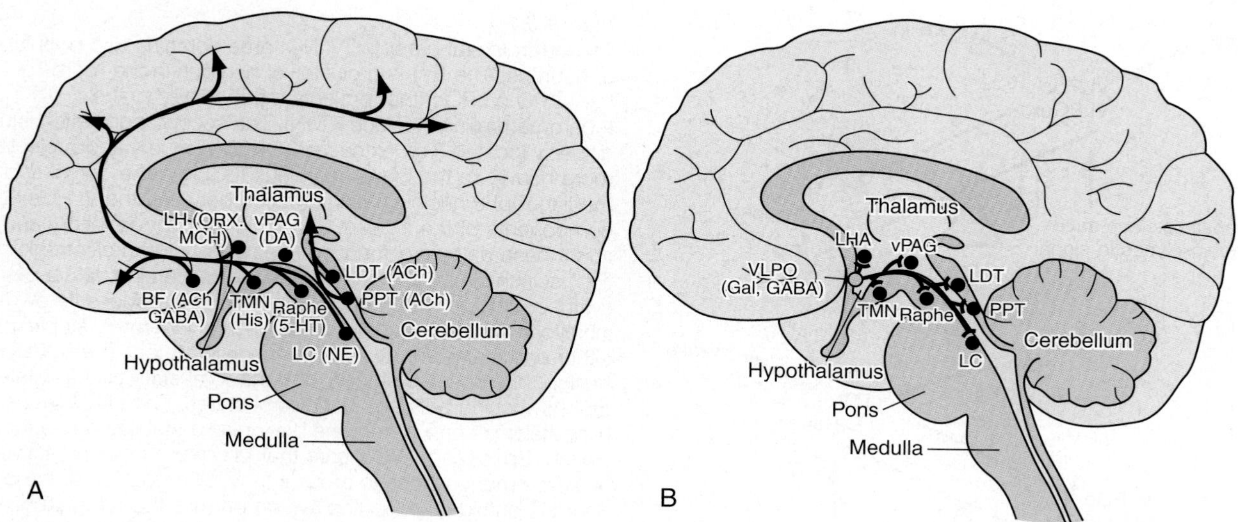

Figure 3.1-3.

A, In the 1970s and 1980s, the neurochemistry of several brainstem "arousal" centers was elaborated. In the contemporary view (A), the ascending arousal system consists of noradrenergic (NE) neurons of the ventrolateral medulla and locus coeruleus (LC), cholinergic neurons (ACh) in the PPT/LDT nuclei, 5-HT serotoninergic neurons in the dorsal raphe nucleus (Raphe), dopaminergic neurons (DA) of the vPAG, and histaminergic neurons (His) of the TMN. These systems produce cortical arousal via two pathways: a dorsal route through the thalamus and a ventral route through the hypothalamus and basal forebrain (BF). The latter pathway receives contributions from the orexin (ORX) and MCH neurons of the lateral hypothalamic (LH) area as well as from GABAergic or cholinergic neurons of the BF. Note that all of these ascending pathways traverse the region at the midbrain-diencephalic junction where von Economo observed that lesions caused hypersomnolence. As shown in A, several putative brainstem arousal centers were identified and characterized nearly 30 years ago. It nevertheless remained unclear for many years how this arousal system was turned "off" so that sleep could be initiated and maintained.

B, Although work by W. J. A. Nauta in 1946 provided support for the concept of sleep-promoting circuitry in the anterior hypothalamus/preoptic area, it was not until the mid-1990s that the identity of this sleep-promoting circuitry was revealed. In these recent investigations (B), it was demonstrated that the VLPO nucleus contains sleep-active cells that contain the inhibitory neurotransmitters GABA and galanin (Gal). The VLPO *(open circle)* projects to all of the main components of the ascending arousal system. Inhibition of the arousal system by the VLPO during sleep is critical for the maintenance and consolidation of sleep. (Additional work has provided support for the concept that an active sleep-promoting area is located near the nucleus of the solitary tract in the medulla. Nevertheless, the presence of sleep-promoting neurons in the medulla remains largely unconfirmed.) 5-HT, 5-hydroxytryptamine; GABA, gamma-amino butyric acid; LDT, laterodorsal tegmental; MCH, melanin-concentrating hormone; PPT, pedunculopontine tegmental; TMN, tuberomammillary nucleus; VLPO, ventrolateral preoptic; vPAG, ventral periaqueductal gray matter.

Figure 3.1-2.

I. In 1935 Bremer uncovered evidence of an ascending arousal system necessary for cortical arousal when he demonstrated that transection of the brainstem at the pontomesencephalic level, that is, cerveau isole, but not the spinomedullary junction, that is, encephale isole, produced coma in anesthetized cats. Bremer hypothesized that the resulting reduction in "cerebral tone" following the cerveau isole was due to interruption of ascending sensory inputs, that is, a passive "deafferentation theory" of sleep. (Adapted from Bremer F: Bulletin de l'Academie Royale de Belgique, 1937, 4.)

II. More than a decade after Bremer's transection experiments, G. Moruzzi (a student of Bremer's) and H. Magoun demonstrated that electrical stimulation of the rostral pontine reticular formation produced a desynchronized EEG (an electrophysiological correlate of the conscious state) in anesthetized cats. Moruzzi and Magoun interpreted their experimental data as evidence for an active "waking center" in the mesopontine reticular formation, essentially refuting the "deafferentation theory" of sleep. Moruzzi and Magoun called this brainstem system the "ascending reticular activating system."

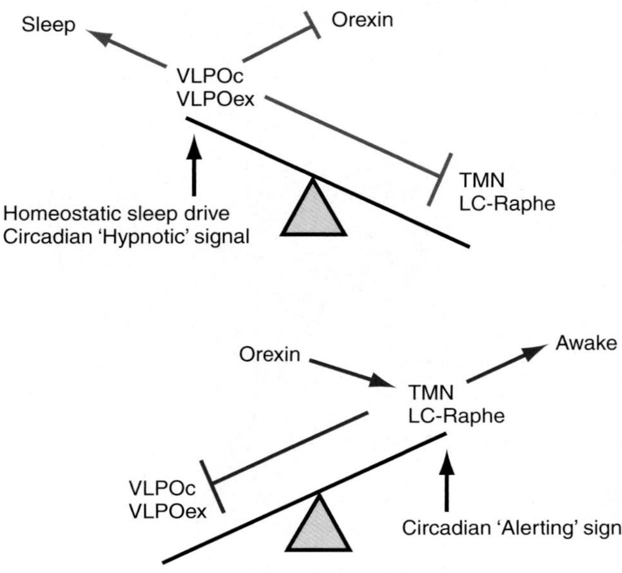

Figure 3.1-4.
The ventrolateral preoptic (VLPO) area contains two populations of neurons. The first is a cluster of neurons in the "core" of the VLPO (VLPOc) that projects most heavily to the tuberomammillary nucleus (TMN). The second population is more diffusely located (i.e., extended VLPO; VLPOex) and projects more heavily to the locus coeruleus (LC) and the dorsal and median raphe nuclei. This interaction between the VLPOex and components of the arousal system is mutually inhibitory and as such these pathways function analogously to an electronic "flip-flop" switch/circuit. By virtue of the self-reinforcing nature of these switches, that is, when each side is firing it reduces its own inhibitory feedback, the flip-flop switch is inherently stable in either end state, but avoids intermediate states. The flip-flop design thus ensures stability of behavioral state and facilitates rapid switching between behavioral states. The LH (lateral hypothalamic) orexin neurons likely play a stabilizing role for the switch. Specifically, it appears that LH orexin neurons actively reinforce monoaminergic arousal tone. The position of the orexin neurons outside the flip-flop switch permits them to stabilize the behavioral state by reducing transitions during both sleep and wakefulness. Narcoleptic humans or animals that lack orexin have increased transitions in both states. (Adapted from Fuller PM, Gooley JJ, Saper CB: Neurobiology of the sleep-wake cycle: Sleep architecture, circadian regulation, and regulatory feedback. J Biol Rhythms 21[6]:482–493, 2006.)

Sleep-Promoting Systems

Neurons of the ventrolateral preoptic (VLPO) system are sleep-active, and loss of VLPO neurons produces profound insomnia and sleep fragmentation (Figs. 3.1-4, 3.1-5).

Sleep Drive

While significant progress has been made in delineating the neuronal circuitry that controls wake and sleep, the basis of "sleep drive" has remained elusive. Sleep drive has been conceptualized as a homeostatic pressure that builds during the waking period and is dissipated by sleep. This homeostatic process, or "sleep homeostat," thus represents the need for sleep (Fig. 3.1-6).

The Control of REM Sleep

REM (rapid eye movement) is a distinct state in which the function of the central nervous system and the autonomic nervous system differs from both wakefulness and NREM (nonrapid eye movement) sleep (Fig. 3.1-7).

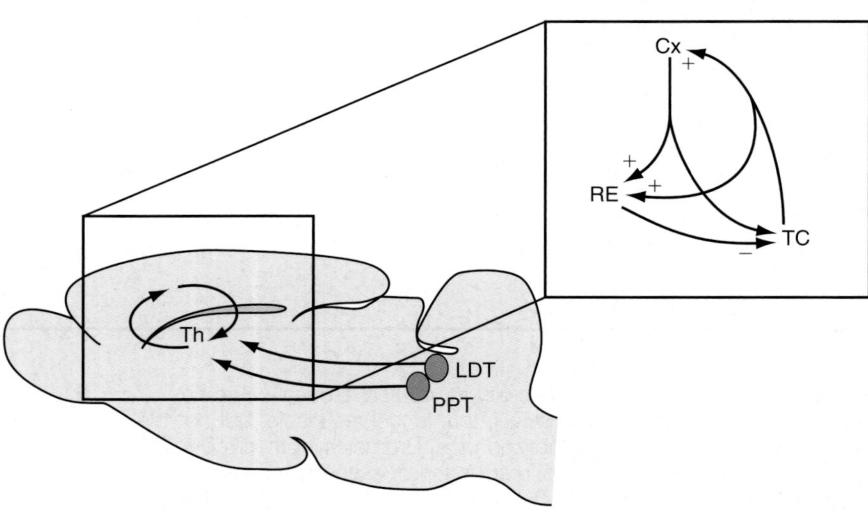

Figure 3.1-5.
During cortical arousal the electroencephalogram (EEG) directly reflects the collective synaptic potentials of inputs largely to pyramidal cells within the neocortex and hippocampus. The thalamocortical (TC) system has been widely considered to be a major source of this activity. The overall level of activity in the TC system, in turn, is thought to be regulated by the ascending arousal system. Today, it is generally accepted that a brainstem cholinergic activating system, located in the pedunculopontine tegmental (PPT) and laterodorsal tegmental (LDT) nuclei *(green circles)*, induces tonic and phasic depolarization effects on TC neurons to produce the low-voltage, mixed frequency, fast activity of the waking and REM sleep EEG. The PPT and LDT cease firing during NREM sleep, which hyperpolarizes the TC neurons to produce two important effects: (1) sensory transmission through the thalamus to the cortex is blocked; and (2) oscillatory activity between TC neurons, cortical neurons (Cx), and reticular thalamus (RE) neurons (see figure inset) is unmasked to manifest several characteristics of the sleep EEG—slow wave activity (0.5–4 Hz) and spindles. Thus, the thalamus appears to be a critical relay for the ascending arousal system for "gating" sensory transmission to the cortex during sleep and wake.

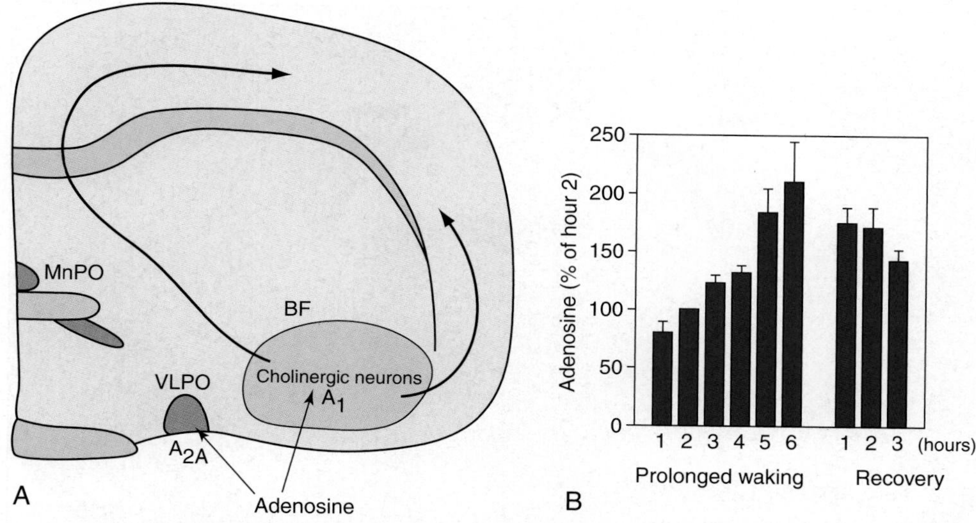

Figure 3.1-6.
The cellular determinant of homeostatic sleep drive is unknown, although a putative endogenous somnogen, adenosine (AD), is thought to play a critical role. **A**, AD is a naturally occurring purine nucleoside. It is hypothesized that AD accumulates during wake and upon reaching sufficient concentrations, inhibits neural activity in wake-promoting circuitry of the basal forebrain (BF) (via A_1 receptors located on BF cholinergic neurons) and, likely, activates sleep-promoting VLPO neurons (via A_{2A} receptors) located adjacent to the BF. A role for adenosine and BF cholinergic neurons in sleep homeostasis has recently been challenged by Blanco-Centurion and colleagues. **B**, Mean BF extracellular AD values by hour during 6 hours of prolonged wakefulness and in the subsequent 3 hours of spontaneous recovery sleep in felines. Microdialysis values in the six animals are normalized relative to the second hour of wakefulness. Mn PO, median preoptic nucleus; VLPO, ventrolateral preoptic area. (Data from Porkka-Heiskanen T, Strecker RE, Thakkar M, et al: Adenosine: A mediator of the sleep-inducing effects of prolonged wakefulness. Science 276[5316]:1265–1268, 1997.)

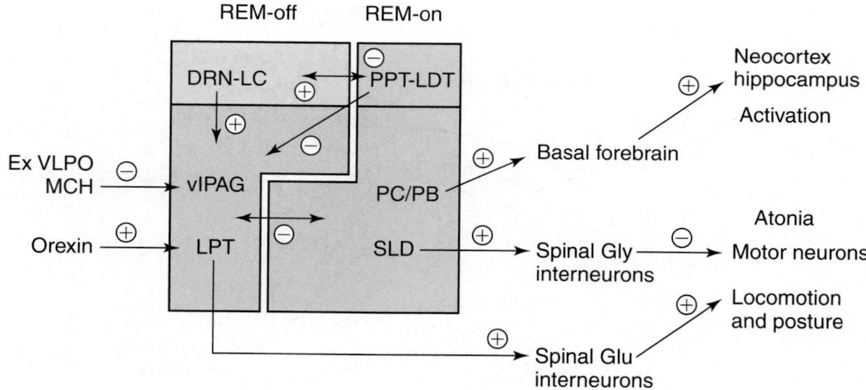

Figure 3.1-7.
In the contemporary REM flip-flop switch model, the REM switch consists of two sides, "REM-on" and "REM-off." The REM-off region is identified by the overlap of inputs from the VLPOex and orexin neurons and melanin-concentrating hormone (MCH) neurons. These REM-off neurons in the ventrolateral periaqueductal gray (vlPAG) and lateral pontine tegmentum (LPT) have a mutually inhibitory interaction with REM-on GABAergic neurons of the ventral sublaterodorsal nucleus (SLD) and the precoeruleus/parabrachial nucleus (PC/PB). Although the cholinergic neurons of the pedunculopontine and laterodorsal tegmental nuclei (PPT-LDT) are REM-on and likely inhibit the LPT, these neurons are not directly inhibited by the LPT and are thus external to the switch. This is also true for the dorsal raphe and noradrenergic locus coeruleus (DRN-LC) neurons that can activate the REM-off area but are not inhibited directly by the SLD. Neurons of the SLD produce atonia during REM sleep through direct glutamatergic spinal projections to interneurons that inhibit spinal motor neurons by both glycinergic and GABAergic mechanisms. Glutamatergic inputs from the REM-on PC region and PB to the medial septum and the basal forebrain appear to play a key role in generating hippocampal and cortical activation during REM sleep. (Adapted from Lu J, Sherman D, Devor M, Saper CB: A putative flip-flop switch for control of REM sleep. Nature 441[7093]:589–594, 2006.)

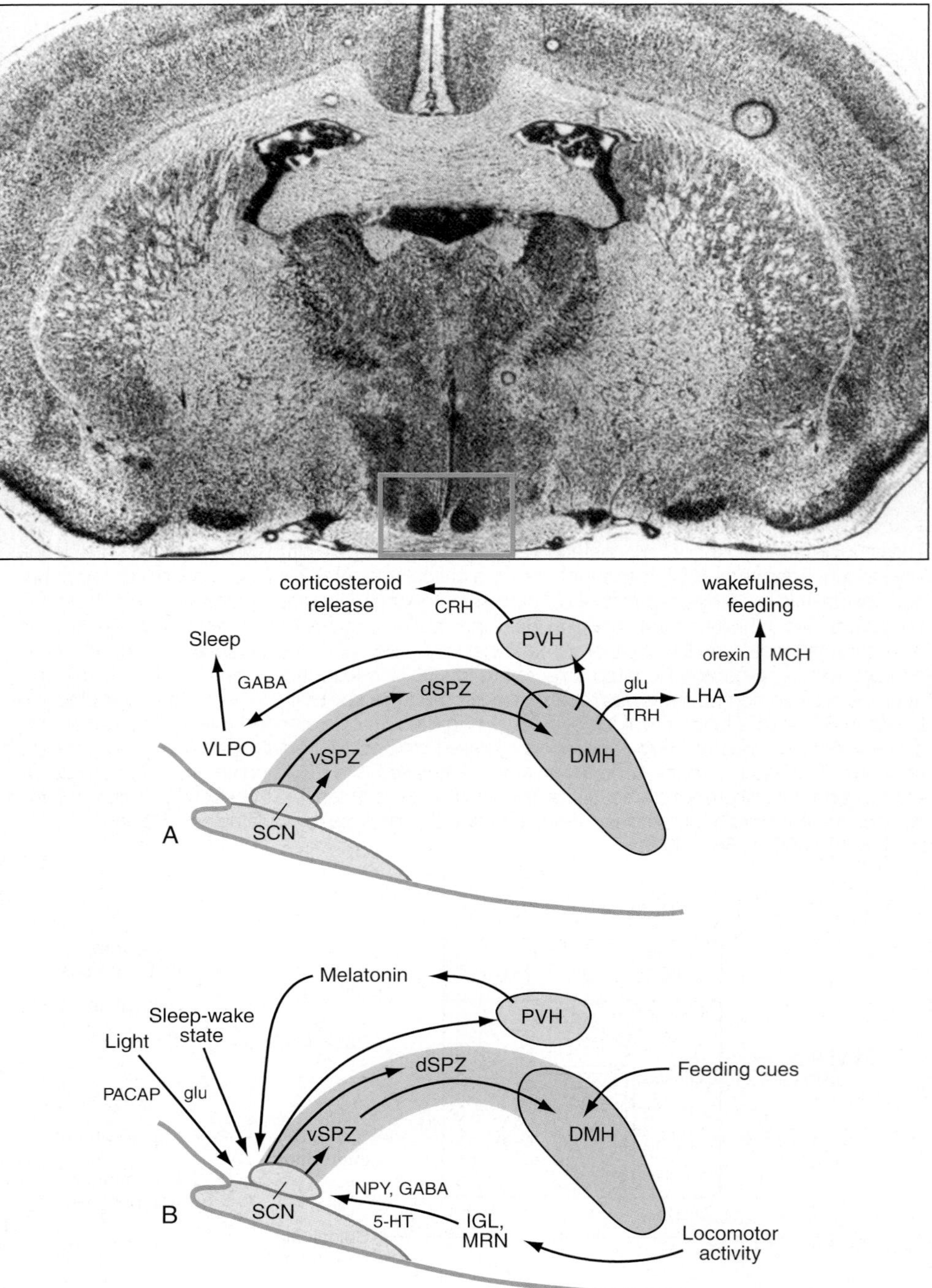

Figure 3.1-8.
At the top of the figure a coronal section of the brain shows the location (box) of the rat SCN. The circadian rhythm of sleep-wake is regulated at multiple levels in the hypothalamus. **A**, The circadian clock in the SCN sends an indirect projection to the DMH via the SPZ, which is critical for the circadian rhythm of sleep-wake. The DMH, in turn, provides rhythmic output to brain regions critical for the regulation of sleep-wake, hormone synthesis and release, and feeding. **B**, This multistage regulation of circadian behavior in the hypothalamus allows for the integration of multiple time cues from the environment to shape daily patterns of sleep-wake. 5-HT, 5-hydroxytryptamine (serotonin); CRH, corticotrophin-releasing hormone; DMH, dorsomedial hypothalamic nucleus; dSPZ, dorsal subparaventricular zone; GABA, gamma-amino butyric acid; glu, glutamate; IGL, intergeniculate leaftlet; LHA, lateral hypothalamic area; MCH, melanin-concentrating hormone; MRN, median raphe nucleus; NPY, neuropeptide Y; PACAP, pituitary adenylate cyclase-activating polypeptide; PVH, paraventricular hypothalamic nucleus; SCN, suprachiasmatic nucleus; SPZ, subparaventricular zone; TRH, thyrotropin-releasing hormone; VLPO, ventrolateral preoptic nucleus; vSPZ, ventral subparaventricular zone. (Adapted from Fuller PM, Gooley JJ, Saper CB: Neurobiology of the sleep-wake cycle: Sleep architecture, circadian regulation, and regulatory feedback. J Biol Rhythms 21[6]:482–493, 2006.)

Control of the Timing of Sleep

In mammals, the circadian clock in the suprachiasmatic nucleus (SCN) of the anterior hypothalamus is critical for establishing the circadian rhythm of sleep-wake. Regulation of sleep-wakefulness by the SCN is evident as the sleep-wake cycle continues on an approximately 24-hour basis even when environmental conditions are constant (i.e., in the absence of environmental time cues), but only if the SCN is intact. In humans, a clear circadian variation in sleep propensity and sleep structure has been demonstrated by uncoupling the rest–activity cycle from the output of the circadian pacemaker (Fig. 3.1-8).

SELECTED READINGS

Basheer R, Strecker RE, Thakkar MM, McCarley RW: Adenosine and sleep-wake regulation. Prog Neurobiol 73(6):379–396, 2004.

Blanco-Centurion C, Xu M, Murillo-Rodriguez E, et al: Adenosine and sleep homeostasis in the basal forebrain. J Neurosci 26(31): 8092–80100, 2006.

Bremer F: Cerveau "isole" et physiologie du sommeil. Comptes Rendus de la Société de Biologie (Paris) 118:1235–1241, 1935.

Bremer F: Preoptic hypnogenic area and reticular activating system. Archives Italiennes de Biologie 111:85–111, 1973.

Edgar DM, Dement WC, Fuller CA: Effect on SCN lesions on sleep in squirrel monkeys: processes in sleep-wake regulation. J. Neuroscienci 13(3):1065–1079, 1993.

Lu J, Sherman D, Devor M, Saper CB: A putative flip-flop switch for control of REM sleep. Nature 441(7093):589–594, 2006.

Morairty S, Rainnie D, McCarley R, Greene R: Disinhibition of ventrolateral preoptic area sleep-active neurons by adenosine: A new mechanism for sleep promotion. Neuroscience 123(2):451–457, 2004.

Moruzzi G, Magoun H: Brainstem reticular formation and activation of the EEG. Electroencephalogr Clin Neurophysiol 1:455–473, 1949.

Nauta WJH: Hypothalamic regulation of sleep in rats: Experimental study. J Neurophysiol 9:285–316, 1946.

Sherin JE, Elmquist JK, Torrealba F, Saper CB: Innervation of histaminergic tuberomammillary neurons by GABAergic and galaninergic neurons in the ventrolateral preoptic nucleus of the rat. J Neurosci 18(12): 4705–4721, 1998.

Sherin JE, Shiromani PJ, McCarley RW, Saper CB: Activation of ventrolateral preoptic neurons during sleep. Science 271(5246):216–219, 1996.

Steriade M, McCormick DA, Sejnowski TJ: Thalamocortical oscillations in the sleeping and aroused brain. Science 262:679–685, 1993.

Von Economo C: Sleep as a problem of localization. J Nerv Ment Dis 71:249–259, 1930.

Kathryn J. Reid, Phyllis C. Zee, and Orfeu Buxton

3.2 Circadian Rhythms Regulation

All living creatures exhibit self-sustaining circadian (near 24-hour) rhythms in physiology and behavior that are regulated by a central clock located in the suprachiasmatic nuclei (SCN) of the hypothalamus. This system is involved in the regulation of many physiological functions including the timing of the production of hormones. The genetics of the circadian system at the cellular level has only recently been understood (Fig. 3.2-1).

The sleep-wake cycle is the most apparent circadian rhythm in humans. Light, physical activity, and melatonin from the pineal gland are the primary synchronizing agents for the human circadian clock. In humans, light is the strongest time giver for the circadian clock. For optimal function, the timing of circadian rhythms needs to be synchronized with the external physical environment and the social- or work-imposed sleep and wake schedules. Circadian rhythm sleep disorders (CRSDs; see Chapter 8) develop when there is disruption of the circadian clock or its entraining pathways, or when the timing of the circadian clock is misaligned with the 24-hour external environment (Figs. 3.2-2, 3.2-3).

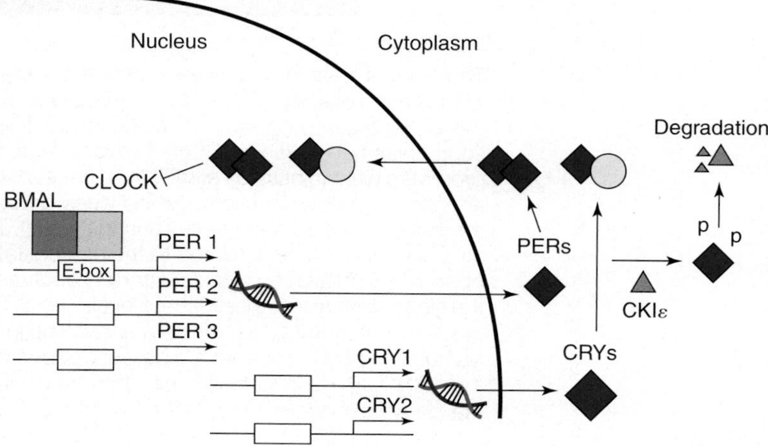

Figure 3.2-1.
The genetic mechanism of the circadian clock is similar in many species, from prokaryotic bacteria to fruit flies to mammals. The key mechanism appears to involve an exquisitely timed transcription and translation feedback loop between nuclear gene expression and their protein products. In mammals, protein dimers of PER and CRY protein bind to dimers of CLOCK and BMAL1 on the E-box for *per* genes and inhibit transcription of the PER and CRY genes. Reduced PER/CRY transcription to mRNAs and translation to proteins subsequently disinhibits CLOCK/BMAL1 binding to the enhancer (E)-box, which leads to renewed transcription of PER and CRY.

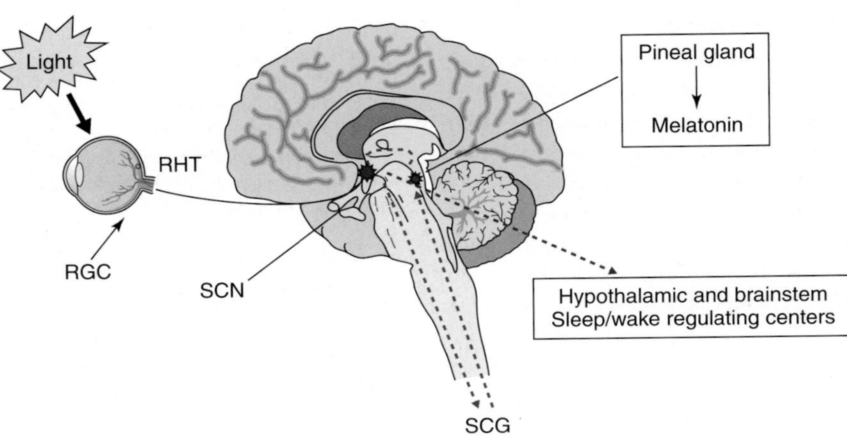

Figure 3.2-2.
Shown here are the basic components of the circadian system. Photic information to the suprachiasmatic nucleus (SCN) is transmitted from the retina via the retinohypothalamic tract (RHT). The retinal ganglion cells (RGC) of the eye, melanopsin containing photoreceptors, provide the primary photic input to the circadian clock, transmitting the signal to the neurons of the SCN. Melatonin is released from the pineal gland at night, and its output is regulated by the SCN via the superior cervical ganglion (SCG). In addition to its ability to synchronize circadian rhythms, melatonin can also promote sleep. Integrated timing information from the SCN is transmitted to sleep-wake centers in the brain. Thus, the sleep-wake cycle is generated by a complex interaction of endogenous circadian and sleep processes, as well as by social and environmental factors.

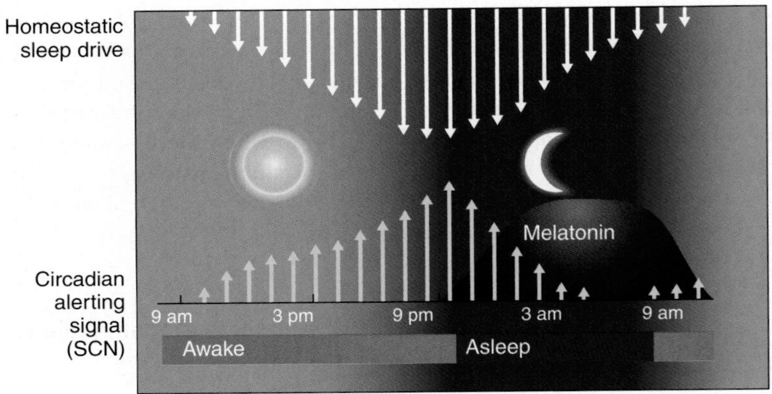

Figure 3.2-3.
There are at least two variables that seem to play a role in the regulation of the timing of sleep. First is the homeostatic sleep drive, which increases the longer a person is awake. The second is timing information from the suprachiasmatic nucleus (SCN). In this two-process model, the SCN promotes wakefulness by stimulating arousal networks. SCN activity appears to oppose the homeostatic sleep drive, and thus the alerting mediated by the SCN increases during the day. The propensity to be awake or asleep at any time is related to the homeostatic sleep drive and the opposing SCN alerting signal. At normal bedtime both the alerting drive and the sleep drive are at their highest level. The SCN has at least two types of melatonin receptors, MT1 and MT2, involved in the regulation of sleep. Stimulation of MT1 receptors is believed to decrease the alerting signal from the SCN, while MT2 stimulation is thought to be involved in synchronizing the circadian system. (Adapted with permission, Takeda Pharmaceuticals.)

Light exposure and exogenous melatonin administration can be used to shift the timing of the circadian clock. Phase response curves to light and other synchronizing agents such as melatonin have been described. Light exposure in the late evening before the core body temperature minimum (Tmin) delays circadian rhythms, and light in the morning after the Tmin advances circadian rhythms. The response to melatonin is the opposite of the response to light; melatonin given in the evening will phase advance the circadian clock, while melatonin in the morning will phase delay the circadian clock.

Circadian phase markers can be used to confirm the diagnosis of circadian rhythm sleep disorders and to determine circadian phase in order to correctly time treatment with light and/or melatonin (see chapter 8). Core body temperature (CBT) can be determined using a rectal thermistor worn for 24 to 28 hours. The CBT minimum (Tmin) usually occurs about 2 to 3 hours before wake time, and it is generally easier to fall asleep on the declining part of the CBT rhythm and to wake on the rising portion. Dim light melatonin onset (DLMO) can be determined from plasma or saliva sampled at regular intervals (30 min) under dim light conditions. The DLMO usually occurs about 2 to 3 hours prior to habitual sleep time in normal controls and in subjects with delayed sleep phase disorder.

SELECTED READINGS

Czeisler CA, Allan JS, Strogatz SH, et al: Bright light resets the human circadian pacemaker independent of the timing of the sleep-wake cycle. Science 233(4764):667–671, 1986.

Czeisler CA, Weitzman E, Moore-Ede MC, et al: Human sleep: Its duration and organization depend on its circadian phase. Science 210 (4475):1264–1267, 1980.

Lewy AJ, Bauer VK, Ahmed S, et al: The human phase response curve (PRC) to melatonin is about 12 hours out of phase with the PRC to light. Chronobiol Int 15(1):71–83, 1998.

Moore RY: A clock for the ages. Science 284(5423):2102–2103, 1999.

Murphy PJ, Campbell SS: Physiology of the circadian system in animals and humans. J Clin Neurophysiol 13(1):2–16, 1996.

Rollag MD, Berson DM, Provencio I: Melanopsin, ganglion-cell photoreceptors, and mammalian photoentrainment. J Biol Rhythms 18(3): 227–234, 2003.

Saper CB, Lu J, Chou TC, et al: The hypothalamic integrator for circadian rhythms. Trends Neurosci 28(3):152–157, 2005.

Van Cauter E, Sturis J, Byrne MM, et al: Demonstration of rapid light-induced advances and delays of the human circadian clock using hormonal phase markers. Am J Physiol 266(6, Pt 1):E953–E963,1994.

3.3 Sleep, A Localized Phenomenon of the Brain

Hans P.A. Van Dongen, David M. Rector, Gregory Belenky, and James M. Krueger

A new paradigm for how the brain is organized to produce sleep posits that sleep regulation is fundamentally a local and use-dependent process. Although specialized brain areas are involved in sleep-wake regulation, there is no evidence that these specific brain nuclei and pathways are necessary for the occurrence of sleep. A telling observation is that for millions of stroke patients and thousands of animal brain-lesion studies, there is not a single report of a postlesion survivor who failed to sleep.

Brain tissue can express sleep regionally, and this may occur spontaneously, without top-down control. When neurobiological substances known to induce sleep are applied unilaterally to the cortex in vivo, they intensify sleep only in the region where these sleep regulatory substances are applied, not in the whole brain. Experiments in intact rats have revealed expression of sleep in even smaller parts of the brain, namely, cortical columns. These are densely interconnected assemblies of neurons thought to be the basic unit of information processing. In the rat experiments, individual cortical columns—specifically, whisker barrels—showed stimulus responses characteristic of sleep, while neighboring columns exhibited wakelike responses. This was observed while the whole organism remained functionally awake. In addition, the local sleep state occurred more frequently when the cortical column

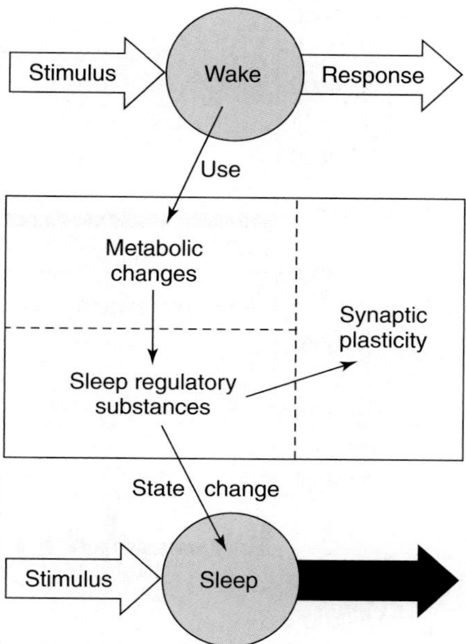

Figure 3.3-1.
Unit of brain circuitry regulating sleep. With continued use of the awake cortical column for stimulus processing, metabolic changes occur that lead to enhanced production of sleep regulatory substances. These induce synaptic plasticity, and render the specific cortical column asleep.

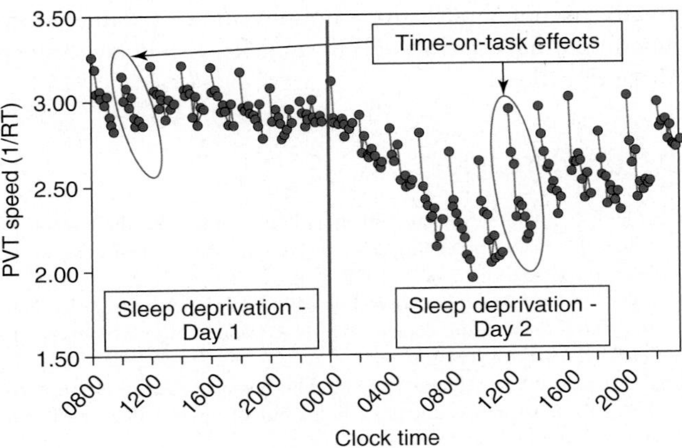

Figure 3.3-2.
Time-on-task effects in human performance. Total sleep deprivation exposes the influence of prior wake duration on the time-on-task effect in a psychomotor vigilance task (PVT). Group-averaged (50 subjects) response speeds are shown for every minute of this 10-minute performance task. Across the period of sleep deprivation, the time-on-task effect (steepness of the performance decline) intensifies, indicating that time awake and time on task interact to degrade waking function. This may be explained in terms of cumulative brain activity, that is, use-dependence. (Adapted from Wesensten NJ, Belenky G, Thorne DR, et al: Modafinil versus caffeine: Effects on fatigue during sleep deprivation. Aviat Space Environ Med 75:520–525, 2004.)

was stimulated more intensively. These findings indicate that sleep regulation is both *local* and *use-dependent* (Fig. 3.3-1).

Experiments in humans, ranging from unilateral somatosensory stimulation and arm immobilization to clever learning paradigms, have also provided evidence of differential, localized expression of sleep. Thus, the same principles of local and use-dependent sleep regulation seen in the rats may apply to human beings as well.

Human waking function is affected by the prior durations of sleep and wakefulness and by time on task. Prior wakefulness magnifies the time-on-task effect (Fig. 3.3-2). Prior wakefulness and time on task both increase cumulative brain activity through repeated use of local circuits. Thus, the interacting effect of wake duration and time on task may reflect use-dependent sleep regulatory mechanisms.

Furthermore, performance during sleep deprivation is unstable across time on task. This phenomenon of wake state instability may be interpreted in terms of prolonged use of the cortical columns involved in executing the task. Consequently, these cortical columns may express local, use-dependent sleep, thereby failing to process information. This would lead to performance instability while the person is otherwise fully awake (Fig. 3.3-3).

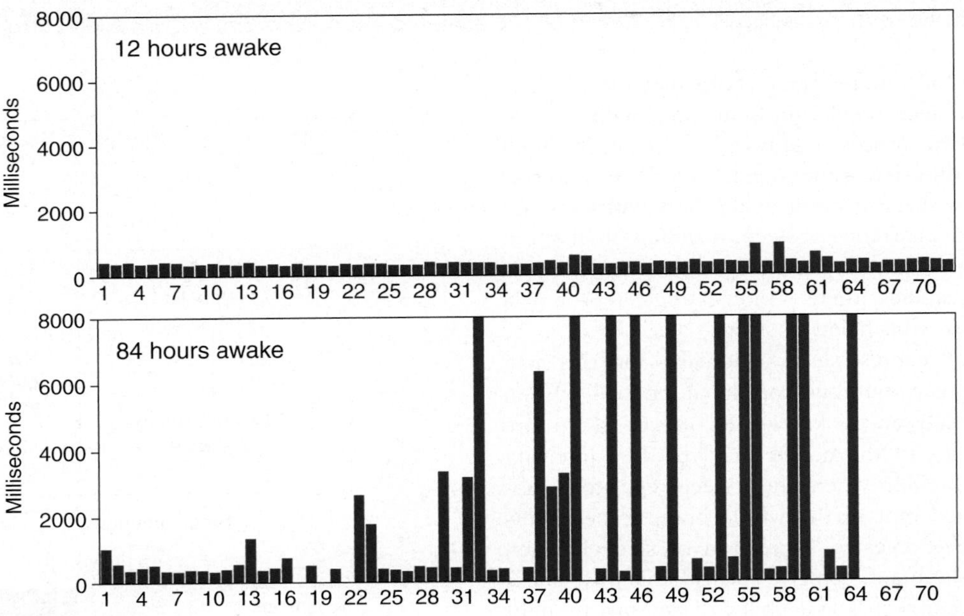

Figure 3.3-3.
Wake state instability. A person's reaction time performance on a psychomotor vigilance test (PVT) is compared at 12 hours of wakefulness *(top)* versus 84 hours of continuous wakefulness *(bottom).* Each panel shows individual reaction times for responding to a visual stimulus appearing at random 2- to 10-second intervals. Note that reaction time variability increases progressively across time on task in the sleep-deprived state. (Adapted from Doran SM, Van Dongen HPA, Dinges DF: Sustained attention performance during sleep deprivation: Evidence of state instability. Arch Ital Biol 139:253–267, 2001.)

The new paradigm of local, use-dependent sleep regulation conceptualizes whole-organism sleep as a bottom-up, self-organizing property of the collective states of cortical columns throughout the brain. This view does not invoke intentional action from specialized neural circuits to initiate or terminate whole-organism sleep, which avoids irresolvable questions as to how such intentional action might itself be triggered and what its purpose might be.

The research was supported by the W.M. Keck Foundation.

SELECTED READINGS

Doran SM, Van Dongen HPA, Dinges DF: Sustained attention performance during sleep deprivation: Evidence of state instability. Arch Ital Biol 139:253–267, 2001.

Kavanau JL: Sleep and dynamic stabilization of neural circuitry: A review and synthesis. Behav Brain Res 63:111–126, 1994.

Koch C: The Quest for Consciousness. Englewood, Colo., Roberts, 2004, pp. 25–34.

Krueger JM, Obál F: A neuronal group theory of sleep function. J Sleep Res 2:63–69, 1993.

Krueger JM, Obál F: Sleep function. Front Biosci 8:d511–d519, 2003.

Rector DM, Topchiy IA, Carter KM, Rojas MJ: Local functional state differences between rat cortical columns. Brain Res 1047:45–55, 2005.

Saper CB, Scammell TE, Lu J: Hypothalamic regulation of sleep and circadian rhythms. Nature 437:1257–1263, 2005.

Tononi G, Cirelli C: Sleep function and synaptic homeostasis. Sleep Med Rev 10:49–62, 2006.

Wesensten NJ, Belenky G, Thorne DR, et al: Modafinil versus caffeine: Effects on fatigue during sleep deprivation. Aviat Space Environ Med 75:520–525, 2004.

Yoshida H, Peterfi Z, Garcia-Garcia F, et al: State-specific asymmetries in EEG slow wave activity induced by local application of TNFα. Brain Res 1009:129–136, 2004.

Pier Luigi Parmeggiani

Physiologic Regulation in Sleep 3.4

Physiologic regulation in mammals varies with the state of the brain and is impacted by arousal and stage of sleep. This is the result of functional dominance of phylogenetically different structures of the brain in different behavioral states.

There is a functional similarity of physiologic events during nonrapid eye movement sleep (NREMS) in different species. During rapid eye movement sleep (REMS) there is variability of such events within and between species. There are nervous system processes that are specific to REMS that result in this autonomic variability and these processes are not related to mental content or homeostatic control.

The basic features of NREMS are active thermoregulation and a decrease in the activity of antigravity muscles. The basic features of REMS are muscle atonia, rapid eye movements, and myoclonic twitches. The basic autonomic feature of NREMS is the functional prevalence of parasympathetic influences associated with quiescence of sympathetic activity. The basic autonomic feature of REMS is the great variability in sympathetic activity associated with phasic changes in tonic parasympathetic discharge.

In NREMS mammals maintain homeostasis at a lower level of energy expenditure compared with quiet wakefulness. In contrast, REMS in all species is characterized by impaired homeostatic activity of physiologic functions (poikilostasis).

The impairment of homeostatic control in REMS is more dramatic and evident in a function, such as temperature regulation in furry animals (Table 3.4-1; Figs. 3.4-1 to 3.4-4), that depends on mechanisms strictly controlled by structures in the diencephalon (preoptic-hypothalamic area).

In functions characterized by more widely distributed control mechanisms, such as respiration (Figs. 3.4-5 to 3.4-7) and circulation (Figs. 3.4-8 and 3.4-9), the features of functional impairment are rather more complex as a result of the persistence of more or less efficient reflex regulation or peripheral autoregulation.

Nevertheless, it is evident that functional changes in REMS depend essentially on the suppression of a highly integrated homeostatic regulation that is operative in NREMS (Fig. 3.4-10). In comparison with REMS, volitional and instinctive drives during active wakefulness may also impose a load on or interfere with homeostatic mechanisms at central and/or effector levels to overwhelm their

Table 3.4-1. Thermoregulatory Responses in Wakefulness and Sleep

RESPONSES	WAKE	NREMS	REMS
Specific			
Behavioral	Locomotion		
	Posture	Posture	
Autonomic	Vasomotion	Vasomotion	
	Piloerection	Piloerection	
	Shivering Tg	Shivering Tg (+)	
	Nonshivering Tg	Nonshivering Tg	
	Thermal Tp	Thermal Tp (+)	
	Sweating	Sweating (+)	Sweating (0,−)
Nonspecific	Vigilance	Arousal	Arousal

Tg, thermogenesis; Tp, tachypnea.

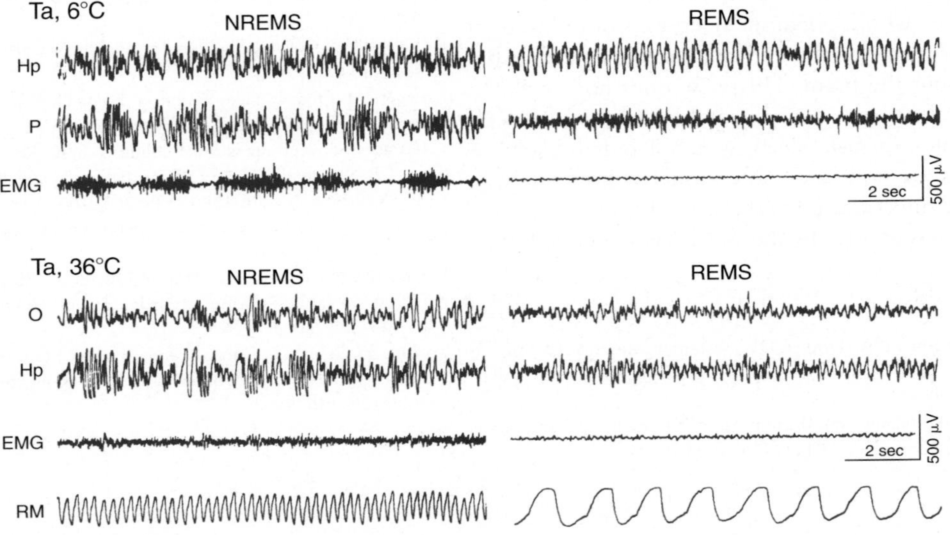

Figure 3.4-1.
Shivering and thermal tachypnea during sleep (cat). Both responses are present in NREMS and absent during REMS. Electrograms: Hp, hippocampus; O, occipital cortex; P, parietal cortex; EMG, neck muscles; RM, respiratory movements; Ta, ambient temperature. (From Parmeggiani PL, Rabini C: Sleep and environmental temperature. Arch Ital Biol 108:369–387, 1970; with permission by Università di Pisa.)

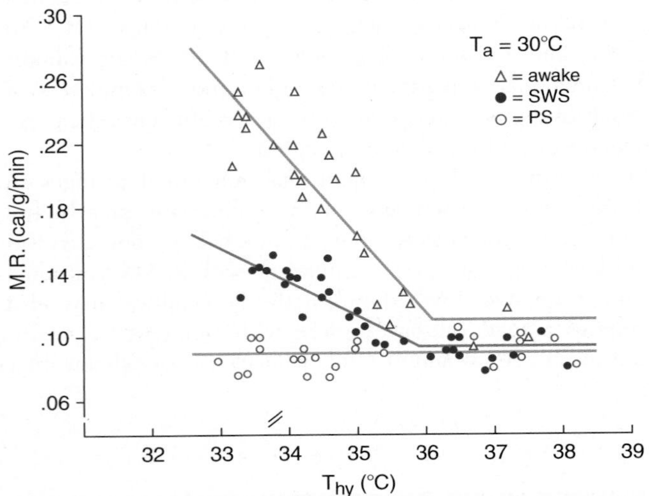

Figure 3.4-2.
Metabolic rate (M.R.) vs. hypothalamic temperature (T_{hy}) during wakefulness, NREMS (SWS) and REMS (PS) at 30° C ambient temperature (T_a) (Kangaroo rat). The effect of the thermal stimulus decreases during NREMS and disappears during REMS. (Adapted from Glotzbach SF, Heller HC: Central nervous regulation of body temperature during sleep. Science 194:537–539, 1976; with permission by AAAS.)

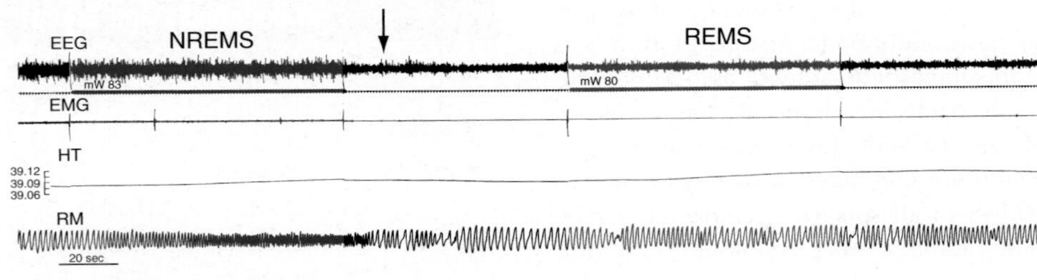

Figure 3.4-3.
Preoptic-anterior hypothalamic diathermic warming elicits tachypnea during NREMS and is ineffective during REMS at neutral ambient temperature (cat). Tachypnea disappears immediately at REMS onset *(arrow)* when hypothalamic temperature is still above threshold. EEG, electroencephalogram; EMG, neck muscle electrogram; HT, hypothalamic temperature (5 mm behind the warming electrode); RM, respiratory movements; mW, milliwatt. (From Parmeggiani PL, Franzini C, Lenzi P, Zamboni G: Threshold of respiratory responses to preoptic heating during sleep in freely moving cats. Brain Res 52:189–201, 1973; with permission by Elsevier.)

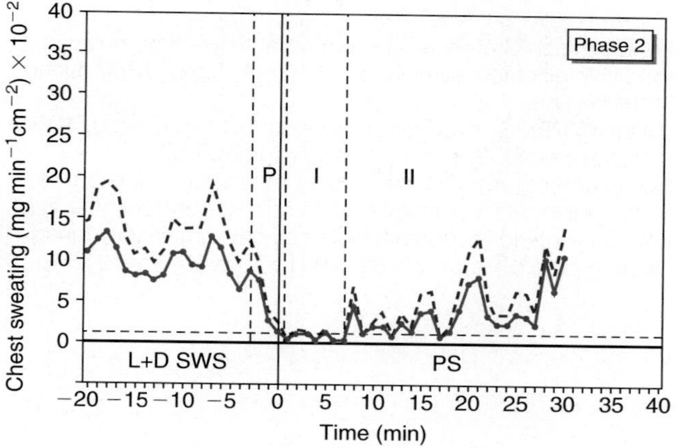

Figure 3.4-4.
Chest sweating drops just before scoring (P) the REMS onset, is fully abolished during the initial part of the episode (I), and slowly and irregularly increases during the rest duration of the episode (human). Means (full curves) ± SEM (dashed curves); L+D SWS, light + deep NREMS; PS, REMS. (Adapted from Dewasmes G, Bothorel B, Candas V, Libert JP: A short-term poikilothermic period occurs just after paradoxical sleep onset in humans: Characterization changes in sweating effector activity. J Sleep Res 6:252–258, 1997; with permission by Wiley-Blackwell.)

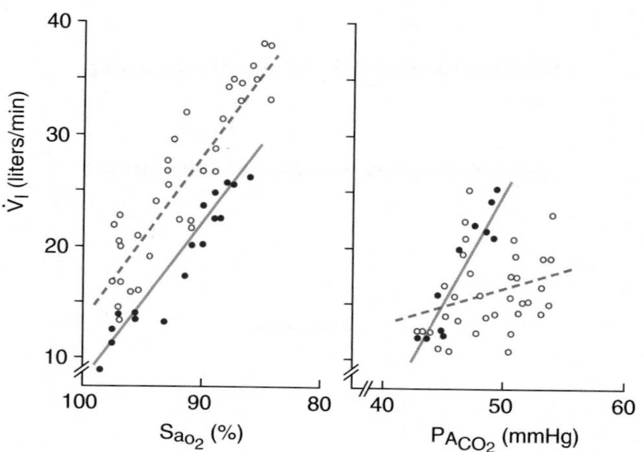

Figure 3.4-5.
Breath-by-breath response of minute volume ventilation ($\dot{V}_I$, L/min) to decreasing arterial O_2 saturation (S_{aO2}) and to increasing alveolar partial pressure of CO_2 (P_{ACO2}) in a sleeping dog. Blue circles, NREMS; red circles, REMS. During REMS, note scatter of data points around calculated linear regression lines and marked decrease of the ventilatory response to hypercapnia. (Adapted from Phillipson EA: Regulation of breathing during sleep. Am Rev Resp Dis 115:217–224, 1977; with permission by American Thoracic Society.)

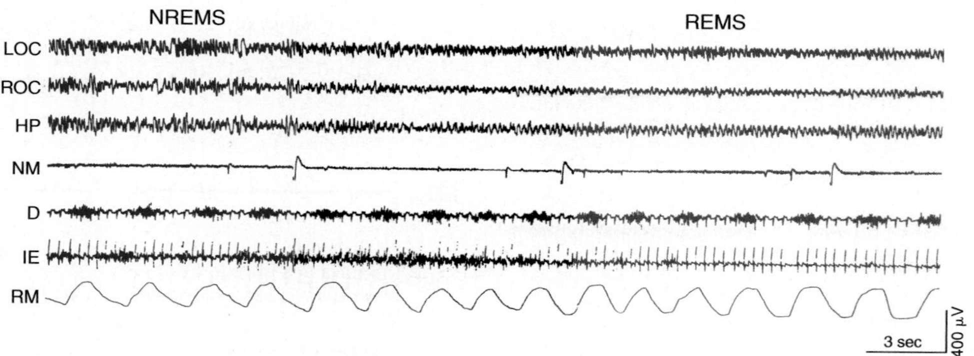

Figure 3.4-6.
Respiratory muscle activity during sleep at ambient thermal neutrality (cat). Postural activity of neck and intercostal muscles disappears during the transition from NREMS to REMS. Respiratory activity of intercostal muscles also disappears whereas that of the diaphragm persists. Electrograms: LOC and ROC, left and right occipital cortex; HP, hippocampus; NM, neck muscles; D, diaphragm; IE, m. intercostalis; RM, respiratory movements. (From Parmeggiani PL, Sabattini L: Electromyographic aspects of postural, respiratory and thermoregulatory mechanisms in sleeping cats. Electroenceph Clin Neurophysiol 33:1–13, 1972, with permission by Elsevier.)

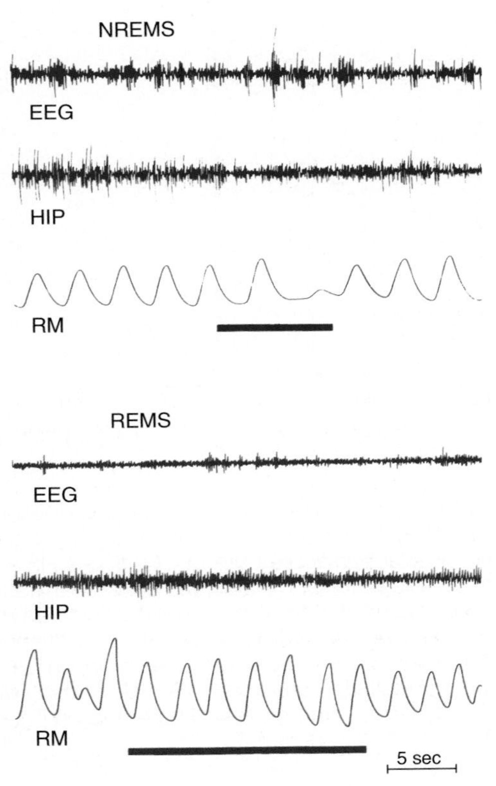

Figure 3.4-7.
Lung inflation-like effect of preoptic-anterior hypothalamic repetitive electrical stimulation (0.13 mA, 5 ms, 10/s) during NREMS (cat).

During REMS, stronger stimulation (0.15 mA, 5 ms, 10/s) is ineffective. EEG, electroencephalogram; HIP, hippocampogram; RM, respiratory movements. (Data from Parmeggiani PL, Calasso M, Cianci T: Respiratory effects of preoptic-anterior hypothalamic electrical stimulation during sleep in cats. Sleep 4:71–82, 1981.)

regulatory power. However, such homeostatic mechanisms are still operative and capable of reestablishing the functional equilibrium that so well characterizes quiet wakefulness and NREMS.

The principles presented here are clinically significant. Compensatory responses such as those that occur in obstructive sleep apnea require the functions present in wakefulness that are lost in sleep. Automatic reflexive control of somatic and autonomic functions allows homeostatic behavior in NREMS without awareness, whereas the impaired homeostasis of REMS elicits physiologic disturbances and can impede compensatory reactions to these disturbances. Figure 3.4-11 summarizes some of the functional changes during sleep.

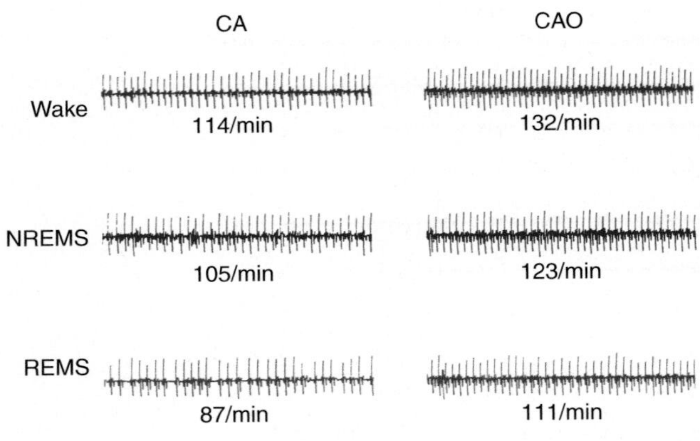

Figure 3.4-8.
CA: spontaneous heart rate (EKG) across wake-sleep states (cat). Note bradyarrhythmia during REMS. CAO: heart rate during bilateral common carotid artery occlusion. Note baroreceptor reflex response during REMS barely exceeding the spontaneous heart rate during NREMS. (Data from Azzaroni A, Parmeggiani PL: Mechanisms underlying hypothalamic temperature changes during sleep in mammals. Brain Res 632:136–142, 1993.)

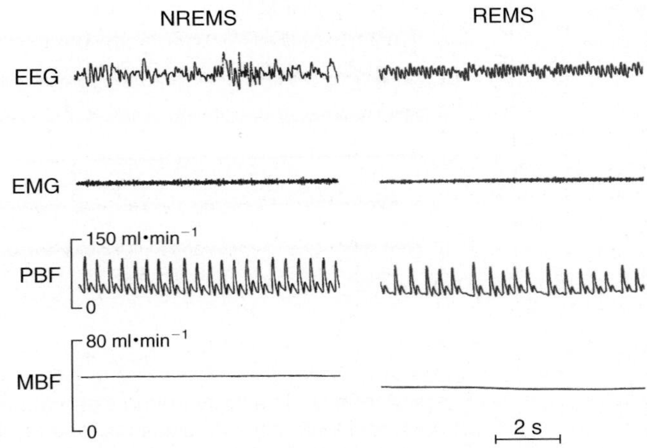

Figure 3.4-9.
The episode of REMS is characterized by bradyarrhythmia, and decreased peak and mean blood flow of common carotid artery (rabbit). EEG, electroencephalogram; EMG, electromyogram; PBF, peak blood flow; MBF, mean blood flow. (Data from Calasso M, Parmeggiani PL: Carotid blood flow during REMS. Sleep 31:701–707, 2008.)

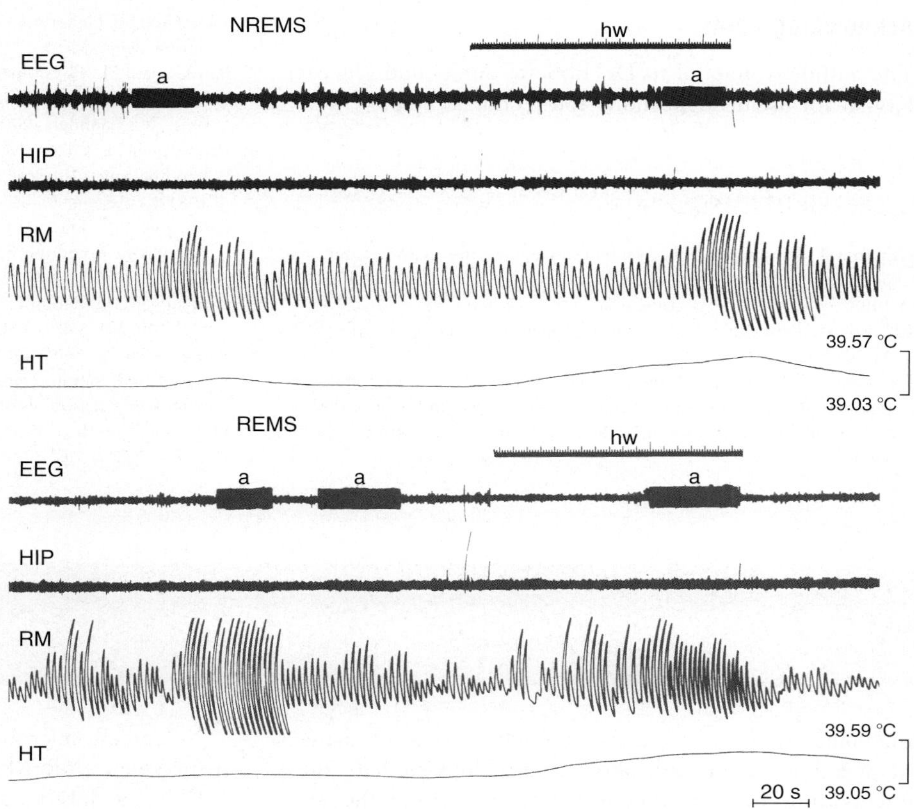

Figure 3.4-10.
Integrative function of preoptic-anterior hypothalamic (PO-AH) structures during sleep (cat). Hyperpnea elicited by PO-AH repetitive electrical stimulation (a: 0.16 mA, 5 ms, 10/s) of one side is enhanced by concomitant diathermic warming of the contralateral area (hw: 0.75 MHz, 70 mW) during NREMS. During REMS, the same procedures are ineffective. Note spontaneous irregular breathing during REMS. EEG, electroencephalogram; HIP, hippocampogram; RM, respiratory movements; HT, hypothalamic temperature; hw, hypothalamic warming. (From Parmeggiani PL, Calasso M, Cianci T: Respiratory effects of preoptic-anterior hypothalamic electrical stimulation during sleep in cats. Sleep 4:71–82, 1981; with permission by the Associated Professional Sleep Societies.)

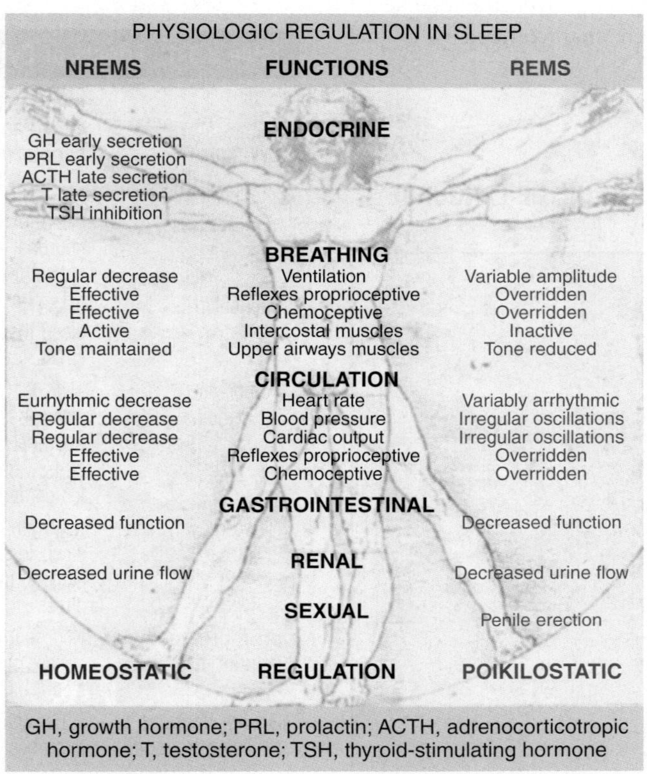

Figure 3.4-11.
Overview of functional changes during sleep.

Acknowledgments

The author is grateful to Dr. Roberto Amici and Dr. Meir Kryger for useful suggestions and technical help.

SELECTED READINGS

Azzaroni A, Parmeggiani PL: Mechanisms underlying hypothalamic temperature changes during sleep in mammals. Brain Res 632:136–142, 1993.

Calasso M, Parmeggiani PL: Carotid blood flow during REMS. Sleep 31:701–707, 2008.

Dewasmes G, Bothorel B, Candas V, Libert JP: A short-term poikilothermic period occurs just after paradoxical sleep onset in humans: Characterization changes in sweating effector activity. J Sleep Res 6:252–258, 1997.

Glotzbach SF, Heller HC: Central nervous regulation of body temperature during sleep. Science 194:537–539, 1976.

Parmeggiani PL: Physiological regulation in sleep. In Kryger MH, Roth T, Dement WC (eds): Principles and Practice of Sleep Medicine. Philadelphia, WB Saunders, 2000, pp. 169–178.

Parmeggiani PL, Calasso M, Cianci T: Respiratory effects of preoptic-anterior hypothalamic electrical stimulation during sleep in cats. Sleep 4:71–82, 1981.

Parmeggiani PL, Franzini C, Lenzi P, Zamboni G: Threshold of respiratory responses to preoptic heating during sleep in freely moving cats. Brain Res 52:189–201, 1973.

Parmeggiani PL, Rabini C: Sleep and environmental temperature. Arch Ital Biol 108:369–387, 1970.

Parmeggiani PL, Sabattini L: Electromyographic aspects of postural, respiratory and thermoregulatory mechanisms in sleeping cats. Electroenceph Clin Neurophysiol 33:1–13, 1972.

Phillipson EA: Regulation of breathing during sleep. Am Rev Resp Dis 115:217–224, 1977.

3.5 *Cytokines, Host Defense, and Sleep*

James M. Krueger, Victor Leyva-Grado, and Stewart Bohnet

Inflammatory states are associated with profound changes in sleep, sleepiness, and fatigue. Cytokines mediate these effects; they form biochemical networks within the brain and immune system. Cytokines are groups of proteins and glycoproteins that behave like hormones and neurotransmitters. The dynamic changes in these chemical entities that occur during normal sleep and over the course of inflammatory diseases have been characterized in animal models (Box 3.5-1; Table 3.5-1)

BOX 3.5-1. ABBREVIATIONS USED IN THE LANGUAGE OF CYTOKINES

- A1AR, adenosine A1 receptor
- CRH, corticotrophin-releasing hormone
- cry, cryptochrome
- EGF, epidermal growth factor
- GABA, gamma-aminobutyric acid
- GHRH, growth hormone releasing hormone
- glu, glutamic acid
- IL1, interleukin-1 beta
- IL10, interleukin-10
- IL1RA, IL1 receptor antagonist
- IL4, interleukin-4
- NF-kB, nuclear factor kappa B
- NGF, nerve growth factor
- NO, nitric oxide
- NOS, nitric oxide synthase
- per, period
- PG, prostaglandins
- sIL1R, soluble IL1 receptor
- sTNFR, soluble TNF receptor
- TNF, tumor necrosis factor alpha

In animals, microbes often enhance nonrapid eye movement sleep (NREMS) while rapid eye movement sleep (REMS) is inhibited. These responses usually begin to occur within a few hours of exposure and last from several days to weeks. Their magnitude, duration, and direction depend on the specific microbe, host species, location of

Table 3.5-1. Effects of Cytokines on Sleep

CYTOKINE	BRAIN STIMULI THAT PROMOTE PRODUCTION/RELEASE	SLEEP EFFECTS: PROMOTES
Interleukin-1 beta	IL1, TNF, NF-kB, sleep loss, microbes, neuronal activity, stress, feeding	NREMS/EEG SWA
Interleukin-6	IL1, TNF, NF-kB, sleep loss, microbes, stress	NREMS
Tumor necrosis factor alpha	TNF, IL1, NF-kB, sleep loss, microbes, neuronal activity, stress, ambient temperature	NREMS/EEG SWA
Nerve growth factor	IL1, TNF, NF-kB, sleep loss, neuronal activity, microbes, stress	NREMS/REMS
Brain-derived neurotrophic factor	Neuronal activity, stress, microbes, sleep loss	NREMS/REMS
Growth hormone releasing hormone	IL1, sleep loss, microbes	NREMS/EEG SWA

Abbreviations: NREMS, nonrapid eye movement sleep; REMS, rapid eye movement sleep; EEG SWA, electroencephalogram slow wave (½-4 Hz) activity.

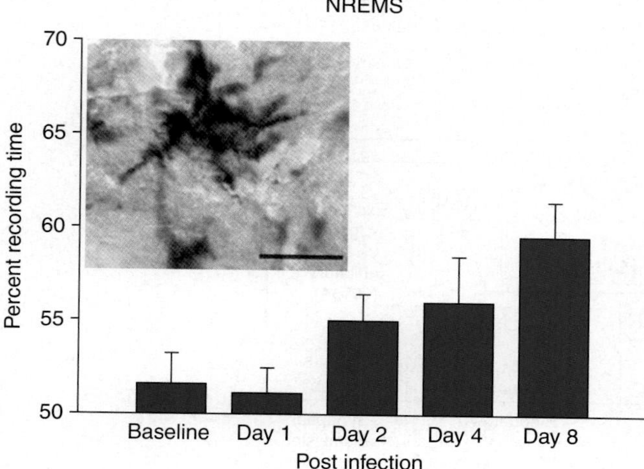

Figure 3.5-1.
Influenza virus infection greatly increases nonrapid eye movement sleep (NREMS). By day 2 after intranasal inoculation of mice with influenza virus NREMS increases. These increases persist for a week or more. The mice recover from the infection after about 2 weeks, and sleep returns toward normal values at that time. The inset shows the detection of viral antigen within the olfactory bulb after inoculation. The cell shown has characteristics of microglia and appears to be activated. Microglia are responsible, in part, for the cellular host defenses in the brain. Such cells likely produce cytokines, and they in turn are involved in sleep regulation.

inflammatory site, and host physiological status, for example, phase of circadian rhythm. Figure 3.5-1 shows the NREMS response of mice induced by intranasal challenge with influenza virus. Although the virus does not replicate within the brain, influenza viral positive and negative sense RNA and viral protein can be detected in the brain within 7 hours. These viral products induce cytokine production locally within brain tissue including the hypothalamus, and these actions probably initiate the acute phase response. The virus also localizes in the lung where it replicates and induces large increases in cytokines.

Systemically produced cytokines also influence brain functions such as sleep (Fig. 3.5-2) and are thought to be responsible for the longer-term maintenance of the acute phase sleep responses.

The molecular steps by which microbes and associated inflammation alter sleep involve the amplification of those mechanisms responsible for physiological sleep (Fig. 3.5-3).

Tumor necrosis factor alpha (TNF) is but one of many such substances that collectively constitute the sleep homeostat, an ultra-complex neuronal and glial biochemical network. Hypothalamic and cerebral cortical levels of TNF mRNA or TNF protein have diurnal variations (2- and 10-fold, respectively) with higher levels associated with greater sleep propensity. Sleep loss is associated with enhanced brain TNF. Central or systemic TNF injection enhances sleep. Inhibition of TNF using the soluble TNF receptor, or anti-TNF antibodies, or a TNF small inhibitory RNA reduces spontaneous sleep. Mice lacking TNF receptors have less spontaneous sleep. Injection of TNF into sleep regulatory circuits, for example, the hypothalamus, promotes sleep. In normal humans, plasma levels of TNF co-vary with electroencephalogram (EEG) slow-wave activity, and in multiple disease states plasma TNF increases in parallel with sleep propensity. Downstream mechanisms of TNF-enhanced sleep include nitric oxide, adenosine, prostaglandins, and activation of nuclear factor kappa B.

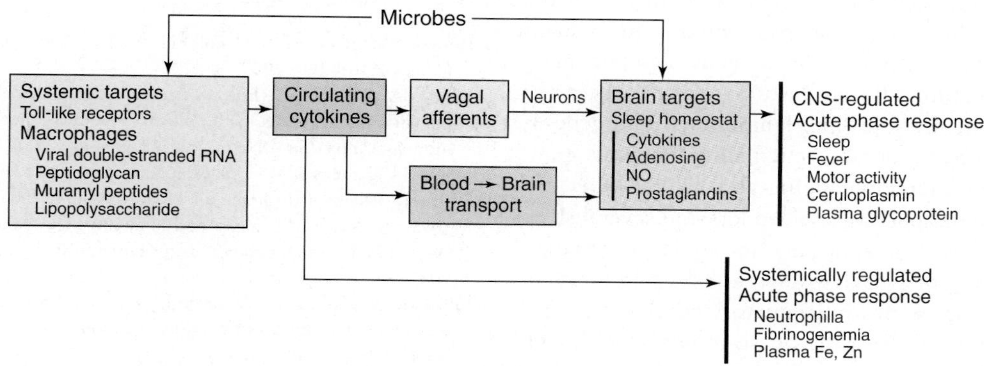

Figure 3.5-2.
Microbes affect sleep via steps involving systemic immunocytes such as macrophages or, if they infiltrate the brain directly, via glia and neurons. Components of bacterial cell walls such as lipopolysaccharide from Gram-negative bacteria, muramyl peptides from either Gram-negative or Gram-positive bacterial peptidoglycan, and double-stranded RNA from viruses interact with toll-like receptors. This interaction leads to enhanced cytokine production. Cytokines released systemically reach the brain via specific blood-to-brain transporters or can signal the brain via vagal nerve afferents. Cytokines released in the brain directly interact with brain targets to enhance sleep. There are several brain-regulated acute phase responses including sleep, fever, social withdrawal, reduced locomotor activity, and some serum proteins. Systemically released cytokines also act on other organs such as the liver and spleen to affect a variety of additional acute phase reactants such as plasma iron and zinc levels.

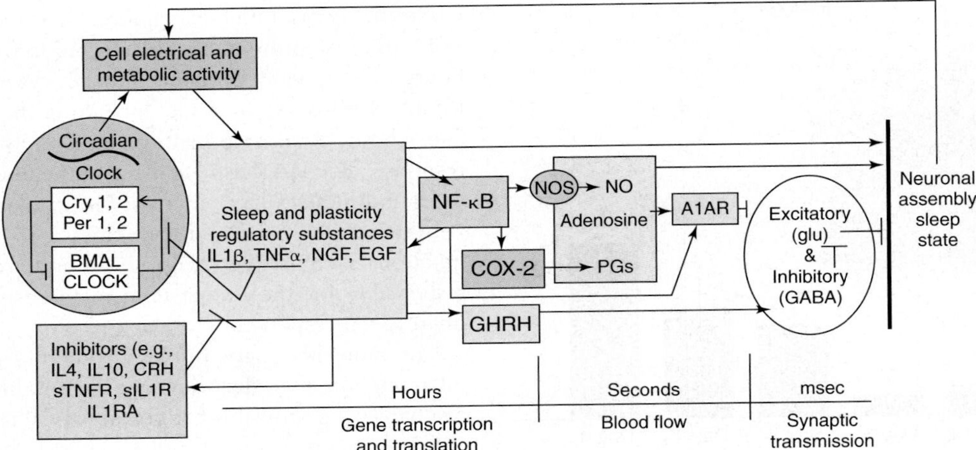

Figure 3.5-3.
Microbes act to amplify the production of many of the components of the sleep homeostat. The cytokines such as IL1, TNF, IL4, IL10, NGF, EGF, and associated soluble and membrane-bound receptors all form part of the sleep biochemical regulatory network. Microbial products affect immunocyte and brain production of these substances. Within brain and immunocytes, adenosine triphosphate (ATP), co-released, for example, during neurotransmission, induces the release of IL1 and TNF from glia. These substances induce their own production and multiple other substances via nuclear factor kappa B activation. These actions are associated with gene transcription and translation and take several hours. Downstream events include well-known immune response modifiers and regulators of the microcirculation such as NO, adenosine, and prostaglandins. They, in turn, affect neurotransmission on an even faster time scale leading to state oscillations within local networks. (See Box 3.5-1 for abbreviations.) (From Krueger JM, Rector DM, Churchill L: Sleep and cytokines. Sleep Med Clinics 2:161–169, 2007.)

That many of the molecules implicated in physiologic sleep regulation (see Fig. 3.5-3) are also known regulatory components in immunocytes suggests an evolutionary link between sleep and host defenses.

Sleep per se may feed back to affect the efficacy of the host defenses. There are numerous studies in humans demonstrating that sleep loss alters many immune parameters, including antibody responses to vaccines, bacterial translocation from the intestine, lymphocyte mitogenesis, phygocytosis, antigen uptake, circulating immune complexes, circulating immunoglobulin, and natural killer cell and T lymphocyte populations. Sleep loss and several sleep pathologies, such as sleep apnea and insomnia, affect circulating levels of certain cytokines such as TNF and interleukin-6; both of these are pro-inflammatory cytokines critical to the development of the acute phase response. Although such findings strongly suggest that sleep plays a role in host defenses, the important question of whether sleep and/or sleep loss alters microbial-associated morbidity or mortality remains unanswered. This is a difficult issue to address because it is not possible to isolate sleep as the independent variable; all physiologic functions vary with state.

SELECTED READINGS

Krueger JM, Rector DM, Churchill L: Sleep and cytokines. Sleep Med Clinics 2:161–169, 2007.

Majde JA, Bohnet SG, Ellis GA, et al: Detection of a mouse-adapted human influenza virus in the olfactory bulb of mice within hours after intranasal infection. J Neurovirol 13:399–409, 2007.

Majde JA, Krueger JM: Links between the innate immune system and sleep. J Allergy Clin Immunol 116:1188–1198, 2005.

Motivala SJ, Irwin MR: Sleep and immunity: Cytokine pathways linking sleep and health outcomes. Curr Direct Psychological Sc 16:21–25, 2007.

Olivadoti M, Toth LA, Weinberg J, Opp MR: Murine gammaherpesvirus 68: A model for Epstein-Barr virus infections and related diseases. Comp Med 57:44–50, 2007.

Opp MR: Sleep and psychoneuroimmunology. Neurol Clin 24:493–506, 2006.

Toth LA, Jhaveri K: Sleep mechanisms in health and disease. Comp Med 53:12–23, 2003.

Dominic Roca, Susie Yim Yeh,
Danny Eckert, and
Atul Malhotra

Control of Breathing 3.6

Normal Sleep

The goal of the respiratory system is to supply oxygen, remove carbon dioxide, and maintain acid-base balance. The primary centers for central respiratory control are located in the pons and medulla (Fig. 3.6-1). These centers receive input from a variety of sources to modulate the respiratory system (Fig. 3.6-2). Oxygen and carbon dioxide levels are two of the main signals that alter the respiratory system (Fig. 3.6-3). Sleep decreases the ventilatory response to hypoxia and hypercarbia. This effect varies with the stage of sleep (Fig. 3.6-4).

Sleep also modifies muscle activation. This is most notable in the upper airway (Fig. 3.6-5). The genioglossus is the best studied of the upper respiratory muscles. It is primarily controlled by the hypoglossal nerve, which receives inputs from a variety of central sites as well as feedback from upper airway mechanoreceptors (Fig. 3.6-6).

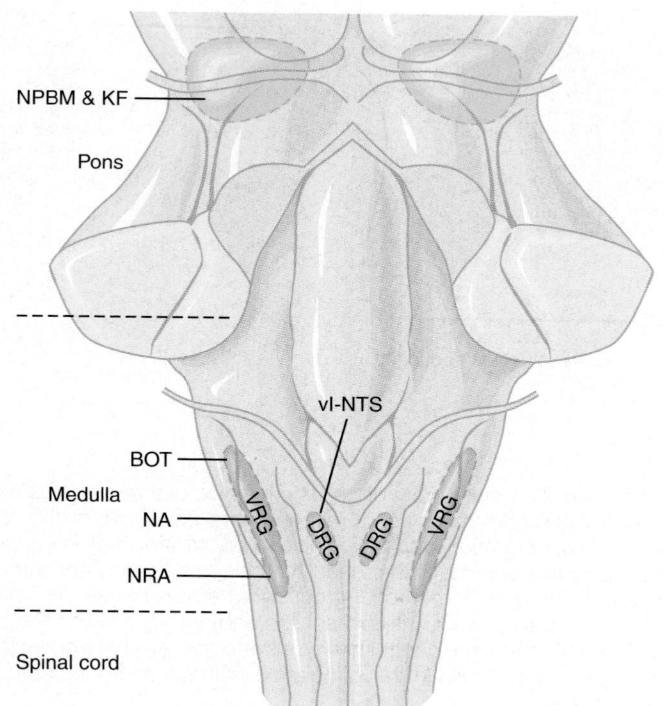

Figure 3.6-1.
Central control of breathing. The central respiratory control centers are located in the pons and medulla. The medulla is the location of the primary respiratory control center. Transections below the medulla cease respiration. The dorsal respiratory group (DRG) contains the ventrolateral nucleus of the tractus solitaries (vl-NTS). This region is thought to be involved in inspiration. The ventral respiratory group (VRG) contains the pre-Botzinger complex (BOT), the nucleus ambiguous (NA), and the nucleus retroambigualis (NRA). These cells fire rhythmically in vitro and respond to hypoxia. They stimulate the phrenic nerve and the hypoglossal nucleus. Some controversy exists regarding the role of the parafacial respiratory group (PRG) and retrotrapezoid nucleus (RTN), including the possibility of more than one oscillator that can drive breathing. (The PRG and RTN are not included in the figure for simplicity.) The pneumotaxic center (which inhibits breathing during inspiration) is located in the nucleus parabrachialis medialis (NPBM) and Kolliker-Fuse (KF) nuclei of the dorsolateral pons. When this area is damaged bradypnea and larger tidal volumes result.

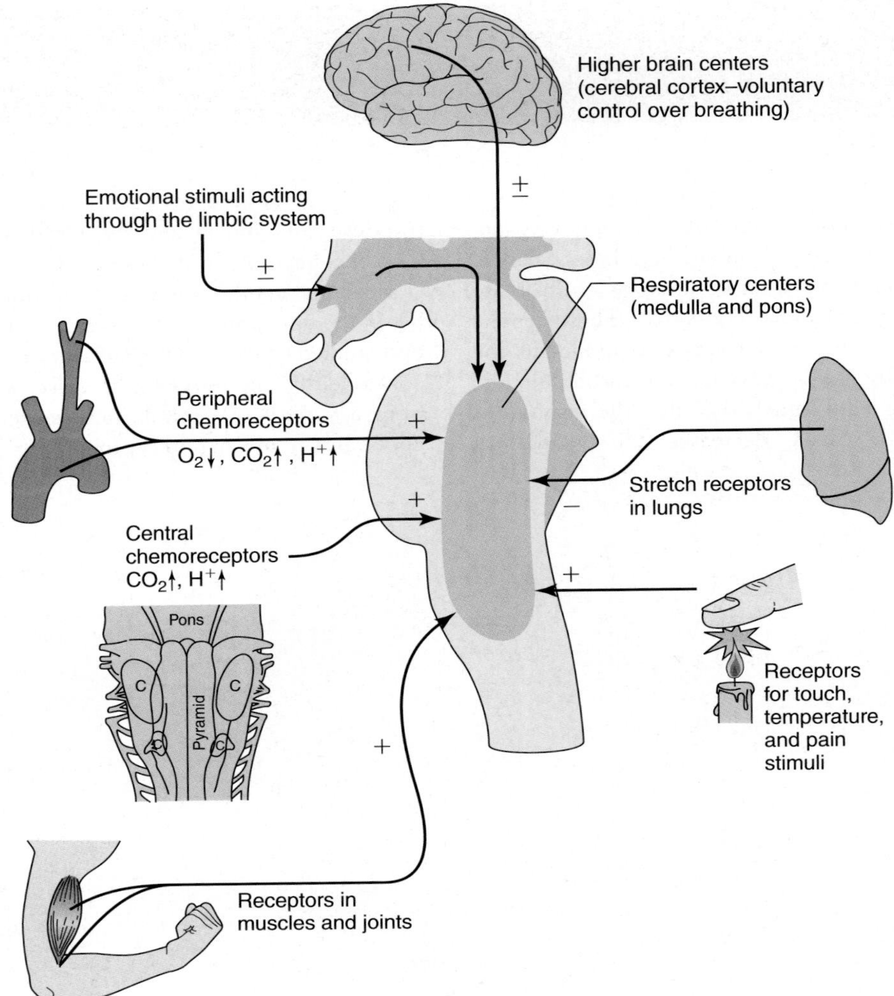

Figure 3.6-2.
Modulators of respiration chemoreceptors. The intrinsic central nervous system respiratory control is modulated by cells responsive to blood chemistry, specifically pCO_2 (and/or H^+ concentration) and pO_2. The primary central chemoreceptors (*C*) are located near the ventral surface of the medulla. The ventral medullary surface and the retrotrapezoid nucleus are two neuronal groups that are extremely sensitive to changes in H^+ concentration. CO_2 is lipid soluble and quickly crosses the blood-brain barrier. The CO_2 that enters the central nervous system is rapidly hydrated and the H^+ concentration rises. This results in the stimulation of these chemoreceptors, and ventilation increases.

The primary peripheral chemoreceptors are the carotid and aortic bodies. The carotid bodies are located at the bifurcation of the common carotid arteries. The aortic bodies are located near the arch of the aorta (but are mainly relevant in nonhuman species). Both sets of chemoreceptors are sensitive to the pO_2 and to a lesser extent pCO_2.

Secondary modulators: The cerebral cortex is responsible for voluntary control of breathing. It sends signals through the corticospinal and corticobulbar tracts. Receptors in the lung are responsible for reacting to lung volume and irritants. They send feedback through the vagus nerve. Proprioceptors in muscles and tendons stimulate respirations, as evidenced by passive movements increasing respiratory rate.

Figure 3.6-3.

Response to hypercapnia and hypoxia. **A**, The rise in ventilation in response to increases in pCO_2 is linear, approximately 2.5 liters/min for each increase in pCO_2. **B**, Ventilation increases as PO_2 falls below 75 mmHg. The response is more dramatic when the PO_2 falls below 55 mmHg. Ventilation increases greater than threefold when the PO_2 has reached 40 mmHg (75% saturation). As evident in the curves there is a rapid response to changes in pCO_2. In comparison, the response to hypoxia is blunted until there is a large decrease in PO_2.

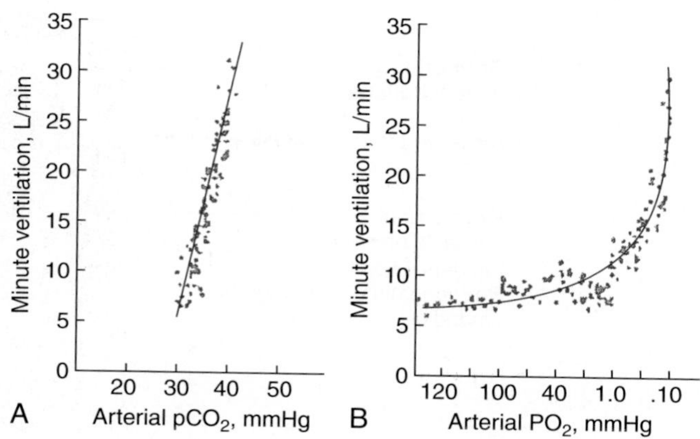

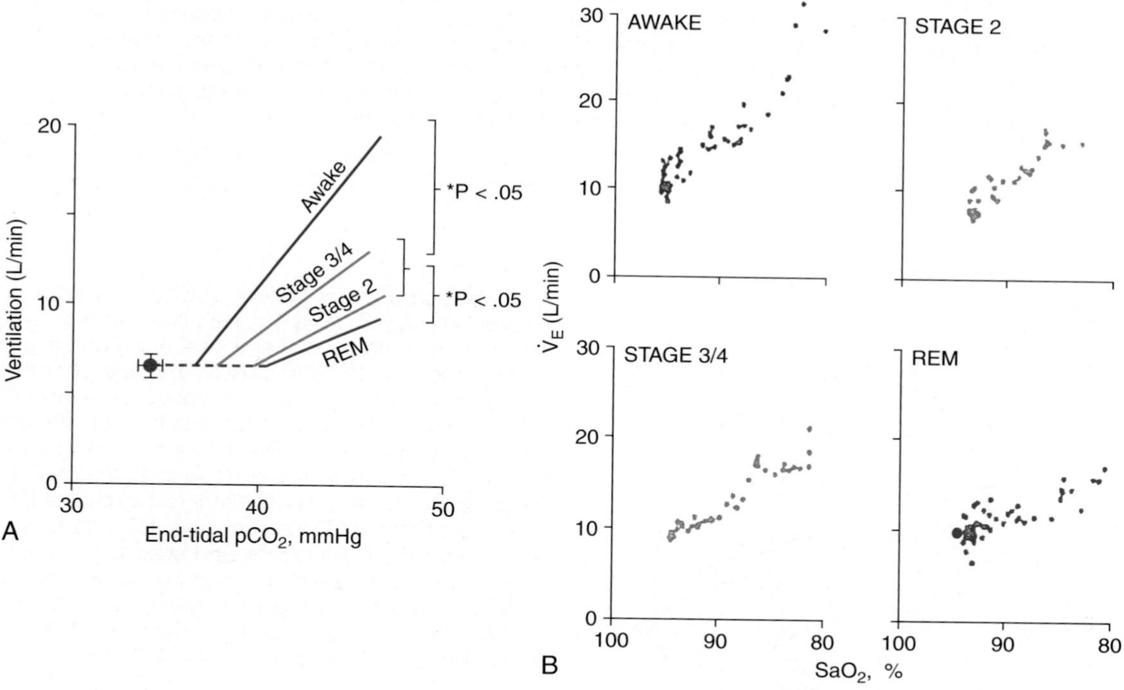

Figure 3.6-4.

The response to hypercapnia and hypoxia is diminished during sleep. **A**, Hypercapnia was induced in 12 healthy subjects using a modified rebreathing technique while recording EEG to assess the subjects' stage of sleep. The graph represents the mean minute ventilation for all 12 subjects. The mean minute ventilation at baseline is indicated. The hypercapnic ventilatory response is reduced in stages 2 and 3/4 compared with wakefulness and further decreased in REM sleep. The blunting of chemoresponsiveness during REM sleep may be a major mechanism whereby many forms of central apnea resolve during REM sleep. Both Cheyne Stokes respirations and high-altitude periodic breathing tend to resolve during REM sleep. This may be secondary to the decrease in chemoresponsiveness associated with REM. ($\dot{V}_E$, expired minute ventilation; *, $P < 0.05$ REM different from stages 2 and 3/4.) **B**, Isocapnic hypoxia was induced in 10 men while recording EEG to assess the subjects' stage of sleep. The graphs are representative data from one subject. The response to hypoxia was blunted in stages 2 and 3/4 and further decreased in REM. (SaO_2, hemoglobin saturation; $\dot{V}_E$, expired ventilation.) (From Douglas NJ, White DP, Weil JV, et al: Hypercapnic ventilatory response in sleeping adults. Am Rev Resp Dis 126(5):758–762, 1982.)

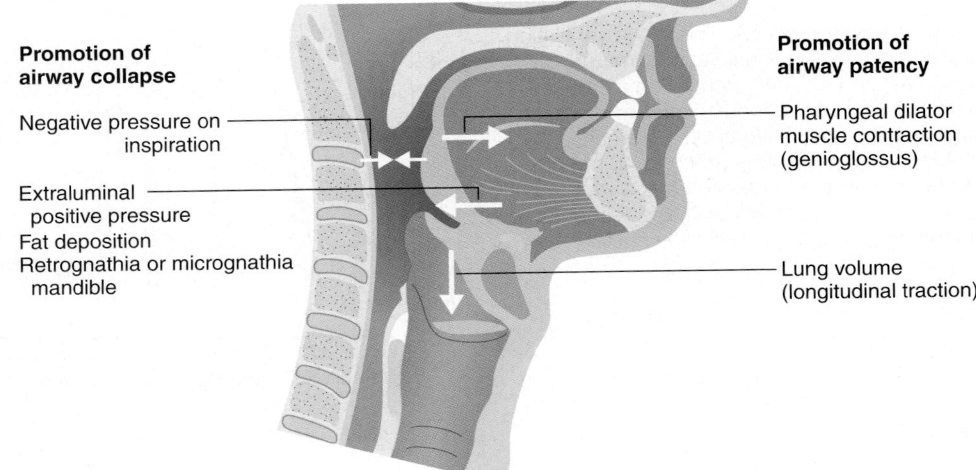

Figure 3.6-5.
The upper airway is vulnerable to collapse. The pharynx comprises predominantly muscle, fat, and connective tissue. This relatively soft structure has a tendency to collapse, as it is devoid of bony support. The recumbent position, especially lying supine, exacerbates this tendency to close. Through reflex-driven protective mechanisms, pharyngeal dilator muscle activity is increased in sleep apnea, likely in compensation for anatomical deficiency. During sleep, reflex activation of pharyngeal muscles is reduced. Inspiration yields a negative airway pressure that creates a collapsing influence on the upper airway. All of these factors tend to compromise the pharynx. As a result, patency requires activation of several muscles including the genioglossus, tensor palatini, and stylopharyngeus. As the lung expands it helps to open the pharynx by longitudinal traction. This balance of forces can be weighted toward collapse by obesity and anatomy (e.g., a small mandible) to result in greater instability and sleep-disordered breathing.

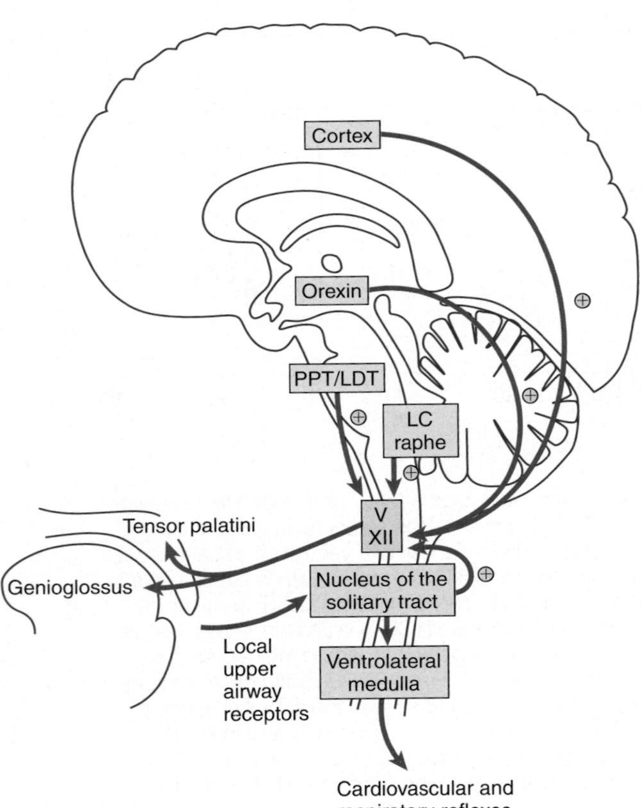

Figure 3.6-6.
The hypoglossal motor system. The hypoglossal nerve controls the genioglossus muscle (tongue). It is involved in many activities including speech and swallowing and is the best-studied pharyngeal dilator muscle. The activity of the hypoglossal nerve is affected by many factors including cortical and brainstem stimulation, breathing pattern, chemoreceptor activation, and input from mechanoreceptors in the pharynx. Several neurochemical systems, such as the cholinergic (from the pedunculopontine and laterodorsal tegmenta [PPT/LDT]), adrenergic (from the locus coeruleus [LC] and subcoeruleus), serotonergic (from the raphe), and orexinergic (from the hypothalamus), modulate sleep and probably have significant roles in modulating genioglossal activity. (Adapted from Eckert DJ, Malhotra A: Pathophysiology of adult obstructive sleep apnea. Proc Am Thorac Soc 5:144–153, 2008.)

Sleep Apnea

Sleep is associated with a number of respiratory disorders (see chapter 11). Obstructive sleep apnea and central sleep apnea are two of the most common.

Obstructive sleep apnea occurs when upper airway patency is compromised (Fig. 3.6-7). This reduction in upper airway patency is the result of a combination of factors including anatomy, dilator muscle activity, arousal

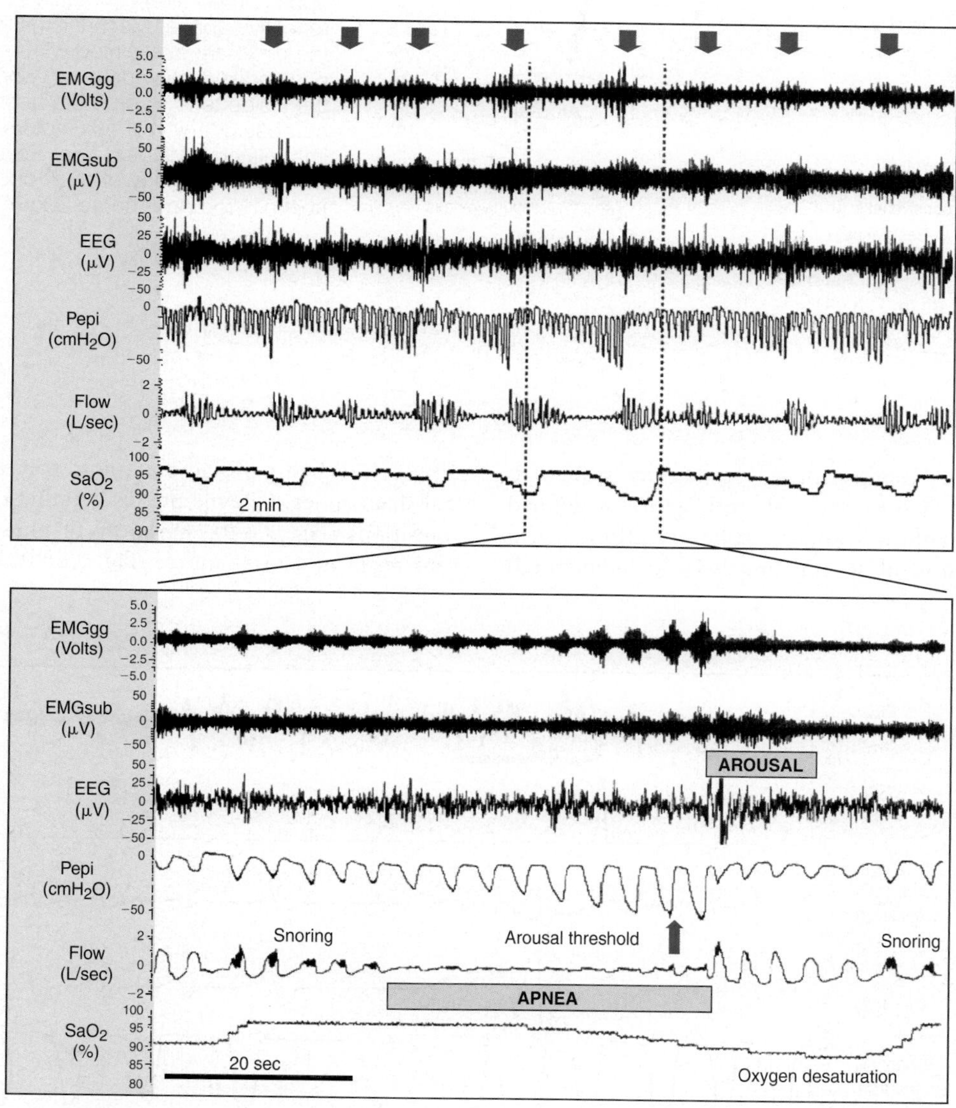

Figure 3.6-7.
Upper airway muscles and arousal threshold. The tracing shows an experimental recording from a patient with obstructive sleep apnea. The cessation of airflow (apnea) leads to both oxygen desaturation and electroencephalogram (EEG) arousal from sleep. Note the progressive increases in genioglossal muscle activity (electromyogram [EMGgg]) that occur with increasing respiratory efforts. Obstructive apnea is characterized by ongoing respiratory efforts in contradistinction to central apnea, in which respiratory effort ceases during attenuated airflow. Respiratory effort leads to swings in intrathoracic pressure that can be estimated with an epiglottic catheter (Pepi). The Pepi is thought to be the primary stimulus for arousal from sleep. Respiratory efforts (as sensed by mechanoreceptors in the chest wall) are thought to yield arousal from sleep. If arousal occurs prematurely (low arousal threshold), then insufficient respiratory stimuli accumulate to activate the genioglossus muscle. On the other hand, if arousal is markedly delayed (high arousal threshold), then profound hypoxemia may develop. Ideally, increases in EMGgg are sufficient to restore airway patency prior to arousal from sleep. (Adapted from Eckert DJ, Malhotra A: Pathophysiology of adult obstructive sleep apnea. Proc Am Thorac Soc 5:144–153, 2008.)

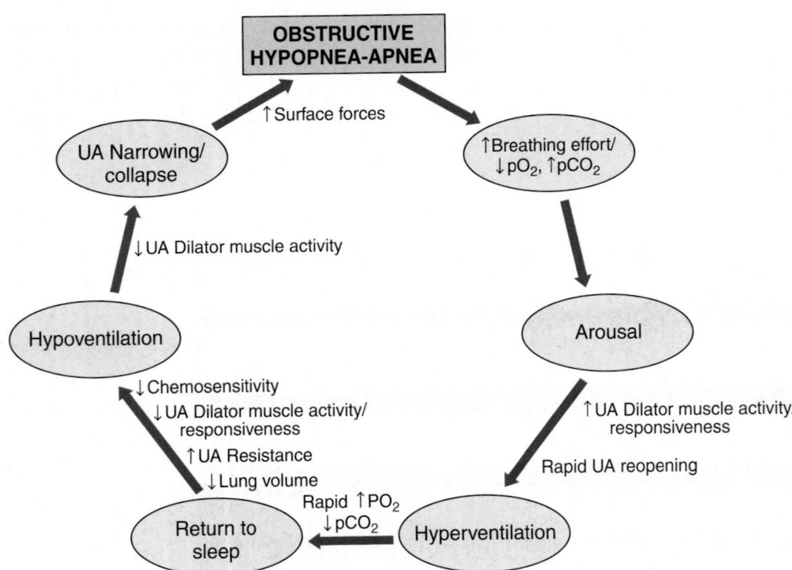

Figure 3.6-8.
The potential cycle of ventilatory instability. Obstructive apnea leads to increases in breathing effort in association with hypoxemia and hypercapnia. Respiratory effort can trigger arousal from sleep with resulting physiologic changes that can restore airway patency and yield hyperventilation. Upon return to sleep, the upper airway (UA) can again collapse, leading to repetitive apnea. Mechanisms listed outside of the circle are associated with restoration of pharyngeal airway patency, whereas those on the inside tend to promote upper airway collapse. Many of these factors can clearly be interrelated. (Adapted from Eckert DJ, Malhotra A: Pathophysiology of adult obstructive sleep apnea. Proc Am Thorac Soc 5:144–153, 2008.)

threshold, and the response of the respiratory system to perturbations (Fig. 3.6-8). Central sleep apnea is defined as an absence of airflow without respiratory effort. It can be the manifestation of several processes including high altitude induced periodic breathing, narcotic induced central sleep apnea, Cheyne Stokes breathing, and sleep-wake transitions (Fig. 3.6-9). A variety of physiologic mechanisms result in central apneas (Fig. 3.6-10).

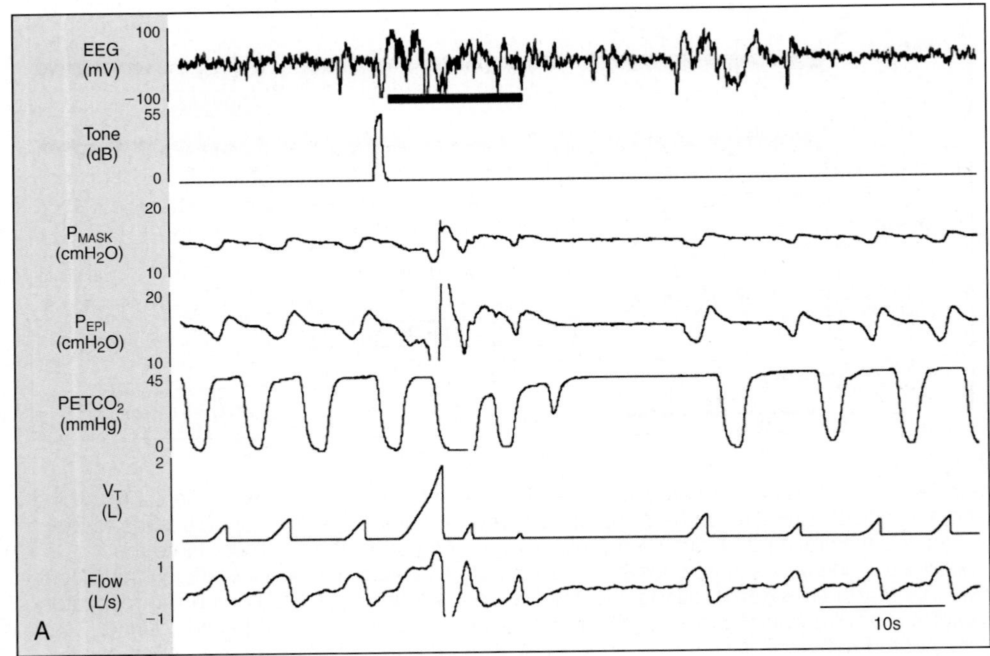

Figure 3.6-9.
Various forms of central apnea. A, An experimentally induced arousal from sleep can yield hyperventilation based on a robust ventilatory response to arousal. The electroencephalogram (EEG) shows an increase in frequency (*underlined portion*) that is typical of arousal. The hyperventilation leads to hypocapnia that can result in apnea if the PCO_2 falls below the CO_2 apnea threshold. The absence of respiratory effort (as seen in the Pepi epiglottic pressure channel) defines central apnea.

(Continued)

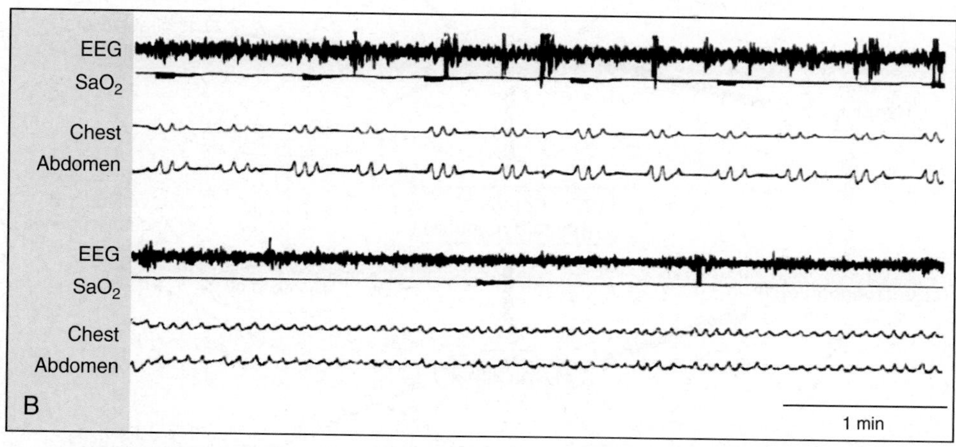

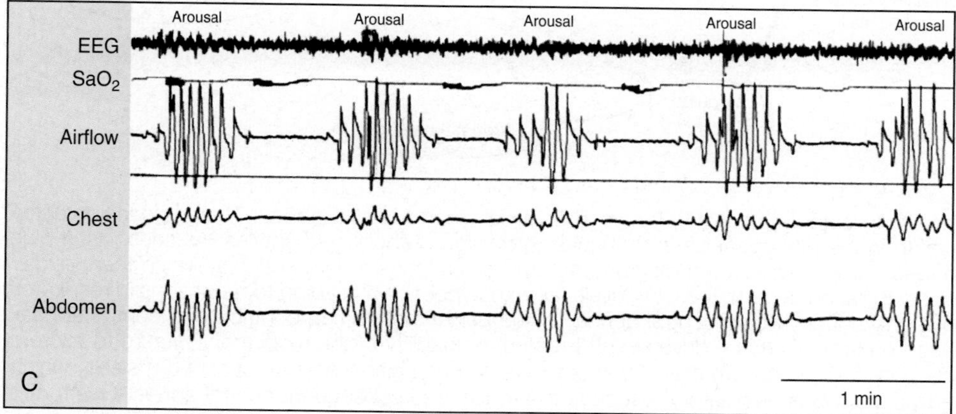

Figure 3.6-9. cont'd

B, Figure shows narcotic-induced central apneas, which occur in up to 50% of patients on chronic narcotic therapy. In the top panel intermittent pauses are observed in the chest and abdominal respiratory belts that occur in central apnea. With reductions in the dose of the narcotic agent, as shown in the lower panel, the breathing pattern is normalized. These graphs illustrate the dose dependence of narcotic-induced central apnea. This breathing pattern is sometimes associated with low respiratory rates (bradypnea). C, Figure shows a crescendo-decrescendo (Cheyne Stokes) pattern in association with central apneas whereby an absence of respiratory effort is seen in association with cessations in airflow. The arousal from sleep typically occurs at the peak of the hyperpnea that corresponds with paroxysmal nocturnal dyspnea complaints in patients. This breathing pattern is seen in between one third and one half of congestive heart failure patients with left ventricular dysfunction. Note the intermittent desaturations that occur delayed in time due to the slow circulation in congestive heart failure. (Adapted from Eckert DJ, Malhotra A: Pathophysiology of adult obstructive sleep apnea. Proc Am Thorac Soc 5:144–153, 2008.)

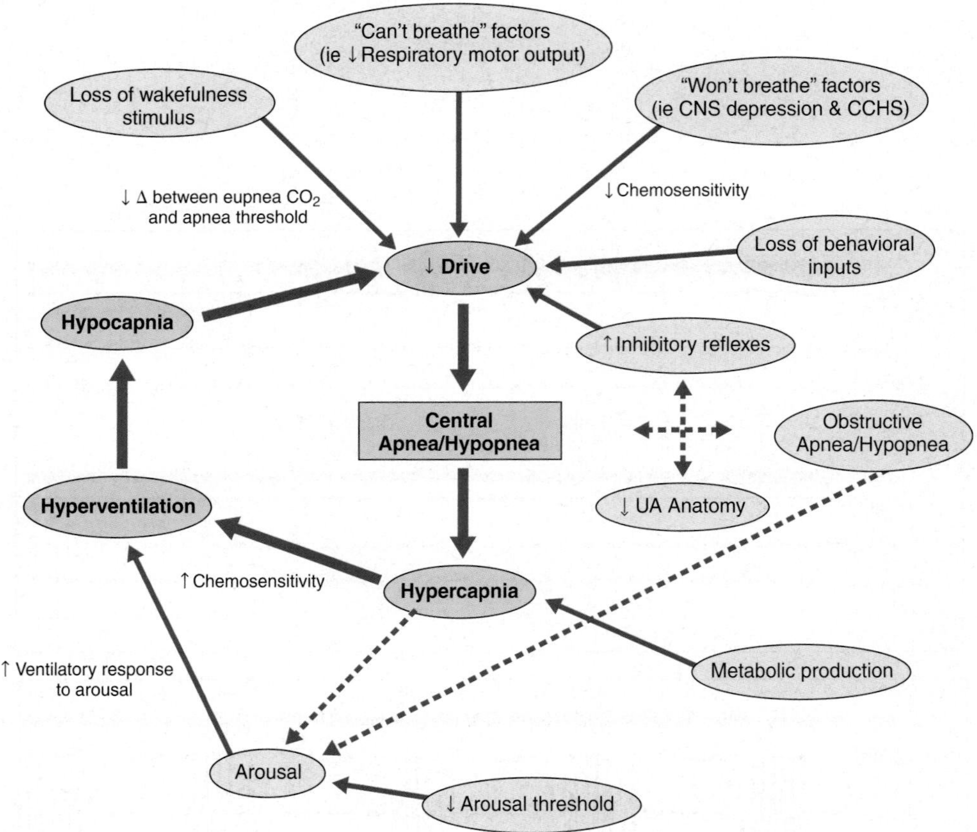

Figure 3.6-10.
The complicated relationship between obstructive and central apnea. There is considerable overlap in the pathogenesis and clinical expression of these two entities. As seen in the blue shaded components of the diagram, central apnea leads to hypercapnia, which then yields hyperventilation. In turn, the CO_2 levels fall with hypocapnia, leading to reductions in respiratory drive and again yielding central apnea. A number of factors can contribute to central apnea based on lack of central drive (won't breathe) or inability of the respiratory system to excrete adequate CO_2 (can't breathe). Obstructive apnea can also lead to arousal from sleep, which can yield a robust ventilatory response to arousal and subsequent central apnea. Obstructive or central apnea can occur during reduced central respiratory drive depending on the prevailing upper airway mechanics. CNS, central nervous system; CCHS, congenital central hypoventilation syndrome. (Adapted from Eckert DJ, Malhotra A: Pathophysiology of adult obstructive sleep apnea. Proc Am Thorac Soc 5:144–153, 2008.)

3.7 Central and Autonomic Regulation in Cardiovascular Physiology

Richard L. Verrier and Ronald M. Harper

Overview

Circulatory homeostasis during sleep requires coordination of two physiologic systems, namely, the respiratory system, which is essential for oxygen and carbon dioxide exchange, and the cardiovascular, which provides blood transport.

Non-rapid eye movement (NREM) sleep, the initial stage, is characterized by relative autonomic stability, with vagus nerve dominance and heightened baroreceptor gain. There is near sinusoidal modulation of heart rate variations, termed *normal respiratory sinus arrhythmia,* due to coupling with respiratory activity and cardiorespiratory centers in the brain (Fig. 3.7-1). Rapid eye movement (REM) sleep is initiated at 90-minute intervals and exhibits a more irregular pattern with periodic surges in heart rate and arterial blood pressure, as well as in other cardiovascular parameters. The challenge to homeostatic regulation is even greater in individuals who have diseased respiratory or cardiovascular systems, particularly in those with apnea or heart failure, or in infants, whose cardiorespiratory control systems may be underdeveloped.

REM sleep induces a near paralysis of accessory respiratory muscles and diminishes descending forebrain influences

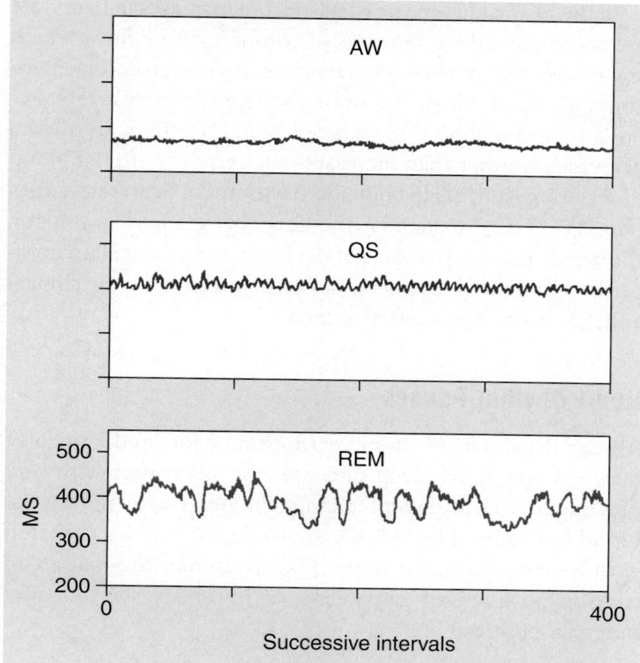

Figure 3.7-1.
The x-axis represents successive heartbeats and the intervals between heartbeats from a healthy 4-month-old infant during non-REM (quiet sleep, or QS), rapid eye movement (REM) sleep, and wakefulness (AW). The y-axis represents time (in milliseconds [MS]) between those heartbeats. Note rapid modulation of intervals during quiet sleep contributed by respiratory variation. Note also lower frequency modulation during REM sleep, and epochs of sustained rapid rate during wakefulness.

on brainstem control regions (see chapter 3.3). Those reorganizations of control during REM sleep have the potential to interfere substantially with compensatory breathing mechanisms that assist arterial blood pressure management and to remove protective forebrain influences on hypo- or hypertension. The significant interaction between breathing and arterial blood pressure is evident in normalization of blood pressure by continuous positive airway pressure in patients with apnea-induced hypertension.

Heart failure patients exhibit severe insular cortex and other brain gray matter loss, preferentially on the right side (Fig. 3.7-2), and impaired functional magnetic resonance signal responses to cold pressor challenges and to Valsalva maneuvers. In addition to an inability to mount appropriate heart rate responses, this injury appears to stem from disordered breathing and accompanying neural circulatory changes during sleep.

Heart Rate Surges

REM-induced accelerations in heart rate consisting of an abrupt, though transitory, 35% to 37% increase in rate, which are concentrated during phasic REM, were observed in canines (Fig. 3.7-3). These marked heart rate surges are accompanied by a rise in arterial blood pressure and are abolished by cardiac sympathectomy. Nerve recordings of sympathetic pathways in human subjects further support the potential involvement of sympathetic activation in REM-associated accelerations in heart rate (Fig. 3.7-4).

Figure 3.7-2.
Areas of gray matter loss *(arrows),* colored-coded by percentage change represented on the color bar, within the insular cortex (i) of heart failure patients (A, $n = 9$) and in the hippocampal region (ii) and cerebellum (iii) of obstructive sleep apnea patients (B, $n = 21$); gray matter loss was calculated from structural MRI scans relative to controls. (**A**, From Woo MA, Macey PM, Fonarow GC, et al. Regional brain gray matter loss in heart failure. J Appl Physiol 95:677–684, 2003. **B**, From Macey PM, Henderson LA, Macey KE, et al. Brain morphology associated with obstructive sleep apnea. Am J Resp Crit Care Med 166:1382–1387, 2002.)

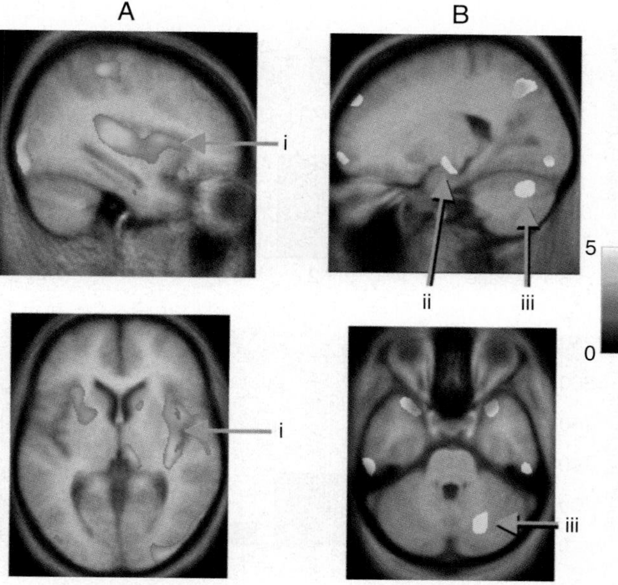

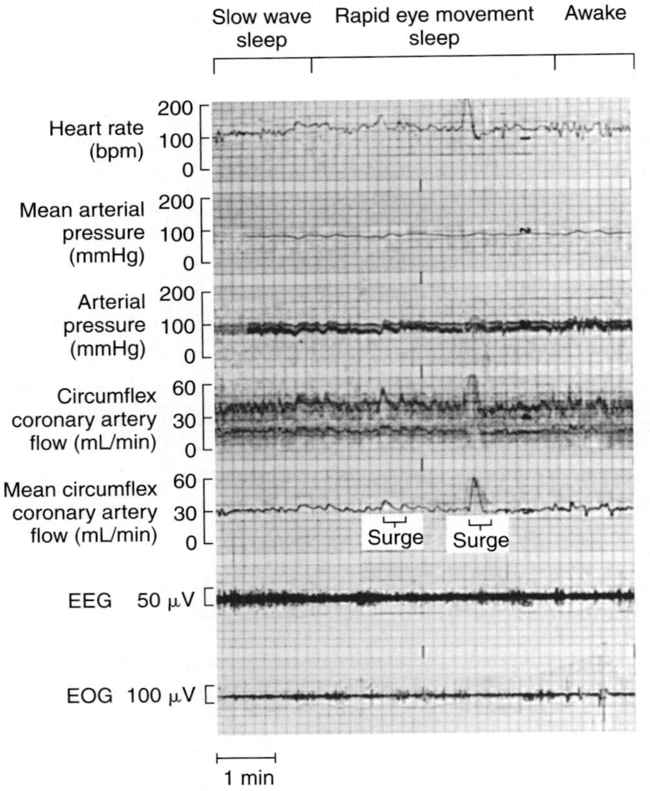

Figure 3.7-3.
Effects of NREM sleep, REM sleep, and quiet wakefulness on heart rate, phasic and mean arterial blood pressure, phasic and mean left circumflex coronary flow, electroencephalogram (EEG), and electro-oculogram (EOG) in the dog. Sleep spindles are evident during NREM sleep, eye movements during REM sleep, and gross eye movements on awakening. Surges in heart rate and coronary flow occur during REM sleep. (From Kirby DA, Verrier RL: Differential effects of sleep stage on coronary hemodynamic function. Am J Physiol 256:H1378–H1383, 1989.)

In the normal heart, the REM-related increases in heart rate are accompanied by increases in coronary blood flow, which are appropriate to the corresponding increase in cardiac metabolic demand. However, during severe coronary artery stenosis (with baseline flow reduced by 60%), there are phasic decreases—rather than increases—in coronary arterial blood flow during REM sleep coincident with these heart rate surges (Fig. 3.7-5). Consequently, the flow changes may not match the metabolic requirements of the heart and can result in myocardial ischemia. This phenomenon could underlie the clinical entity known as "nocturnal angina."

Heart Rhythm Pauses

Abrupt decelerations in heart rhythm occur predominantly during tonic REM sleep and are not associated with any preceding or subsequent change in heart rate or arterial blood pressure (Fig. 3.7-6). In some individuals afflicted with genetically based long QT_3 syndrome, the pause can trigger cycle-length dependent arrhythmias such as torsades de pointes.

Physiologic Mechanisms Underlying Nocturnal Cardiac Events

The physiologic mechanisms described provide a conceptual framework for understanding a number of cardiac syndromes that have increased prevalence during sleep (Table 3.7-1). See also chapter 13.

Summary

Sleep states exert a major impact on cardiorespiratory function. This is a direct consequence of the significant variations in brain states that occur in the normal cycling

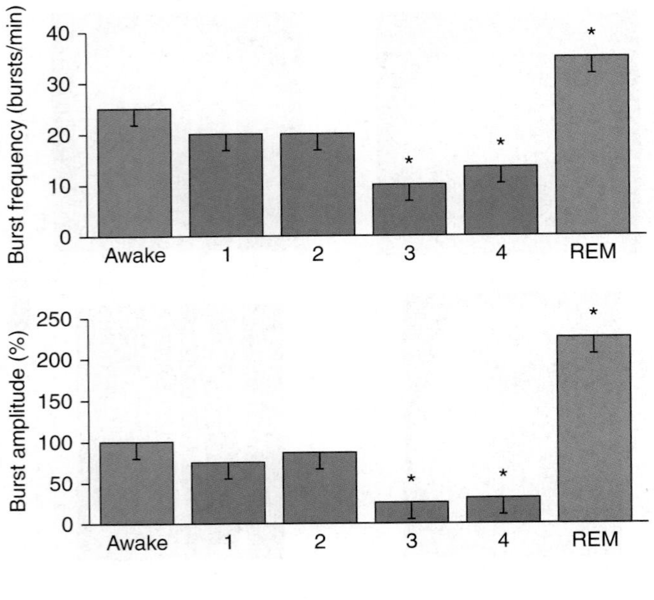

Figure 3.7-4.
Sympathetic burst frequency and amplitude during wakefulness, NREM sleep (eight subjects), and REM sleep (six subjects). Sympathetic activity was significantly lower during stages 3 and 4 (*$P < 0.001$). During REM sleep, sympathetic activity increased significantly ($P < 0.001$). Values are means ± SEM. (Adapted from Somers VK, Dyken ME, Mark AL, et al: Sympathetic nerve activity during sleep in normal subjects. N Engl J Med 328:303–307, 1993. Copyright ©1993 Massachusetts Medical Society. All rights reserved.)

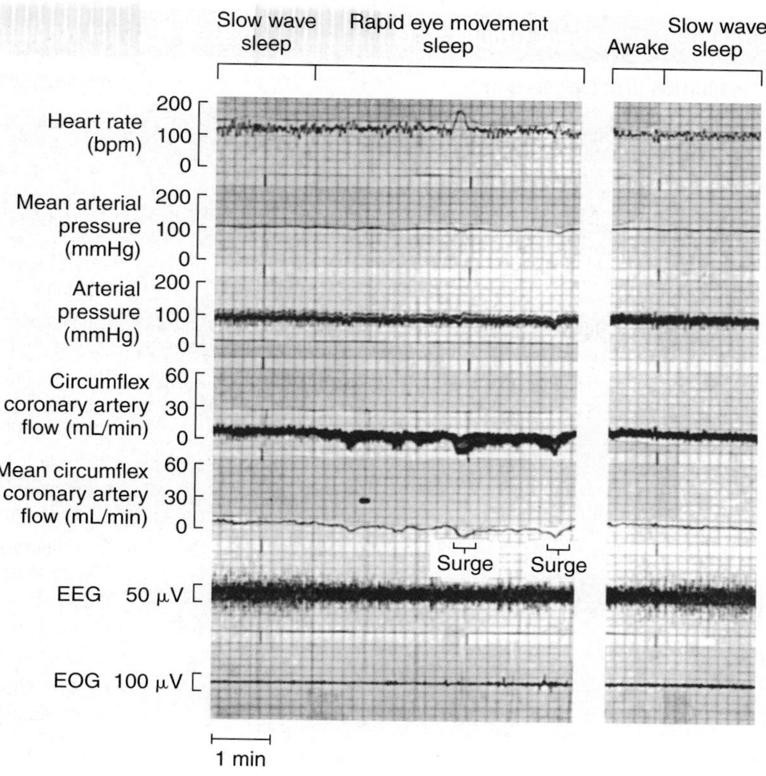

Figure 3.7-5.
Effects of sleep stage on heart rate, mean and phasic arterial blood pressures, and mean and phasic left circumflex coronary artery blood flow in a typical dog during stenosis. Note phasic decreases in coronary flow occurring during heart rate surges while the dog is in REM sleep. EEG, electroencephalogram; EOG, electro-oculogram. (From Kirby DA, Verrier RL: Differential effects of sleep stage on coronary hemodynamic function during stenosis. Physiol Behav 45:1017–1020, 1989.)

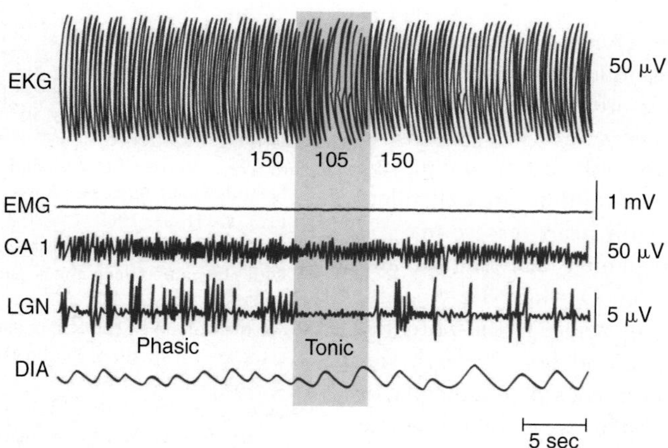

Figure 3.7-6.
Representative polygraphic recording of a primary heart rate deceleration during tonic REM sleep. During this deceleration, heart rate decreased from 150 to 105 bpm, or 30%. The deceleration occurred during a period devoid of ponto-geniculo-occipital (PGO) spikes in the lateral geniculate nucleus (LGN) or theta rhythm in the hippocampal (CA 1) leads. The deceleration is not a respiratory arrhythmia, as it is independent of diaphragmatic (DIA) movement. The abrupt decreases in amplitude of hippocampal theta (CA 1), PGO waves (LGN), and respiratory amplitude and rate (DIA) are typical of transitions from phasic to tonic REM. EKG, electrocardiogram; EMG, electromyogram. (From Verrier RL, Lau RT, Wallooppillai U, et al: Primary vagally mediated decelerations in heart rate during tonic rapid eye movement sleep in cats. Am J Physiol 43:R1136–R1141, 1998.)

Table 3.7-1. Patient Groups at Potentially Increased Risk for Nocturnal Cardiac Events

INDICATION (U.S. CASES/YEAR)	POSSIBLE MECHANISM
Nocturnal angina, ischemia, myocardial infarction (~250,000), lethal arrhythmias or cardiac arrest at night (~47,500)	The nocturnal pattern suggests a sleep state–dependent autonomic trigger or respiratory distress. • Nondemand ischemia and angina peak between midnight and 6:00 A.M. • Nocturnal onset of myocardial infarction is more frequent in older and sicker patients and carries higher risk of congestive heart failure.
Atrial fibrillation (2.5 million)	29% of episodes occur between midnight and 6:00 A.M. Respiratory and autonomic mechanisms are suspected.
Family report of highly irregular breathing, excessive snoring, or apnea in patients with coronary disease (5–10 million patients with apnea)	Patients with hypertension or atrial or ventricular arrhythmias should be screened for sleep apnea.
Long QT_3 syndrome, Brugada syndrome, and sudden nocturnal death syndrome (SUNDS)	The profound cycle-length changes associated with sleep may trigger pause-dependent torsades de pointes in these patients, who have an associated, genetic basis for arrhythmias.
Near-miss or siblings of sudden infant death syndrome (SIDS) victims	"Crib death" commonly occurs during sleep with characteristic cardiorespiratory symptoms. Passive smoking (including during gestation) increases the incidence of SIDS deaths.
Patients on cardiac medications (13.5 million patients with cardiovascular disease)	Beta-blockers and calcium channel blockers that cross the blood-brain barrier may increase nighttime risk, as poor sleep and violent dreams may be triggered. Medications that increase the Q–T interval may conduce to pause-dependent torsades de pointes during the profound cycle-length changes of sleep. Because arterial blood pressure is decreased during nonrapid eye movement sleep, additional lowering by antihypertensive agents may introduce a risk of ischemia and infarction due to lowered coronary perfusion.

between NREM and REM sleep. Dynamic fluctuations in central nervous system variables influence heart rhythm, arterial blood pressure, coronary artery blood flow, and ventilation. Whereas REM-induced surges in sympathetic and parasympathetic nerve activity with accompanying significant surges and pauses in heart rhythm are well tolerated in normal people, patients with heart disease may be at heightened risk for life-threatening arrhythmias and myocardial ischemia and infarction. During NREM sleep, in the severely compromised heart, there is the potential for hypotension that can impair blood flow through stenotic coronary vessels to trigger myocardial ischemia or infarction. Damage to central brain areas that regulate autonomic activity and that coordinate upper airway and diaphragmatic action can lead to enhanced sympathetic outflow, increasing risk in heart failure, and contributing to hypertension in obstructive sleep apnea. Coordination of cardiorespiratory control is especially pivotal in infancy, when developmental immaturity can compromise function and pose special risks. Throughout sleep, the coexistence of coronary disease and apnea is associated with heightened risk of cardiovascular events due to the challenge of dual control of the respiratory and cardiovascular systems.

SELECTED READINGS

Javaheri S: Effects of continuous positive airway pressure on sleep apnea and ventricular irritability in patients with heart failure. Circulation 101:392–397, 2000.

Kirby DA, Verrier RL: Differential effects of sleep stage on coronary hemodynamic function. Am J Physiol 256 (Heart Circ Physiol 25): H1378–H1383, 1989.

Macey PM, Henderson LA, Macey KE, et al: Brain morphology associated with obstructive sleep apnea. Am J Resp Crit Care Med 166:1382–1387, 2002.

Rowe K, Moreno R, Lau RT, et al: Heart rate surges during REM sleep are associated with theta rhythm and PGO activity in cats. Am J Physiol 277:R843–R849, 1999.

Shamsuzzaman AS, Gersh BJ, Somers VK: Obstructive sleep apnea: Implications for cardiac and vascular disease. JAMA 290:1906–1914, 2003.

Verrier RL, Harper RM, Hobson JA: Central and autonomic mechanisms regulating cardiovascular function. In Kryger MH, Roth T, Dement WC (eds): Principles and Practice of Sleep Medicine, 4th ed. Philadelphia, WB Saunders, 2005, pp. 192–202.

Verrier RL, Josephson ME: Cardiac arrhythmogenesis during sleep: Mechanisms, diagnosis, and therapy. In Kryger MH, Roth T, Dement WC (eds): Principles and Practice of Sleep Medicine, 4th ed. Philadelphia, WB Saunders, 2005, pp. 1171–1179.

Verrier RL, Mittleman MA: Sleep-related cardiac risk. In Kryger MH, Roth T, Dement WC (eds): Principles and Practice of Sleep Medicine, 4th ed. Philadelphia, WB Saunders, 2005, pp. 1161–1170.

Woo MA, Macey PM, Fonarow GC, et al: Regional brain gray matter loss in heart failure. J Appl Physiol 95:677–684, 2003.

Carlo Franzini

Sleep and Blood Flow 3.8

Blood flow to the tissues throughout the body is related to activity of the autonomic nervous system (ANS) and metabolic demands. Arousal state (wakefulness, W; non-rapid eye movement sleep, NREMS; and rapid eye movement sleep, REMS) plays a prominent role, being associated with changes in both ANS activity and metabolic demands.

Cerebral blood flow (CBF) mostly decreases during NREMS, becoming lower than it was during W, and rises again markedly in REMS. Positron emission tomography studies showed the spatial and temporal dimension of CBF changes during sleep. During REMS, blood flow (BF) increases in the pontine tegmentum, dorsal mesencephalon, thalamic nuclei, amygdalae, and anterior cingulate and enthorinal cortices. On the contrary, a significant negative correlation was found between the occurrence of NREMS and regional CBF in the central core structures (pons, mesencephalon, thalamus) (Fig. 3.8-1A).

No significant correlation was found between the changes in CBF and those in BF to the extra-cerebral head structures in the different states of the wake-sleep cycle.

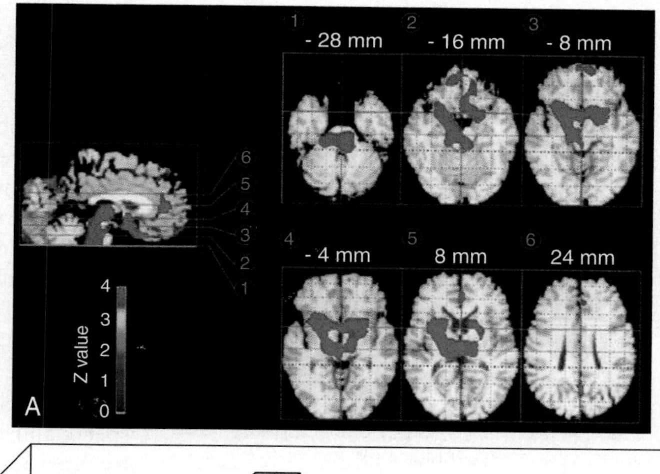

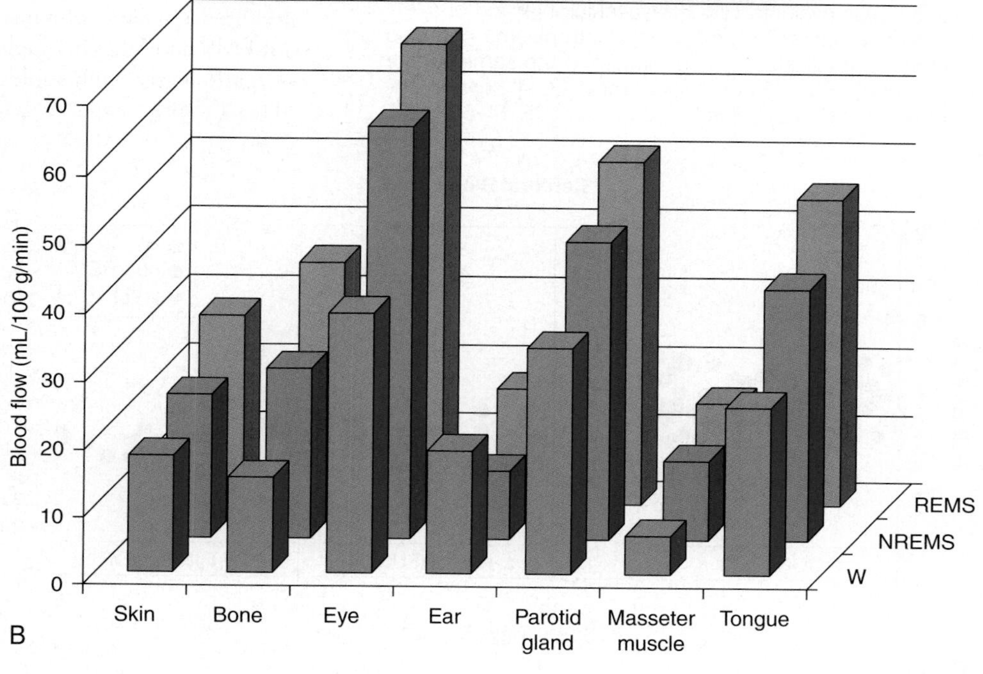

Figure 3.8-1.
A, Midsagittal and transverse sections showing brain areas (in red) where activity was significantly and negatively correlated with NREMS in humans. B, Blood flow (mL/100 g/min) in different extra-cranial head structures during the wake-sleep cycle in rats. No statistically significant differences were found among wake-sleep states. (A, From Maquet P, Degueldre C, Delfiore G, et al: Functional neuroanatomy of human slow wave sleep. J Neurosci 17:2807–2812, 1997. B, Adapted from Zoccoli G, Bach V, Cianci T, et al: Brain blood flow and extra-cerebral carotid circulation during sleep in rat. Brain Res 641:46–50, 1994.)

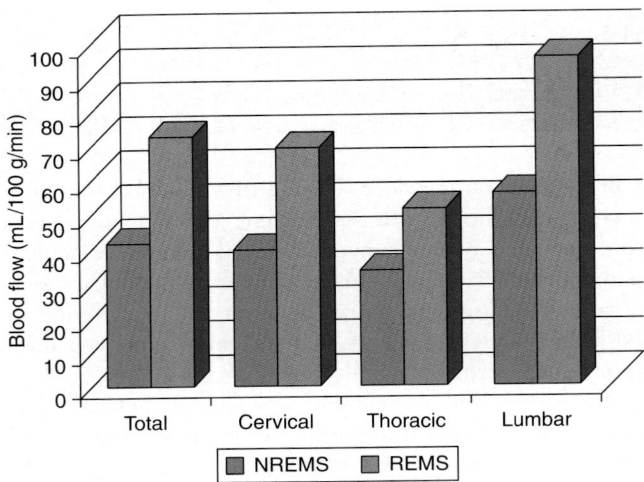

Figure 3.8-2.
Regional spinal cord blood flow during NREMS and REMS in rats. (Adapted from Zoccoli G, Bach V, Nardo B, et al: Spinal cord blood flow changes during the sleep-wake cycle in rat. Neurosci Lett 163:173–176, 1993.)

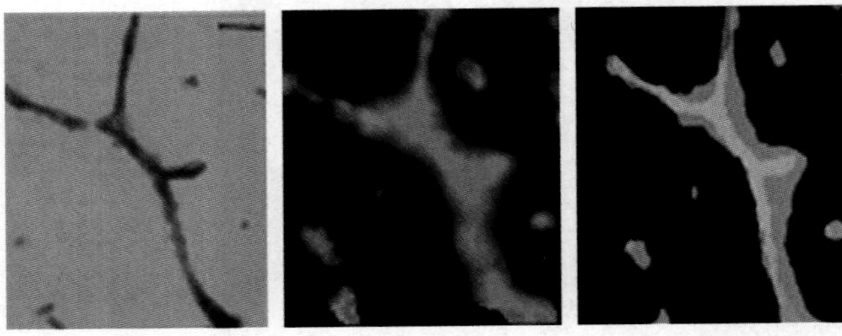

Figure 3.8-3.
Pictures showing capillary profiles in the rat cerebral cortex. Histochemical staining of the capillary endothelia identified the anatomical population *(left panel).* The perfused capillary network was evaluated by intravascular injection of a fluorescent marker *(central panel).* Both plasma perfused and anatomical capillaries were evaluated in the same section *(right panel).* Bar: 25 μm. (From Franzini C: Il cervello che dorme. Le Scienze, Scientific American 338:44–50, 1996.)

This suggests independent regulation of brain and external carotid circulation (Fig. 3.8-1B).

Spinal cord BF also increases in REMS with respect to NREMS. The similar trends of BF changes in brain and spinal cord indicate that the sleep process involves a modulation of the activity in the entire central nervous system (Fig. 3.8-2).

The regulation of cerebral circulation aims to match BF to the metabolic needs of brain activity at a regional level (flow-metabolism coupling). The adult brain relies mainly on glucose for its energy metabolism. To be transported into the brain, blood glucose must cross the blood-brain barrier (BBB) through stereospecific membrane carriers. Glucose flux depends mainly on glucose concentration, the surface area (S) of the capillary network, and the capillary permeability (P) to glucose. The product of BBB surface area and permeability to glucose (PS product) does not change between W and REMS, while CBF significantly increases during REMS. The capillary surface area S, measured as the fraction of cerebral capillaries perfused by plasma, is constant in the different wake-sleep states. These data indicate that changes in BBB permeability to glucose are negligible during sleep-related brain activation (Fig. 3.8-3).

The inhibition of nitric oxide (NO) synthase with the nonselective inhibitor *N*-nitro-L-arginine (L-NNA) led to the conclusion that NO is the major, although not the only, determinant of CBF differences occurring across the wake-sleep states (Fig. 3.8-4A).

The regulation of the cerebral circulation protects the brain from arterial pressure fluctuations (autoregulation). Autoregulation operates during sleep: cerebral vasodilation in response to acute hypotension occurs in all wake-sleep states, albeit with reduced efficacy in REMS. Both the speed and the magnitude of the vasoactive response to hypotension are diminished in REMS compared with NREMS and W. This suggests that the cerebral circulation is particularly vulnerable to hypotension during REMS (Fig. 3.8-4B).

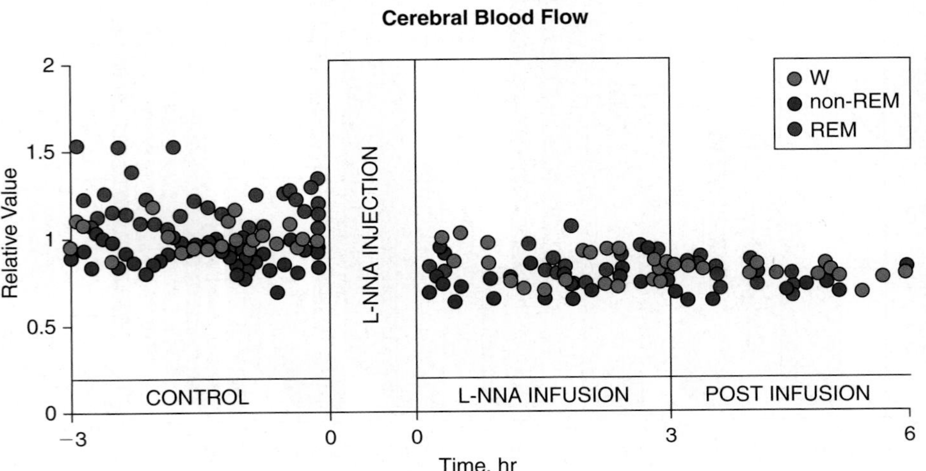

Figure 3.8-4.
A, Cerebral blood flow (CBF) recorded in lambs in spontaneous wake-sleep states during consecutive experimental periods of (a) control, (b) *N*-nitro-L-arginine (L-NNA) infusion, and (c) post infusion recovery period. Values are averaged over 1 minute of recording and normalized for each animal to the mean value recorded in wakefulness (W) during the control period. The normal sleep-related difference of CBF is abolished after L-NNA infusion.

(Continued)

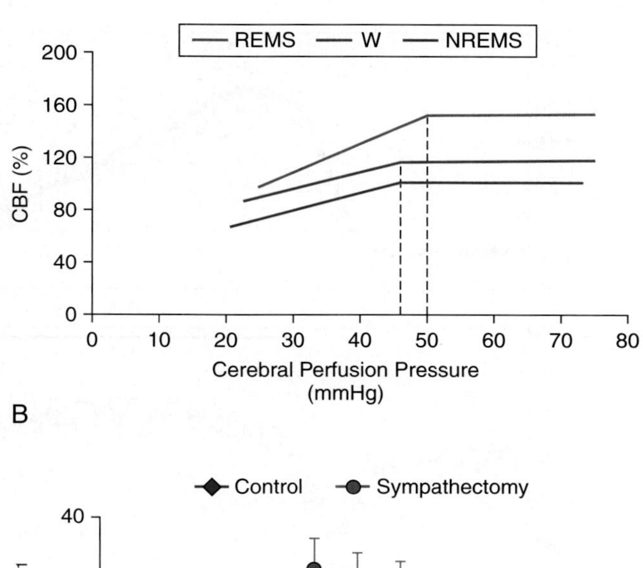

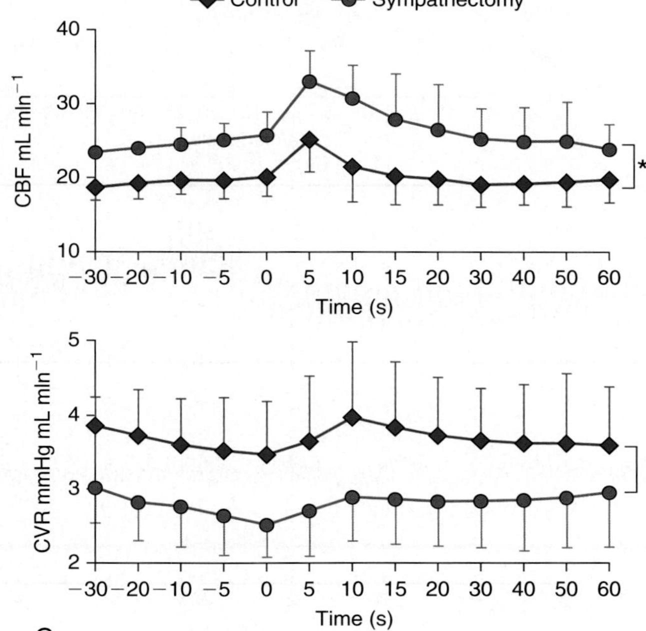

Figure 3.8-4. cont'd

B, Average autoregulation curves in lambs during wakefulness (W), NREMS, and REMS. Data were normalized to the baseline value recorded for each lamb in NREMS. The sleep-dependent differences in CBF are maintained across all levels of cerebral perfusion pressure. The position of the breakpoint of the autoregulation curve is shifted to the right in REMS relative to that in W and NREMS. In REMS, the slope of the descending limb of the autoregulation curve is also steeper than in either NREMS or W. Both higher breakpoint and greater slope of the autoregulation curve may place the brain in danger of ischemia and hypoxia should hypotension occur during REMS. **C**, Coherent averages of cerebral blood flow (CBF) and cerebral vascular resistance (CVR) during the spontaneous surges of arterial pressure in REMS in lambs. Time 0 corresponds to the onset of the arterial pressure upswing. After bilateral removal of the superior cervical ganglia, CBF is significantly greater and CVR is significantly lower throughout the surge episode. (**A**, Adapted from Zoccoli G, Grant DA, Wild J, Walker AM: Nitric oxide inhibition abolishes sleep-wake differences in cerebral circulation. Am J Physiol (Heart Circ Physiol) 280:H2598–H2606, 2001. **B**, Adapted from Grant DA, Franzini C, Wild J, et al: Autoregulation of the cerebral circulation during sleep in newborn lambs. J Physiol 564:923–930, 2005. **C**, Adapted from Loos N, Grant DA, Wild J, et al: Sympathetic nervous control of the cerebral circulation in sleep. J Sleep Res 14:275–283, 2005.)

The study of cerebral circulation after removal of the superior cervical ganglia revealed that the extrinsic sympathetic innervation of the brain significantly constricts the cerebral circulation and reduces CBF during W, NREMS, and REMS (Fig. 3.8-4C).

Pressure surges occur during REMS in humans and animal models, and is thus a remarkably robust feature of this sleep state. The pressure surges during REMS in the last part of the night may contribute to the increased incidence of acute cardiovascular events, which is observed in the early morning hours after awakening. Heart rate increases during the pressure surges in REMS. This pattern of hypertension and tachycardia contrasts with the operating logic of the arterial baroreflex, suggesting a central autonomic regulation (Fig. 3.8-5).

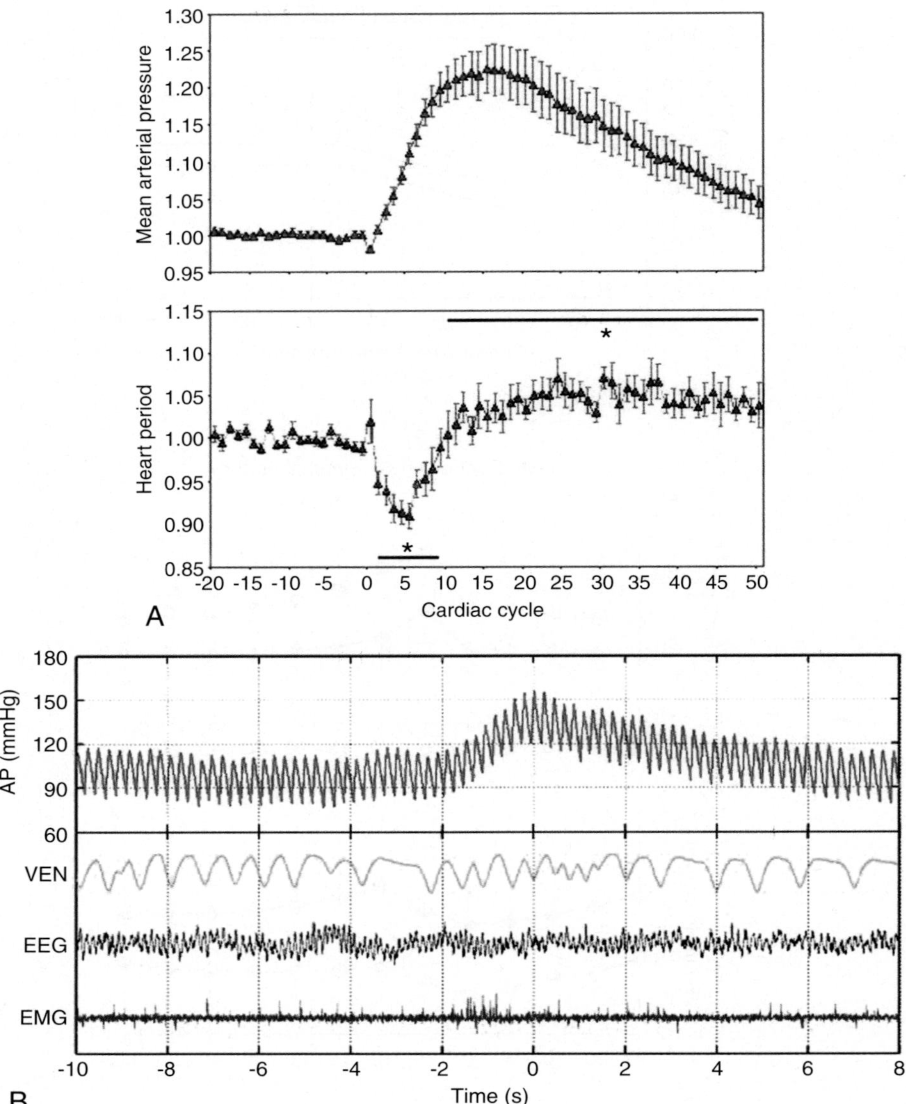

Figure 3.8-5.
A, Coherent averages of heart period (HP) and mean arterial pressure (MAP) during phasic blood pressure surges in REMS in lambs. Values of HP and MAP were divided by their respective baseline values. Time 0 corresponds to the cardiac cycle at the onset of the pressure surges. HP decreased at the onset of the pressure surges. B, Recordings during a surge of arterial pressure (AP) during REMS in rat. Ventilation (VEN) showed a prominent variability throughout the pressure surge. The electroencephalogram (EEG) displayed a prevalent theta rhythm, which accelerated before the surge peak. The electromyogram (EMG) indicated muscle atonia, which was interrupted by a muscle twitch. (A, Adapted from Silvani A, Asti V, Bojic T, et al: Sleep-dependent changes in the coupling between heart period and arterial pressure in newborn lambs. Pediatr Res 57:108–114, 2005. B, Adapted from Berteotti C, Franzini C, Lenzi P, et al: Surges of arterial pressure during REM sleep in spontaneously hypertensive rats. Sleep 31:111–117, 2008.)

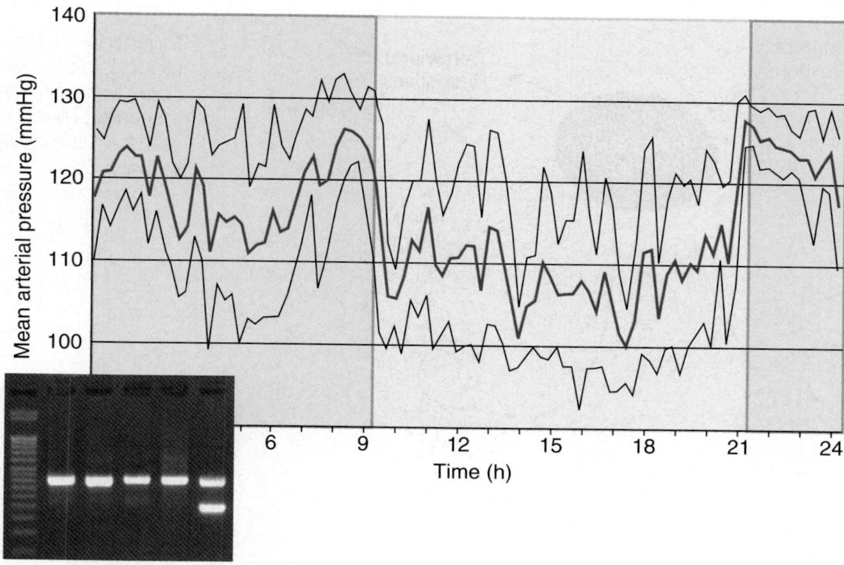

Figure 3.8-6.
Circadian profile of mean arterial pressure (MAP) in a C57Bl6/J mouse. Lines indicate mean ± standard deviation of MAP over 7 recording days (lights on from 09.00 to 21.00). The circadian MAP profile results from the circadian rhythm of wakefulness and NREMS and the sleep-dependent changes in MAP. The inset shows the results of a gel electrophoresis of DNA, which is used to evidence genetic differences between mouse strains in studies of functional genomics.

C57Bl6/J mice are the most commonly used control strain in studies of functional genomics. Research on functional genomics is supported by the growing availability of mouse mutant lines, which include models of human disease such as Alzheimer's disease and narcolepsy. Genetic differences between mouse strains may be evidenced with techniques of molecular biology such as DNA amplification and gel electrophoresis. Differences in the sleep structure or the physiologic hemodynamic pattern within sleep states may underlie many of the derangements in cardiovascular control that are associated with genetic mutations in mice (Fig. 3.8-6).

SELECTED READINGS

Berteotti C, Franzini C, Lenzi P, et al: Surges of arterial pressure during REM sleep in spontaneously hypertensive rats. Sleep 31:111–117, 2008.

Franzini C: Il cervello che dorme. Le Scienze, Scientific American 338: 44–50, 1996.

Grant DA, Franzini C, Wild J, et al: Autoregulation of the cerebral circulation during sleep in newborn lambs. J Physiol 564:923–930, 2005.

Loos N, Grant DA, Wild J, et al: Sympathetic nervous control of the cerebral circulation in sleep. J Sleep Res 14:275–283, 2005.

Maquet P, Degueldre C, Delfiore G, et al: Functional neuroanatomy of human slow wave sleep. J Neurosci 17:2807–2812, 1997.

Maquet P, Péters J-M, Aerts J, et al: Functional neuroanatomy of human rapid-eye-movement sleep and dreaming. Nature 383:163–166, 1996.

Silvani A: Physiological sleep-dependent changes in arterial blood pressure: Central autonomic commands and baroreflex control. Clin Exp Pharmacol Physiol 35:987–994, 2008.

Silvani A, Asti V, Berteotti C, et al: Sleep-related brain activation does not increase the permeability of the blood-brain barrier to glucose. J Cereb Blood Flow Metab 25:990–997, 2005.

Silvani A, Asti V, Bojic T, et al: Sleep-dependent changes in the coupling between heart period and arterial pressure in newborn lambs. Pediatr Res 57:108–114, 2005.

Zoccoli G, Bach V, Cianci T, et al: Brain blood flow and extracerebral carotid circulation during sleep in rat. Brain Res 641:46–50, 1994.

Zoccoli G, Bach V, Nardo B, et al: Spinal cord blood flow changes during the sleep-wake cycle in rat. Neurosci Lett 163:173–176, 1993.

Zoccoli G, Grant DA, Wild J, et al: Nitric oxide inhibition abolishes sleep-wake differences in cerebral circulation. Am J Physiol (Heart Circ Physiol) 280:H2598–H2606, 2001.

Éva Szentirmai, Levente Kapás, and James M. Krueger

3.9 Interactive Regulation of Sleep and Feeding

The regulations of sleep and food intake are closely related. The mechanisms responsible for food-seeking behavior and the control of sleep are coordinated by partly overlapping hypothalamic neuronal systems. These systems receive information about the energy status of the body through hunger, adiposity, and satiety signals arising from the periphery and the central nervous system (Fig. 3.9-1). These signals include hormones and neuromodulators, such as ghrelin, cholecystokinin (CCK), and leptin (Table 3.9-1).

Central administration of ghrelin stimulates wakefulness, food intake, and growth hormone release in rodents. In rats, plasma and hypothalamic ghrelin levels increase in response to sleep deprivation. The wake-promoting effect of ghrelin involves the activation of hypothalamic orexinergic and neuropeptide Y (NPY)-ergic mechanisms. Ghrelin

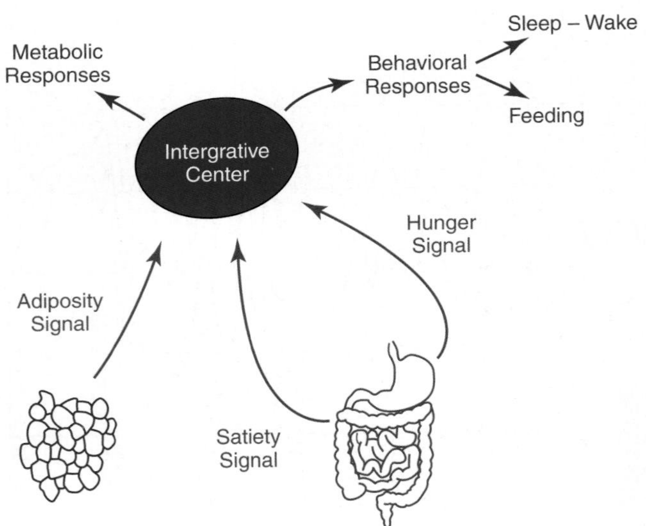

Figure 3.9-1.
Mounting evidence supports the idea that mechanisms responsible for feeding behavior and the control of sleep are coordinated by partly overlapping hypothalamic neuronal systems. These systems receive information about the energy status of the body through hunger, adiposity, and satiety signals.

also stimulates the hypothalamo-pituitary-adrenal axis by stimulating corticotroph-releasing hormone (CRH) secretion in the paraventricular nucleus (Fig. 3.9-2). NPY, orexin, and CRH have wakefulness-promoting effects. The hypothalamic NPY-orexin-ghrelin network plays an important role in integrating circadian, visual, and metabolic signals (Fig. 3.9-3). The ghrelin gene also codes for another biologically active peptide, obestatin; it has the opposite effects on both food intake and sleep as ghrelin. In humans, the effects of ghrelin on sleep are less clear. Systemic repeated bolus injections of ghrelin during the night enhance stage IV sleep and suppress rapid eye movement sleep (REMS) in male healthy subjects, although ghrelin is ineffective in women. Epidemiologic studies suggest a relationship between sleep duration and plasma ghrelin levels. Habitual short sleep duration and sleep restriction to 4 hours per night are associated with elevated ghrelin plasma levels and increased hunger, suggesting that chronic sleep curtailment is a risk factor for obesity.

CCK elicits the complete behavioral sequence of the satiety syndrome, including the cessation of feeding, increased sleep, decreased motor activity, and social withdrawal. These actions are mediated by peripheral targets, since central injections of CCK do not suppress feeding or promote sleep. While the feeding-suppressive effects of CCK are mediated by the vagus nerve, sleep induction appears to be independent of the vagus nerve and pancreatic insulin. Animals that lack CCK-1 receptors do not show any gross alteration in their baseline sleep pattern, suggesting that in the absence of CCK signaling through the peripheral receptor subtype, normal sleep-wake activity can be maintained.

Leptin also suppresses feeding and it stimulates metabolism. Circulating leptin enters the brain via saturable transport mechanisms. Leptin receptors are expressed in various hypothalamic nuclei and in the brainstem. Via these receptors, leptin stimulates melanocyte-stimulating hormone secretion and suppresses NPY-producing cells;

Table 3.9-1. Relationship between Sleep and Ghrelin, Leptin, and CCK Plasma and Hypothalamic Levels

	GHRELIN	LEPTIN	CHOLECYSTOKININ
Effect of acute sleep deprivation	Elevated plasma and hypothalamic levels	Reduced diurnal amplitude	n.a.
Relation to chronic short sleep duration in humans	Elevated plasma levels	Reduced plasma levels	n.a.
Effects on sleep	Humans: no effect or increased sleep Rodents: central administration induces wakefulness	Increases NREMS, decreases REMS	Peripheral administration increases NREMS, central injection no effect
Sleep in knockout (KO) animals	Normal diurnal rhythm, fragmented sleep in ghrelin and ghrelin receptor KO mice	Attenuated diurnal rhythm of sleep, increased and fragmented NREMS	CCK-1 receptor deficient rats have normal sleep-wake activity
Plasma levels in sleep disorders	Enhanced nocturnal ghrelin levels in night eating syndrome	Reduced levels in narcolepsy and in night eating syndrome	n.a.

CCK, cholecystokinin; NREMS, nonrapid eye movement sleep; REMS, rapid eye movement sleep; n.a., not available

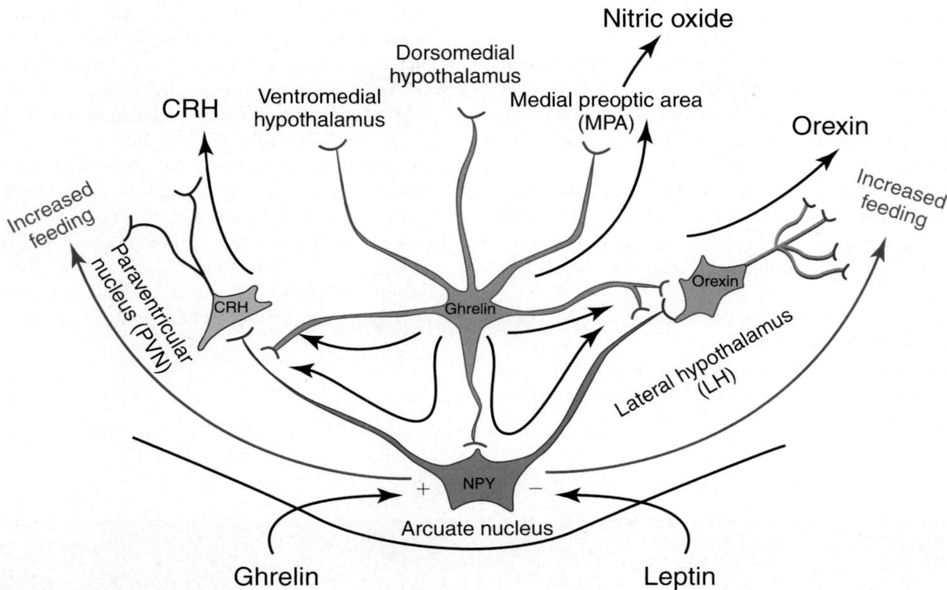

Figure 3.9-2.
Hypothalamic ghrelin-, orexin-, and neuropeptide Y (NPY)-ergic neurons form a well-characterized circuit that is implicated in the regulation of food intake and sleep. Circulating ghrelin and leptin can modulate the activity of the circuit through NPY in the arcuate nucleus. Ghrelin promotes wakefulness when injected to the lateral hypothalamus (LH), paraventricular nucleus (PVN), or medial preoptic area (MPA). Ghrelin administration and ghrelinergic neurons activate orexinergic cells in the LH and NPY-containing cells in the arcuate nucleus. In the PVN, ghrelin facilitates corticotroph-releasing hormone (CRH) release indirectly through the stimulation of NPY-ergic neurons. Ghrelin microinjection into the LH may promote wakefulness through the stimulation of orexin release. In the PVN, ghrelin indirectly facilitates CRH release that leads to increased wakefulness. In the MPA, ghrelin's wakefulness-promoting effect might be mediated by nitric oxide (NO). Several actions of ghrelin are NO-dependent, and NO-ergic mechanisms are implicated in sleep regulation.

two of the main effects that underlie leptin's satiety effects. The effects of leptin itself on sleep are less understood. Leptin plasma levels peak at night in humans; this diurnal rhythm appears to be entrained by eating. Sleep deprivation suppresses the nocturnal rise in leptin. Obese, leptin-deficient mice have increased amounts of nonrapid eye movement sleep (NREMS), but sleep appears to be more fragmented. Injection of leptin in rats both stimulates NREMS and suppresses REMS, whereas in mice it only stimulates NREMS.

Figure 3.9-3.
The hypothalamic ghrelin-orexin-neuropeptide Y (NPY) circuit receives and integrates metabolic, circadian, and visual signals. The activation of the circuit has two main parallel outputs in rodents: increased wakefulness and increased feeding activity.

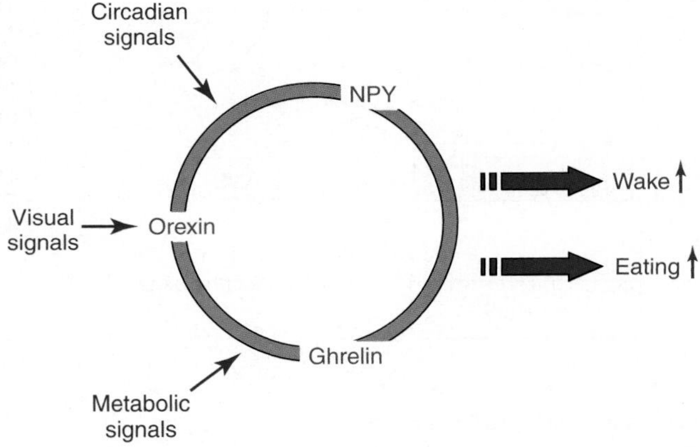

SELECTED READINGS

Kapás L, Obál F Jr, Alföldi P, et al: Effects of nocturnal intraperitoneal administration of cholecystokinin in rats: Simultaneous increase in sleep, increase in EEG slow-wave activity, reduction of motor activity, suppression of eating, and decrease in brain temperature. Brain Res 438(1-2):155–164, 1988.

Kapás L, Obál F Jr, Farkas I, et al: Cholecystokinin promotes sleep and reduces food intake in diabetic rats. Physiol Behav 50(2):417–420, 1991.

Laposky AD, Shelton J, Bass J, et al: Altered sleep regulation in leptin-deficient mice. Am J Physiol Regul Integr Comp Physiol 290(4): R894–R903, 2006.

Mansbach RS, Lorenz DN: Cholecystokinin (CCK-8) elicits prandial sleep in rats. Physiol Behav 30(2):179–183, 1983.

Sinton C, Fitch T, Gershenfeld HK: The effects of leptin on REM sleep and slow wave delta in rats are reversed by food deprivation. J Sleep Res 8:197–203, 1999.

Spiegel K, Tasali E, Penev P, et al: Sleep curtailment in healthy young men is associated with decreased leptin levels, elevated ghrelin levels, and increased hunger and appetite. Ann Intern Med 141:846–850, 2004.

Szentirmai E, Kapás L, Krueger JM: Ghrelin microinjection into forebrain sites induces wakefulness and feeding in rats. Am J Physiol Regul Integr Comp Physiol 292:R575–R585, 2007.

Szentirmai E, Kapás L, Sun Y, et al: Spontaneous sleep and homeostatic sleep regulation in ghrelin knockout mice. Am J Physiol Regul Integr Comp Physiol 293(1):R510–R517, 2007.

Szentirmai E, Krueger JM: Obestatin alters sleep in rats. Neurosci Lett 14;404(1-2):222–226, 2006.

Weikel JC, Wichniak A, Ising M, et al: Ghrelin promotes slow-wave sleep in humans. Am J Physiol Endocrinol Metab 284(2):E407–E415, 2003.

3.10 Endocrine Physiology

Rachel Leproult, Karine Spiegel, and Eve Van Cauter

Overview of Endocrine Physiology

CENTRAL MECHANISMS CONTROLLING PITUITARY HORMONE SECRETION OVER THE 24-HOUR DAY

There are two interacting time-keeping processes in the central nervous system that can be affected by synchronizing factors.

The activity of these processes controls the 24-hour profiles of hypothalamo-pituitary hormones. Pulsatile activity of hypothalamic releasing and/or inhibiting factors affects the function of the pituitary gland. In addition, the autonomic nervous system (ANS) can affect the activity of the peripheral endocrine organs (Fig. 3.10-1).

Process S	Sleep homeostat	Effects depend on the amount of prior wakefulness.
Process C	Circadian rhythmicity	Effects depend on time of day, irrespective of whether there is sleep or wakefulness. Generated by pacemaker in the suprachiasmatic nuclei (SCN) of the hypothalamus.
Modulating factors	These can synchronize or desynchronize the systems.	Light, body position, stress, food intake, and exercise can affect the patterns of pituitary hormone release.

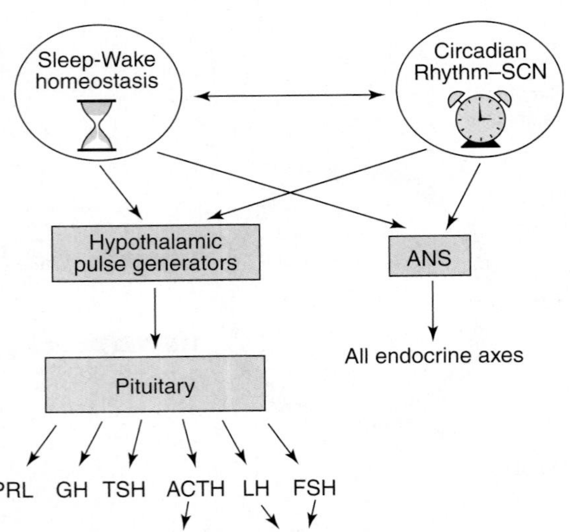

Figure 3.10-1.
Schematic representation of the central mechanisms involved in the control of temporal variations in pituitary hormone secretions over a 24-hour cycle. ACTH, adrenocorticotropic hormone; ANS, autonomic nervous system; FSH, follicle-stimulating hormone; GH, growth hormone; LH, luteinizing hormone; PRL, prolactin; SCN, suprachiasmatic nuclei; TSH, thyroid-stimulating hormone. (Adapted from Van Cauter E, Copinschi G: Endocrine and other biological rhythms. In Degroot LJ, Jameso JL [eds]: Endocrinology, 5th ed, vol 1. Philadelphia: Elsevier Saunders, pp. 341–372, 2006.)

TEMPORAL VARIATIONS OF PLASMA LEVELS OF HORMONES

Levels of hormones can be related to whether the person is asleep, the time of day, and whether sleep deprivation is present. In Figure 3.10-2 data are shown from a protocol in which male subjects are studied for 53 hours, which includes 8 hours of nocturnal sleep from 11:00 P.M. until 7:00 A.M.; 28 hours of continuous wakefulness, which includes a night of total sleep deprivation; and daytime recovery sleep from 11:00 A.M. until 7:00 P.M., beginning 12 hours out of phase with the usual bedtime.

From these studies one can conclude: (a) *growth hormone* secretion is primarily controlled by the sleep-wake homeostasis and is maximal during slow wave sleep; (b) *cortisol* secretion is almost entirely related to clock time (circadian rhythm), and its level is minimally affected by sleep or sleep deprivation; (c) secretion of thyroid-stimulating hormone (*TSH*) is controlled by both sleep homeostasis and circadian rhythmicity; and (d) sleep-onset, no matter when it occurs, has a stimulatory effect on the release of *prolactin*.

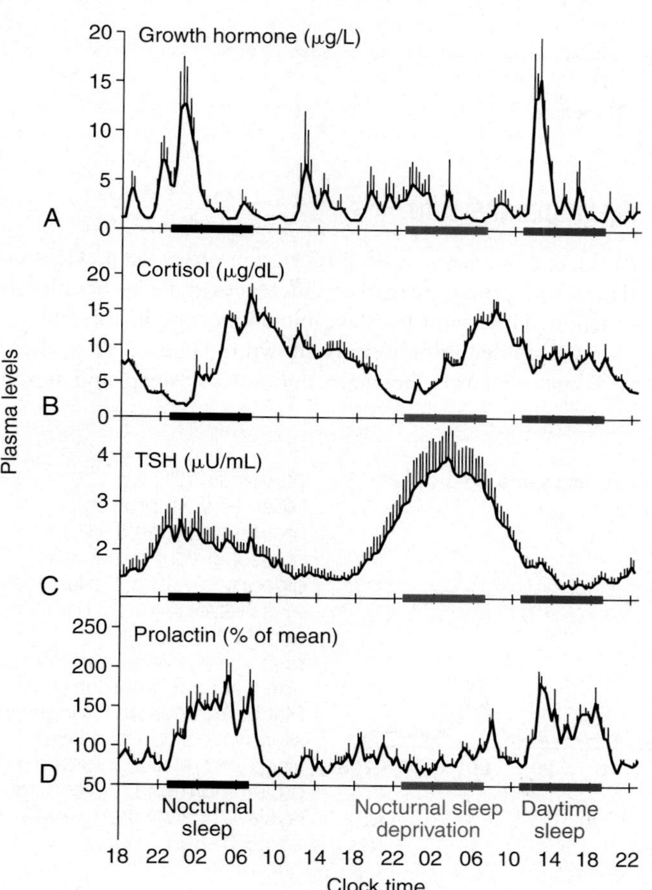

Figure 3.10-2.
Mean (+SEM) hormonal profiles obtained in a protocol designed to delineate the respective contributions of the circadian rhythmicity and the sleep-wake homeostasis. The effects of the circadian modulation can be observed in the absence of sleep and the effects of sleep can be observed at an abnormal circadian time. (Adapted from Van Cauter E, Spiegel K: Circadian and sleep control of hormonal secretions. In Zee PC, Turek FW [eds]: Regulation of sleep and circadian rhythms, Lung Biology in Health and Disease [Lenfant C, series ed], vol 133. New York: Marcel Dekker, Inc., pp. 397–426, 1999.)

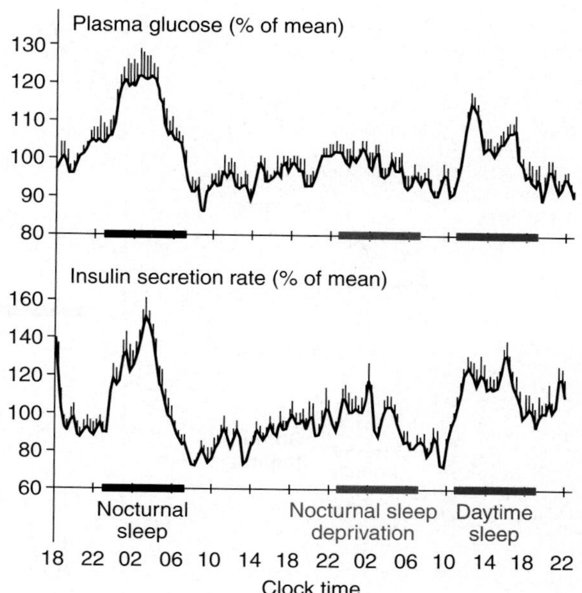

Figure 3.10-3.
Mean (+SEM) profiles of glucose and insulin secretion in a group of normal young men studied over 53 hours including 8 hours of usual nocturnal sleep, 28 hours of continuous wakefulness including one night of sleep deprivation, and a daytime recovery sleep period. (Adapted from Van Cauter E, Blackman JD, Roland D, et al: Modulation of glucose regulation by circadian rhythmicity and sleep. J Clin Invest 88:934–942, 1991.)

GLUCOSE REGULATION AND HUNGER

In the study illustrated in Figure 3.10-3, the subjects were fasting and caloric intake was in the form of an intravenous glucose infusion at a constant rate. Despite the fact that exogenous glucose input was constant, the levels of glucose and insulin secretion rate increased during sleep, returned to baseline in the morning, then gradually increased during the day, the latter suggesting a circadian effect. During daytime sleep glucose and insulin also increase. Thus, there is both a sleep and a circadian effect on glucose regulation and insulin secretion.

Leptin, a satiety hormone (produced by fat cells), and ghrelin, a hunger hormone (produced by gastric cells), demonstrate diurnal variation (see also chapter 3.9). The 24-hour variation in leptin levels depends on when meals are taken; levels are low in the morning, increase gradually during the day, and are highest at night. Ghrelin is also high at night. During the daytime, ghrelin levels decrease after eating, then increase in anticipation of the next meal (Fig. 3.10-4).

Examples of Conditions that Impact Hormones and Metabolism

AGING

With aging there is a reduction in the amount of slow-wave sleep. Since growth hormone (GH) secretion is maximal in slow-wave sleep, a reduction in GH levels during sleep is apparent in older people (Fig. 3.10-5).

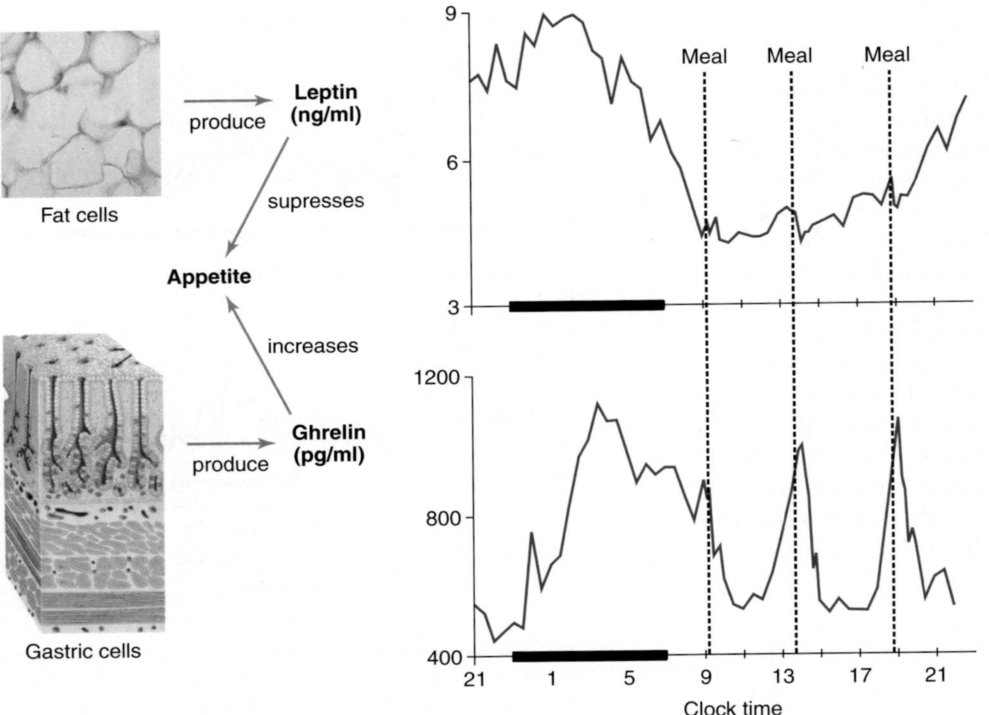

Figure 3.10-4. Individual 24-hour profiles of leptin and ghrelin. The black bars represent the bedtimes. Identical meals were presented at 5-hour intervals. (From unpublished individual data.)

DISEASE STATES THAT REDUCE SLOW WAVE SLEEP

In untreated sleep apnea syndrome (see chapter 11) sleep is fragmented and there is a reduction in slow-wave sleep. Nocturnal growth hormone levels are also reduced but are increased with CPAP (continuous positive airway pressure) treatment (Fig. 3.10-6).

SLEEP DEPRIVATION

At the end of a week of sleep restriction versus sleep extension (Fig. 3.10-7), there are marked differences in the 24-hour levels of leptin. This might translate into an increase in appetite.

In the epidemiologic study shown in Figure 3.10-8, there is a linear relation between duration of sleep and leptin

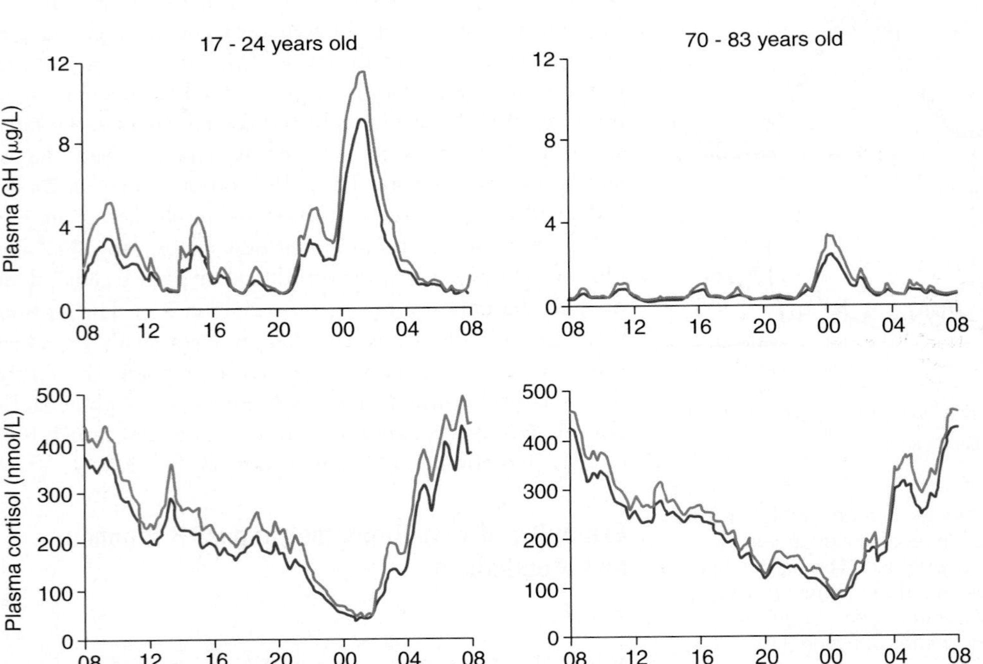

Figure 3.10-5. Mean (+SEM) profiles of growth hormone (GH) and cortisol in young men and older men with a similar body mass index (24.1$\pm$0.6 kg/m^2 and 24.1$\pm$0.8 kg/m^2, respectively). (Adapted from Van Cauter E, Leproult R, Plat L: Age-related changes in slow wave sleep and REM sleep and relationship with growth hormone and cortisol levels in healthy men. JAMA 284:861–868, 2000.)

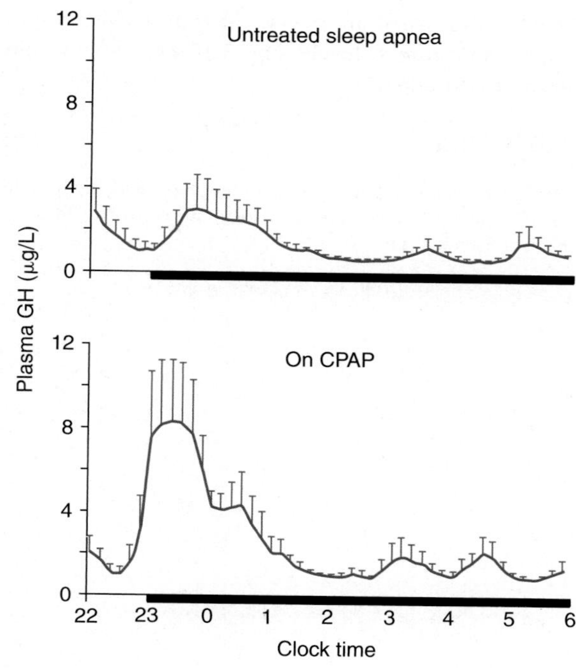

Figure 3.10-6.
Nocturnal profiles (mean + SEM) growth hormone (GH) before and after continuous positive airway pressure (CPAP) treatment. (Adapted from Saini J, Krieger J, Brandenberger G, et al: Continuous positive airway pressure treatment. Effects on growth hormone, insulin and glucose profiles in obstructive sleep apnea patients. Horm Metab Res 25[7]:375–381, 1993.)

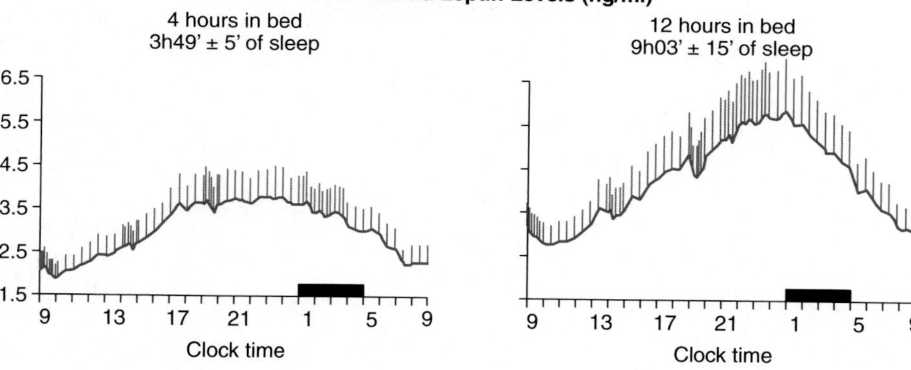

Figure 3.10-7.
Mean (+SEM) leptin profiles at the end of one week of sleep restriction (4 hours in bed per night) and at the end of one week of sleep extension (12 hours in bed per night). (Adapted from Spiegel K, Leproult R, L'Hermite–Balériaux M: Impact of sleep duration on the 24-hour leptin profile: Relationships with sympatho-vagal balance, cortisol and TSH. J Clin Endocrinol Metab, 89[11]:5762–5771, 2004.)

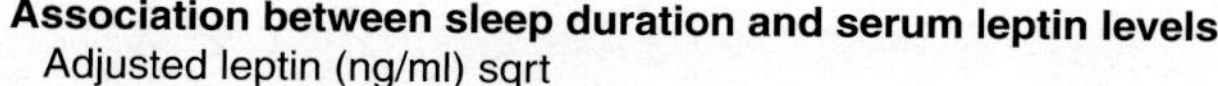

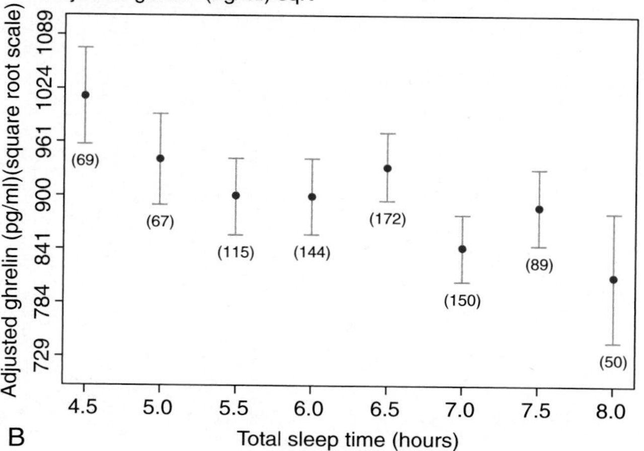

Figure 3.10-8.
Relationship between sleep duration and serum leptin (A) and ghrelin levels (B). (Adapted from Taheri S, Lin L, Austin D: Short sleep duration is associated with reduced leptin, elevated ghrelin, and increased body mass index. PLoS Med 1[3]:e62, 2004.)

levels (Fig. 3.10-8A) and an inverse relation between duration of sleep and ghrelin levels (Fig. 3.10-8B). This would result in increased appetite.

SELECTED READINGS

Van Cauter E, Copinschi G: Endocrine and other biological rhythms. In Degroot LJ, Jameson JL (eds): Endocrinology, 5th ed, vol 1. Philadelphia, Elsevier Saunders, pp. 341–372, 2006.

Van Cauter E, Holmback U, Knutson K, et al: Impact of sleep and sleep loss on neuroendocrine and metabolic function. Horm Res 67(1):2–9, 2007.

Van Cauter E, Leproult R, Plat L: Age-related changes in slow wave sleep and REM sleep and relationship with growth hormone and cortisol levels in healthy men. JAMA 284:861–868, 2000.

Van Cauter E, Spiegel K: Circadian and sleep control of hormonal secretions. In Zee PC, Turek FW (eds): Regulation of Sleep and Circadian Rhythms, vol 133 of Lung Biology in Health and Disease (Lenfant C, ed). New York, Marcel Dekker, 1999, pp. 397–426.

CHAPTER 4

NORMAL SLEEP

Alon Y. Avidan

All organisms have periods of activity and inactivity. This is true for organisms ranging from viruses to the most complex of mammals. Such a finding, which is pervasive in all living organisms, suggests that sleep is basic to life (Box 4-1). In this chapter we review normal sleep and the impact of sleep deprivation. In chapter 17 are reviewed the technical aspects of recording and the staging of sleep.

BOX 4-1. WHAT IS SLEEP?

- Sleep has been defined behaviorally as a reversible state of perceptual disengagement from and unresponsiveness to the environment.
- Sleep is a complex state in which there occur changes in physiologic and behavioral processes compared with wakefulness.
- Sleep is physiologic, necessary, temporary, reversible, and cyclic.

The Staging of Sleep

All animals sleep, and they generally assume a posture that is instantly recognizable as sleeping or resting (Fig. 4-1).

However, when inspecting the animal, we cannot really tell if the animal is actually asleep; in addition, there are different "depths" of sleep. Using techniques that record the electrical activity of the nervous system, we can now categorize by stage the depth of sleep in humans and other species. Recently, the rules for the staging of human sleep have been updated by the American Academy of Sleep Medicine (AASM). This is a time of transition, and, where important, we include information and examples of the classic rules, as well as the updated ones. A huge and monumental knowledge base has been developed using the classic rules, and so it seems appropriate to include information about them. In contrast, pediatric rules had not been rigorously defined by consensus; for pediatrics, therefore, where relevant, we focus on the scoring rules developed by the AASM.

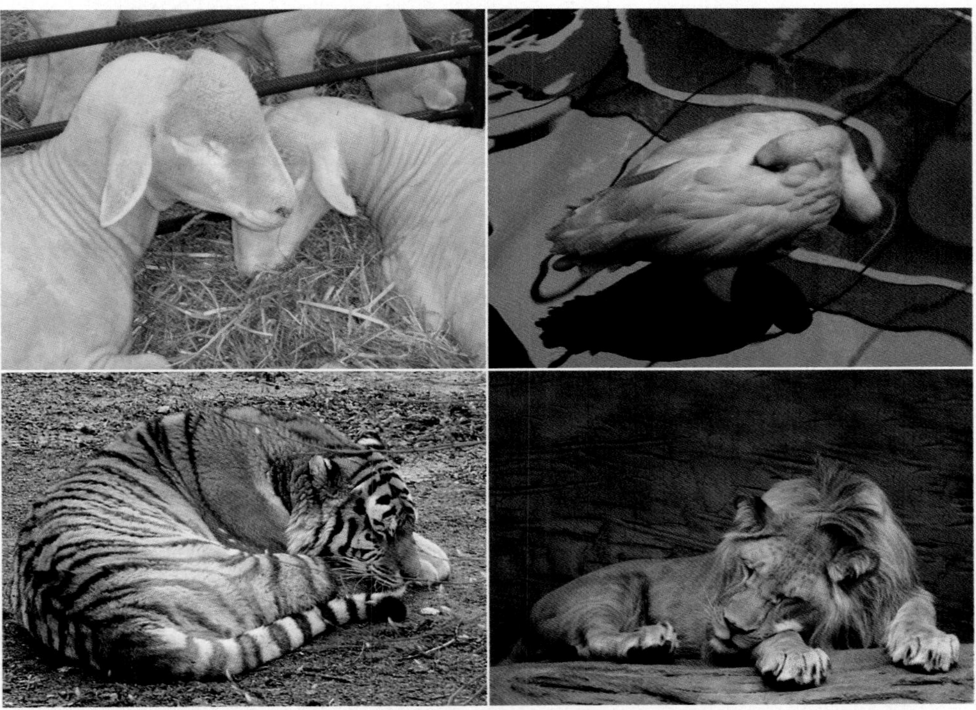

Figure 4-1.
Animals assume a recognizable posture when sleeping.

Sleep staging uses the frequency, amplitude, and pattern of data obtained by means of electroencephalography (brainwave activity), electro-oculography (eye movements), and electromyography (muscle tone), which together score the record as stage W, N1, N2, N3, or R. Examples of 30-second fragments are shown in Figures 4-2 through 4-6. The technical details and scoring rules are reviewed in chapter 17. See Table 4-1.

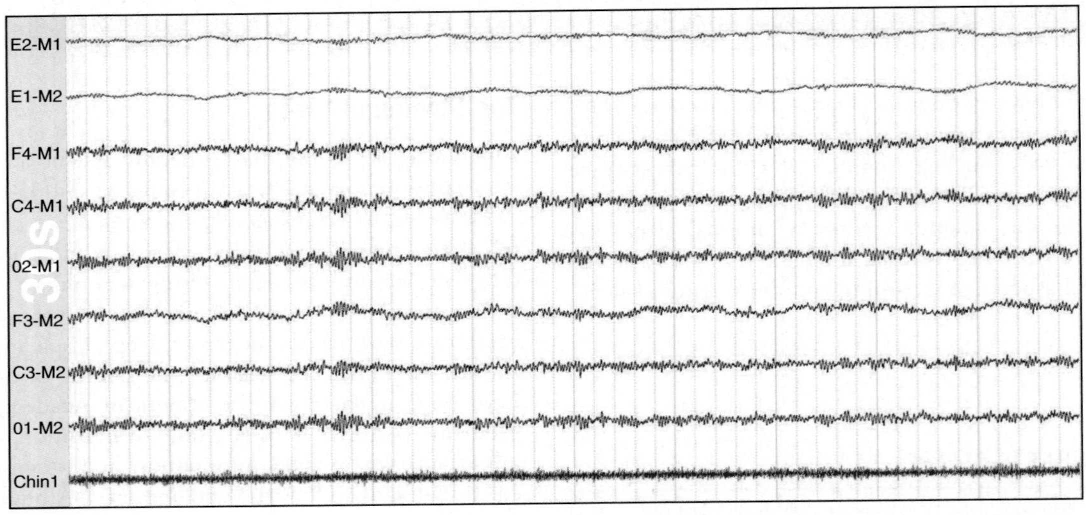

Figure 4-2.
Stage W (wakefulness). This fragment is a 30-second epoch. The two top channels represent the channels that monitor eye movements. The next six channels are used to record the EEG. The first three of these (F_4-M_1, C_4-M_1, O_2-M_1) are the ones recommended for scoring sleep. The others are backups in case electrodes malfunction. The bottom channel is the chin EMG. The key finding that indicates this is wakefulness is the presence of alpha rhythm over the occipital region (monitored by the O leads) occupying more than 30 seconds of the epoch. See chapter 17, Table 17-2, for technical details and definitions of the waves seen in sleep. Figures 4-3 to 4-6 use the same montage.

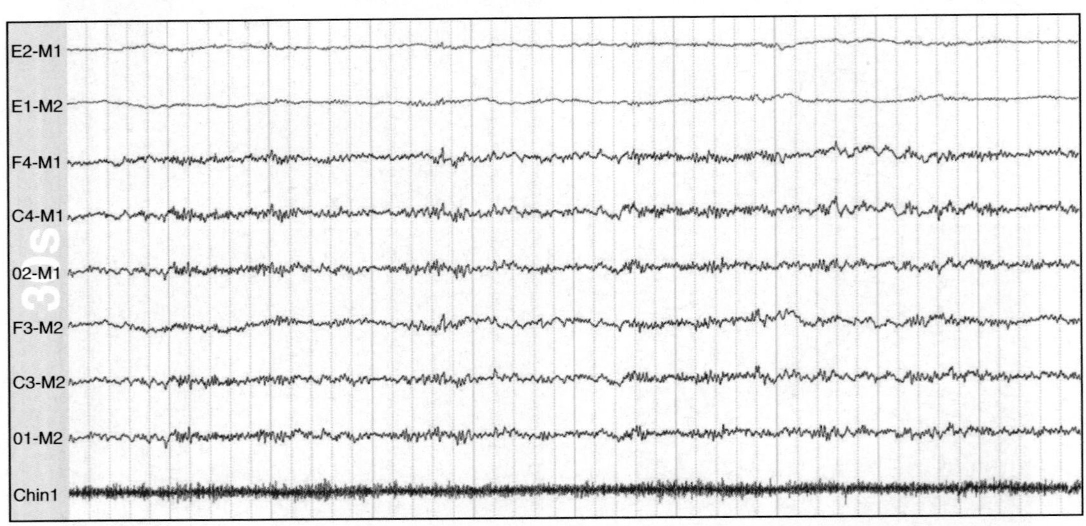

Figure 4-3.
Stage N1. This is stage N1 because a mixed frequency, low-amplitude pattern has replaced the alpha rhythm for more than 50% of the epoch.

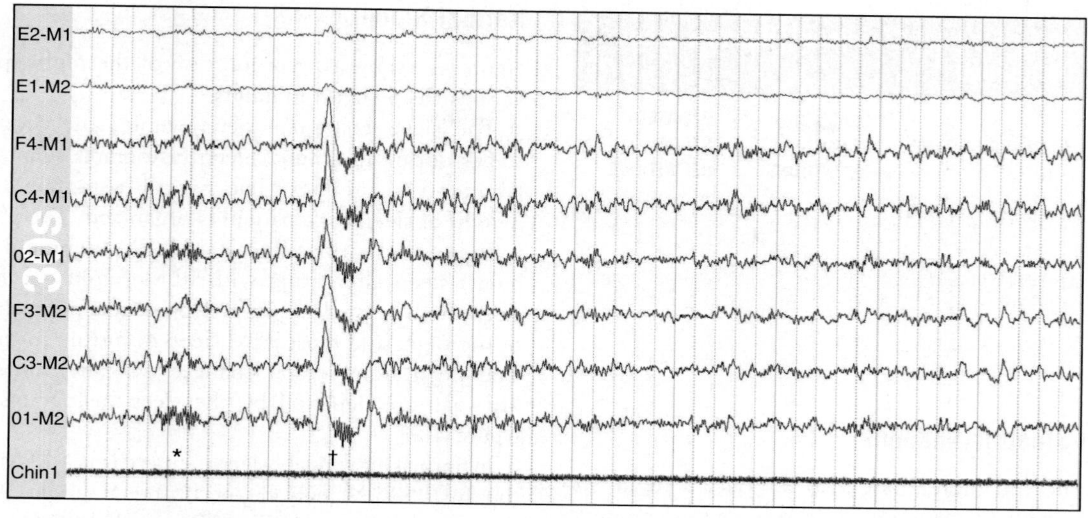

Figure 4-4.
Stage N2. A train of sleep spindles (*) toward the beginning of the epoch is followed shortly by a K complex (†).

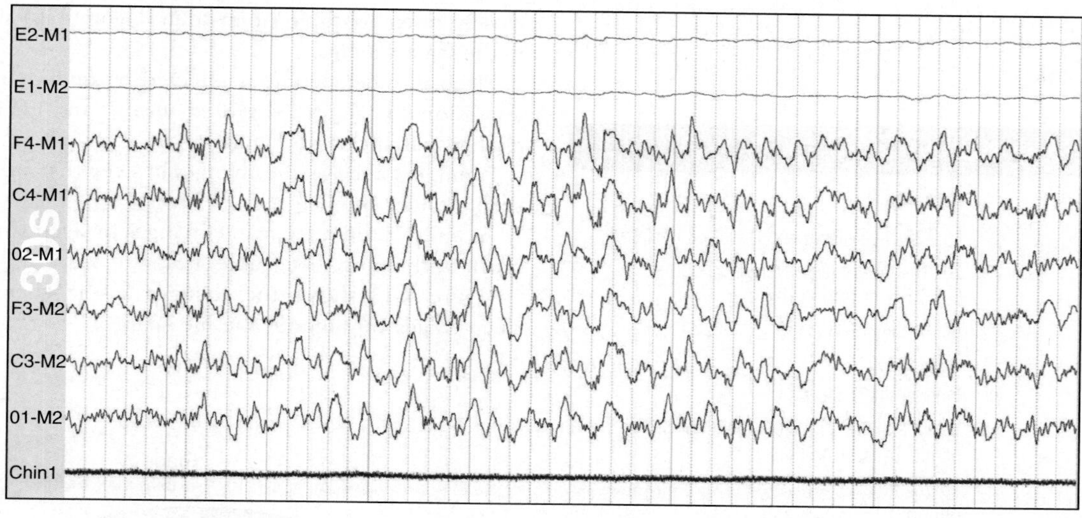

Figure 4-5.
Stage N3. This is stage N3 because more than 20% of the epoch consists of slow-wave activity.

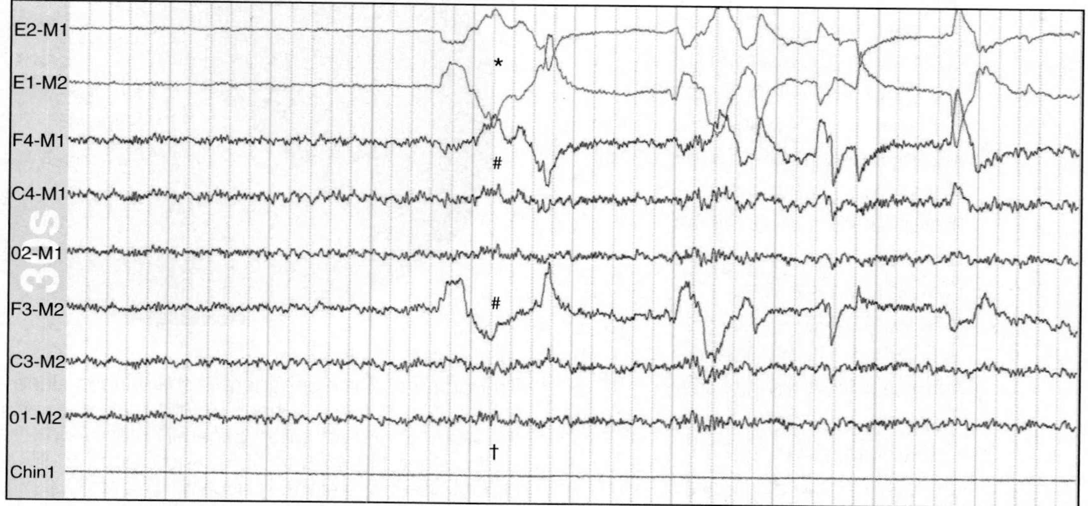

Figure 4-6.
Stage R. There are rapid eye movements (*) and a mixed-frequency, low-amplitude EEG; muscle tone (chin EMG) is absent (†). Note that some of the activity of the eyes has spilled over into the two frontal (F) leads (#).

Table 4-1. Sleep Staging: Classic vs. Updated Stage Definitions

TERMS USED TO DESCRIBE TYPE OF SLEEP		CLASSIC STAGE DEFINITIONS	UPDATED STAGE DEFINITIONS
NREM	"Light sleep"	1	N1
		2	N2
	"Deep sleep" or slow-wave sleep	3 } 4 }	N3
REM	REM sleep, dreaming sleep, paradoxical sleep	REM	R

How Much Sleep Is Enough?

To sustain life, no more than 3 to 5 hours a night are required; however, this amount of sleep leads to sleepiness, impaired performance, and reduced executive functions. To sustain optimal alertness throughout the day, the requirement varies across individuals. For some persons, 5 hours is enough; for others 10 hours. The mean is 7 to 8 hours for adults (Table 4-2).

Table 4-2. Sleep Stages

AGE	FINDINGS
In utero	80% "active sleep" at 30 weeks' gestation
Newborns	16–18 hours sleep every 24 hours; 5–10 hours during daytime Active sleep—50% Quiet sleep Indeterminate sleep Establishment of major nocturnal sleep period by 3–4 months
One year	13–15 hours every 24 hours; 2–3 hours during daytime naps 30% REM sleep
Two years	12–14 hours; 1.5–2.5 hours during daytime naps 25% REM sleep (fixed)
Three to five years	11–13 hours sleep every 24 hours; 0–2.5 hours during daytime nap(s)
Five to twelve years	9–12 hours every 24 hours; usually no naps
Teenage years	8–9 hours every 24 hours; usually no naps
Second to seventh decade	Marked decline in amplitude of SWS Gradual decline in amount of SWS Other stages remain relatively fixed
Older adults (>65 years of age)	Decreased nocturnal sleep Increased napping Increased difficulty falling asleep Increased difficulty staying asleep Lighter sleep Increased awakening Changes in timing/depth/melatonin secretion

SWS, slow-wave sleep.

Normal Sleep

Figure 4-7 shows the proportion of the night spent in the various sleep stages in adults.

The sleep histogram demonstrates the progression of stages during the night. Sleep histograms summarize sleep laboratory recordings. The typical histogram shows how a night of sleep for a patient is organized. The y-axis corresponds to the various stages of NREM (nonrapid eye movement) sleep alternating with REM (rapid eye movement) sleep, with most slow-wave sleep occurring in the first part of the night and most REM sleep occurring in the last part. The sleep architectural changes typically seen across the life span are depicted by the sleep histograms shown in Figure 4-8.

In normal individuals, sleep is entered via NREM sleep, with the first NREM episode occurring at about 90 minutes; thereafter NREM and REM alternate about every 90 minutes. Figure 4-9 shows that the slow waves in stage N3 in a child often have a very high amplitude; the other stages more closely resemble those of an adult. Figure 4-10 shows REM in the same patient.

Sleep in older people is affected by underlying medical conditions, changes related to vision, and environmental changes, as shown in Figure 4-11.

Figure 4-12 shows the changes in sleep that are frequently seen in older people.

As a result there are many changes in sleep structure that occur with aging. See Table 4-3.

Figure 4-13 shows the changes in the quantity of the sleep stages throughout the life span.

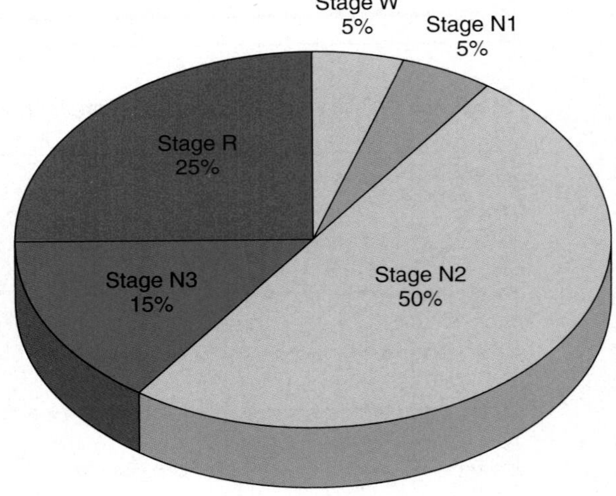

Figure 4-7.
Proportion of the night spent in the various sleep stages in adults. Wakefulness in sleep usually makes up less than 5% of the night. Stage N1 sleep generally makes up 2% to 5% of sleep, stage N2 45% to 55%, and stage N3 3% to 15%. NREM sleep, therefore, is usually 75% to 80% of sleep. Stage R sleep is usually 20% to 25% of sleep, occurring in three to six discrete episodes.

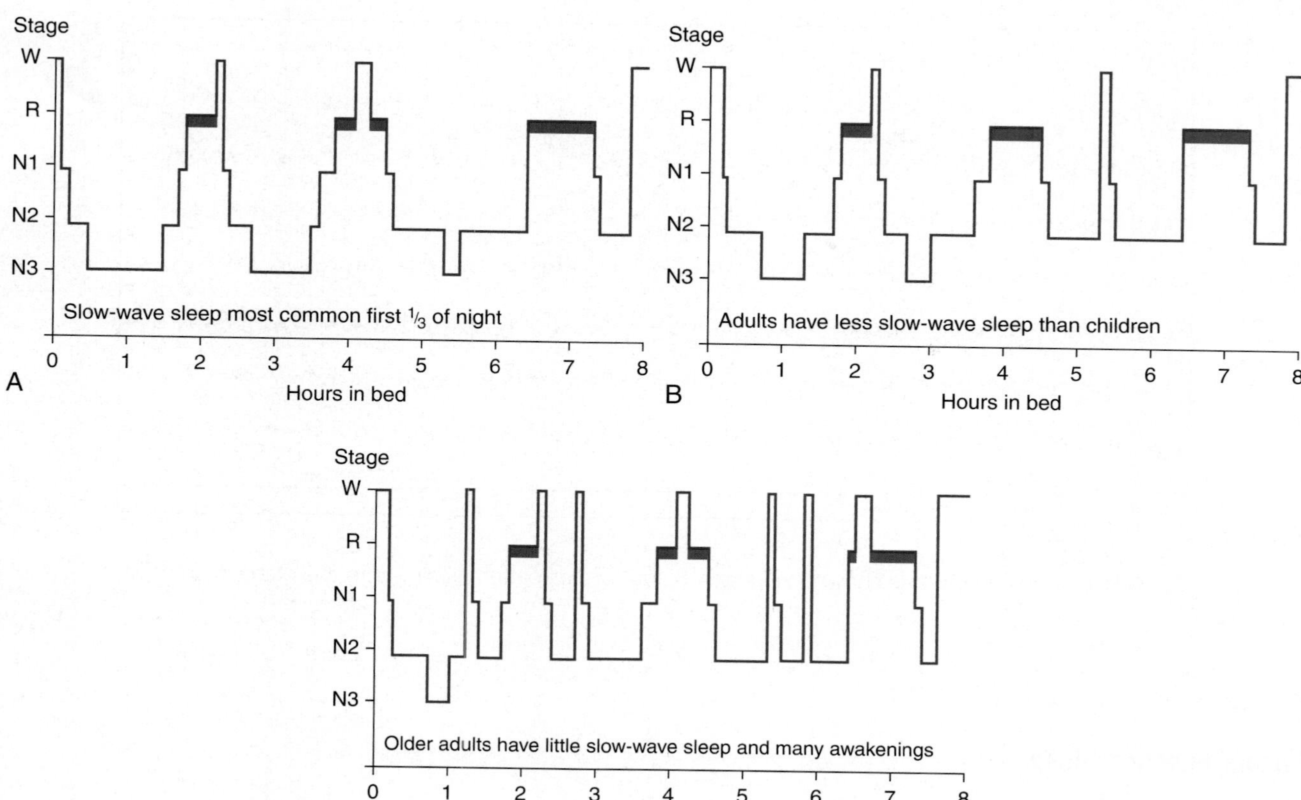

Figure 4-8.
These illustrative histograms of a child (A), a young to middle-aged adult (B), and an older adult (C) show the changes in sleep with aging. Slow-wave sleep is maximal in children and decreases with aging. It is minimal or absent in the elderly (C). The same holds true for REM sleep, which diminishes to a lesser extent and becomes more fragmented with aging. Older adults also have prolonged sleep latency when compared with younger subjects, more frequent arousals, and reduced sleep efficiency [(total sleep time ÷ total recording time) × 100].

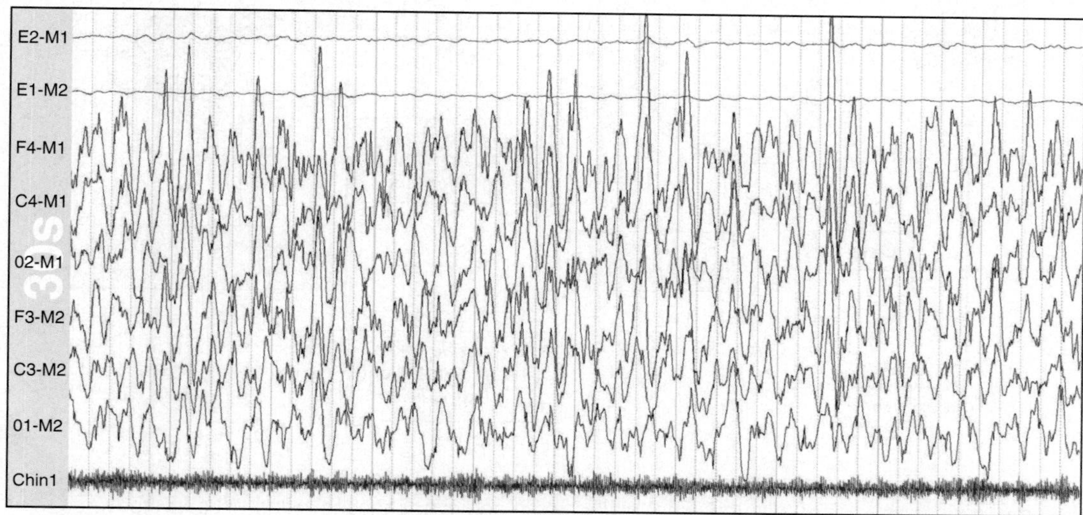

Figure 4-9.
Stage N3 in a child. This epoch is obtained from the record of a 10-year-old boy. Notice the very high amplitude of the slow waves.

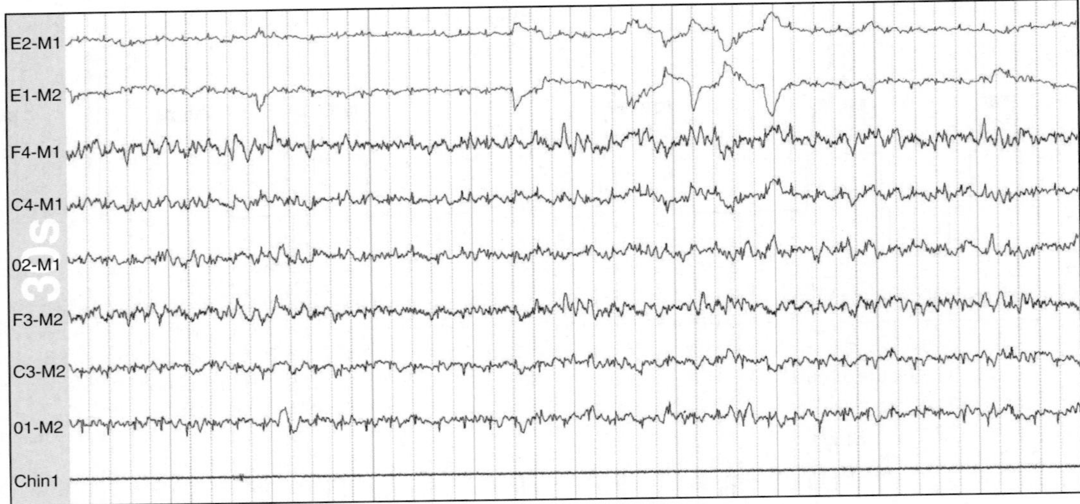

Figure 4-10.
Stage R in the same child as shown in Figure 4-9. The overall pattern is similar to this stage in an adult.

Factors Affecting Sleep

There are many diseases, medications, lifestyle choices, and habits that can adversely impact sleep (Table 4-4).

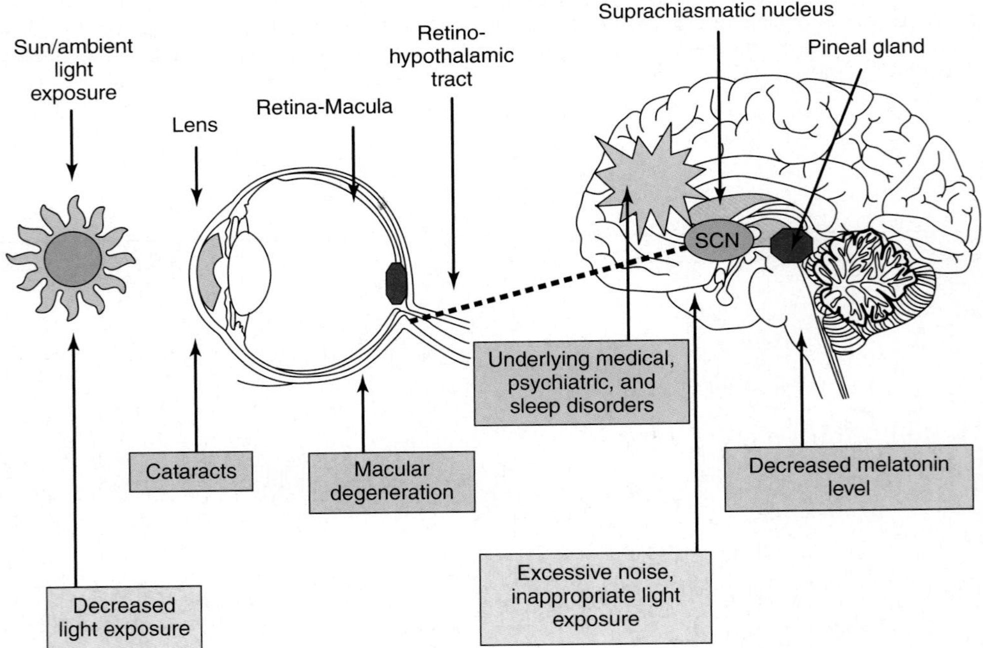

Figure 4-11.
Sleep in older people is affected by underlying medical, psychiatric, and sleep disorders that can cause arousal and disrupt sleep *(pink box).* In addition, changes in the visual system *(blue boxes)* and changes in light exposure and other environmental factors can result in circadian rhythm changes *(tan boxes).* (From Avidan AY: Clinical neurology of insomnia in neurodegenerative and other disorders of neurological function. Rev Neurol Dis 4:21–34, 2007.)

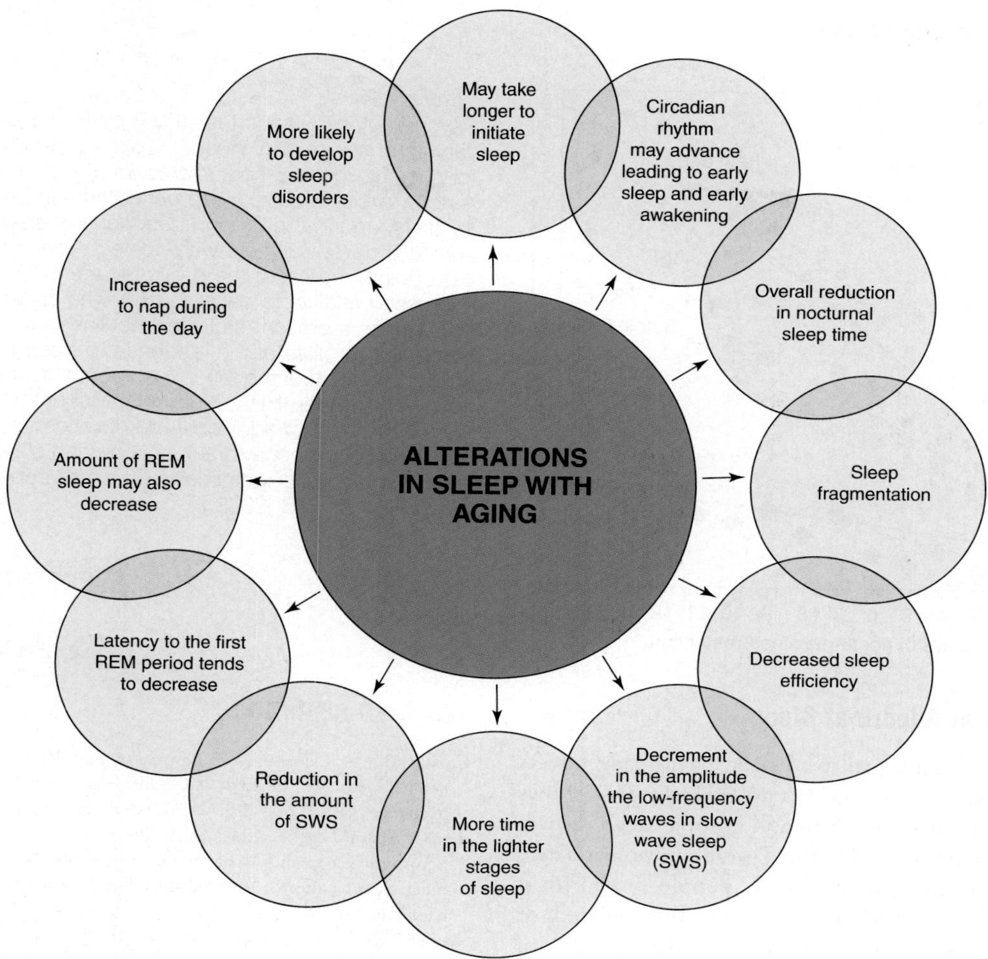

Figure 4-12.
There are many changes in sleep that occur with aging. REM, rapid eye movement; SWS, slow-wave sleep.

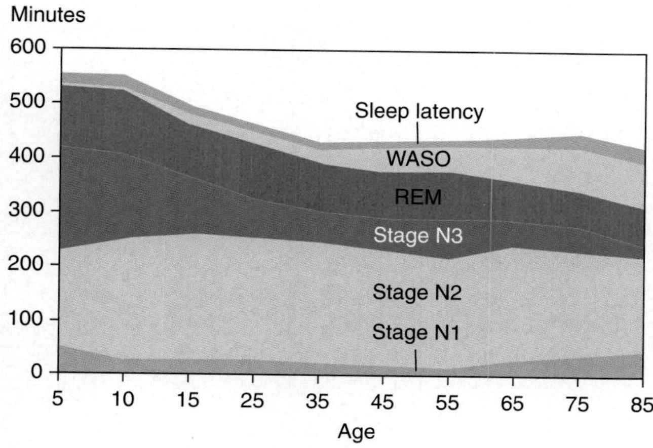

Figure 4-13.
Changes in sleep stages with age. WASO, wake after sleep onset. (Modified from Ohayon M, Carskadon MA, Guilleminault C, et al: Meta-analysis of quantitative sleep parameters from childhood to old age in healthy individuals: Developing normative sleep values across the human lifespan. Sleep 27:1255–1273, 2004.)

Table 4-3. Sleep Through the Life Span

INCREASE	DECREASE
Sleep latency	REM sleep (%)
Arousals, awakenings, stage shifts	Sleep efficiency
Stages 1, 2	Slow-wave sleep % (worse in men)
Napping	Slow-wave sleep amplitude
Resistance to sleepiness, sleep deprivation	
Phase advancement	

Table 4-4. Factors Affecting Sleep

	EXAMPLES	SEE CHAPTER
Medical diseases	Heart failure, COPD	Chapters 5,11,13
Psychiatric diseases	Depression, schizophrenia	Chapter 16
Sleep disorders	Sleep apnea, narcolepsy	Chapters 10,11
Medications	Antidepressants	Chapters 5,16
Habits	Alcohol, caffeine	Chapter 5
Lifestyle	Voluntary sleep restriction, shift work	Chapter 7

COPD, chronic obstructive pulmonary disease.

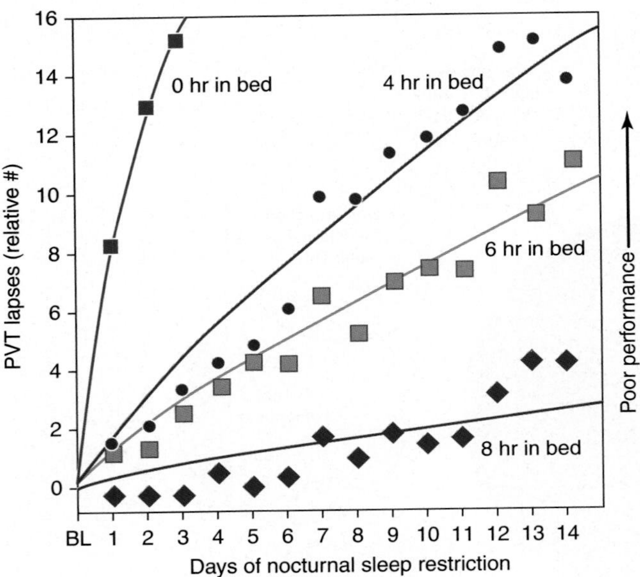

Figure 4-14.
Psychomotor vigilance task (PVT) performance lapses under varying doses of daily sleep. Displayed are group averages for subjects in the 8-hour *(diamond)*, 6-hour *(light square)*, and 4-hour *(circle)* chronic sleep period time in bed (TIB) across 14 days, and in the 0-hour *(dark square)* sleep condition across 3 days. Subjects were tested every 2 hours each day; data points represent the daily average (07:30 to 23:30) expressed relative to baseline (BL). The curves through the data points represent statistical nonlinear, model-based, best-fitting profiles of the response to sleep deprivation for subjects in each of the four experimental conditions. (Adapted from Van Dongen HPA, Maislin G, Mullington JM, et al: The cumulative cost of additional wakefulness: Dose-response effects on neurobehavioral functions and sleep physiology from chronic sleep restriction and total sleep deprivation. Sleep 26:117–126, 2003.)

Consequences of Abnormal Sleep

Abnormal quantity and quality of sleep have many effects on the nervous system. As one example, Figure 4-14 shows the effect of 3 nights of no sleep and chronic sleep restriction on results obtained with the Psychomotor Vigilance Task. Notice that after about a week, people in bed for 4 and 6 hours a night had many lapses—they missed or ignored visual cues to perform the task. The impact of the consequences of abnormal sleep on a person and society is covered in chapter 7.

SELECTED READINGS

Carskadon MA, Dement, WC: Normal human sleep: An overview. In Kryger MH, Roth T, Dement WC (eds): Principles and Practice of Sleep Medicine. New York, Elsevier Saunders, 2005, pp 13–23.

Iber C, Ancoli-Israel S, Chesson A, Quan SF: The AASM Manual for the Scoring of Sleep and Associated Events: Rules, Terminology, and Technical Specifications. Westchester, Ill., American Academy of Sleep Medicine, 2007.

Shepard JW, Atlas of Sleep Medicine. Armonk, N.Y., Futura, 1991.

Walczak T, Chokroverty S: Electroencephalography, electromyography and electrooculography: General principles and basic technology. In Chokroverty S (ed): Sleep Disorders Medicine, 2nd ed. Boston, Butterworth-Heinemann, 1999.

CHAPTER 5

PHARMACOLOGY

Wallace Mendelson

Pharmacologic agents are often taken by patients to help them fall asleep, or to be more alert during the daytime. Such compounds are among the most widely used medications.

Drugs with Hypnotic Properties

Drugs listed here are those that have a specific indication for sleep granted by the U.S. Food and Drug Administration. Later sections will deal with antihistamines, which are sold over-the-counter to aid sleep, and prescription compounds that are not specifically indicated for sleep but which in practice are often used "off label" for this purpose. Older agents including chloral hydrate, barbiturates, and ethchlorvynol are not presented here because of their very limited current use, but the interested reader is referred to *The Use and Misuse of Sleeping Pills* by W. B. Mendelson.

The modern era of hypnotic pharmacology began in the 1960s with the introduction into the United States of the benzodiazepines, or "Valium-like" compounds, which dominated the market until the development of the newer nonbenzodiazepine agents in the 1990s (Table 5-1).

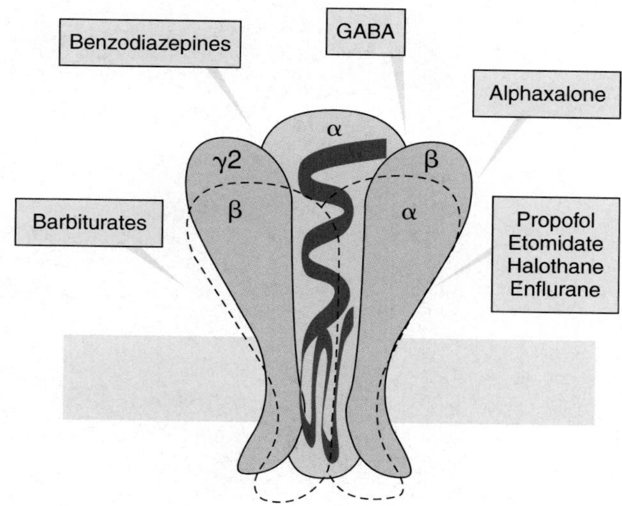

Figure 5-1.
Schematic representation of the GABA-A receptor complex: The sites at which a variety of sedative/hypnotics and anesthetics act are indicated. (Adapted from Rudolph U, Mohler H: Analysis of GABAA receptor function and dissection of the pharmacology of benzodiazepines and general anesthetics through mouse genetics. Annu Rev Pharmacol Toxicol 44:475–498, 2004.)

Table 5-1. Drugs Often Used for Sleep

	USUAL DOSE	RAPID ONSET	HALF-LIFE (H)	DAYTIME (HANG-OVER) EFFECTS	WORKS SELECTIVELY TO ENHANCE GABA	SAFETY
Zopiclone	7.5 mg	+	3.5–6	?Yes	√	√
Zolpidem	10 mg	++	1.5–3	No	√	√
Zaleplon	10 mg	++	1–2	No	√	√
Temazepam	20 mg		5–12	?Yes	√	√
Loprazolam	1 mg		5–13	?Yes	√	√
Lormetazepam	1 mg	+	8–10	?Yes	√	√
Nitrazepam	5–10 mg	+	20–48	Yes	√	√
Lorazepam	0.5–1 mg	+	10–20	Yes	√	√
Diazepam	5–10 mg	+	20–60	Yes	√	√
	15–30 mg		5–20	Yes	√	√
Alprazolam	0.5 mg	+	9–20	Yes	√	√
Clonazepam	0.5–1 mg	+	18–50	Yes	√	√
Chloral hydrate/ betaine	0.7–1 g	+	8–12	?Yes	X	X
Chlormethiazole	192 mg	+	4–8	?Yes	X	X
Barbiturates		+		Yes	X	X
Promethazine	25 mg		7–14	?Yes	X	X/√

All except promethazine, which is an antihistamine and does not have a U.S. indication as a sleep aid, act by modulating the function of the GABA-A receptor complex. Zopiclone (as well as eszopiclone, its S-isomer), zolpidem, and zaleplon are sometimes referred to as the "Z drugs," newer nonbenzodiazepines that act at the GABA-A receptor.

Data from Wilson S, Nutt DJ: Sleep Disorders. New York, Oxford University Press, 2008.

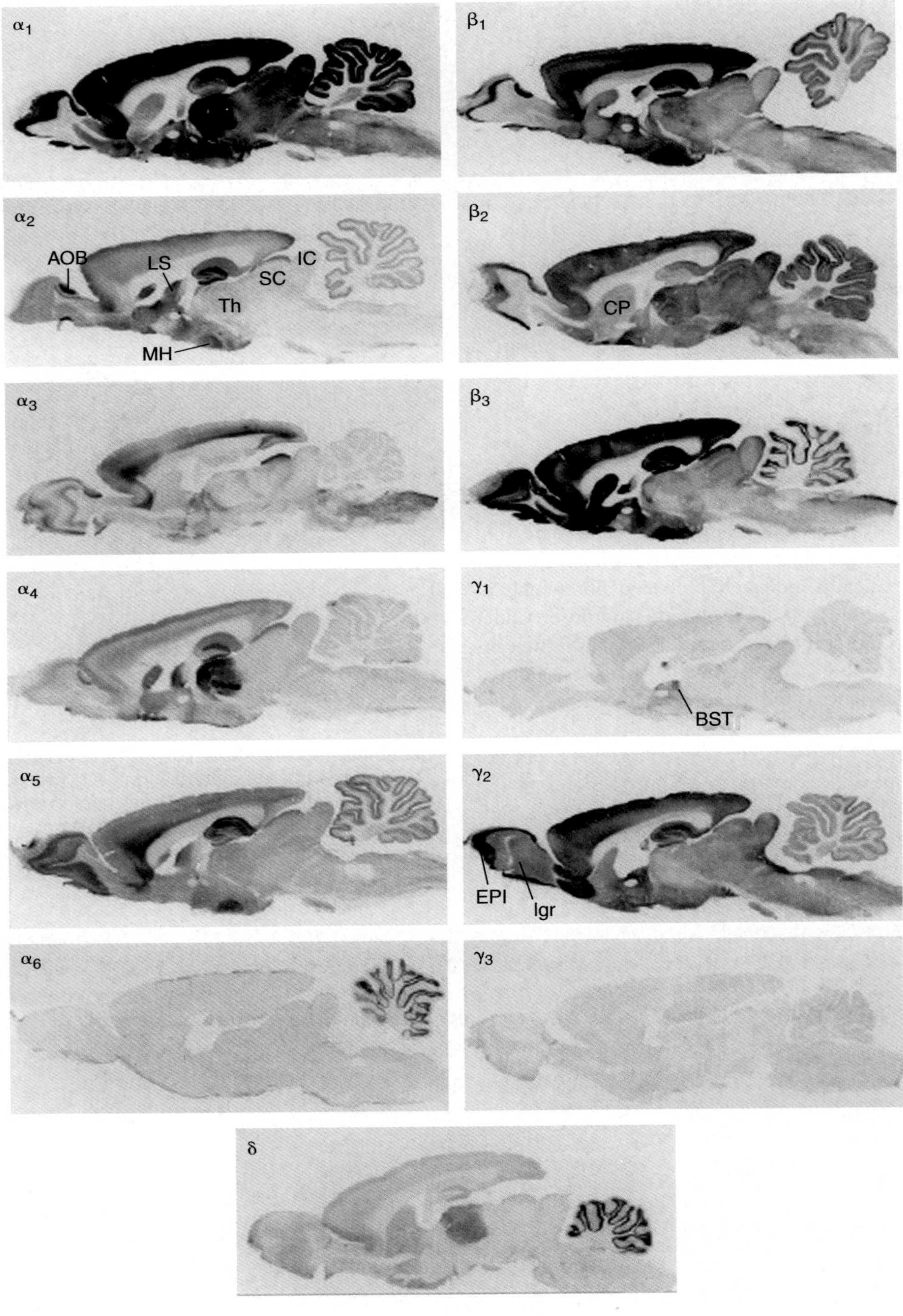

Figure 5-2.
Immunocytochemical distribution of GABA-A receptor subunits α1–α6, β1–β3, γ1–γ3, and δ in sagittal sections. The α-1 subunit, which is thought to be associated with sleep induction as well as memory effects, is found throughout the brain, although in varying concentrations in different regions. α types 2–6 are localized in more specific brain regions. Some hypnotics, notably eszopiclone, also have significant activity at the α-3 subunit. Scale bar = 2 mm. AOB, accessory olfactory bulb; BST, bed nucleus of stria terminalis; CP, caudoputamen; IC, inferior colliculus; LS, lateral septal nucleus; MH, medial hypothalamic nuclei; SC, superior colliculus; Th, thalamus. (Adapted from Pirker S, Schwarzer C, Wieselthaler A, et al: GABA-A receptors: Immunocytochemical distribution of 13 subunits in the adult rat brain. Neuroscience 101:815–850, 2000.)

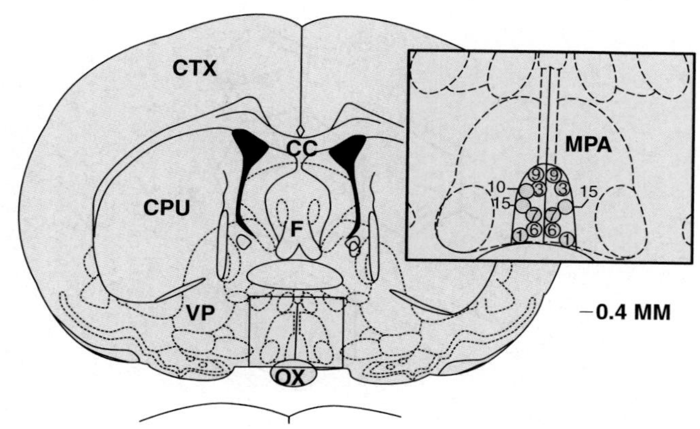

Figure 5-3.
Typical injection sites of triazolam into the medial preoptic area in rats. This produced shortened sleep latency and increased total sleep, while injections into surrounding areas had no effect. CC, corpus callosum; CPU, caudate putamen; CTX, cortex; F, fornix; MPA, medial preoptic area, OX, optic chiasm, VP, ventral pallidum. (Adapted from Mendelson WB, Monti D: Effects of triazolam and nifedipine injections into the medial preoptic area on sleep. Neuropsychopharmacology 8:227–232, 1993.)

All of the currently U.S.-approved agents, with the exception of ramelteon, which is presented later, act by modulating the function of the GABA-A receptor complex. This complex comprises five glycoprotein subunits, each of which comes in multiple isoforms (Fig. 5-1).

Hypnotic activity resulting from GABA agonist compounds appears to be related to action at the alpha-1 and possibly alpha-3 isoforms. Distribution of the alpha isoforms is seen in Figure 5-2.

The neuroanatomical site of action of hypnotics has not been fully elucidated. Among the important sites for agents that act at the GABA-A receptor are the medial preoptic area (MPA) and ventrolateral preoptic area of the hypothalamus. Microinjections of a variety of agents, including triazolam, pentobarbital, ethanol, adenosine, and propofol, into the MPA induce sleep in animal studies (Fig. 5-3).

Ramelteon, in contrast to most available hypnotics, is thought to act at melatonin types I and II receptors located in the suprachiasmatic nucleus of the hypothalamus.

Figure 5-4 illustrates triazolam, as representative of the benzodiazepines; Table 5-2 details triazolam's effects on sleep.

Table 5-2. Effects of Triazolam on Polygraphic Measures of Sleep in a 4-Week Trial

		TRIAZOLAM 0.25 MG				
	PLACEBO	WEEK 1	WEEK 2	WEEK 3	WEEK 4	P VALUE
Total sleep time (min)	314.8 ± 17.0	364.5 ± 12.0[a]	351.5 ± 11.8[a]	348.0 ± 14.3[a]	366.8 ± 11.5[a]	<0.01
Sleep latency (min)	53.6 ± 12.5	24.9 ± 9.2[a]	19.0 ± 4.0[a]	32.3 ± 6.4[a]	26.9 ± 9.1[a]	<0.05
REM latency (min)	129.2 ± 20.5	152.6 ± 23.4	118.4 ± 15.8	125.7 ± 20.3	140.5 ± 18.8	NS
Sleep efficiency (%)	76.0 ± 4.2	89.7 ± 2.0[a]	85.4 ± 2.2[a]	82.4 ± 3.2	89.1 ± 2.3[a]	<0.01
Stage 1 (min)	7.0 ± 1.5	3.4 ± 0.6	5.7 ± 1.3	5.1 ± 1.2	4.2 ± 0.8[a]	<0.05
Stage 2 (min)	70.0 ± 2.6	78.8 ± 3.6	76.7 ± 1.8	78.3 ± 2.6	74.4 ± 3.0	NS
Stage 3 (min)	8.5 ± 2.7	6.5 ± 2.4	4.2 ± 1.4	4.6 ± 2.0	5.0 ± 1.5	NS
REM sleep (min)	17.5 ± 3.5	17.4 ± 3.7	21.0 ± 6.6	14.4 ± 2.8	22.6 ± 4.8	NS
Wake time after initial sleep onset (min)	45.9 ± 12.9	16.0 ± 4.2[a]	37.9 ± 9.2	34.8 ± 8.4	16.5 ± 4.5[a]	<0.05
No. of awakenings (total)	58.9 ± 10.6	43.9 ± 8.2	49.5 ± 7.1	57.1 ± 10.9	59.6 ± 11.2	NS
No. of awakenings > 3 min	8.4 ± 2.0	4.9 ± 0.9	4.8 ± 0.7	6.6 ± 1.6	5.9 ± 1.5	NS

It can be seen that triazolam decreases polygraphic sleep latency and increases total sleep at all time points. Subjective reports indicated an increase in reported total sleep throughout the study, but a shortened sleep latency only for the first 2 weeks. One implication of this might be that patient complaints of tolerance to a hypnotic's effects may be dependent on what the predominant symptom is for the patient—total amount of sleep, or time it takes to fall asleep.

[a]Differs from placebo condition by at least $p < 0.05$ (Least Significant Difference Test).
NS, not significant.
Data from Mendelson WB: Subjective vs. objective tolerance during long-term administration of triazolam. Clin Drug Invest 10:276–279, 1995.

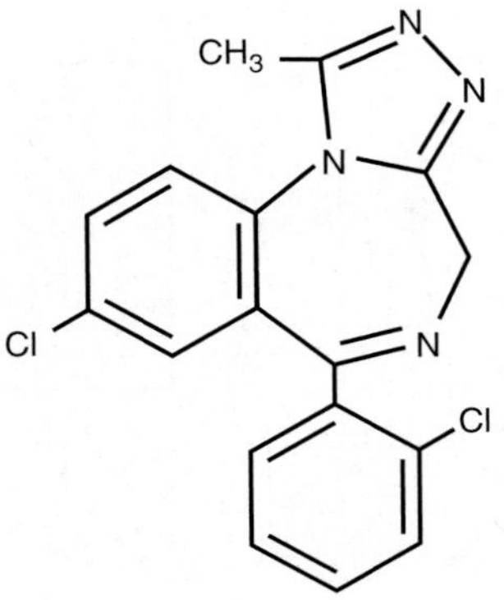

Figure 5-4.
Structure of triazolam.

ZOLPIDEM AND ZOLPIDEM EXTENDED-RELEASE FORMULATION

The newer nonbenzodiazepine GABA-A agonists, beginning with zolpidem in the early 1990s, are more selective in their binding to alpha isoform subtypes than are the benzodiazepines, as seen in Figures 5-5 and 5-6.

Zolpidem comes in its original form, now generic in the United States, as well as in a modified-release two-layer tablet that contains both the original compound and a slower-release preparation (Ambien CR) (Figs. 5-7, 5-8).

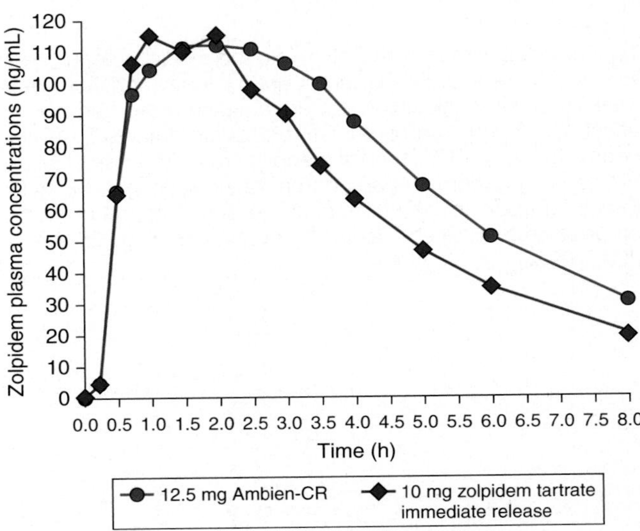

Figure 5-7.
Plasma concentrations following administration of zolpidem two-layer, modified-release 12.5 mg, and zolpidem 10 mg. Note the higher plasma concentrations of the modified-release preparation in the second half of the night. (Data from Amin J, Lee A, Gerlovin M, German D (eds): Monthly Prescribing Reference: Diagnosis and Treatment of Insomnia. Prescribing Reference, 2006. Available at www.empr.com.)

ZOPICLONE AND ESZOPICLONE (Figs. 5-9, 5-10, 5-11)

ZALEPLON (Figs. 5-12, 5-13)

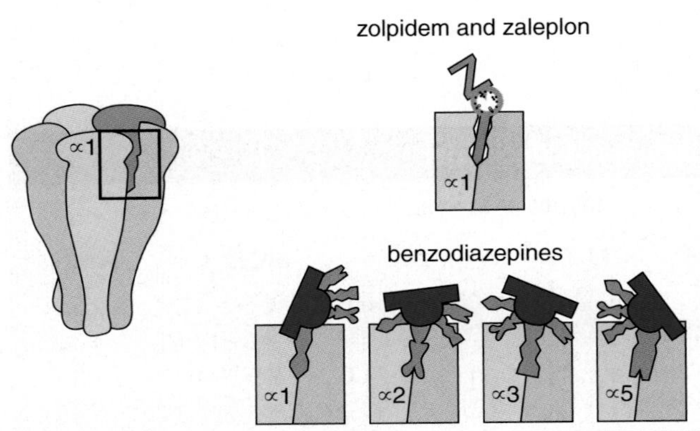

Figure 5-5.
Binding of benzodiazepines, zolpidem, and zaleplon to the alpha-subunit of the GABA receptor. The benzodiazepines such as triazolam and estazolam bind to all of the α-unit isoforms of the GABA-A receptor complex, which may explain why they have a wide range of pharmacologic effects in addition to sleep induction. The newer nonbenzodiazepine GABA receptor agonists such as zolpidem have relatively greater selectivity for the α-1 subunit, which may correspond to their higher ratio of sleep/nonsleep effects. (Adapted from Sleep: Excessive Sleepiness. San Diego, Calif., NEI Press, 2005, copyright Neuroscience Education Institute, with permission.)

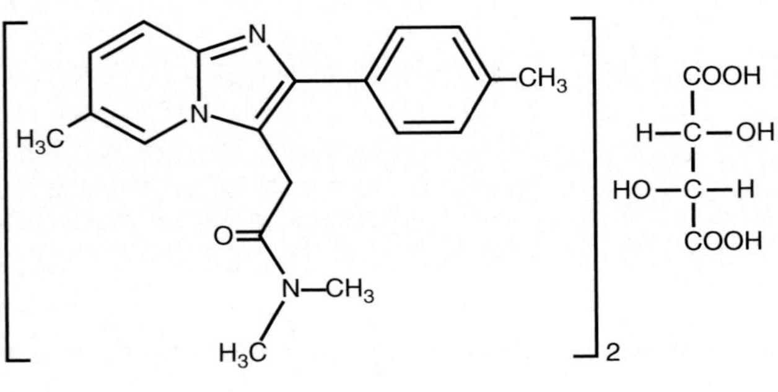

Figure 5-6.
Structure of zolpidem.

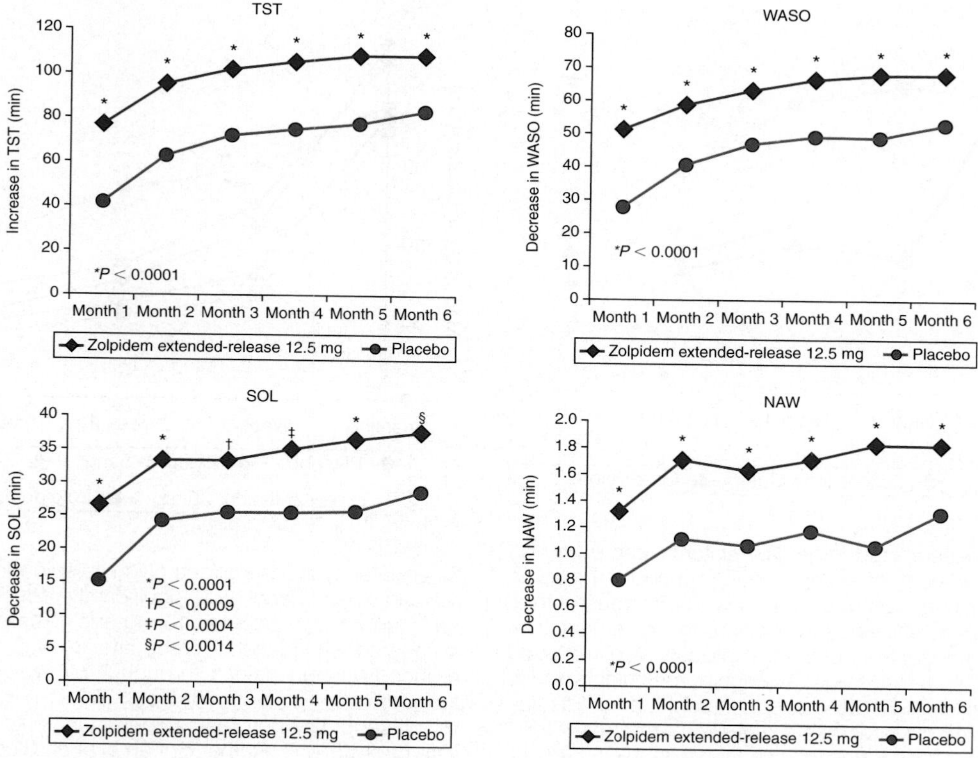

Figure 5-8.
Sample efficacy data for zolpidem modified-release 12.5 mg given 3–7 nights per week over 6 months. Data are taken from a patient morning questionnaire. Abbreviations: NAW, number of nocturnal awakenings; SOL, sleep onset latency; TST, total sleep time; WASO, wake after sleep onset. (Data from Krystal A, Erman M, Zammit GK, et al: Long-term efficacy and safety of zolpidem extended-release 12.5 mg, administered 3 to 7 nights per week for 24 weeks, in patients with chronic primary insomnia. Sleep, 31:79–90, 2008.)

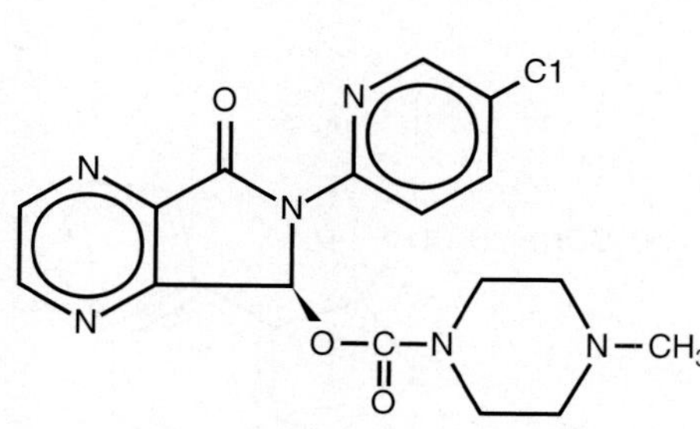

Figure 5-9.
Structure of eszopiclone, the S-isomer of racemic zopiclone. (From data on file, Sepracor Inc.)

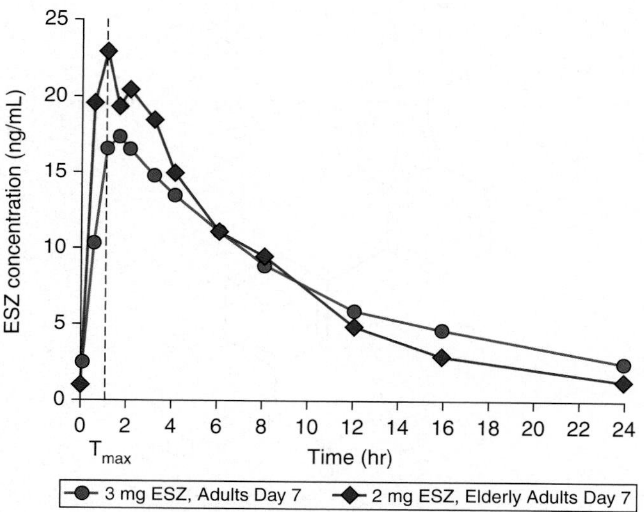

Figure 5-10.
Pharmacokinetics of eszopiclone (ESZ) 2 mg and 3 mg. (From data on file, Sepracor Inc.)

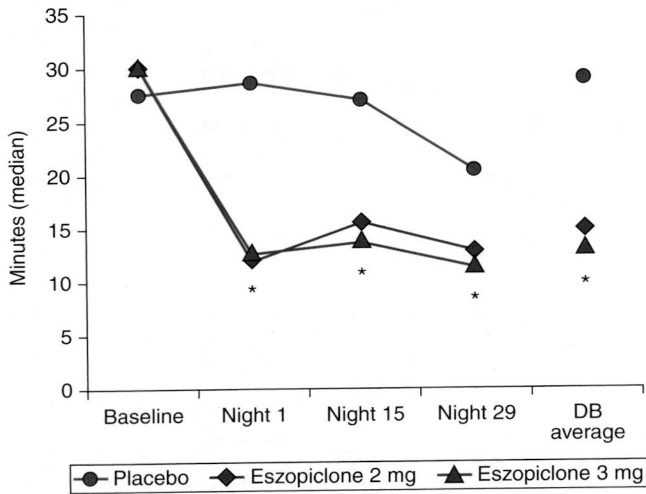

Figure 5-11.
Polygraphically measured latency to persistent sleep on nights 1, 15, and 29 in a study of eszopicione 2 mg and 3 mg given to insomniacs for one month. Both doses also increased total sleep time and sleep efficiency throughout the treatment period. The 3-mg dose, but not the 2-mg dose, also improved sleep maintenance. DB average, average across nights 1, 15, 29 (Data from Zammit GK, McNabb LJ, Caron J, et al: Efficacy and safety of eszopiclone across six-weeks of treatment for primary insomnia. Curr Med Res Opin 20:1979–1991, 2004.)

RAMELTEON

Ramelteon has a different mechanism of action than do all other hypnotics on the market in the United States at the time of this writing. It has little affinity for GABA-A receptors, but rather acts as an agonist at melatonin types I and II receptors. It has been hypothesized that the anatomical site of action is the suprachiasmatic nucleus (SCN), at which agonism at the type I receptors may decrease the waking signal from the SCN. Agonism at the type II receptors

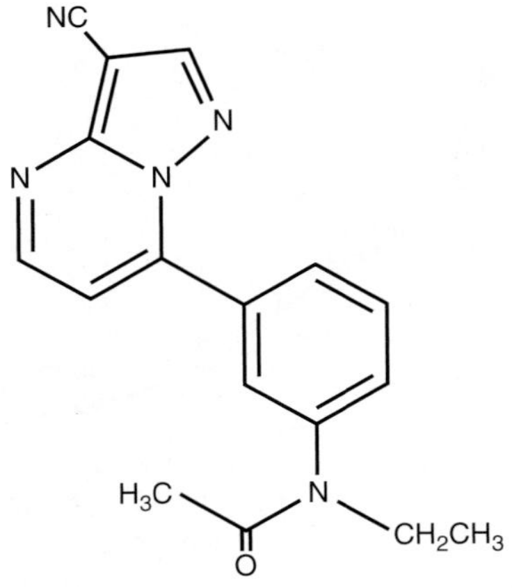

Zaleplon

Figure 5-12.
Structure of zaleplon.

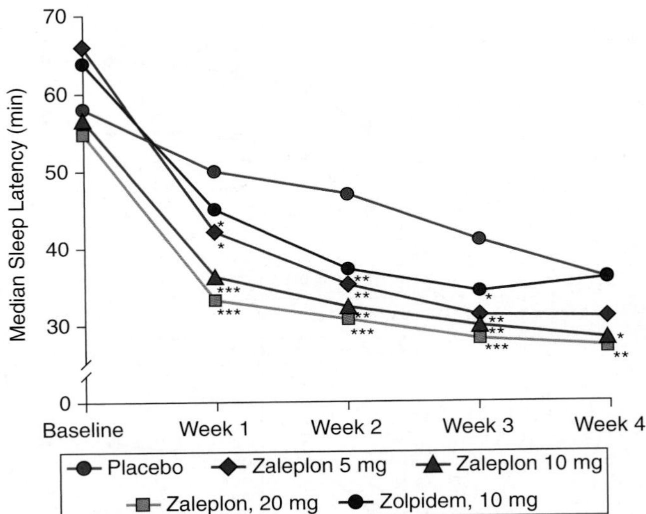

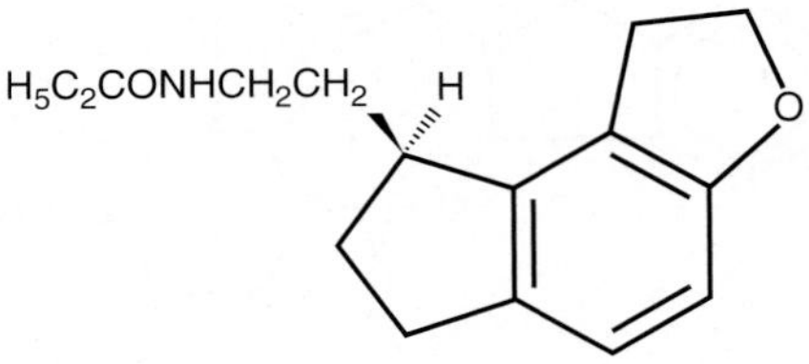

Figure 5-13.
Sleep latency in insomniacs given zaleplon for 28 nights. Median sleep latency was significantly reduced during weeks 1 through 4 with zaleplon 10 mg and zaleplon 20 mg, compared with placebo. Sleep latency was significantly reduced during weeks 1 through 3 with zaleplon 5 mg, and zolpidem 10 mg (*$p \leq .05$, **$p \leq .01$, ***$p \leq .001$). Zaleplon vs. placebo: Dunnett test; zolpidem vs. placebo: F test. (Data from Elie R, Ruther E, Farr I, et al: Sleep latency is shortened during 4 weeks of treatment with zaleplon, a novel nonbenzodiazepine hypnotic. J Clin Psychiat 60:536–544, 1999.)

has been hypothesized to alter the clocklike functions of the SCN (Figs. 5-14, 5-15).

DIPHENHYDRAMINE

This compound is the most common ingredient in over-the-counter sleep aids. Its limited benefits for sleep should be balanced against its potential anticholinergic side effects and rapid onset of tolerance (Tables 5-3, 5-4).

SEDATING ANTIDEPRESSANTS

In practice, these agents, particularly trazodone, are used off-label as sleep aids. Though clinically found to be sedating in the daytime, the limited studies available on trazodone when given at night to insomniacs suggest limited effectiveness and rapid development of tolerance (Figs. 5-16, 5-17; Box 5-1).

Figure 5-14.
Structure of ramelteon.

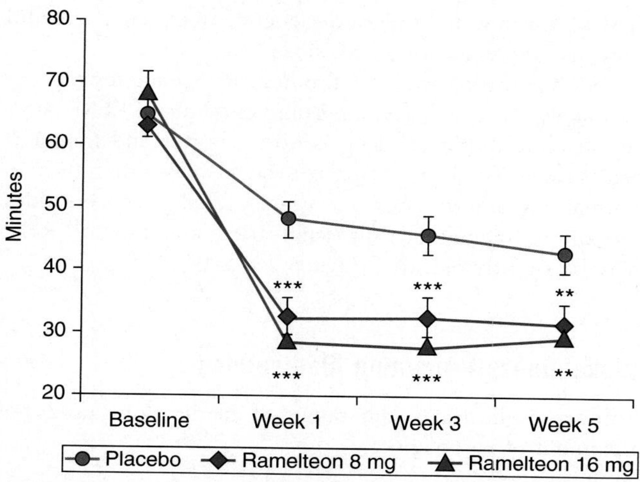

Figure 5-15.
Polygraphic latency to persistent sleep in insomniacs who received ramelteon 8 mg and 16 mg and placebo for 5 weeks. For comparisons of ramelteon dose and placebo: ***$p \leq .001$, **$p \leq .010$. (Data from Zammit G, Erman M, Wang-Weigand S, et al: Evaluation of the efficacy and safety of ramelteon in subjects with chronic insomnia. J Clin Sleep Med 3:495–504, 2007.)

Table 5-3. Commonly Used Over-the-Counter Agents

DRUG (TRADE NAME)	USUAL HYPNOTIC DOSE	TERMINAL ELIMINATION HALF-LIFE (H)
Diphenhydramine (Nytol, Sleep-Eze, Sominex)	25–50 mg/day	2.4–9.3 h
Doxylamine (Unisom Nighttime)	25 mg/day	10 h
Diphenhydramine in Combination (Anacin PM, Excedrin PM, Tylenol PM)	25–50 mg/day	2.4–9.3 h
Melatonin	1–2 mg/day	0.5-1 h

Data from Kupfer DJ, Reynolds CF: Management of insomnia. New Engl J Med 336:341–346, 1997.

Table 5-4. Studies of Diphenhydramine on Nocturnal Sleep

REFERENCE	SUBJECTS	DESIGN	RESULTS
Borbely, *Int J Clin Pharmacol Ther Toxicol*, 1988	10 normal volunteers	Single-dose 50–75 mg, PBO-controlled; self-report, actigraphy	No differences from PBO in subjective measures of sleep
Sunshine, *J Clin Pharmacol*, 1978	1295 post-partum	12.5, 25, 50 mg, PBO-controlled; self-report	No change in sleep latency, sleep duration, morning alertness vs. PBO
Teutsch, *Clin Pharm Ther*, 1975	VA patients	PBO-controlled, 50, 150 mg; self-report	50 mg difference from PBO on subjective responses

PBO, placebo; VA, Veterans Administration.

$C_{19}H_{22}ClN_5O - HCl$

Figure 5-16.
Structure of trazodone.

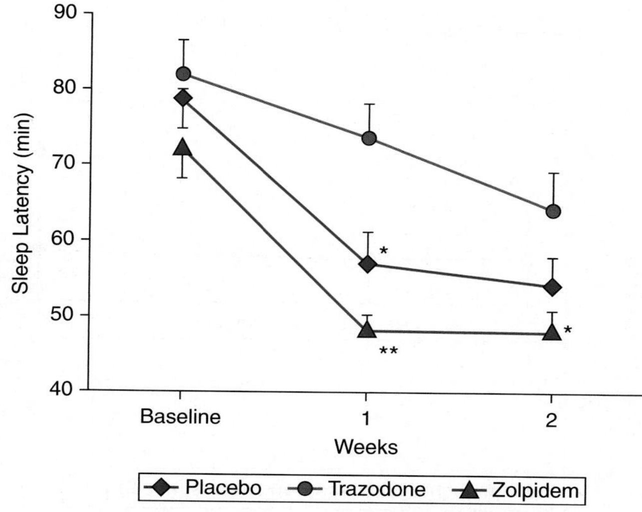

Figure 5-17.
Effects on self-reported sleep onset time in insomniacs given 2 weeks of trazodone 50 mg, zolpidem 10 mg, and placebo. Note that at week 1 the reduction in sleep latency by trazodone was significantly less effective than that of zolpidem, and that at week 2 the effect of trazodone on sleep latency was no longer significantly different from placebo. (Data from Walsh JK, Erman M, Erwin CW, et al: Subjective hypnotic efficacy of trazodone and zolpidem in DSMIII-R primary insomnia. Human Psychopharmacol 13:191–198, 1998.)

BOX 5-1. CHARACTERISTICS OF TRAZODONE

- Heterocyclic antidepressant that inhibits serotonin uptake
- Chemically and pharmacologically distinct from SSRIs
- Functions as a blocker of 5-HT and alpha-1 adrenergic receptors, which may account for side effects of falls and priapism
- The active metabolite meta-chlorophenylpiperazine
- (*m*-CCP) may be responsible for some side effects

5-HT, serotonin; m-CCP, m-chlorophenypiperazine; SSRIs, selective serotonin reuptake inhibitors.
Data from James SP, Mendelson WB: The use of trazodone as a hypnotic: A critical review. J Clin Psychiat 65:752–755, 2004.

ETHANOL

Ethanol is the most widely used psychotropic agent; the average American consumes the equivalent of 38 six-packs of beer, 12 bottles of wine, and two quarts of distilled spirits annually. In some population studies it has been shown to be the most common substance used to promote sleep. This is of some concern because of exposure to the risk of ethanol dependence; moreover, acute oral ingestion of ethanol is unsatisfactory as a hypnotic. Although sleep latency may be shortened, the rapid metabolism leads to disturbance in the second half of the night characterized by increased arousals. In normal volunteers, rapid eye movement (REM) sleep is suppressed, at least in the first half of the night. In alcohol-dependent patients, ethanol may also increase slow-wave sleep.

Alcohol withdrawal syndromes are characterized by extremely disrupted sleep and high amounts of REM. After the acute withdrawal, sleep is often shorter and fragmented; slow-wave sleep is often low and may not return to normal amounts for up to 2 years. (REM) sleep episodes are often fragmented, although total amounts of REM may be slightly elevated (Figs. 5-18, 5-19).

H–C(H)(H)–C(H)(H)–OH

Figure 5-18.
Structure of ethanol.

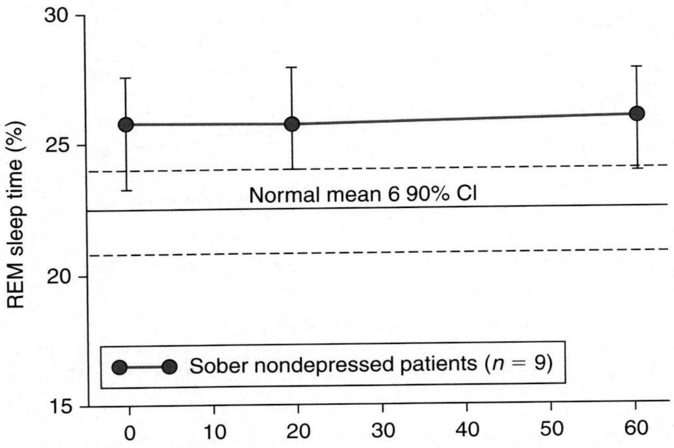

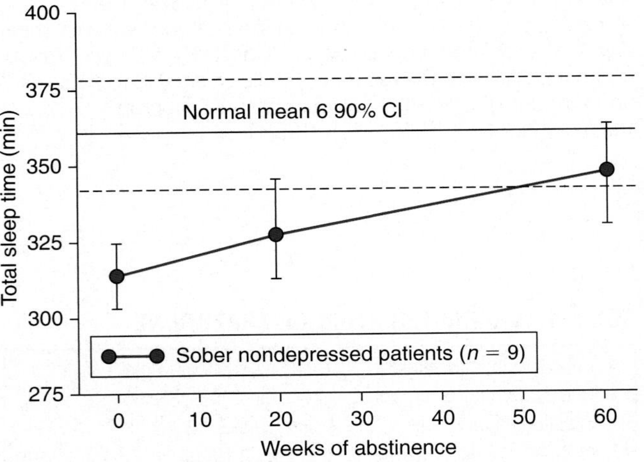

Figure 5-19.
REM sleep and total sleep in recovering alcoholic males. Note that both measures differ from age-matched healthy control subjects for most of the recovery period. Values for the patients are mean ± standard error of the mean, and for healthy control subjects, mean 90% confidence interval (CI). (Data from Drummond SPA, Gillin JC, Smith TL, DeModena A: The sleep of abstinent pure primary alcoholic patients: Natural course and relationship to relapse. Alcohol Clin Exp Res 22:1796–1802, 1998.)

Wakefulness-Promoting Medications

Table 5-5 illustrates the range of medications used for treatment of narcolepsy.

Table 5-5. Medications Used in Treatment of Narcolepsy

Excessive daytime sleepiness/Irresistible episodes of sleep*	
• *First-line treatments*	
• Armodafinil	150 or 250 mg in one A.M. dose
• Modafinil	100–400 mg/day in two doses
• Sodium oxybate	6–9 g/night in two doses
• *Second-line treatments*	
• Methylphenidate	10–60 mg/day
• *Third-line treatments*	
• Amphetamines	15–60 mg/day
• Pemoline	18.75–112.50 mg/day
• Phenelzine	60–90 mg/day
• Selegiline	10–40 mg/day
Cataplexy	
• *First-line treatments*	
• Sodium oxybate	4.5–9 g/night in two doses
• *Second-line treatments*	
• Clomipramine	10–75 mg/day
• Fluoxetine	20–60 mg/day
• Fluvoxamine	25–200 mg/day
• Venlafaxine	150–375 mg/day
• *Third-line treatments*	
• Phenelzine	60–90 mg/day
• Selegiline	10–40 mg/day
• Amphetamines	15–60 mg/day
Poor sleep	
• *First-line treatments*	
• Sodium oxybate	3–9 g/night
• *Second-line treatments*	
• Modafinil	100–400 mg/day in two doses
• *Third-line treatments*	
• Triazolam	0.25 mg/night
Note that hypnotics are sometimes used as a minor part of treatment, for purposes of consolidating nocturnal sleep.	

*Behavioral treatments are always advisable.
Data from Mamelak M: Improving outcomes in narcolepsy. Psychiatric Times Reporter (Suppl), Dec. 2007.

Table 5-6. Clinical Characteristics of Stimulants

MEDICATION BRANDS	AVAILABLE STRENGTHS (mg)	DOSE RANGE (mg)	WEEKLY DOSE INCREMENTS (OR AS TOLERATED)	APPROXIMATE DURATION IN HOURS	SCHEDULE	POSSIBLE AND SELECTED COMMON SIDE EFFECTS
Focalin	2.5, 5, 10	5–40	5	5	tid	Insomnia, rebound, irritability, anxiety, decreased appetite, late night binging, headache, dysphoria, anger, excitability, dry mouth, absence of normal fatigue, and mild elevation of blood pressure and heart rate
Focalin XR	5, 10, 15, 20	5–40	5	12	qd or bid	
Adderall	5, 7.5, 10, 12.5, 15, 20, 30	5–40	6	6	tid	
Adderall XR	5, 10, 15, 20, 25, 30	5–40	12	12	qd	
Atomoxetine	10, 18, 25, 40, 60	Titrate up to 1.2–1.4 mg/kg	0.3 mg/kg until at full dose or 100 mg, whichever is less	Once patient has stabilized and responded, medication wear-off is not obvious	qd or bid, can be given in the evening	Somnolence or insomnia, irritability, dysphoria, sexual dysfunction, urinary retention, constipation, stomachache, nausea, decreased appetite, and elevation of blood pressure or heart rate

These are clinical suggested uses. Some of the higher doses would be off-label and should be considered only with appropriate caution. Duration of action is approximate and may vary with the demands on the patient later in the day.
bid, twice a day; qd, every day; tid, three times a day.
From Weiss M, Hunter J, Gibbins C: Management of ADHD in adults. In "Perspectives in Psychiatry: A clinical update," Psychiatric Times (Suppl.), Dec. 2007.

AMPHETAMINES AND RELATED COMPOUNDS

Table 5-6, taken from a paper on attention-deficit/hyperactivity disorder (ADHD), describes the characteristics of the traditional stimulants methylphenidate and amphetamines (Fig. 5-20).

The site of action of these compounds is not entirely clear. There are at least two major pathways that promote wakefulness. One ascends from brainstem structures such as the dorsal raphe and locus coeruleus, receiving afferents from the basal forebrain and tuberomammillary bodies of the hypothalamus, and then continues on to the cortex. The second ascends from the brainstem to the thalamus, where it particularly affects neurons related to relaying sensory data. It seems likely that the function of one or both of these pathways is affected by wakefulness-promoting drugs.

MODAFINIL

Modafinil and its R-enantiomer, armodafinil, are used to promote wakefulness in treated obstructive sleep apnea patients with residual sleepiness, shift work disorders, and narcolepsy. In the latter, it has little effect on cataplexy. Its mechanism of action is shown in Figures 5-21 and 5-22 and in Table 5-7.

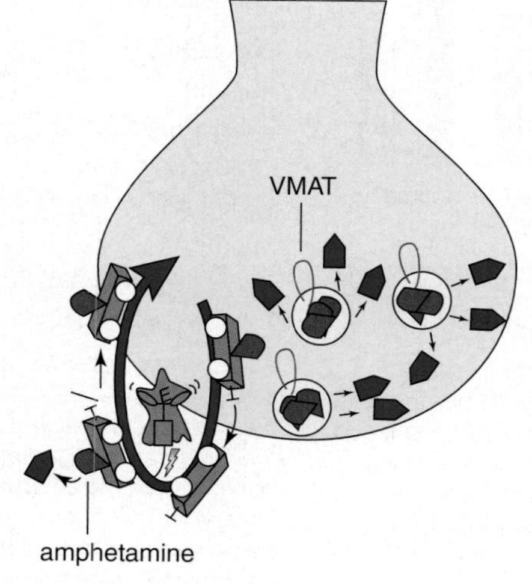

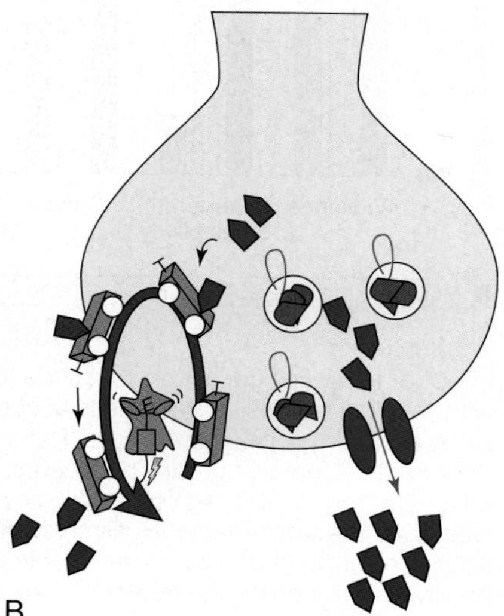

Figure 5-20. Mechanism of action of stimulants. **A**, In addition to binding to the dopamine transporter (DAT), amphetamine enters neurons and binds to the vesicular transporter (VMAT), ultimately producing displacement of dopamine from synaptic vesicles and enhanced dopamine release into the synaptic space. **B**, Modafinil also alters DAT function such that dopamine leaves the neuron instead of entering it. (Adapted from Sleep: Excessive Sleepiness. San Diego, Calif., NEI Press, 2005, copyright Neuroscience Education Institute, with permission)

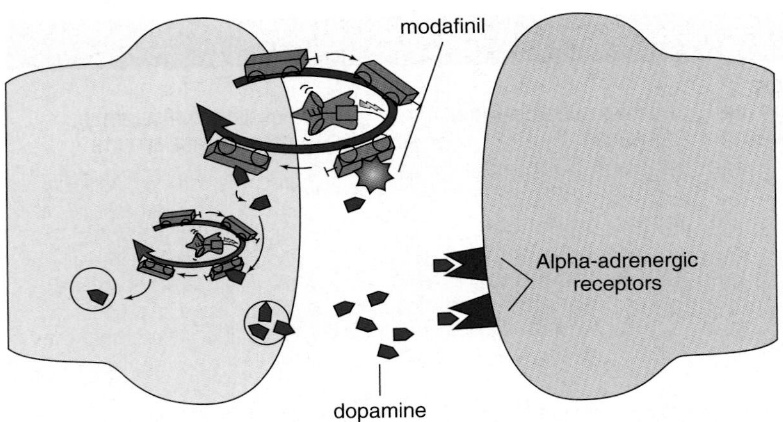

Figure 5-21.
Although the mechanism is not fully elucidated, modafinil binds to the dopamine transporter (DAT) and requires its presence as well as that of alpha-adrenergic receptors, in particular alpha 1. Modafinil does not need the norepinephrine transporter or dopamine receptors postsynaptically. It is thought that the increase in synaptic dopamine following blockade of DAT increases alpha receptor activity and ultimately produces downstream effects on transmitters including glutamate and histamine. (Adapted from Sleep: Excessive Sleepiness. San Diego, Calif., NEI Press, 2005, copyright Neuroscience Education Institute, with permission.)

SODIUM OXYBATE

This compound can be used to improve nocturnal sleep in narcoleptics with a goal of improving daytime wakefulness, as well as reducing cataplexy. Its dependence potential and very short half-life (requiring patients to wake up at night for a middle-of-the-night dose) need to be balanced against its benefits in improving sleep continuity and in consolidating REM sleep (Fig. 5-23).

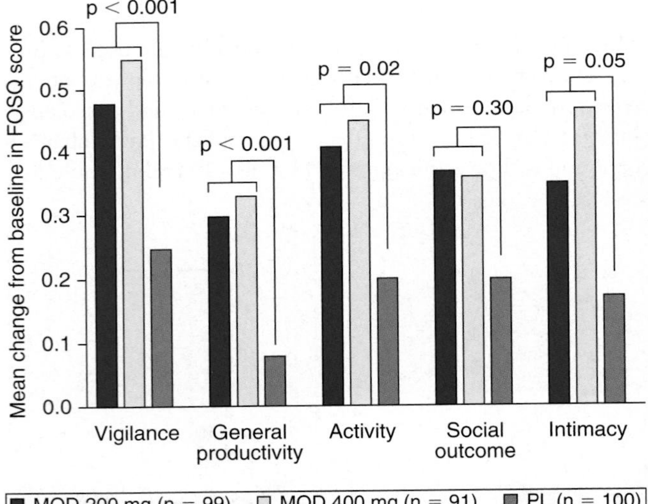

Figure 5-22.
Effect of modafinil (MOD) on functional outcome in patients with residual excessive sleepiness associated with obstructive sleep apnea/hypopnea syndrome. Patients in this randomized, double-blind, parallel group, multicenter study received oral MOD 200 mg or 400 mg once daily or placebo (PL) for 12 weeks. (Data from Black JE, Hirshkowitz M: Modafinil for treatment of residual excessive sleepiness in continuous positive airway pressure–treated obstructive sleep apnea/hypopnea syndrome. Sleep 28[4]:464–471, 2005.)

CAFFEINE

Caffeine, a xanthine derivative, is probably the most widely consumed stimulant. It acts primarily as a nonspecific antagonist for adenosine receptors. Since cholinergic neurons in the basal forebrain are under tonic inhibition by adenosine, it is thought that caffeine indirectly reduces this inhibition and hence increases some aspects of central nervous system cholinergic function. Caffeine has a half-life of 3.5 to 5 hours. Very large doses equivalent to 12 cups of coffee per day can produce a syndrome that includes agitation, tremors, and, not surprisingly, sleep disturbance (Fig. 5-24).

Table 5-7. Pharmacokinetics (Mean Values) of Oral Modafinil 200 mg in Six Healthy Men Following a Single Dose (Day 1) and Once-Daily Administration for 7 Days

PARAMETER	DAY 1	DAY 7
C_{max} (μg/mL)	4.8	6.4
t_{max} (h)	2.3	2.7
AUC_∞ (μg • h/mL)	74.0	
AUC_τ (μg • h/mL)		79.0
V/F (L/kg)	0.8	0.8
$t_{1/2}$ (h)		17.0
CL/F (mL/min)	46.0	44.0
CL_R (mL/min)	2.3	

AUC_∞, area under the plasma concentration-time curve from time zero to infinity; AUC_τ, AUC across one dosing interval; C_{max}, peak plasma concentration; CL/F, apparent oral plasma clearance; CL_R, renal clearance; $t_{1/2}$, elimination half-life; t_{max}, time to C_{max}; V/F, apparent volume of distribution.
Data from Wong YN, Simcoe D, Hartman LN, et al: A double-blind, placebo-controlled, ascending-dose evaluation of the pharmacokinetics and tolerability of modafinil tablets in healthy male volunteers. J Clin Pharmacol 39(1):30–40, 1999.

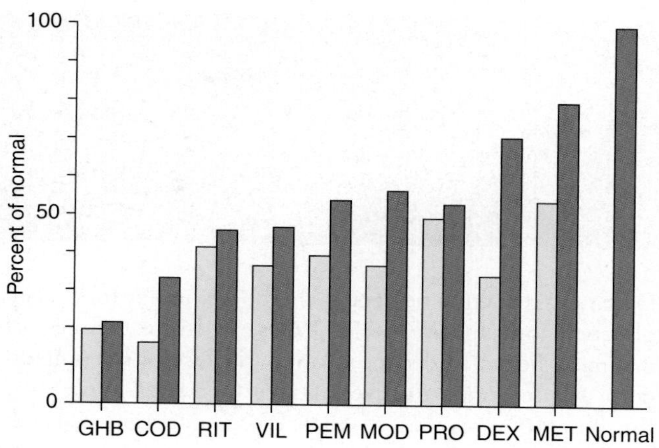

Figure 5-23.
Relative efficacy of drugs for treating narcolepsy presented in terms of percentage of normal levels of sleepiness. The lightest shading denotes baseline values. The darkest shading denotes treatment values, or the normal values *(extreme right)*. A comparison among drugs in a blind protocol has not been performed. COD, codeine; DEX, dextroamphetamine; GHB, gamma-hydroxybutyrate; MET, methylphenidate; MOD, modafinil; PEM, pemoline; PRO, protriptyline; RIT, ritanserin; VIL, viloxazine. (Data from Mitler MM, Hajdukovic R: Relative efficacy of drugs for the treatment of sleepiness in narcolepsy. Sleep 14:218–220, 1991.)

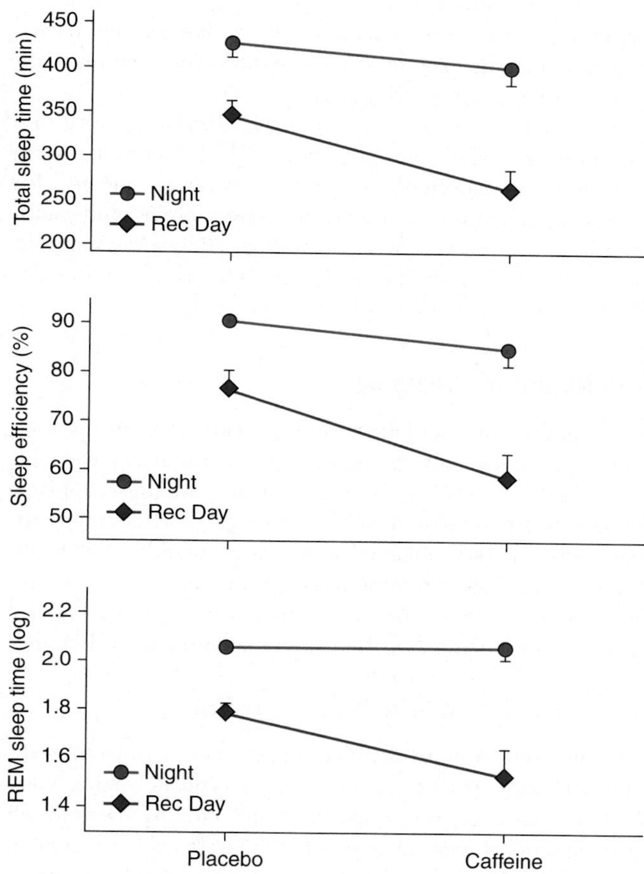

Figure 5-24.
Effects of caffeine on sleep in two groups of moderate caffeine consumers. One group was studied at habitual bedtime, the other during daytime recovery sleep after one night of sleep deprivation. In both groups, subjects received 100 mg of caffeine 3 hours before bedtime and a second 100 mg 1 hour before bedtime. It can be seen that caffeine had a greater effect on recovery sleep. (Data from Carrier J, Fernandez-Bolanos M, Robillard R, et al: Effects of caffeine are more marked on daytime recovery sleep than on nocturnal sleep. Neuropsychopharmacology 32:964–972, 2007.)

SELECTED READINGS

Amin J, Lee A, Gerlovin M, German D (eds): Monthly Prescribing Reference Diagnosis and Treatment of Insomnia. Prescribing Reference, 2006. Available at www.empr.com.

Angier N: An ancient medicine, New York Times, Dec. 11, 2007.

Mendelson WB: The Use and Misuse of Sleeping Pills. New York, Plenum Press, 1980.

Mendelson WB: Hypnotic medications: Mechanisms of action and pharmacologic effects. In Kryger MH, Roth T, Dement WC (eds): Principles and Practice of Sleep Medicine. Philadelphia, Elsevier Saunders, 2005, pp. 444–451.

Rudolph U, Mohler H: Analysis of GABAA receptor function and dissection of the pharmacology of benzodiazepines and general anesthetics through mouse genetics. Annu Rev Pharmacol Toxicol 44:475–498, 2004.

CHAPTER 6

DREAMING

Tore A. Nielsen

Dreaming remains a neglected and poorly understood sleep phenomenon. In the early 1970s, scientific studies of dreaming began to decline relative to those of sleep medicine, and remained relatively scarce thereafter. Only over the past 10 years has a gradual rise in dream research become perceptible.

A major obstacle to a thriving dream science has been a lack of consensus on the nature and phenomenology of dreaming. Dreaming encompasses a largely uncharted range of human experiences, with numerous genres, subtypes, variants, and deviations.

Following Aserinsky and Kleitman's 1953 discovery of a link between rapid eye movement (REM) sleep and vivid dreaming, researchers possessed objective means for detecting dreaming, collecting accurate samples, and establishing a definitive phenomenology. Polysomnography-based sampling of dreaming reports became the gold standard for research studies of all kinds.

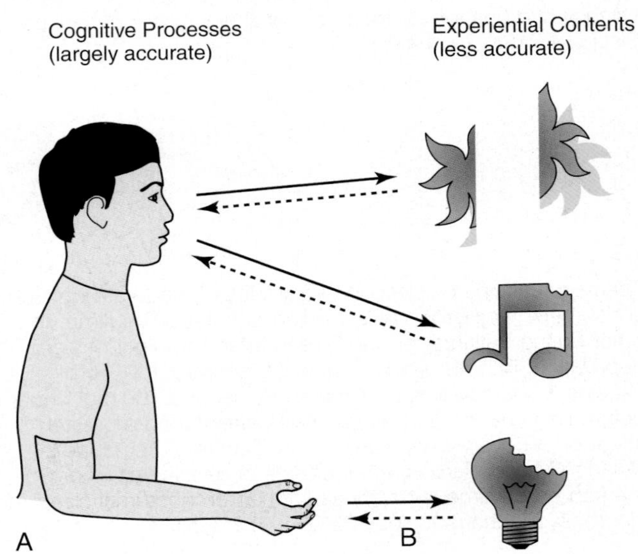

Figure 6-1.
Dreaming simulates waking reality accurately in some respects and inaccurately in others. **A**, Waking cognitive processes such as perception and feeling are reliably simulated, producing an accurate sense of a self that interacts with other characters and objects (*solid arrows*). **B**, The experiential contents of wakefulness are not reliably simulated. Dream portrayals of the characters, scenes, and objects of waking life are often flawed (*dashed arrows*).

The Nature of Dreaming

Dreaming is the simulation, during sleep, of both the cognitive processes and the experiential contents of wakefulness (Fig. 6-1). With some exceptions, waking cognitive processes are simulated quite thoroughly, while experiential contents are simulated much less accurately. The result is a reproduction of reality in which one feels to be present, actively perceiving and interacting with a virtual world whose components are often novel, unfamiliar, or bizarre.

SIMULATION OF COGNITIVE PROCESSES

The apparent flow of dreamed experience is indistinguishable in many respects from that of typical waking state experience (Table 6-1, upper section). Judging by the high prevalences of various measures, rudimentary perceptual activities such as seeing and hearing are reliably simulated. Activities such as smelling, tasting, and feeling pain, although much less prevalent, are nonetheless perceived as quite realistic when they occur. The subjective self is present in 95% of dreams, is perceived to be normally oriented within 3D space, and is felt to be viewing the dream scene from an egocentric point of view much more often (89%) than from a third person point of view (11%). When present, the self is felt to be participating in actions most (94%) of the time. Dream movements appear to be self-initiated and to respect the mechanical forces of the 1G earth gravitational field. The self's interactions with a succession of settings, objects, and other living beings are experienced as normal most of the time. The fundamental perceptual background of this flow display relative constancy, for example, size and shape are only rarely distorted relative to reality, that is, in 12.7% and 8.4% of dreams, respectively.

Emotional sequences are also reliably simulated. When present in laboratory REM dreams, subjects judge emotions to be appropriate to the dreamed situation most (84%) of the time.

Different cognitive processes are simulated with variable frequency (see Table 6-1, lower section). Thinking is relatively lifelike, with a high prevalence of internal commentary. Moderate prevalences are seen for choice, reflection, self-reflection, and self-consciousness, low prevalences for volition and inference. Two distinctly rare processes are the abilities of knowing one is hallucinating and appreciating dream contents as bizarre. Both lacunae likely help prevent the interruption of sleep.

Table 6-1. Prevalence of Common Cognitive and Perceptual Processes Present During Dreaming

PERCEPTUAL AND COGNITIVE PROCESSES	PRESENT IN % DREAM REPORTS
Perceptual processes	
Perceptual activity	95
Self-participating action	94
Self-motion	90
Egocentric orientation	89
Object size/shape preserved	87–92
Emotion	84–87
Cognitive processes	
Internal commentary	90–92
Focused attention	76
Self-reflection	53
Reflection	40–70
Choice	40–53
Self-consciousness	35–53
Volition	20–40
Inference	20–30

Basic perception-like processes (seeing, hearing, acting, emoting) are almost ubiquitous whereas higher-level cognitive processes (choosing, inferring) are more variably present.

Table 6-2. Prevalence of Some Dream Contents Is Low Despite Their High Prevalence in Waking Life

SELECT DREAM CONTENTS	PRESENT IN % DREAM REPORTS
Complete episodic memories	1.7
Money	1
Tools	1
Food/drink	2
Smells	1
Tastes	1
Using computer	4
Reading	7
Looking in mirror	16
Attending movie	17

The simulation of waking processes is reliable but by no means perfect. Many simulation "failures" contribute to dreaming's notoriety as strange and surrealistic. For example, fallibility of orientation simulation (manifesting as anomalies of dreamed gravity) produces the familiar illusions of falling, flying, and floating. Such exceptions are frequent when proprioceptive systems are disrupted during REM sleep with external stimulation or because of vestibular disease.

SIMULATION OF EXPERIENTIAL CONTENT

Even though cognitive processes are simulated quite reliably, the specific experiential contents of waking experience are not. As shown in Table 6-2, dreams do not replay personal memories and are not clearly a form of autobiographical or episodic narrative. Only a small fraction (1.7%) of dream reports describe complete episodic memories, consisting of an ensemble of locations, objects, actions, and characters. The episodic element most frequently absent from dreams is location (16% prevalence). However, the absence of some common objects is also striking: money and tools, food or drink, smells and tastes all occur in at best 1% to 2% of reports.

Dreaming also frequently fails to simulate many prominent classes of waking behavior. About 90% of subjects "never" or "hardly ever" dream about reading, writing, typing, or calculating even though an average of 6 hours a day is spent on such activities. The dramatic absence of episodic replays in dreams contrasts markedly with the nightmares of individuals with post-traumatic stress disorder (PTSD), which replay detailed traumatic memories.

If dreaming does not simulate the most common waking experience (episodic memories), it does consistently refer to components of such memories ("episodic referencing") in a disjunctive fashion. This is demonstrated when subjects, presented with salient pre-sleep stimuli such as emotionally charged films or ego-threatening tasks, report partial references to them in subsequent dreams. One common form of episodic referencing, Freud's well-known day residue effect, is the recurrence of features of the sleep laboratory (34% of dreams). A lesser known phenomenon is the referencing of events occurring approximately a week earlier, the "dream-lag effect."

More general instances of fragmented episodic referencing consist in the appearance of an individual's friends, acquaintances, and family members. Dreamed characters, excluding the self, are more often familiar than they are unfamiliar in both children's dreams (70% vs. 30%, respectively) and adults' dreams (52% vs. 48%).

Dream contents are not only a rehash of episodic features. They also draw upon dissociated elements of generalized knowledge, or semantic memories of meanings and general facts that are not connected to episodic experiences and usually not temporally tagged. Semantic references occur in 16% to 50% of studies, and more often (66% to 72%) if abstract self-references are included.

In sum, dreaming simulates the process or flow of experience quite dependably but produces only inexact, partial simulations of experiential contents. The result is a sustained illusion of first-hand experience in which out-of-context episodic elements such as people, places, and objects are combined with semantic elements such as facts and general knowledge in novel and unexpected ways. The dreamer's perceptions, thoughts, and feelings about these events nonetheless remain largely as they would during the waking state. It may be this juxtaposition of accurate experiential process and selective, reorganized episodic and semantic content that underlies the surreal quality of dreaming and that is responsible for frequent attributions about its "bizarre" or "distorted" nature.

Dreaming in Sleep Medicine

WHY ASSESS A PATIENT'S DREAMS?

Dreaming is disturbed in a variety of neurologic, psychiatric, and sleep-disordered conditions. Knowledge of the nature of a dreaming disturbance may provide clues to disease etiology, pathology, diagnosis, prognosis, and treatment. As the role of sleep and dreaming in memory functions becomes clearer, an equally important rationale for assessing dream disturbances may be to evaluate cognitive deficits suffered by sleep-disordered patients.

DREAM DISTURBANCE CONTINUUM

One pathophysiological factor seemingly implicated in the panoply of dream disturbances concerns the abnormal simulation of waking experience (previous section). It is descriptively convenient to characterize dreaming disturbances along a continuum of experiential simulation, one end of which reflects simulation attenuation, or dream experience impoverishment, the other simulation augmentation, or intensified dream realism (Fig. 6-2).

Three types of disturbance characterize attenuation (Table 6-3). The most extreme, global cessation of dreaming, involves a complete, albeit usually temporary, disappearance of dream recall and affects primarily neurologic patients. Less extreme forms of attenuation are impoverished dreaming,

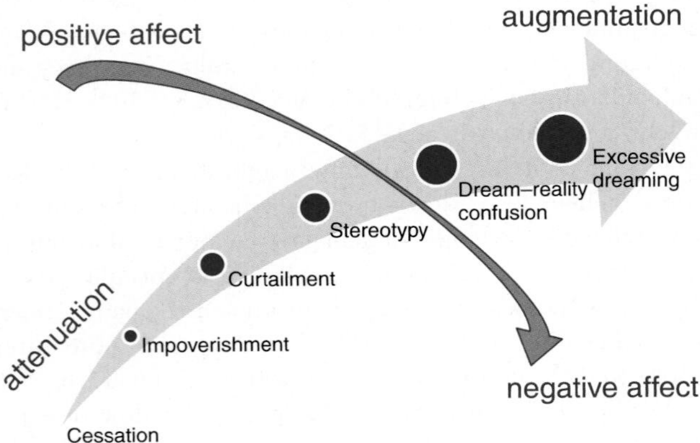

Figure 6-2.
The dream disturbance continuum. Reality simulation during dreaming varies between extremes of attenuation and augmentation. This dimension is largely independent of the dream's emotional valence (positive to negative), but reality augmentation is usually associated with a parallel increase in emotional intensity, regardless of its valence.

Table 6-3. Dreaming Disturbances Characterized by Simulation Attenuation

	CONDITIONS	FEATURES
Global cessation of dreaming	• Charcot-Wilbrand syndrome • Frontal lobotomy • Parietal lobe lesions	• Total loss of dream recall • Often suddenly after illness/medical procedure
Dream impoverishment	• Alexithymia • PTSD • Brain syndromes	• Reduction in dream recall, vividness, or complexity
Dream curtailment	• Dream interruption insomnia	• Repeated awakenings early in REM sleep episodes

PTSD, post-traumatic stress disorder.

or a reduction in the recall, vividness, or complexity of dreaming, and dream curtailment, or the shortening of dreaming episodes as a result of early spontaneous awakenings from REM sleep. Dream impoverishment is observed among alexithymic patients, PTSD victims, and some brain syndromes, and dream curtailment in cases of dream interruption insomnia (DII). As many DII patients have past histories of nightmares, dream curtailment may be an involuntary preemptive prevention of the production of nightmares.

Studies of dream phenomenology are not definitive but suggest that dream impoverishment involves primarily attenuation of process simulation, that is, reduction in the vividness of dreamed perceptual activity or emotion.

Three types of disturbance also characterize the augmentation end of the continuum (Table 6-4). Dream stereotypy, or the recurrence of particular contents, occurs in conditions such as REM sleep behavior disorder (RBD; violent, defensive content), epilepsy (aura-related content), PTSD (trauma-related content), and migraine and cardiac disease (symptom-related content). Except for RBD, in which violent dream content is strangely unrelated to waking state aggression, the content anomalies in these conditions involve atypical "episodic replays" to various degrees. Repetitive content may also characterize excessive dreaming, for example, brain-damaged patients who report increases in dream frequency and vividness or recurrence of the same dream content throughout the night. For both dream–reality confusion and excessive dreaming there occurs a heightening of process simulation to the point that dream experience is partially or totally confused with reality. Patients spending prolonged time in an intensive care unit (ICU) frequently experience "ICU dream delirium," or persistent horrific nightmares that combine the reality of the ICU with macabre dream content; these may have lasting traumatic effects. Total confusion of dreaming and reality may occur among actively or borderline psychotic individuals and may precipitate violent acting out.

Table 6-4. Dreaming Disturbances Characterized by Simulation Augmentation

	CONDITIONS	FEATURES
Dream stereotypy	• RBD/Parkinsonism • Epilepsy • PTSD • Migraine • Cardiac disease	• Recurrence of content • May incorporate medical symptoms, e.g., aura, angina, pain
Dream–reality confusion	• ICU dream delirium • Postpartum infant distress • Existential dreams • Psychotic dream aggression	• Dream vivification • Banal or everyday content may be confused with actual events
Excessive dreaming	• Epic dreaming • Brain damage • Drug withdrawal	• Seems to continue through sleep; may involve vivification, banal or repetitive content

ICU, intensive care unit; PTSD, post-traumatic stress disorder; RBD, REM behavior disorder.

NIGHTMARES

The most common dream disturbance, nightmares (Fig. 6-3), comprises a range of dream phenomena that also vary in reality simulation intensity. The latter covaries with the intensity of negative dreamed emotions. Mildly apprehensive dreams are quite common and may be only somewhat more realistic than normal dreams. Anxiety dreams and bad dreams are also common and disturbingly realistic, but not to the point of disturbing sleep with awakenings. Even more extreme are nightmares per se, which are intensely realistic and produce awakenings. Most extreme are the replicative nightmares of PTSD patients.

Enhanced dream realism is also frequently disturbed in many sleep disorders, including narcolepsy, sleep paralysis, and RBD, or after severe sleep fragmentation as endured by postpartum mothers. In such conditions, vividly realistic, even pseudo-hallucinatory, dreams are commonplace and frequently accompanied by a vivid sense of the presence of someone in the bedroom. In Video 2, a female patient afflicted with RBD relates some of the intense realism of her dreams of enduring knife attacks.

The nature and frequency of dreaming may be altered dramatically by drugs and alcohol. Catecholaminergic agents (e.g., reserpine, thioridazine, levodopa), beta-blockers (betaxolol, metoprolol, propranolol), some barbiturates, nonbenzodiazepine hypnotics (zolpidem), atypical antidepressants (bupropion), selective serotonin reuptake inhibitors (paroxetine, fluvoxamine), and tricyclic antidepressants all can induce nightmares and bizarre dreaming. The therapies most often associated with nightmares are sedative/hypnotics, beta-blockers, and amphetamines. Alcoholic patients report vivid dreams and nightmares post-withdrawal, sometimes lasting for weeks, which can lead to resumed drinking. Withdrawal is associated with an increase in REM sleep "pressure" which predicts early relapse.

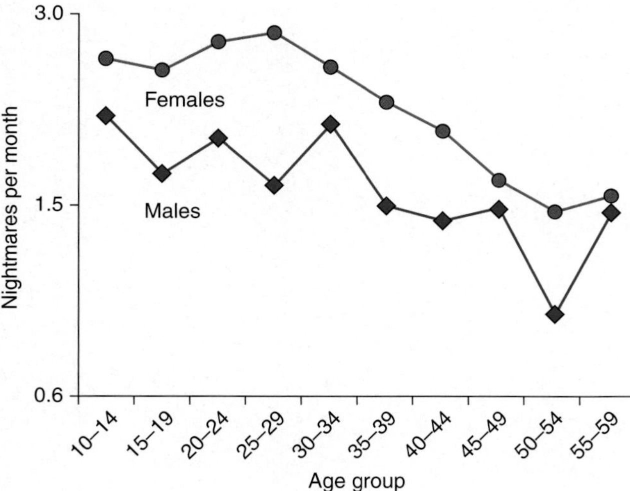

Figure 6-3.
Nightmare frequency by gender and age. Estimates of typical monthly nightmare frequency reported by 4573 male and 19,266 female respondents to an Internet questionnaire. Males and females differ significantly ($p < .05$, 2-tailed t-test) at all age strata except 45–49 and 55–59.

Treatment

Nightmares are highly responsive to various cognitive-behavioral treatments, including desensitization, operant procedures, hypnosis, analysis, story line alteration, and "face and conquer" approaches. Such success suggests that the treatments may be effective in treating other kinds of dream disturbance. Careful screening is necessary to determine that the underlying cause is not organic (e.g., RBD), traumatic (PTSD), or substance-induced. Successful drug therapies are available for RBD (Clonazepam) and PTSD (Prazosin) but have not been tested widely with other dream disturbances.

Video Examples

Chapters 19 and 20 contain video clip images of patients with RBD.

SELECTED READINGS

Arkin AM, Antrobus JS: The effects of external stimuli applied prior to and during sleep on sleep experience. In Ellman SJ, Antrobus JS (eds): The Mind in Sleep, 2nd ed. New York, Wiley, 1991, pp. 265–307.

Fosse MJ, Fosse R, Hobson JA, et al: Dreaming and episodic memory: A functional dissociation? J Cogn Neurosci 15:1–9, 2003.

Halliday G: Direct psychological therapies for nightmares: A review. Clin Psychol Rev 7:501–523, 1987.

Nielsen TA: Disturbed dreaming in medical conditions. In Kryger M, Roth N, Dement WC (eds): Principles and Practice of Sleep Medicine, 4th ed. St. Louis, Mo., Elsevier Saunders, 2005, pp. 936–945.

Nielsen TA, Stenstrom P: What are the memory sources of dreaming? Nature 437:34–38, 2005.

Nielsen TA, Zadra AL: Nightmares and other common dream disturbances. In Kryger M, Roth N, Dement WC (eds): Principles and Practice of Sleep Medicine, 4th ed. St. Louis, Mo., Elsevier Saunders, 2005, pp. 926–935.

Nielsen TA, Zadra AL, Simard V, et al: The typical dreams of Canadian university students. Dreaming 13:211–235, 2003.

Snyder F: The phenomenology of dreaming. In Madow L, Snow LH (eds): The Psychoanalytic Implications of the Psychophysiological Studies on Dreams. Springfield, Ill., Charles C Thomas, 1970, pp. 124–151.

Solms M: The Neuropsychology of Dreams. Mahwah, NJ, Lawrence Erlbaum Associates, 1997.

Spoormaker VI, Schredl M, Bout JV: Nightmares: From anxiety symptom to sleep disorder. Sleep Med Rev 10:19–31, 2005.

Thompson DF, Pierce DR: Drug-induced nightmares. Ann Pharmacother 33:93–98, 1999.

IMPACT, PRESENTATION, AND DIAGNOSIS

CHAPTER 7

Michael Zupancic, Leslie Swanson, Todd Arnedt, and Ron Chervin

Impact

Disordered sleep is common, and its effect on health and well-being has become increasingly recognized over the past several decades. Sleep apnea, for example, affects about 5% of adults and probably about 20% of older people. Unfortunately, the public, patients, and health care professionals often fail to recognize and diagnose these common, treatable disorders. Many catastrophic disasters with devastating effects have been attributed to disordered sleep or sleepiness (Fig. 7-1).

Many people around the world experience chronic sleep deprivation because they devote less time to sleep than needed, and therefore experience daytime sleepiness, which affects their productivity, ability to learn, and ability to drive safely. National surveys have shown that one third of drivers in the United States have fallen asleep at the wheel (Boxes 7-1, 7-2).

Most adolescents are sleep deprived. They cannot obtain the required 9 hours of nocturnal sleep because of their circadian tendency to have a late bedtime and early start time in school. Extracurricular activities and social and scholastic obligations also encroach on their sleep time (Box 7-3).

BOX 7-1. DANGERS OF DROWSY DRIVING

The U.S. National Highway Safety Administration conservatively estimates that each year driver fatigue causes:

- Over 100,000 police-reported crashes
- At least 4% of fatal crashes
- Over 1550 deaths
- 71,000 injuries
- 12.5 billion dollars in monetary losses

BOX 7-2. EXAMPLES OF IMPACT OF SLEEP PROBLEMS ON WORKPLACE PRODUCTIVITY

- Over one fourth of employees fell asleep or became very sleepy at work.
- Over 1 in 10 employees arrived late to work due to sleepiness.
- Insomnia, which affects up to 30% of adults, is associated with increased absenteeism.

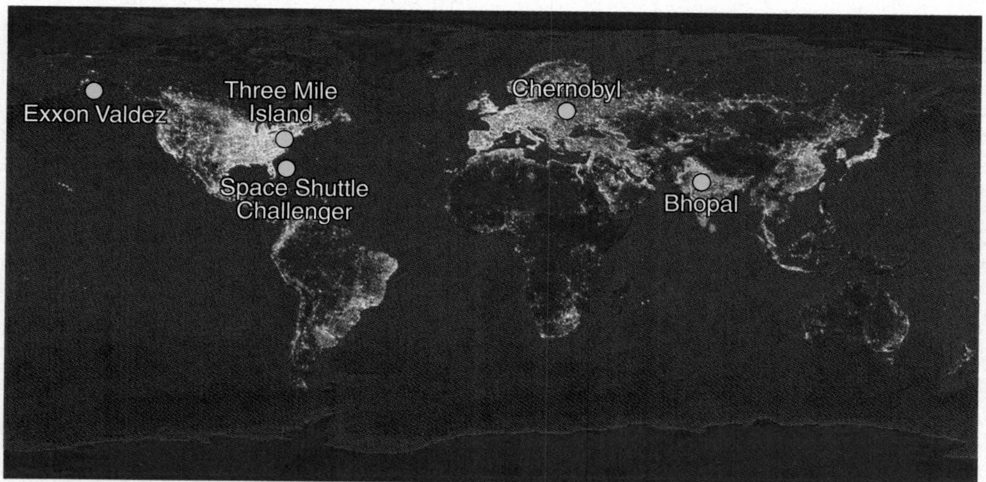

Figure 7-1.
Disasters where sleepiness has been implicated. Three Mile Island Nuclear Meltdown (March 28, 1979), Bhopal Pesticide Release Disaster (December 3, 1984), Space Shuttle Disaster (January 28, 1986), Chernobyl Nuclear Power Plant Explosion (April 26, 1986), and Exxon Valdez Oil Spill (March 24, 1989).

BOX 7-3. IMPACT OF SLEEP PROBLEMS ON ADOLESCENTS

- One in 10 high school seniors have nodded off while driving over a 1-year period.
- Half of adolescents admitted to driving drowsy over the past year with 11% driving drowsy 1-2 times a week.
- Over one fourth of teenagers have had an accident or near accident because of drowsy driving.
- 28% of high school students admit to falling asleep at least once a week while in school.

Presentation and Diagnosis

MAGNITUDE AND SIGNIFICANCE OF SLEEP DISORDERS

Although numerous population-based surveys have shown that sleep disorders are common, they most often remain undiagnosed (Fig. 7-2). Failure to correctly recognize, diagnose, and treat someone with a sleep disorder increases health care costs. This is likely due to their sleep disorder causing or worsening their other medical disorders, such as obstructive sleep apnea (OSA) worsening hypertension, or sleep disorder symptoms are incorrectly diagnosed as another disorder, such as a mood disorder. As shown in Figure 7-3, a Canadian study showed that 181 patients with untreated OSA sought heath care more frequently and spent nearly twice as many nights in the hospital, resulting in higher costs, than matched controls for 10 years prior to being diagnosed with this disease.

CLINICAL EVALUATION

Accurate and detailed clinical histories and physical exams of patients with disordered sleep are the cornerstones to proper evaluation, diagnosis, and treatment. Patients' complaints fall most often into one or more of the categories shown in Box 7-4.

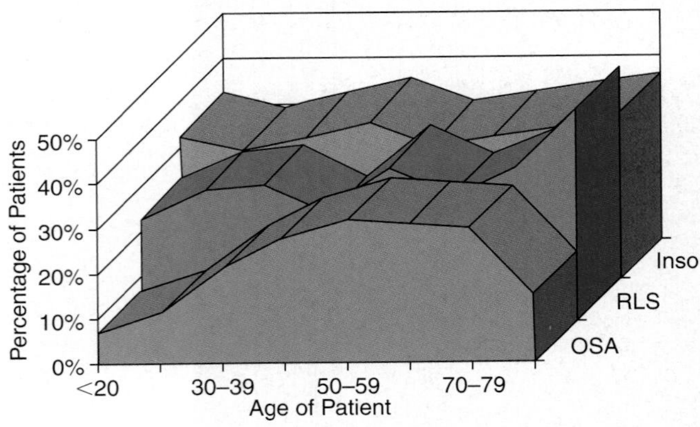

Figure 7-2.
The percentage of patients in a primary practice with symptoms of sleep disorders. Most were undiagnosed. Inso, insomnia; OSA, obstructive sleep apnea; RLS, restless legs syndrome. (Adapted from Kushida CA, Nichols DA, Simon RD, et al: Symptom-based prevalence of sleep disorders in an adult primary care population. Sleep Breath 4[1]:9–14, 2000.)

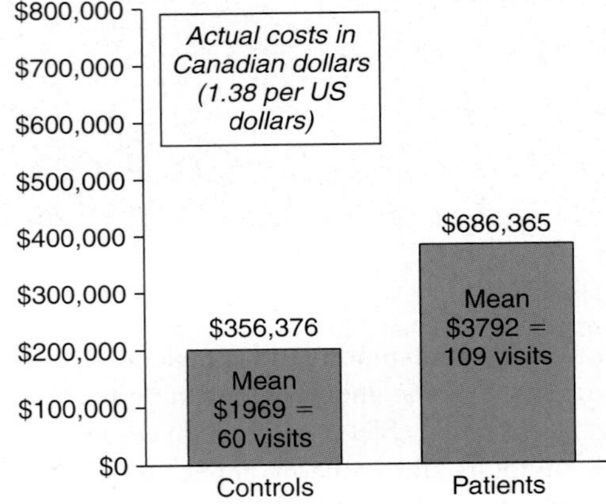

Figure 7-3.
Utilization of health care is high in the decade prior to the diagnosis of sleep apnea. (Ronald J, Delaive K, Roos L, Manfreda J, et al: Health care utilization in the 10 years prior to diagnosis in obstructive sleep apnea syndrome patients. Sleep 22[2]:225–229, 1999.)

BOX 7-4. PATIENTS' COMPLAINTS

- Histories very suggestive of obstructive sleep apnea (snoring, witnessed apneas, sleepiness)
- Problems falling asleep or staying asleep (insomnia)
- Excessive sleepiness (idiopathic hypersomnia, narcolepsy, sleep deprivation)
- Abnormal movements, sensations, or behaviors during sleep

History of the present illness

A history should include the onset of symptoms and their evolution over time and associations (e.g., weight change, new comorbidities, precipitating factors, new medications).

Sleep-disordered breathing

Sleep-disordered breathing is prevalent and can worsen many other sleep disorders. It is important to ask every patient about its symptoms (Box 7-5).

BOX 7-5. SLEEP-DISORDERED BREATHING SYMPTOMS

Questions to ask patients that may point to the presence of sleep breathing disorders:

- Snoring frequency and loudness?
- Witnessed apneas while sleeping?
- Daytime sleepiness, tiredness, lack of energy, fatigue?
- Unrefreshing sleep?
- Snore/gasp arousals?
- Nocturnal headaches?
- Nocturnal sweating?
- Excessive movement in bed?
- Nocturia?
- Dry mouth or water by bedside?

Insomnia

To properly evaluate patients with insomnia, the duration of insomnia and any triggers should also be queried (Boxes 7-6 and 7-7). The answers to these simple questions are often clues to the practitioner about the cause of insomnia or excessive daytime sleepiness, such as circadian rhythm disorders or the insufficient sleep syndrome. Those with insomnia often report fatigue rather than sleepiness.

Excessive sleepiness

Excluding sleep-disordered breathing, the most important causes of hypersomnolence include insufficient sleep syndrome, long sleeper syndrome, narcolepsy, and idiopathic hypersomnia (Box 7-8). Patients with insufficient sleep syndrome or long sleeper syndrome typically have an irregular sleep schedule between workdays and weekend days. They achieve restful sleep and normal daytime alertness when able to go to bed and awaken in response to their bodies' natural tendencies. The daily requirement of 10 or more hours of nocturnal sleep to meet this need is consistent with long sleep syndrome.

Patients with narcolepsy (see chapter 10.1) frequently describe disrupted nocturnal sleep but are refreshed upon morning awakening, whereas those with idiopathic hypersomnia often describe themselves as deep sleepers but awake unrefreshed and experience a prolonged sleep inertia lasting several hours. Despite the amount of sleep patients with either idiopathic hypersomnia or narcolepsy obtain, they remain excessively sleepy during wakeful hours.

Cataplexy, the abrupt loss of muscle tone lasting less than a minute, triggered by positive strong emotions, is a common feature of narcolepsy and occurs in two thirds of these patients. The axial muscles are most frequently involved and consciousness is retained during cataplectic attacks. The presence of knee buckling when telling or hearing a joke is highly suggestive of cataplexy and is seen in the majority of patients with this disease. Sleep paralysis is the perception of being paralyzed when awakened from sleep (sometimes during a dream). Hyponogogic and hypnopompic hallucinations refer to the symptoms of vivid dream imagery on sleep onset and on awakening. These symptoms are common in narcoleptics. Information about naps can be helpful in diagnosis (Box 7-9).

BOX 7-6. SCREENING QUESTIONS REGARDING INSOMNIA

Questions to ask patients with insomnia:

- Sleep schedule and daytime energy level during week, weekends, and vacation?
- Sleep environment and hygiene?
- Latency to falling asleep and number/duration of nocturnal awakenings?
- Quality of sleep?
- Attitude toward sleep?
- Thoughts while awake in bed?
- Next-day consequences of poor sleep?
- Duration of symptoms and triggers?
- Presence of comorbidities?
- Medications used?

BOX 7-7. CHRONIC INSOMNIA EXPLANATORY QUESTIONS

When evaluating factors that may make insomnia persist, the following should be explored:

- What are the patient's attitudes and thought content before and after entering the bedroom?
- Does the patient look forward to going to bed or become anxious on entering the bedroom?
- Does the patient view sleep as a nightly battle, become frustrated at his or her inability to fall asleep, then ruminate and make a catastrophe out of the impact he or she believes his or her poor night's sleep will have on the next-day activities, such as do those with psychophysiologic insomnia?
- Does the patient have behaviors that not only disrupt nocturnal sleep but can condition him or her to view the bedroom as a place of mental activity rather than a place of rest?
- Review the patient's sleep hygiene for factors that will exacerbate insomnia (excessive caffeine or exercise close to bedtime).

BOX 7-8. HYPERSOMNOLENCE EVALUATION

Questions to ask when evaluating disorders of excessive sleepiness:

- The questions to rule out sleep breathing disorders in Box 7-5
- Sleep schedule, level of alertness on awakening, sleep quality?
- Episodes of muscle weakness with strong emotions (cataplexy)?
- Sleep paralysis?
- Are naps long or short? Are naps refreshing or not refreshing?

Sleep behaviors

When evaluating a patient with a parasomnia (see chapter 12), it is important to obtain information on the behavior, age when it first appeared, and time of the sleep period

BOX 7-9. NAPS IN HYPERSOMNIA

- Narcoleptics frequently take short (10 to 30 minutes) intentional or unintentional naps that improve daytime alertness and are described as refreshing. Patients often dream during naps.
- Patients with idiopathic hypersomnia frequently nap for hours and describe the naps as unrefreshing. They do not note an obvious improvement in alertness and do not dream during the naps.
- Patients with sleep apnea also have unrefreshing daytime sleep episodes and do not dream during the naps.

BOX 7-10. PARASOMNIA EVALUATION/HISTORY

Questions to ask when evaluating abnormal behaviors:

- Describe any abnormal noises or behaviors during sleep.
- Age at first occurrence?
- Does behavior occur during the first half or second half of the sleep period?
- Does the patient recall vivid dreaming during parasomnia?
- Are the behaviors repetitive?

in which it occurred. A detailed account of the behavior from the patient's bed partner is extremely helpful in making the correct diagnosis; moreover, any injuries resulting from the parasomnia are important to note (Box 7-10).

The clinician should first attempt to categorize the behavior as either a rapid eye movement (REM) or non-REM (NREM) parasomnia. NREM parasomnias typically begin in childhood, occur during the first third of the sleep period, and are rarely remembered by the patient. REM parasomnias usually begin after the age of 50, occur in the second half of the sleep period, and the behavior correlates with a vivid dream that the patient is able to recall if awakened. Nocturnal seizures are distinguished from REM and NREM parasomnias by their stereotyped nature, presence of daytime seizures, and presence of tongue biting and incontinence.

Impact of disorder on patient

The impact that disordered sleep has on one's daily life must be assessed when evaluating all study participants, and should include effects on driving, work, mood, and family. The duration and effect these complaints have on each patient's personal and professional lives should also be attained.

Medical history (Box 7-11)

As an example, patients with Parkinson's disease (see chapter 10.4) are apt to be excessively sleepy, not only because of central nervous system dysfunction but often because of prolonged nocturnal awakenings due to bradykinesia, limiting their ability to achieve a comfortable position in bed.

BOX 7-11. SLEEP MEDICINE COMPLETE MEDICAL HISTORY

Medical history should cover:

- Coexisting medical and psychiatric disorders
- Current and past medications
- Social history
  - Occupation
  - Use of alcohol, tobacco, and caffeine
  - Use of illicit drugs
- Family history

Up to 25% of those with Parkinson's disease have REM behavior disorder.

Medications can contribute to disordered sleep. Diuretics administered at night can disrupt sleep by causing nocturnal urination. Propranolol often causes disturbing nightmares. Tricyclic antidepressants can cause REM behavior disorder, and nonsedating antidepressants taken in the evening can contribute to insomnia. Narcotic pain medications can contribute to daytime somnolence as a result of their sedating central nervous system activity, but they can also disrupt sleep by causing central sleep apnea.

A social history can contribute to a determination of the cause of disordered sleep. The frequency, amount, and timing of alcohol consumption can impact sleep. Alcohol causes one to fall asleep quickly, but the result is a lighter, disrupted sleep during the second half of the sleep period. Alcohol also worsens OSA. Tobacco is a stimulant and can contribute to insomnia when taken before bedtime or in the middle of the night.

Family history is a critical component of the evaluation. People who have a first-degree relative with OSA are twice as likely to have this disease.

PHYSICAL EXAM

A complete physical exam is required to evaluate the patient with disordered sleep, as shown in Box 7-12. A detailed HEENT (head, eyes, ears, nose, and throat) exam is required when evaluating for sleep-disordered breathing (Box 7-13). This is reviewed in greater detail in chapters 11.1, 11.2, and 11.3.

Complete cardiovascular and pulmonary exams are preformed to evaluate for pathology that can either contribute to or be a consequence of disordered sleep. See chapter 13. Peripheral edema may be a clue to heart failure, which is a known consequence of untreated OSA. Conversely, people with heart failure frequently have disrupted sleep from central sleep apnea.

A full neurologic exam is indicated when evaluating specific sleep conditions such as restless legs syndrome and insomnia. It is also important to evaluate mood and other psychiatric disorders as these frequently coexist and can contribute to daytime sleepiness and disrupted nocturnal sleep.

BOX 7-12. THE MINIMUM PHYSICAL EXAM IN PATIENTS WITH SLEEP DISORDERS

- Height, weight, body mass index, blood pressure
- General appearance and level of alertness
- HEENT exam
- Cardiovascular exam
- Pulmonary exam
- Extremity exam
- Neurologic exam

BOX 7-13. SLEEP APNEA UPPER AIRWAY EXAM

The HEENT exam should include:

- Neck circumference. A neck circumference over 43 cm is a common finding in adults with obstructive sleep apnea (OSA).
- Skeletal features such as maxillary deficiency and retrognathia, which may cause OSA.
- Nasal airway to evaluate nasal airflow, the internal and external nasal valves, nasal turbinates, or the presence of a deviated nasal septum, since nasal obstruction contributes to sleep-disordered breathing and also hinders treatment with continuous positive airway pressure.
- Oral exam (see chapter 11.1)
  Mallampati score should be noted, as higher scores are correlated with having OSA.
  An erythematous uvula due to vibrational trauma from snoring is a common finding in a patient with OSA.
  Scalloping of the tongue suggests the oral cavity is too small.
  The presence and size of tonsils should be recorded because surgical outcomes are generally better in OSA patients with large tonsils.
  A high, arched hard palate is a common finding in patients with OSA and indicates the oral cavity is too narrow.

SELF-ADMINISTERED INSTRUMENTS HELPFUL IN EVALUATION OF SLEEP DISORDERS

Sleep diaries

Sleep diaries provide subjective information on a patient's sleep-wake patterns and are widely used in both clinical and research settings. Typical entries include bedtime, rise time, estimate of sleep latency, frequency of nighttime awakenings, estimate of time spent awake after sleep initiation, naps, caffeine intake, use of sleep aids, and ratings of sleep quality and level of fatigue, from which summary scores are calculated.

An example of a sleep diary from the National Sleep Foundation is shown in Figure 7-4. Research has demonstrated modest to poor correlations between sleep diaries and objective measures (e.g., overnight polysomnography or actigraphy), with total sleep time underestimated and sleep latency overestimated in diaries versus objective measurement. Thus, diaries are a good representation of patients' perception of their sleep, but may not accurately reflect objective sleep parameters.

DAY 1 DAY________ DATE________

COMPLETE IN MORNING	I went to bed last night at: ____ PM/AM	I got out of bed this morning at: ____ AM/PM	Last night, I fell asleep in: ____ Minutes	I woke up during the night: # of Times ____ # of Minutes ____	When I woke up for the day, I felt: ☐ Refreshed ☐ Somewhat refreshed ☐ Fatigued	Last night I slept a total of: ____ Hours	My sleep was disturbed by: *(List any mental, physical or environmental factors)* ____ ____

COMPLETE AT THE END OF THE DAY	I consumed caffeinated drinks in the: ☐ Morning ☐ Afternoon ☐ Evening ☐ Not applicable	I exercised at least 20 minutes in the: ☐ Morning ☐ Afternoon ☐ Evening ☐ Not applicable	Approximately 2–3 hours before going to bed, I consumed: ☐ Alcohol ☐ A heavy meal ☐ Not applicable	Medication(s) I took during the day: ____ ____ ____ ____	About 1 hour before going to sleep, I did the following activity: ____ ____ ____

0 Wide Awake 1 2 3 4 Falling Asleep

Record with a "0, 1, 2, 3, or 4" which face most represents how sleepy you feel at the given time.

Morning (6am–12pm)	Afternoon (12pm–6pm)	Evening (6pm–12am)	Night (12–6am)
☐ Time:____	☐ Time:____	☐ Time:____	☐ Time:____

DAY 2 DAY________ DATE________

COMPLETE IN MORNING	I went to bed last night at: ____ PM/AM	I got out of bed this morning at: ____ AM/PM	Last night, I fell asleep in: ____ Minutes	I woke up during the night: # of Times ____ # of Minutes ____	When I woke up for the day, I felt: ☐ Refreshed ☐ Somewhat refreshed ☐ Fatigued	Last night I slept a total of: ____ Hours	My sleep was disturbed by: *(List any mental, physical or environmental factors)* ____ ____

COMPLETE AT THE END OF THE DAY	I consumed caffeinated drinks in the: ☐ Morning ☐ Afternoon ☐ Evening ☐ Not applicable	I exercised at least 20 minutes in the: ☐ Morning ☐ Afternoon ☐ Evening ☐ Not applicable	Approximately 2–3 hours before going to bed, I consumed: ☐ Alcohol ☐ A heavy meal ☐ Not applicable	Medication(s) I took during the day: ____ ____ ____ ____	About 1 hour before going to sleep, I did the following activity: ____ ____ ____

0 Wide Awake 1 2 3 4 Falling Asleep

Record with a "0, 1, 2, 3, or 4" which face most represents how sleepy you feel at the given time.

Morning (6am–12pm)	Afternoon (12–6pm)	Evening (6pm–12am)	Night (12–6am)
☐ Time:____	☐ Time:____	☐ Time:____	☐ Time:____

Figure 7-4.
National Sleep Foundation sleep diary.

Epworth Sleepiness Scale

Using the following scale, circle the *most appropriate number* for each situation.

0 = would doze *less than once a month*
1 = *slight* chance of dozing
2 = *moderate* chance of dozing
3 = *high* chance of dozing

Situation	Chance of Dozing
Sitting and reading	0 1 2 3
Watching TV	0 1 2 3
Sitting, inactive in a public place (in a theater or in a meeting)	0 1 2 3
As a passenger in a car for an hour without a break	0 1 2 3
Lying down to rest in the afternoon (when circumstances permit)	0 1 2 3
Sitting and talking to someone	0 1 2 3
Sitting quietly after a lunch without alcohol	0 1 2 3
In a car, while stopped for a few minutes in the traffic	0 1 2 3

Add the 8 numbers you have circled **TOTAL** ________

Figure 7-5.
The Epworth Sleepiness Scale. (Adapted from Johns MW: A new method for measuring daytime sleepiness: The Epworth Sleepiness Scale. Sleep 14[6]:540–545, 1991.)

Epworth Sleepiness Scale

The Epworth Sleepiness Scale, as seen in Figure 7-5, is a tool patients can quickly fill out and is a subjective measure of sleepiness. A total score of 10 or above indicates excessive daytime sleepiness. A score of 16 is commonly reported in narcoleptics, whereas a score of 6 is the population norm. Subjects with insomnia often have scores within the normal values.

Berlin Apnea Questionnaire

The Berlin Apnea Questionnaire helps identify patients at risk for the sleep apnea syndrome and is often used in research to estimate the frequency of OSA. This questionnaire has a sensitivity of 0.86 and a specificity of 0.77 for correctly diagnosing OSA (as compared with polysomnography) in those patients who fall into the high-risk category (Fig. 7-6).

SELECTED READINGS

Anic-Labat S, Guilleminault C, Kraemer HC, et al: Validation of a cataplexy questionnaire in 983 sleep-disordered patients. Sleep 22(1): 77–87, 1999.

Knab B, Engel RR: Perception of waking and sleeping: Possible implications for the evaluation of insomnia. Sleep 11(3):265–272, 1988.

National Sleep Foundation. Sleep in America Polls, 2006, 2008.

Ozminkowski RJ, Wang S, Walsh JK: The direct and indirect costs of untreated insomnia in adults in the United States. Sleep 30:263–273, 2007.

Rosen RC, Zozula R, Jahn EG, Carson JL: Low rates of recognition of sleep disorders in primary care: Comparison of a community-based versus clinical academic setting. Sleep Med 2(1):47–55, 2001.

Sateia MJ, Doghramji K, Hauri PJ, Morin CM: Evaluation of chronic insomnia: An American Academy of Sleep Medicine review. Sleep 23 (2):243–308, 2000.

Young T, Evans L, Finn L, Palta M: Estimation of the clinically diagnosed proportion of sleep apnea syndrome in middle-aged men and women. Sleep 20(9):705–706, 1997.

Modified Berlin Apnea Questionnaire

Start here

BOX A: Category 1 SNORING
- ☐ Do you snore?
- ☐ Is snoring louder than talking?
- ☐ Is snoring present more than at least 3–4 times a week?
- ☐ Has snoring ever bothered others?
- ☐ Has anyone noticed the stopping of breathing during sleep more than at least 3–4 times a week?

___ Add up the number of positive answers
✓ If more than 2 this category is positive.

BOX B: Category 2 SLEEPINESS
- ☐ Are you tired or fatigued after waking up more than 3–4 times a week?
- ☐ During the day are you tired or fatigued more than 3–4 times a week?
- ☐ Do you have any trouble staying awake driving?

___ Add up the number of positive answers
✓ If 2 or more, this category is positive.

BOX C: Category 3 RISK FACTORS
- ☐ Do you have high blood pressure?
- ☐ Is your BMI more than 30 or is your neck collar size more than 17 inches?
- ☐ Do you have a very small jaw or a large overbite?

___ Add up the number of positive answers
✓ If 2 or more, this category is positive.

End here

BOX D: FILL THIS IN LAST: Check positive categories
- ☐ Category 1 SNORING
- ☐ Category 2 SLEEPINESS
- ☐ Category 3 RISK FACTORS

___ Add up the number of positive answers
✓ If 2 or more, the chance that apnea is present is high.

Figure 7-6.
Modified Berlin Apnea Questionnaire. (Based on Netzer NC, Stoohs RA, Netzer CM, et al: Using the Berlin Questionnaire to identify patients at risk for obstructive sleep apnea syndrome. Adapted from Ann Intern Med 131[7]:485–491, 1999.)

CIRCADIAN RHYTHM SLEEP DISORDERS

CHAPTER 8

Kathryn J. Reid and Phyllis C. Zee

Circadian rhythm sleep disorders are sleep disorders where there is a misalignment between the timing of the sleep-wake cycle and the circadian clock or an alteration in the circadian clock that results in insomnia, sleepiness, and impaired daytime function. Circadian disorders of sleep include delayed sleep phase type, advanced sleep phase type, free-running sleep type, irregular sleep-wake type, shift work type, and jet lag type.

Delayed Sleep Phase Disorder

Delayed sleep phase disorder (DSPD) is characterized by difficulty in falling asleep and waking at the desired time and excessive daytime sleepiness. This disorder is relatively common in adolescents with a reported prevalence of approximately 7% and, in the general population, of about 0.17%. Individuals with delayed sleep phase disorder typically have a delayed sleep-wake cycle with sleep onset between 2 and 6 A.M. and wake time between 10 A.M. and 2 P.M. (Fig. 8-1).

In addition to a delay in the sleep-wake cycle there is a delay in other circadian rhythm phase markers such as core body temperature and the dim light melatonin rhythm (Fig. 8-2). Endogenous melatonin can serve as a useful marker for the timing of circadian rhythms (Fig. 8-3).

Treatment for delayed sleep phase disorder is aimed at realigning the sleep-wake cycle to the conventional or desired time; this can be achieved in several ways. Behavioral interventions should be used initially to improve sleep. For example, patients with DSPD should be encouraged to practice good sleep hygiene and to avoid excessive light exposure in the evening, which may perpetuate or even exacerbate the delay in the sleep-wake cycle. Chronotherapy can also be used This requires patients to

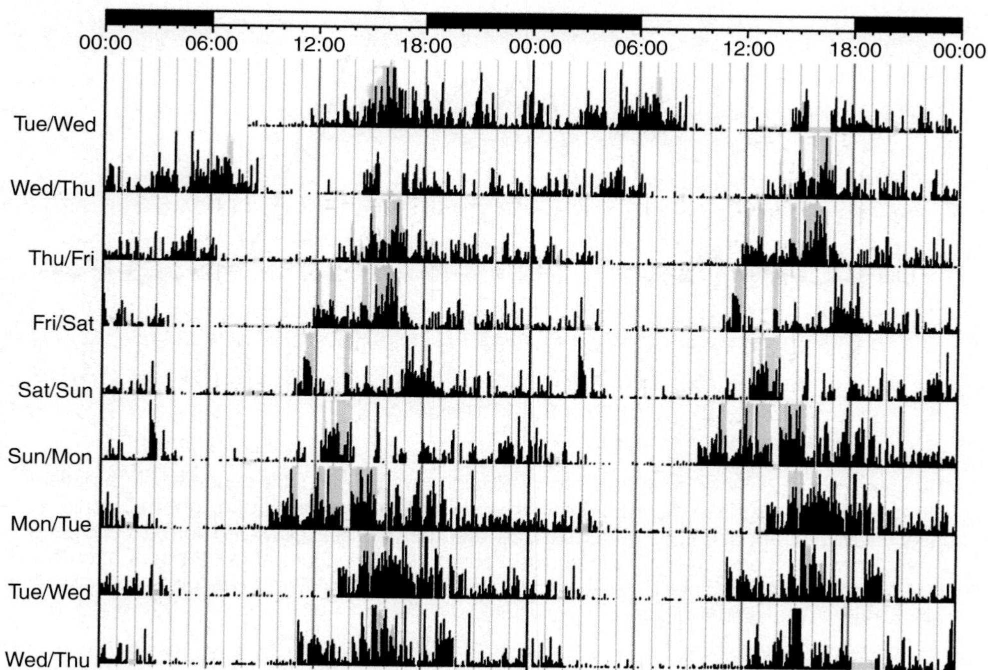

Figure 8-1.
An example of the rest-activity cycle in a patient with delayed sleep phase disorder recorded with wrist activity monitoring. The dark lines indicate activity and the yellow bars indicate light level. Where the black lines are absent it is inferred the patient is asleep. The data are plotted twice to make it easier to see the rest-activity cycle over several days. Time is plotted across the x-axis and is between midnight and midnight over 2 days. The y-axis indicates the day of the week. For this individual the average sleep onset is at about 4 A.M. and the wake time is around 12 P.M.

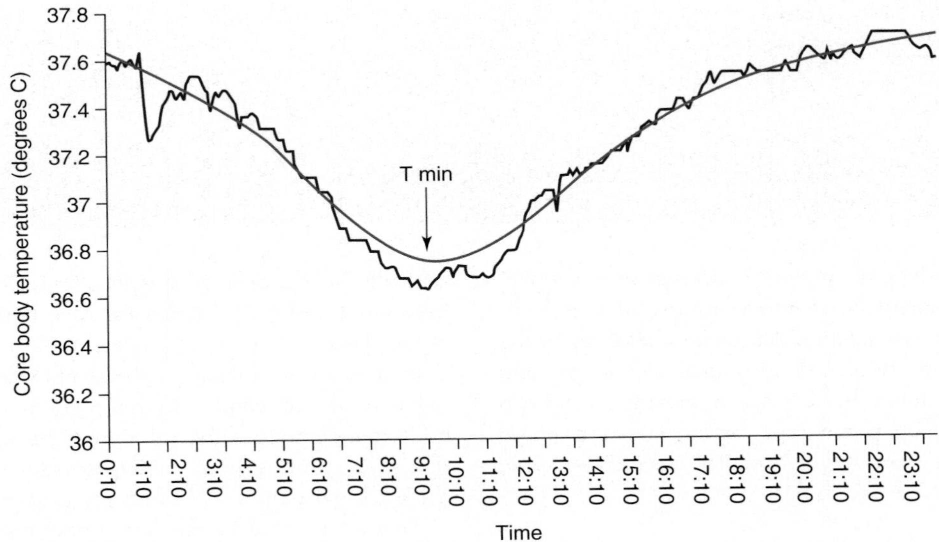

Figure 8-2.
An example of a 24-hour core body temperature (CBT) rhythm in an individual with delayed sleep phase disorder. Time is indicated on the x-axis and temperature in degrees Celsius on the y-axis. The T_{min} occurs at about 9 A.M. The declining portion of the CBT rhythm begins at about 3 A.M., and the rising portion of the CBT rhythm begins at about 11 A.M. This would make it difficult for this person to fall asleep earlier than 3 A.M. and to wake before 11 A.M., and if he did wake before 11 A.M. in order to get to work or class he would most likely feel extremely sleepy as his CBT would still be low.

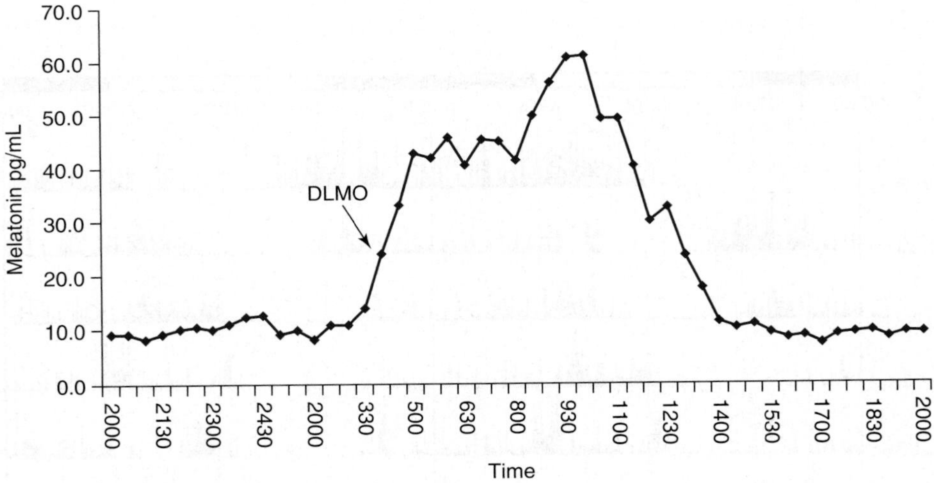

Figure 8-3.
An example of a 24-hour melatonin profile obtained under dim light conditions in a patient with delayed sleep phase disorder. The arrow indicates the time of dim light melatonin onset (DLMO) at about 3 A.M., which is much later than normal (DLMO in normal controls is usually between 8 and 10 P.M.). Since sleep onset usually occurs about 2 hours after the DLMO, this person may not be sleepy until around 2 A.M., making it difficult to fall asleep earlier than 4 A.M. even if desired.

progressively delay their sleep and wake time by 3 hours every few days until they reach their desired sleep time. Another alternative is manipulating the circadian clock with light or exogenous melatonin, which should be used in conjunction with good sleep hygiene practices. Bright light exposure in the morning can be used to phase-advance the timing of the circadian clock and the sleep-wake cycle. Bright light exposure of 2500 lux for approximately 2 hours in the morning starting at 6 A.M. has been successful in phase-advancing the sleep-wake cycle. Melatonin in the evening 5 to 7 hours prior to habitual sleep time has been shown to phase-advance the sleep-wake cycle and improve quality of life in patients with DSPD.

Advanced Sleep Phase Disorder

Advanced sleep phase disorder is characterized by a difficulty staying awake in the evening and waking too early in the morning before the desired time (Fig. 8-4). Dim light melatonin levels can also be used to assess the circadian clock and the degree of phase-advance in patients with advanced sleep phase disorder (Fig. 8-5).

Treatment for advanced sleep phase disorder typically involves using bright light to phase-delay the circadian clock and the sleep-wake cycle. Bright light exposure for several hours in the evening after 8 P.M. has been used successfully to phase-delay circadian rhythms and reduce feelings of sleepiness in the evening. Hypnotic medications can also be used to maintain sleep in the early morning.

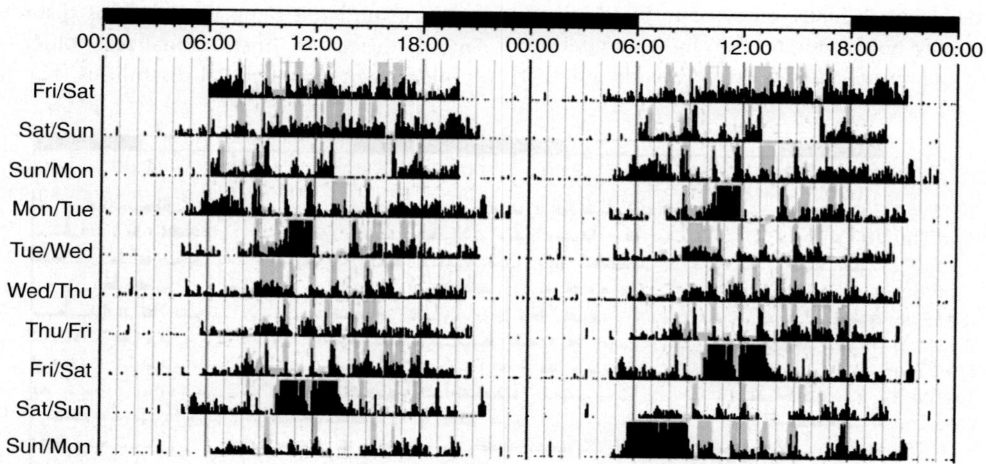

Figure 8-4.
An example of the rest-activity cycle in a patient with advanced sleep phase disorder recorded with wrist activity monitoring. This patient has a sleep onset time ranging between 8 and 9 P.M. and a wake time between 4 and 5 A.M. on most days.

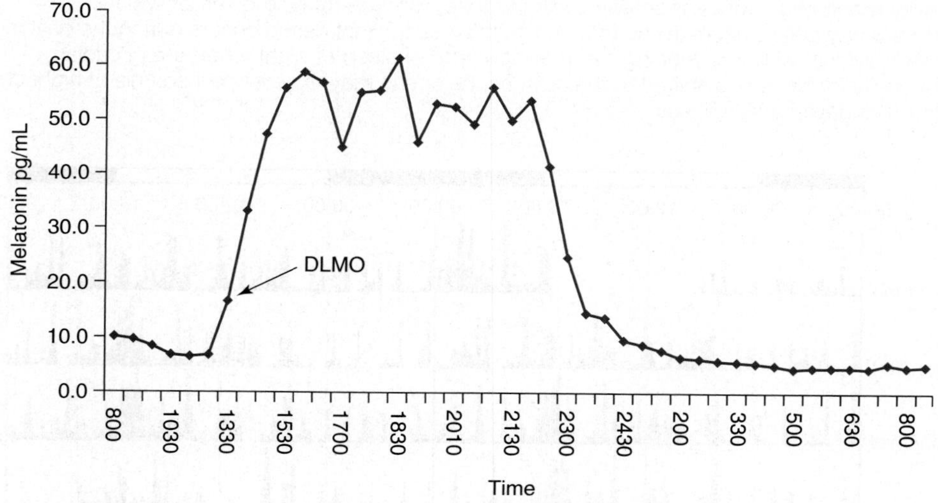

Figure 8-5.
This 24-hour profile of melatonin levels indicates that this patient has a dim light melatonin onset (DLMO) at about 2 P.M. *(arrow)*, which is much earlier than normal (8 to 10 P.M.). Since sleep onset usually occurs about 2 hours after the DLMO, this person will likely be very sleepy at around 4 in the afternoon.

Free-running Disorder/Nonentrained Disorder

Free-running disorder is characterized by a progressive delay in the circadian clock and the sleep-wake cycle that results in insomnia and sleepiness depending on when sleep is attempted in relation to the phase of the circadian clock. This disorder is most commonly seen in blind individuals but has also been reported after brain injury and in normal-sighted individuals (Fig. 8-6).

Treatment of free-running disorder depends on the timing of the circadian clock relative to the desired bedtime. Since this disorder is usually reported in blind individuals who may or may not have circadian light perception, melatonin is most commonly used to treat this disorder. If the patient free-runs, treatment usually starts when the patient's sleep-wake cycle has reached the desired time. At this point, melatonin is given about an hour before desired bedtime, in conjunction with keeping a regular sleep and work schedule to try to entrain the sleep-wake cycle to the desired time.

Irregular Sleep-Wake Disorder

Patients with irregular sleep-wake disorder have at least three sleep periods across the day and night and lack a single consolidated sleep period. This disorder is most commonly seen in institutionalized older adults and in children with intellectual disabilities (Fig. 8-7).

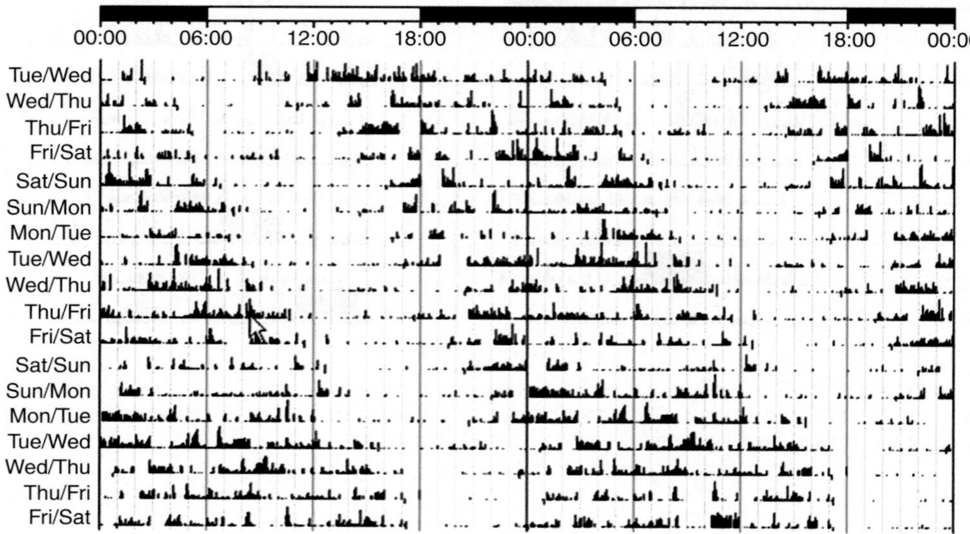

Figure 8-6.
An example of the rest-activity cycle in a patient with free-running disorder recorded with wrist activity monitoring. The rest-activity cycle in those with free-running disorder typically progressively delays each day so that at certain times the rest period occurs during the daytime. If the individual with free-running disorder attempts to sleep at night when the circadian propensity for sleep has shifted to the daytime, he or she may experience insomnia at night and excessive daytime sleepiness.

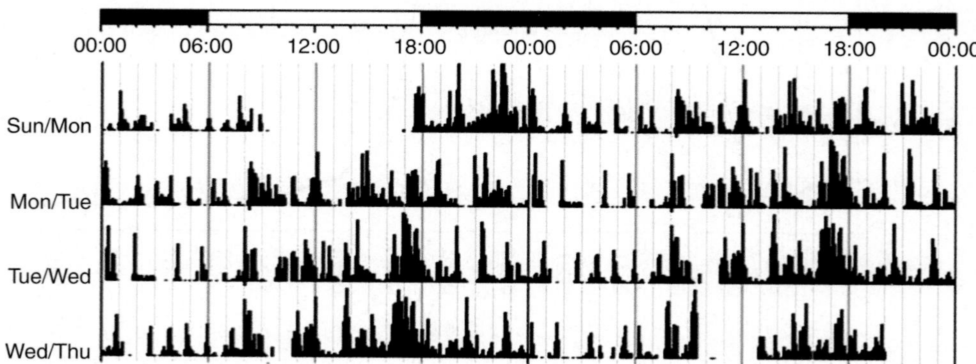

Figure 8-7.
An example of the rest-activity cycle in a 75-year-old woman with irregular sleep-wake disorder recorded with wrist activity monitoring. Unlike the other rest-activity cycles shown there is no consolidated sleep period; instead, there are multiple short naps/sleeps across the 24-hour period.

Treatment for irregular sleep-wake disorder aims to consolidate the nocturnal sleep period. Several approaches have been used, including increasing the exposure to circadian zeitgebers such as light and activity levels. In children with intellectual disabilities melatonin administration has been successful.

Shift Work Sleep Disorder

Shift work sleep disorder is characterized by insomnia and sleepiness that is associated with the work schedule. This sleep disturbance should not be better explained by another current sleep disorder, medical or neurologic disorder, mental disorder, medication use, or substance use disorder. The prevalence of shift work sleep disorder is estimated to be about 10% of the night and rotating shift work population (Fig. 8-8).

Treatment for shift work sleep disorder aims to phase-shift (usually delay) the circadian clock so that the patient is able to be alert at night and sleep during the day. This can be achieved in several ways. It is recommended that night workers try to avoid bright light on the commute home from work, as light at this time will phase-advance the circadian clock. Bright light exposure during the first part of the night shift has been successful in improving alertness at night due to the immediate alerting effects of light, as well as phase-delaying the circadian clock. Alternatively, symptoms are treated using stimulants to keep people alert at night while they are working and hypnotics to help them sleep during the day.

Jet Lag Sleep Disorder

Jet lag sleep disorder is characterized by a complaint of insomnia or excessive daytime sleepiness associated with transmeridian jet travel across at least two time zones, which is associated with impaired daytime function, general malaise, or somatic symptoms such as gastrointestinal disturbance within 1 to 2 days of travel. This sleep disturbance should not be better explained by another current sleep disorder, medical or neurologic disorder, mental disorder, medication use, or substance use disorder. The most commonly reported symptoms of jet lag include disturbed sleep and fatigue during the day.

Jet lag can be treated by speeding the adjustment of the circadian clock to the new time zone or by treating the symptoms of insomnia and sleepiness. An example of how to speed the phase adjustment to an eastward flight is described in Figure 8-9. It has even been recommended that, if possible, the adjustment to the new time zone start prior to departure. Table 8-1 provides a summary of the clinical presentation, preferred sleep-wake times, and treatment options for each of the circadian rhythm sleep disorders.

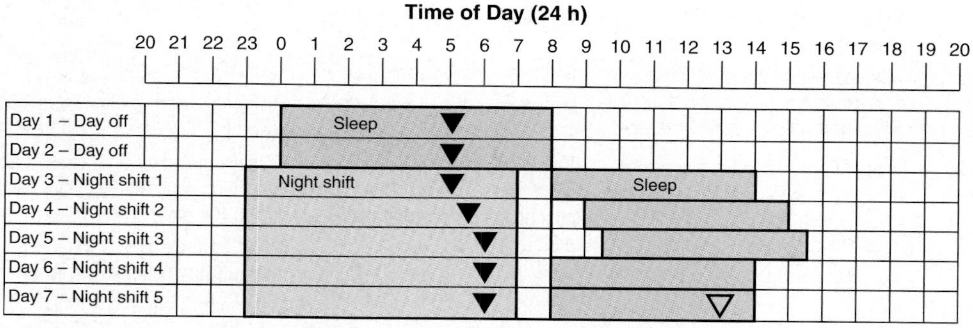

Figure 8-8.
This figure illustrates changes in the timing of the circadian clock in a typical night worker. Sleep periods are represented by the purple bars. Night shift work periods are represented by the pink bars. The triangles represent the timing of the T_{min}. The black triangles show where the T_{min} is likely to be on each day. The open triangle shows where the T_{min} needs to phase-delay to for complete re-entrainment to occur. The symptoms caused by the misalignment between the daytime sleep period and the circadian clock will diminish greatly if the T_{min} falls within the daytime sleep period. Because the circadian clock does not shift quickly, the shift worker is sleeping during the day when the core temperature rhythm is high. As a result, night workers do not typically sleep as long during the day, so that the daytime sleep periods are only about 6 hours long. (Adapted from Reid KJ, Burgess HL: Circadian sleep disorders. Primary Care: Clinics in Office Practice 32[2]:449–473, 2005.)

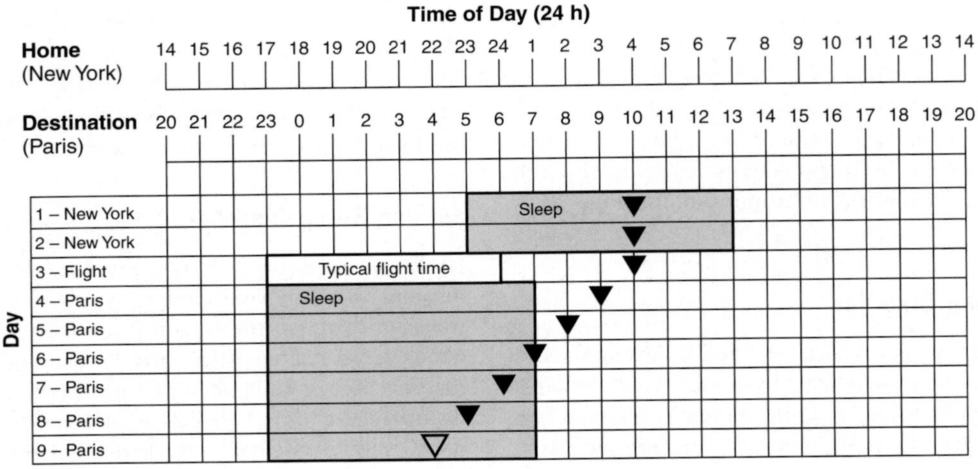

Figure 8-9.
This figure illustrates the circadian misalignment that will occur following an eastward flight from New York to Paris. The purple bars represent sleep times. The home and transitional T_{mins} are shown as black triangles. The open triangle represents the new timing of the T_{min} once full re-entrainment is achieved. In this figure, the T_{min} is advancing at a rate of 1 hour per day and jet lag will be felt for approximately 4 to 5 days. A faster rate of phase advancing, at, say, about 1.5 hours per day, might occur if every day the traveler received minimal light in the 3 hours before his or her T_{min} (by sleeping or wearing dark sunglasses) and maximal light in the 3 hours after his or her T_{min} (by going outside to receive light). Exogenous melatonin, if taken 10 to 12 hours before the T_{min}, could also help hasten the phase advance. (Adapted from Reid KJ, Burgess HL: Circadian sleep disorders. Primary Care: Clinics in Office Practice 32[2]:449–473, 2005.)

Table 8-1. Summary of the Clinical Presentation, Preferred Sleep-Wake Times, and Treatment Options for Each of the Circadian Rhythm Sleep Disorders

CIRCADIAN RHYTHM SLEEP DISORDER	CLINICAL PRESENTATION	PREFERRED SLEEP-WAKE TIMES	TREATMENT OPTIONS
Delayed sleep phase disorder	Difficulty falling asleep at the desired time Difficulty waking up in the morning Morning sleepiness	Bedtime: 2–6 A.M. Waketime: 10 A.M. – 1 P.M.	Bright light therapy: 2000–2500 lux for 2–3 hr starting from 6 A.M.; dark goggles from 4 P.M. to dusk (optional) Melatonin: 0.3–3 mg at night, 5–7 hr before habitual sleep time
Advanced sleep phase disorder	Early evening sleepiness Waking up too early in the morning	Bedtime: 6 to 9 P.M. Waketime: 2 to 5 P.M.	Bright light therapy: 2500 lux for 4 hr starting from 8 P.M. or 4000 lux for 2–3 hr starting from 8–9 P.M.
Free-running disorder/ Nonentrained disorder	Alternating periods of insomnia and excessive sleepiness or both, with short asymptomatic periods	Bedtime: delayed each day Waketime: delayed each day	Sleep hygiene Melatonin: 10 mg 1 hr before bedtime; maintenance dose of 0.5 mg 1–2 hr before desired bedtime
Irregular sleep-wake disorder	Insomnia or excessive sleepiness	Irregular pattern of sleep and wake times with no consolidated nocturnal sleep period	Increase circadian time cues such as social interaction, physical activities, and light exposure during the day Bright light therapy: 2500–3000 lux for 2 hr in the morning has been shown to be effective Melatonin: 3 mg at 6:30 P.M.
Shift work sleep disorder	Difficulty falling asleep or maintaining sleep associated with the work schedule Sleepiness at work		Bright light therapy: 5000–10,000 lux beginning early during night shift and terminating 2 hr before end of shift (continuous or intermittent); avoidance of morning bright light with dark goggles Melatonin: 1–3 mg before bedtime Wake-promoting agents: caffeine (avoid caffeine close to bedtime) or modafinil Strategic short naps: during work if allowed
Jet lag sleep disorder	Sleep initiation and maintenance insomnia Daytime sleepiness Decreased performance Gastrointestinal complaints		Timed light exposure: on eastward flights, minimize morning light and maximize afternoon light; on westward flights, stay awake while it is light out Melatonin: 2–5 mg before bedtime upon arrival; repeat up to 4 nights Hypnotics: zolpidem 10 mg, up to 3 nights

SELECTED READINGS

Drake CL, Roehrs T, Richardson G, et al: Shift work sleep disorder: Prevalence and consequences beyond that of symptomatic day workers. Sleep 27(8):1453–1462, 2004.

Hayakawa T, Uchiyama M, Kamei Y, et al: Clinical analyses of sighted patients with non-24-hour sleep-wake syndrome: A study of 57 consecutively diagnosed cases. Sleep 28(8):945–952, 2005.

Lack L, Wright H: The effect of evening bright light in delaying the circadian rhythms and lengthening the sleep of early morning awakening insomniacs. Sleep 16(5):436–443, 1993.

Lockley SW, Skene DJ, James K, et al: Melatonin administration can entrain the free-running circadian system of blind subjects. J Endocrinol 164(1):R1–R6, 2000.

Nagtegaal JE, Kerkhof GA, Smits MG, et al: Delayed sleep phase syndrome: A placebo-controlled cross-over study on the effects of melatonin administered five hours before the individual dim light melatonin onset. J Sleep Res 7(2):135–143, 1998.

Okawa M, Mishima K, Hishikawa Y, et al: Circadian rhythm disorders in sleep-waking and body temperature in elderly patients with dementia and their treatment. Sleep 14(6):478–485, 1991.

Reid KJ, Burgess HJ: Circadian rhythm sleep disorders. Prim Care 32(2): 449–473, 2005.

Rosenthal NE, Joseph-Vanderpool JR, Levendosky AA, et al: Phase-shifting effects of bright morning light as treatment for delayed sleep phase syndrome. Sleep 13(4):354–361, 1990.

Sateia M (ed): The International Classification of Sleep Disorders: Diagnostic and Coding Manual, 2nd ed. Westchester, Ill., American Academy of Sleep Medicine, 2005.

Schrader H, Bovim G, Sand T: The prevalence of delayed and advanced sleep phase syndromes. J Sleep Res 2(1):51–55, 1993.

Weitzman ED, Czeisler CA, Coleman RM, et al: Delayed sleep phase syndrome: A chronobiological disorder with sleep-onset insomnia. Arch Gen Psychiatry 38(7):737–746, 1981.

CHAPTER 9

INSOMNIA

Meir Kryger and Thomas Roth

Introduction

The term *insomnia* refers to a symptom. It also refers to disorders, as defined in several diagnostic systems, in which the presenting features include difficulty sleeping at night and impaired functioning during the day (Box 9-1).

The daytime consequences of insomnia include impaired cognitive function, fatigue or tiredness, depressed mood or irritability, and, in adults, impaired performance at work, and, in children, poor performance in school.

Patients with insomnia are often evaluated in sleep disorder centers. In the diagnosis and management of such cases polysomnography (PSG) is not routinely indicated, unless the insomnia is thought to be comorbid with specific conditions in which diagnostic findings with PSG might help guide management.

BOX 9-1. CRITERIA FOR DEFINING INSOMNIA

- Difficulty falling asleep, *or*
- Difficulty staying asleep, *or*
- Early-morning awakening, *or*
- Nonrefreshing or nonrestorative sleep.

With daytime consequences or distress lasting at least 1 month despite opportunity and circumstances to sleep.

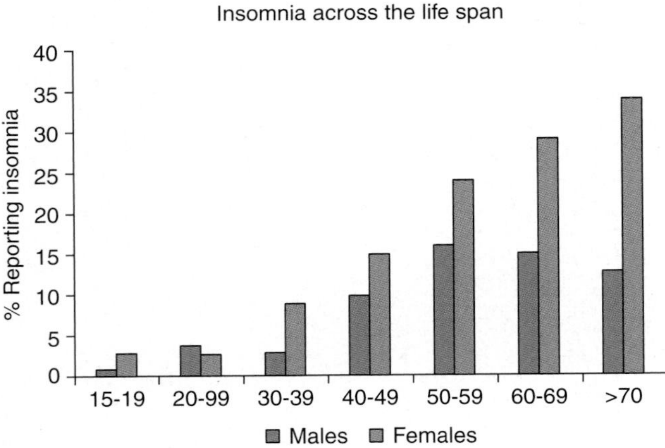

Figure 9-1.
The percentages of men and women who report insomnia. Insomnia is more common in women than in men in all age groups. (Based on data and adapted from Ohayon MM, Caulet M, Guilleminault C: How a general population perceives its sleep and how this relates to the complaint of insomnia. Sleep 20[9]:715–723, 1997.)

Classification

There is a great deal of confusion about the classification of insomnia, because there are at least three diagnostic classifications in widespread use, and the various classifications are inconsistent in their terminology. The three classifications are the *International Classification of Sleep Disorders: Diagnostic and Coding Manual* (2nd ed.) (*ICSD-2*), the *Diagnostic and Statistical Manual of Mental Disorders* (4th ed.) (*DSM-IV*), and the *International Statistical Classification of Diseases* (*ICD*). Adding to the confusion is a document produced by a National Institutes of Health state-of-the-art consensus conference on insomnia, which produced new definitions. This conference codified in general terms two types of insomnia, insomnia that is *comorbid* (i.e., associated with another medical or psychiatric condition, which is the case 80% to 90% of the time), and *primary insomnia,* the suggested term to be used when there is no coexisting disorder. In this chapter we focus on patients with insomnia symptoms who are evaluated most often in sleep disorder centers.

Epidemiology

About 30% to 40% of adults have some degree of disturbed sleep during the year. About 10% to 13% meet diagnostic criteria for insomnia. The most important risk factors for insomnia are gender and age (Fig. 9-1). Of patients with insomnia the most common complaints are nonrefreshing sleep and frequent awakenings. Patients often have more than one symptom (Fig. 9-2).

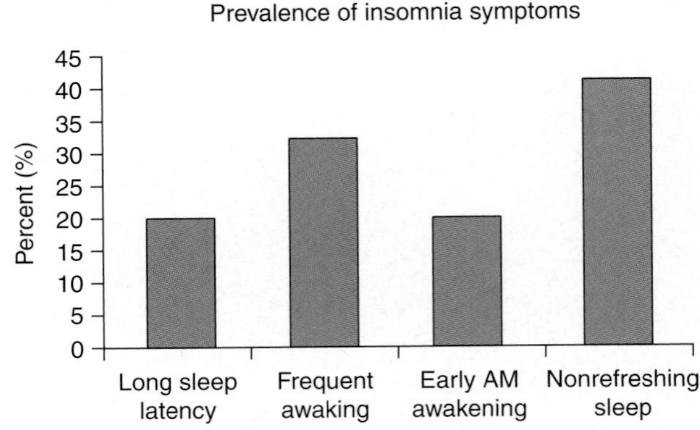

Figure 9-2.
Of the main insomnia symptoms the most common is nonrefreshing sleep. Note that the prevalences add up to more than 100%; therefore many patients have more than one insomnia symptom. (Adapted from Ancoli-Israel S, Roth T: Characteristics of insomnia in the United States: Results of the 1991 National Sleep Foundation Survey: I. Sleep 22[Suppl 2]:S347–S353, 1999.)

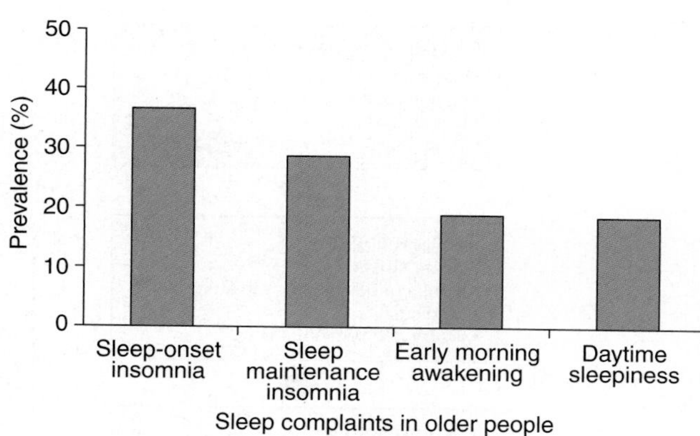

Figure 9-3.
Complaints about sleep are common in an older community dwelling sample of 1050 people. The most common main complaint was difficulty falling asleep. Approximately 2 years later, the same cohort was surveyed (see Fig. 9-4). (Data from Ganguli M, Reynolds CF, Gilby JE: Prevalence and persistence of sleep complaints in a rural older community sample: The MoVIES project. J Am Geriatr Soc 44:778–784, 1996.)

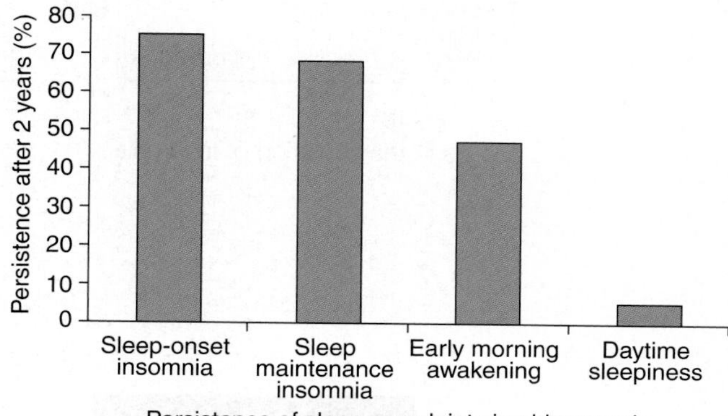

Figure 9-4.
Complaints about sleep, especially insomnia, persist in older people after 2 years. This is also true in younger people with insomnia. (Data from Ganguli M, Reynolds CF, Gilby JE: Prevalence and persistence of sleep complaints in a rural older community sample: The MoVIES project. J Am Geriatr Soc 44:778–784, 1996.)

The most common sleep complaint of older patients is sleep-onset insomnia (Fig. 9-3). Insomnia tends to persist for years. When patients were surveyed after 2 years, it was found that most continued to suffer from insomnia (Fig. 9-4).

Pathophysiology of Insomnia

Insomnia was once thought to be a symptom secondary to another condition, and that the other condition was the primary disorder (e.g., depression, COPD) and caused the difficulty falling asleep or the awakenings and arousals. Although no single model explains all insomnia, some theories and models are helpful. Spielman's 3P model is useful in helping us understand the evolution of insomnia.

Predisposing factors	What makes people more prone to develop insomnia? Physiologic and cognitive hyper-responsivity, the key pathophysiologic factor in insomnia
Precipitating factors	What acute events trigger insomnia? Medical, psychiatric, sleep, and circadian disorders, as well as life stressors
Perpetuating factors	What keeps insomnia from resolving? Behavioral and cognitive maladaptive responses to disturbed sleep

The factors form the basis of a more complex model for explaining the evolution of insomnia (Fig. 9-5).

One of the underlying assumptions of current theories is that insomnia patients are in a state of hyperarousal over the 24-hour period and that this hyperarousal leads patients to develop sleep disturbances when stressed. This may also be the basis for why not all patients with certain medical conditions (e.g., COPD) will develop insomnia and leads to a better understanding of comorbid insomnia as a concept. According to this view, the insomnia often predates the comorbid condition and is not fully resolved when the comorbid condition is resolved.

Imaging studies suggest that the hyperaroused brain of insomnia patients does not reduce its metabolic rate with sleep (Fig. 9-6). Research also supports the notion that the hyperarousal state results in measurable changes in physiologic systems, not just the nervous system (Fig. 9-7).

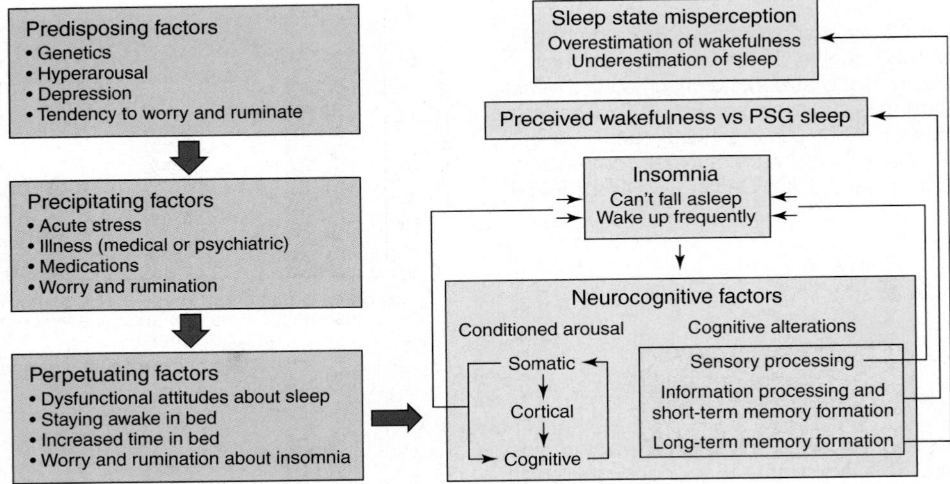

Figure 9-5.
Steps in the evolution of insomnia.

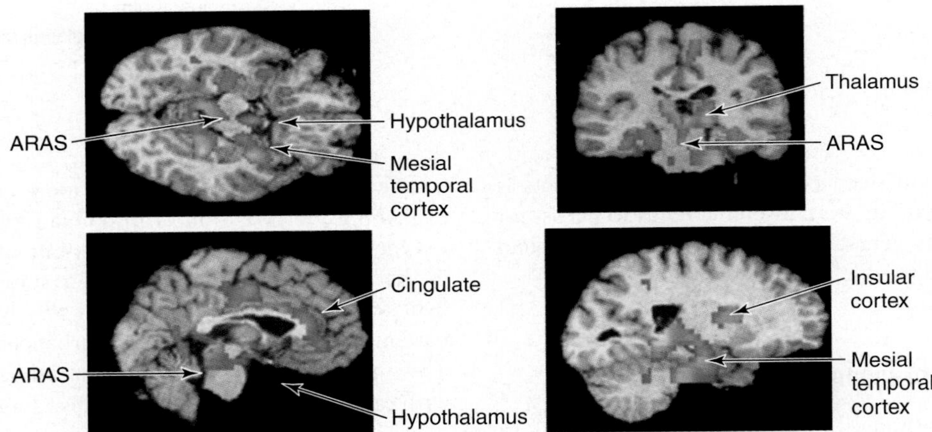

Figure 9-6.
Hyperarousal in insomnia. The red and yellow areas show that regions of the brain that are normally wake-promoting do not decrease their metabolic rate with sleep. ^{18}F (fluorodeoxyglucose) positron emission tomography was used to evaluate regional glucose metabolism in the brain. This suggests that the brains of patients with insomnia are hyperaroused. ARAS, ascending reticular activating system. (Nofzinger EA, Buysse DJ, Germain A, et al: Functional neuroimaging evidence for hyperarousal in insomnia. Am J Psychiatry 161[11]:2126–2128, 2004.)

Types of Insomnia

The insomnia features described in Box 9-1 are found in three groups of patients (Fig. 9-8):

A. *Comorbid insomnia*. Patients in whom a medical or psychiatric condition coexists with the insomnia.

B. *Primary sleep disorders*. Patients in whom the primary sleep disorder may include symptoms of insomnia.

C. *Primary insomnia*. Patients in whom insomnia exists in the absence of a psychiatric or medical disorder.

Figure 9-7.
Studies have documented a hyperarousal state in insomnia patients. There are increases in cortisol (hypothalamic-pituitary activation), increases in heart rate response (sympathetic nervous system activation), an increased 24-hour metabolic rate, and changes indicating increased metabolic rate in regions of the brain promoting wakefulness.

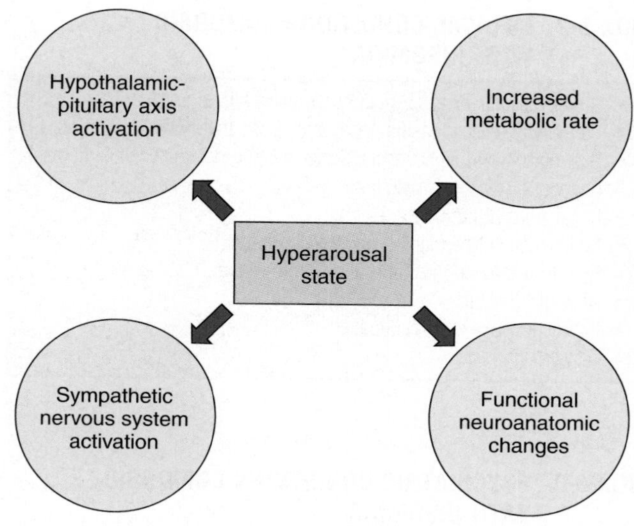

Figure 9-8.
Approximate distribution of types of insomnia. Those with primary insomnia make up but a small portion of the population of people with insomnia. (Data from Ford DE, Kamerow DB: Epidemiologic study of sleep disturbances and psychiatric disorders: An opportunity for prevention? JAMA 262[11]:1479–1484, 1989.)

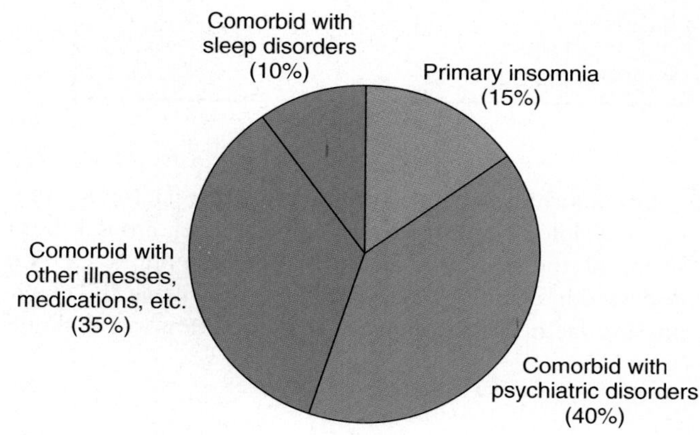

COMORBID INSOMNIA

Comorbid insomnia refers to patients who have a medical or psychiatric condition and who also have insomnia symptoms (Fig. 9-9). Some of the diseases that frequently have comorbid insomnia are listed in Boxes 9-2 and 9-3. The term *secondary insomnia,* previously used to refer to such conditions, is not always accurate. The implication when using that term is that when the disease is treated the insomnia always resolves. Typically that does not happen. For example, in patients successfully treated for depression, insomnia is the most common refractory symptom.

Figure 9-9.
In a study of 3445 patients with chronic medical conditions a substantial proportion of patients with common comorbidities had mild or severe insomnia even in the absence of depression. The mean age of the studied population of patients was 54 years. (Data from Katz DA, McHorney CA: Clinical correlates of insomnia in patients with chronic illness. Arch Intern Med 158:1099–1107, 1998.)

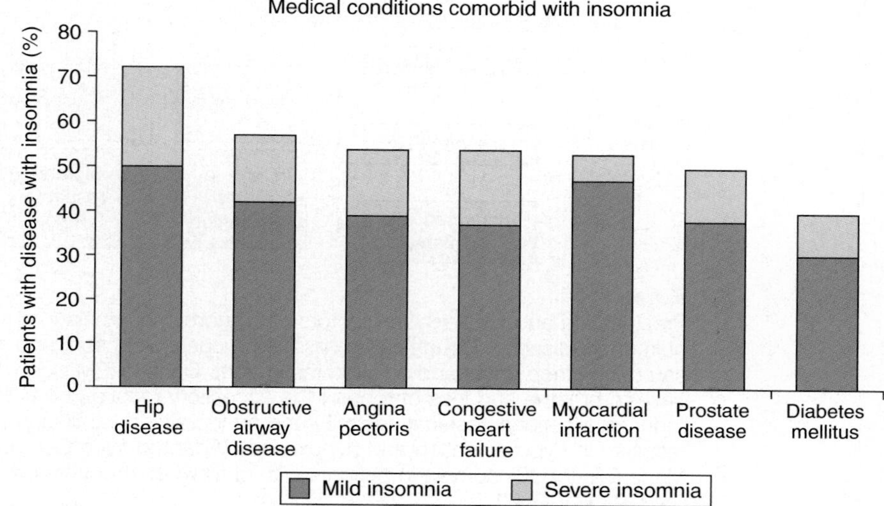

BOX 9-2. MEDICAL CONDITIONS COMORBID WITH INSOMNIA

- Cardiovascular disease (congestive heart failure and stroke)
- Pulmonary disease (asthma, chronic obstructive pulmonary disease)
- Gastrointestinal (peptic ulcer disease, gastroesophageal reflux disease)
- Endocrine (diabetes mellitus)
- Renal (renal failure)
- Neurologic (Alzheimer's, Parkinson's disease)
- Pain from any source (arthritis, fibromyalgia)
- Urologic (nocturia)
- Perimenopause and menopause
- Cancer

BOX 9-3. PSYCHIATRIC CONDITIONS COMORBID WITH INSOMNIA

- Anxiety disorder
- Depression
- Schizophrenia
- Alcohol and drug abuse

In comorbid insomnia, the precipitating factor is often the physiologic consequence (typically an arousal from sleep) of the comorbid disorder. An example is COPD, discussed in chapter 11.3. Figure 9-10 shows that the precipitating factor for insomnia in this condition is a biologic response to the disorder that disturbs sleep (e.g., cough, dyspnea), and that with treatment, some of the COPD perpetuating factors may be resolved, only to be replaced by other perpetuating factors, for example, medications (bronchodilators and corticosteroids) and some of the psychophysiologic factors mentioned above. Thus, in some individuals (those predisposed to insomnia), the COPD-related arousal will lead to insomnia, whereas in those not so predisposed, the COPD will result in only a brief arousal with a rapid return to sleep.

Similarly, in congestive heart failure (Fig. 9-11), the abnormal breathing pattern can initiate insomnia. Therapy for heart failure may improve the breathing pattern, but the low cardiac output state could still be associated with increased catecholamine levels that could interfere with sleep and cause hyperarousal.

Sleep difficulties are present in most patients with psychiatric disorders, and, indeed, it is estimated that about 40% of all patients with insomnia have a coexisting psychiatric problem (see Box 9-3). These sleep complaints of insomnia patients are related to both their disease and the treatment of their disease (see chapter 16). Anxiety disorder is the most common disease comorbid with insomnia seen in clinical practice (Fig. 9-12).

In depressed patients (Fig. 9-13) and in patients with primary insomnia one may find evidence of hyperarousal in the sleep electroencephalogram (EEG) (Fig. 9-14). At times medications can alter the hypnogram of patients with depression (Fig. 9-15).

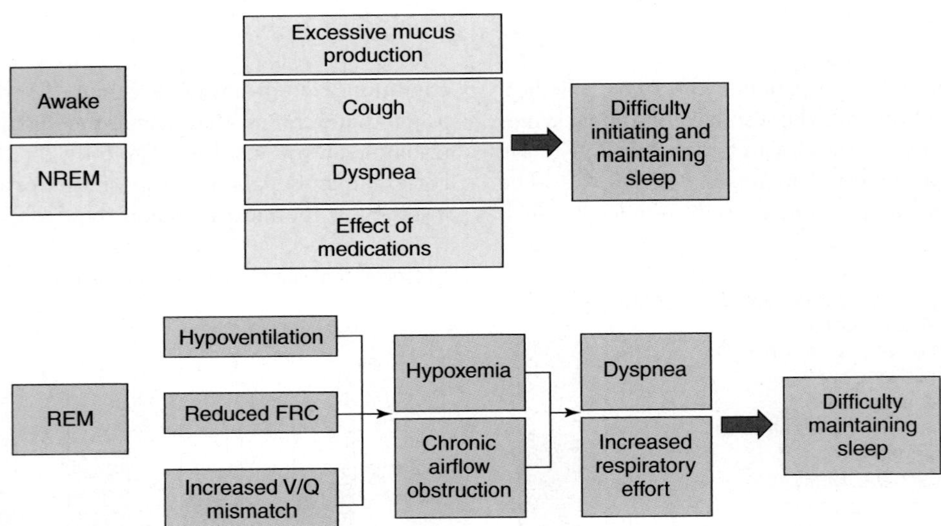

Figure 9-10.
Precipitating and perpetuating factors of comorbid insomnia in chronic obstructive pulmonary disease. Coughing, excessive mucus production, and effects of medications can delay sleep onset and awaken the patient. During REM sleep there is a blunting of the drive to breathe and loss of tone of the accessory respiratory muscles, which leads to reduced functional residual capacity and an increased ventilation-perfusion mismatch resulting in hypoventilation and hypoxemia. (Adapted from George CF, Bayliff CD: Management of insomnia in patients with chronic obstructive pulmonary disease. Drugs 63:379–387, 2003.)

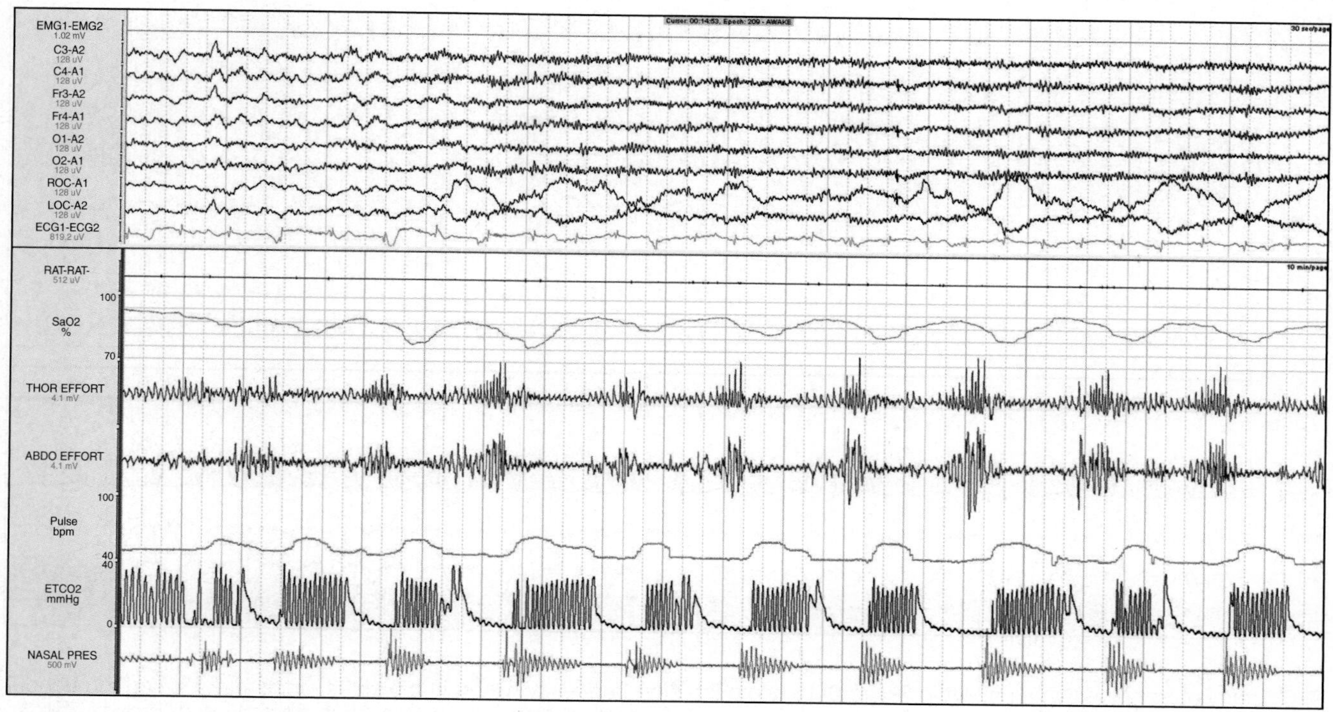

Figure 9-11.
The top panel is an epoch of 30 seconds showing wakefulness. The bottom is 10 minutes. This patient had congestive heart failure and awake Cheyne Stokes breathing episodes with quite significant oxygen desaturations. Note the small blips in the end-tidal CO_2 during some of the apneic/hypopneic episodes. These are cardiogenic oscillations. This patient was not able to achieve persistent sleep despite severe sleepiness because he kept waking up during the hyperpneic episodes.

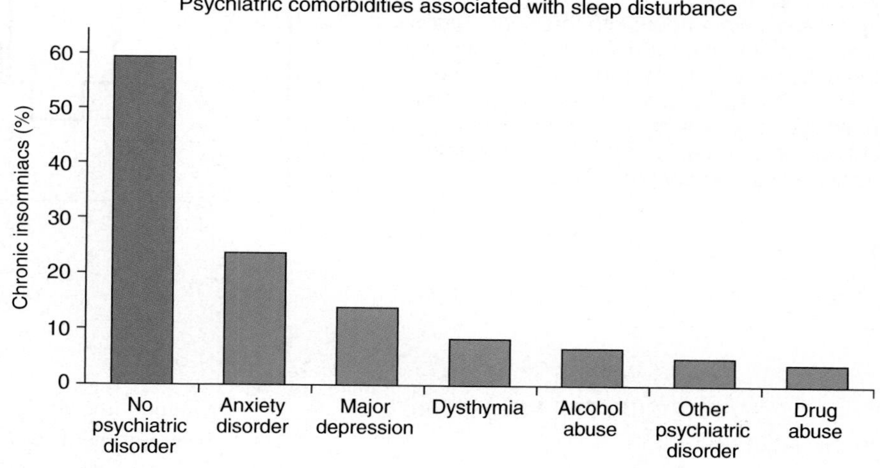

Figure 9-12.
Psychiatric comorbidities associated with insomnia. Insomnia is found in most psychiatric disorders. About 40% of chronic insomniacs have comorbid psychiatric disease. Anxiety disorders are the most common psychiatric comorbidities associated with insomnia, followed by depression. (Data from Ford DE, Kamerow DB: Epidemiologic study of sleep disturbances and psychiatric disorders: An opportunity for prevention? JAMA 262[11]:1479–1484, 1989.)

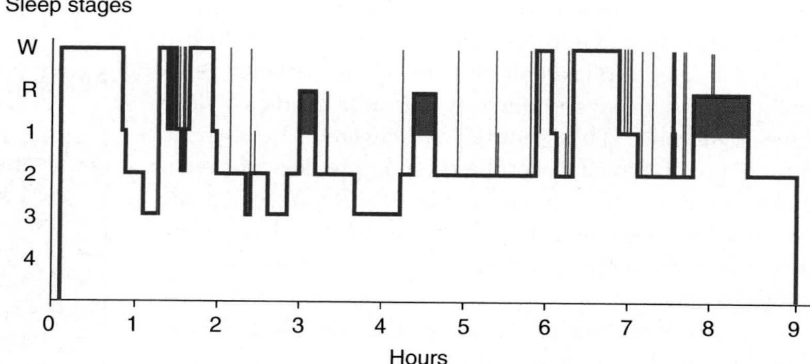

Figure 9-13.
Hypnogram of sleep onset and sleep maintenance insomnia in a 23-year-old male patient with untreated depression. Note the long sleep latency and several prolonged episodes of wakefulness during sleep. Depression cannot be diagnosed from a sleep study.

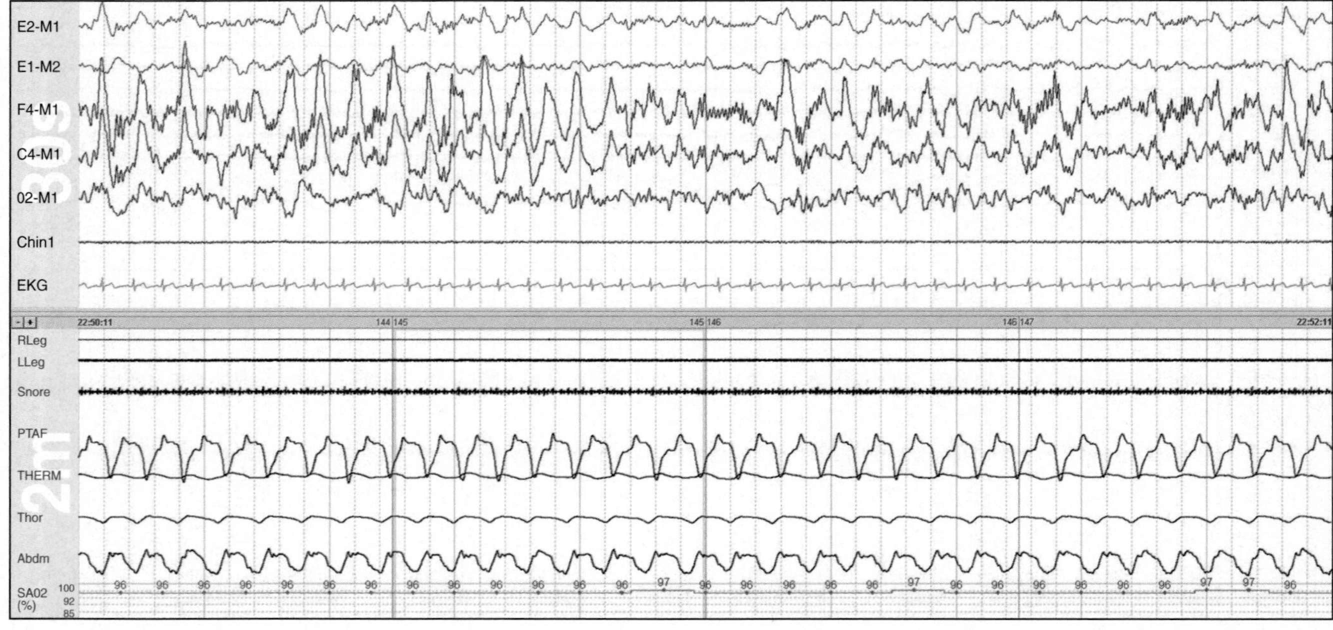

Figure 9-14.
PSG fragment from the same patient in Figure 9-13. Note the high-frequency waves in the alpha range interspersed throughout the EEG. Although this finding is not uncommon, it is not specific or diagnostic for depression or other sleep disorders. This may be a manifestation of hyperarousal.

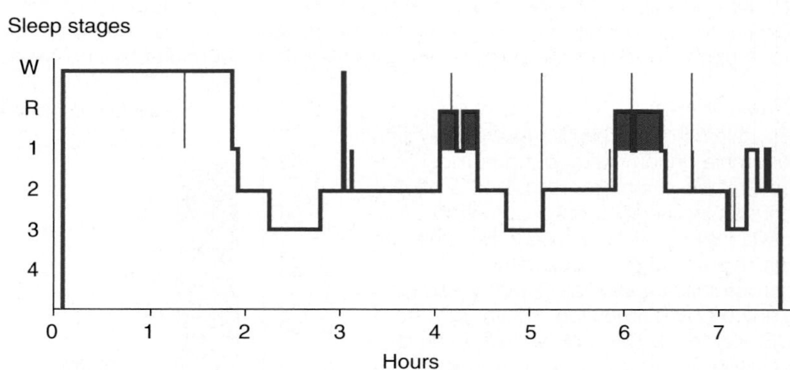

Figure 9-15.
PSG fragment in a depressed patient complaining of insomnia who is being treated with an antidepressant. Notice that the first REM episode occurs 4 hours into the night. This is likely related to the REM-suppressing effects of the antidepressant. Note the very long sleep latency. Once asleep the patient did not have prolonged awakenings. In some patients antidepressant medications can cause motor restlessness (see chapter 16).

PRIMARY SLEEP DISORDERS PRESENTING WITH INSOMNIA

Several primary sleep disorders often have insomnia as the presenting complaint. This is a classic symptom in patients with restless legs syndrome (see chapter 10.2). Disturbed sleep is a feature of narcolepsy, and many patients, especially women, have insomnia as a manifestation of sleep apnea syndrome. These entities are covered elsewhere in this volume. Delayed sleep phase syndrome does not technically fit the criteria for insomnia because, although the patients may complain of difficulty in falling asleep, when they are given ample opportunity to sleep, their sleep is in fact normal.

It is also important to remember that circadian rhythm disorders, such as phase advance and delay syndromes and shift work, virtually always present with insomnia symptoms (Box 9-4). Patients with sleep apnea may present with insomnia, giving them a characteristic hypnogram and overnight oximetry (Fig. 9-16).

BOX 9-4. PRIMARY SLEEP DISORDERS THAT MAY PRESENT WITH INSOMNIA

- Movement disorder (e.g., restless legs syndrome, periodic limb movements in sleep)
- Obstructive sleep apnea syndrome
- Narcolepsy
- Central sleep apnea syndrome
- Cheyne Stokes respiration
- Delayed sleep phase syndrome

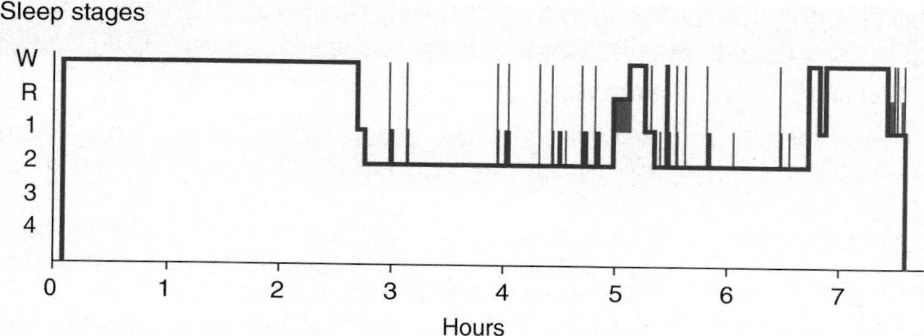

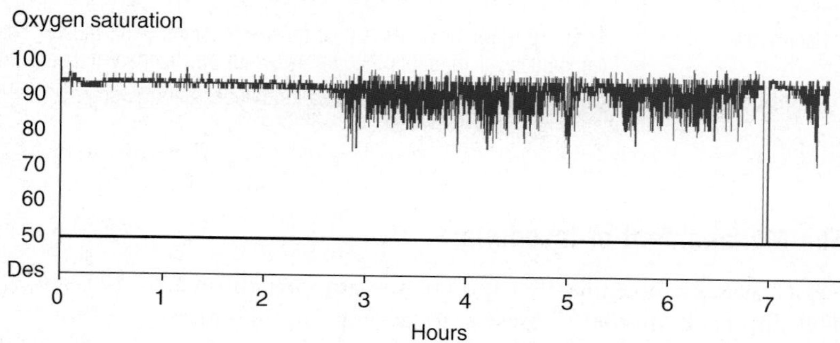

Figure 9-16.
Hypnogram and overnight oximetry in a patient complaining of insomnia who also has obstructive sleep apnea. Notice the very long sleep latency during which time oxygen saturation is stable. Once asleep the large changes in oxygen saturation caused by back-to-back apneas are apparent. The SaO_2 is lowest in the brief episodes of REM sleep. The patient has a prolonged awakening toward morning.

PRIMARY INSOMNIA

Primary insomnia, the term suggested by the National Institutes of Health consensus conference, means insomnia without a coexisting disorder. The insomnia disorders as classified by ICSD-2 are listed in Table 9-1 in the order of how often they are seen in the sleep disorder centers.

Polysomnograms are not generally done in cases of primary insomnia, except for paradoxical insomnia, in which the findings are usually normal. In the other diagnostic categories are long sleep latency, increased wake after sleep onset, increased awakenings during the night, and evidence of arousal on EEG (see Fig. 9-14). The hypnogram is useful in getting a snapshot of the entire night of such patients (Fig. 9-17).

Table 9-1. Primary Insomnia Types

CATEGORY	ESSENTIAL DIAGNOSTIC FEATURES
Psychophysiologic insomnia	Hyperarousal and learned sleep-preventing associations that result in a complaint of insomnia
Inadequate sleep hygiene	Insomnia caused by lifestyle and activities that interfere with sleep
Idiopathic insomnia	Lifelong insomnia often begun during infancy or early childhood
Paradoxical insomnia	Complaint of severe insomnia that occurs without object evidence of abnormal sleep; such patients typically have little daytime impairment; also called "sleep state misperception"
Adjustment sleep disorder	Insomnia related to an identifiable stressor; usually short term

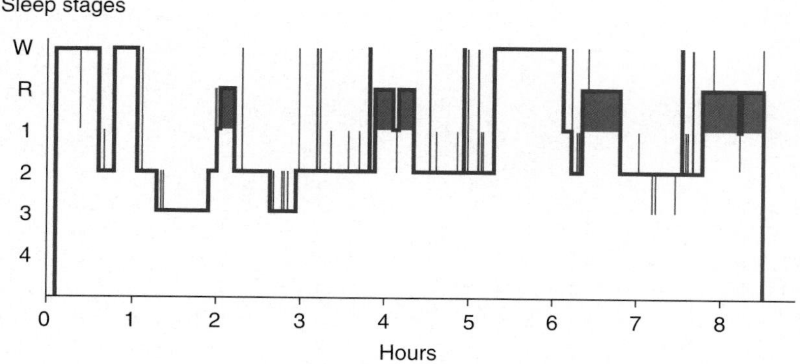

Figure 9-17.
PSG fragment in a 34-year-old male patient complaining of long-standing insomnia. There are no medical comorbidities or psychopathology. He has sleep-onset and middle-of-the-night insomnia, and many awakenings during the night.

Table 9.2. Components of Cognitive-Behavioral Therapy

TECHNIQUE	INVOLVES	TREATS
Sleep hygiene education	**Review:** diet, exercise, alcohol, and environmental factors that may help or interfere with sleep; importance of regular bedtime and setime and the negative effects of long naps	Lifestyle and behaviors that are hurdles to good quality sleep
Stimulus control	**Teach patient to:** go to bed only when sleepy; get out of bed when unable to sleep and when sleepy stop all sleep-incompatible activities (e.g., TV in bed, using computer electronics before bedtime)	The learned associations of bed with wakefulness
Sleep restriction	**Emphasize:** the importance of reducing time in bed to actual sleep time	Disrupted and fragmented sleep related to too much time in bed
Relaxation	**Teach patient how to:** reduce muscle tensions (e.g., muscle relaxation techniques) or thoughts that will not shut off (imagery training, meditation)	Increased hyperarousal (physiologic, cognitive, or emotional)
Cognitive	**Correct:** the inaccurate beliefs and attitudes about insomnia	Incorrect information and misconceptions that are perpetuating the problem

The Management of Insomnia

Most cases of insomnia that require therapy are chronic. The approach in these cases is to attempt to minimize the perpetuating factors. In comorbid insomnia we treat the comorbid condition while also focusing on the behavioral and psychological perpetuating factors. The modification of the behavioral factors sometimes can be quite simple (improving sleep hygiene, reducing caffeine intake, etc.), but in many cases, a more formal cognitive-behavioral intervention is helpful (Table 9-2). If a cognitive-behavioral intervention is not available, or if the patient still has severe insomnia after the cognitive-behavioral intervention has been tried, then the use of hypnotics is considered (see chapter 5). In any case, in all patients sleep hygiene should be reviewed and discussed.

SELECTED READINGS

American Psychiatric Association. Diagnostic and Statistical Manual of Mental Disorders, 4th ed. Washington, D.C., American Psychiatric Association, 1994.

Breslau N, Roth T, Rosenthal L, Andreski P: Sleep disturbance and psychiatric disorders: A longitudinal epidemiological study of young adults. Biol Psychiatry 39(6):411–418, 1996.

Chang PP, Ford DE, Mead LA, et al: Insomnia in young men and subsequent depression: The Johns Hopkins Precursors Study. Am J Epidemiol 146(2):105–114, 1997.

Ford DE, Kamerow DB: Epidemiologic study of sleep disturbances and psychiatric disorders: An opportunity for prevention? JAMA 262 (11):1479–1484, 1989.

Katz DA, McHorney CA: The relationship between insomnia and health-related quality of life in patients with chronic illness. J Fam Pract 51 (3):229–235, 2002.

Leshner A: National Institutes of Health State of the Science Conference statement on Manifestations and Management of Chronic Insomnia in Adults, June 13–15, 2005. Sleep 28(9):1049–1057, 2005.

Nofzinger EA, Buysse DJ, Germain A, et al: Functional neuroimaging evidence for hyperarousal in insomnia. Am J Psychiatry 161(11):2126–2128, 2004.

Ohayon MM: Epidemiology of insomnia: What we know and what we still need to learn. Sleep Med Rev 6(2):97–111, 2002.

Perlis ML, Smith MT, Andrews PJ, et al: Beta/Gamma EEG activity in patients with primary and secondary insomnia and good sleeper controls. Sleep 24(1):110–117, 2001.

Vgontzas AN, Bixler EO, Lin HM, et al: Chronic insomnia is associated with nyctohemeral activation of the hypothalamic-pituitary-adrenal axis: Clinical implications. J Clin Endocrinol Metab 86(8):3787–3794, 2001.

NEUROLOGIC DISORDERS

CHAPTER 10

Alon Y. Avidan

10.1 Narcolepsy and Idiopathic Hypersomnia

Introduction

The first clue that a patient has severe hypersomnia is the image of the patient fast asleep waiting to be seen by the doctor (Fig. 10.1-1). When one sees a patient like this, one starts to formulate an image of the patient, what other symptoms they may have, and what etiologies may be responsible. If the patient is overweight and snoring, the focus will be on a sleep breathing disorder (see chapter 11.2). If the patient is an adolescent or young adult, the focus of etiologies switches to sleep deprivation, circadian rhythm disorders, and narcolepsy. In this chapter we review hypersomnia of central origin, that is, diseases in which abnormalities in the central nervous system lead to the symptom of falling asleep at the wrong time in the wrong place. The two most common hypersomnias of central origin are narcolepsy and idiopathic hypersomnia. In this chapter we mention others but focus on the most commonly seen clinical entities. Hypersomnias caused by other conditions are covered elsewhere in this volume.

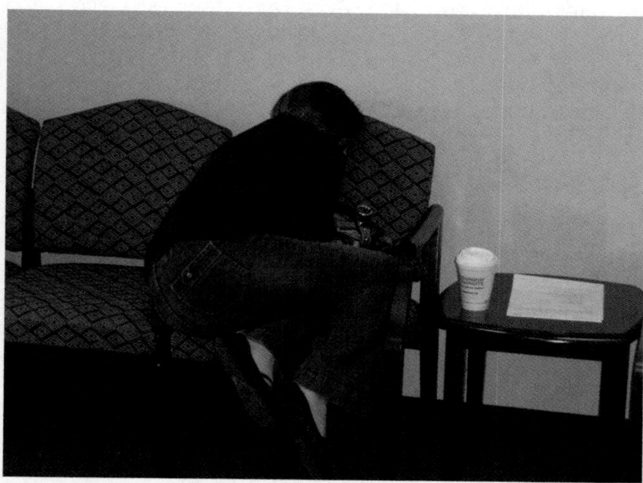

Figure 10.1-1.
This 29-year-old woman had about a 10-year history of narcolepsy that had not been previously diagnosed. The photo was taken at 2:19 in the afternoon. Notice the cup of coffee by her side.

Epidemiology of Narcolepsy

The prevalence rate of narcolepsy is about 1 in 4000 in North America and Europe. The prevalence is much higher in countries such as Japan (1 in 600) and much lower in countries such as Israel (1 in 500,000). The U.S prevalence is estimated to be between 0.03% and 0.07%. Out of the 125,000 Americans who suffer from narcolepsy, only 35% (43,000) are diagnosed and are receiving medical treatment. Male to female prevalence is equal. Symptoms usually appear in the teens or twenties, but the diagnosis often lags behind and is generally made in mid-life. Onset after age 55 or prior to age 10 is rare.

Definition of Narcolepsy

Narcolepsy is defined as a pentad of symptoms that include excessive daytime sleepiness (EDS), disturbed nocturnal sleep, cataplexy, hypnagogic hallucinations, and sleep paralysis; the latter three are abnormal manifestations of rapid eye movement (REM) sleep intrusion into wakefulness. (Box 10.1-1 summarizes these symptoms along with some additional associated factors.) Recently REM sleep behavior disorder (RBD) has been seen with increased frequency in adults with narcolepsy. The condition is defined

BOX 10.1-1. MAJOR NARCOLEPSY SYMPTOMS

These five symptoms make up the narcolepsy pentad.

- *Excessive sleepiness:* Patients are not relieved by adequate amounts of sleep. Sleepiness persists throughout the day.
- *Cataplexy:* A sudden loss of postural tone is brought on by emotion, particularly laughter. Cataplexy is virtually pathognomonic for narcolepsy.
- *Sleep paralysis:* Sleep paralysis occurs at the onset of sleep or on awakening.
- *Hypnagogic hallucinations:* Dream imagery occurs at the onset or end of sleep.
- Fragmented nocturnal sleep

Associated symptoms include:

- REM sleep behavior disorder
- Automatic behavior
- Obesity

by the abnormal augmentation of limb or chin electromyogram (EMG) tone during REM sleep associated with dream enactment (see chapter 10.5).

Definition of Idiopathic Hypersomnia

Idiopathic hypersomnia (IH) is a clinically related variant of narcolepsy in which the associated hypersomnia is often manifested by a prolonged sleep period and long unrefreshing naps. Unlike narcolepsy, however, the disorder lacks REM sleep abnormalities or cataplexy. IH may follow central nervous system infection and trauma and may be seen following other illnesses, including Guillain-Barré syndrome, mononucleosis, and atypical viral pneumonia. Currently, little is known about the underlying pathophysiology of idiopathic hypersomnia and no animal model is currently available for studying this disorder. Figure 10.1-2 contrasts between IH and narcolepsy. While the two disorders share several underlying common features, including severe sleepiness as the primary symptom, the main difference between the two conditions is the absence of REM intrusion phenomena such as cataplexy in IH.

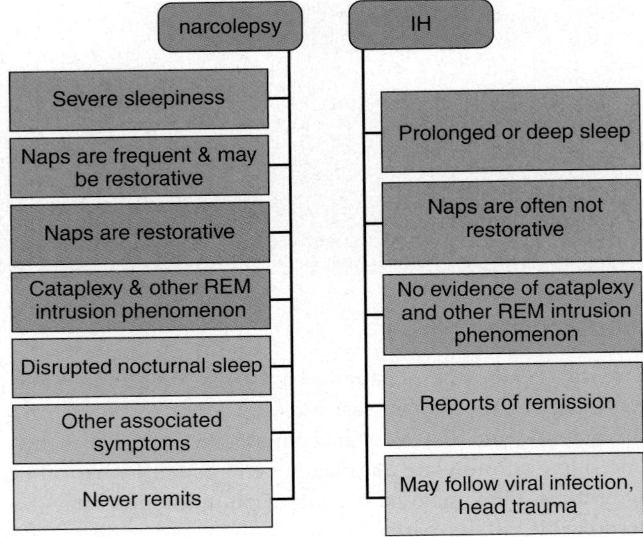

Figure 10.1-2.
Comparison of narcolepsy and idiopathic hypersommic (IH).

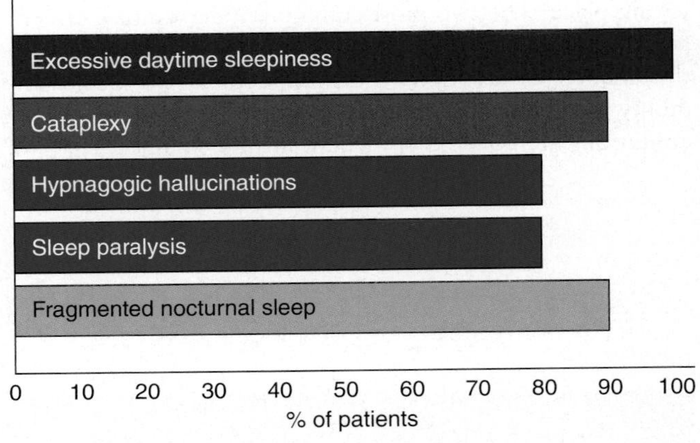

Figure 10.1-3.
Estimated upper range of the frequency of narcolepsy symptoms.

Narcolepsy Symptoms

Box 10.1-1 summarizes the symptoms of narcolepsy. Excessive daytime sleepiness, or EDS, is the initial symptom of narcolepsy. It occurs in all patients and is regarded as the sine qua non of narcolepsy. The majority of patients who suffer from narcolepsy cannot overcome the sleepiness, and it represents the most disabling feature of narcolepsy. Manifestations of REM sleep intrusion (cataplexy, hypnagogic hallucinations, sleep paralysis) occur at more widely varying prevalence rates. Whereas all patients with narcolepsy experience EDS, cataplexy affects 60% to 100% of patients, hypnagogic hallucinations occur in 15% to 80%, sleep paralysis in 17% to 80%, and fragmented nighttime sleep in 60% to 90% (Fig. 10.1-3). About 40% to 50% of patients may also experience automatic behaviors. Cataplexy is characterized by sudden episodes of bilateral skeletal muscle weakness or paralysis triggered by intense emotions such as laughter (most common trigger), anger, grief, fear, embarrassment, excitement, and sexual arousal (Fig. 10.1-4). Cataplexy, which occurs in the majority of narcolepsy patients (about 70%), is a unique feature of narcolepsy and its presence is virtually diagnostic of narcolepsy. Attacks last seconds to minutes, may be localized to specific body areas, or may involve skeletal muscle groups, but never compromise respiration or consciousness. The frequency of cataplexy varies from several times daily to less than once per month. Patients may stagger and fall or slump into a chair. Twitching around the face or eyelids may accompany the weakness. Figure 10.1-5 demonstrates muscle groups affected in cataplexy.

Sleep paralysis is an episode lasting a few seconds or minutes of inability to move during the sleep onset or upon awakening. It usually ends spontaneously or after mild sensory stimulation.

Hypnagogic (drowsiness preceding sleep) and hypnopompic (drowsiness preceding wakefulness) hallucinations are visual. Dreamlike hallucinations are the rule, although there may be auditory or tactile hallucinations (Fig. 10.1-6). Automatic behaviors, which may be due to chronic sleepiness, represent amnesic episodes associated with semipurposeful activity. These episodes may occur during monotonous or repetitive activities, last for seconds to 30 minutes or more, and may be associated with brief lapses of speech or irrelevant words or remarks.

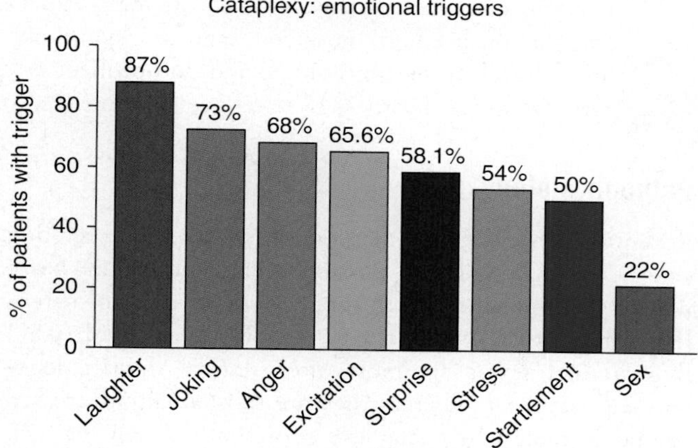

Figure 10.1-4.
The most specific way to establish cataplexy is to ask about triggering factors. These data from a study that included 63 patients with clearly established narcolepsy demonstrate the emotional triggers that most frequently provoke an episode of cataplexy. The most common emotional trigger is laughter, whereas the most specific trigger is joking. (Adapted from Anic-Labat S, Guilleminault C, Kraemer HC, et al: Validation of a cataplexy questionnaire in 983 sleep-disordered patients. Sleep 22[1]:77, 1999.)

ICSD-2

The ICSD-2, or *International Classification of Sleep Disorders: Diagnostic and Coding Manual,* 2nd edition, classifies conditions characterized by primary hypersomnolence into a single category entitled "Hypersomnias of central origin not due to a circadian rhythm disorder, sleep related breathing disorder, or other case of disturbed nocturnal sleep," as summarized in Box 10.1-2.

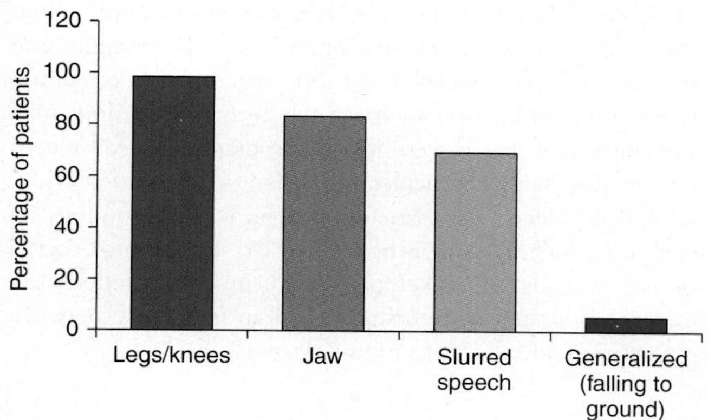

Figure 10.1-5.
Muscle groups affected in cataplexy. Most patients experience partial episodes consisting of unbuckling at the knees or legs. Very rarely do episodes generalize to compromise posture and cause the patient to fall. (Adapted from Anic-Labat S, Guilleminault C, Kraemer HC, et al: Validation of a cataplexy questionnaire in 983 sleep-disordered patients. Sleep 22[1]:77, 1999.)

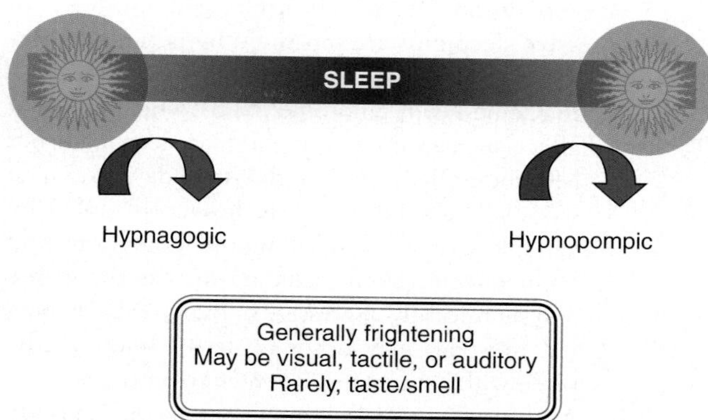

Figure 10.1-6.
Hypnagogic (drowsiness preceding sleep) and hypnopompic (drowsiness preceding wakefulness) hallucinations.

I. *Narcolepsy with cataplexy:* Narcolepsy with cataplexy is characterized by excessive daytime sleepiness and cataplexy.
II. *Narcolepsy without cataplexy:* Narcolepsy without cataplexy is similar to narcolepsy with cataplexy in most clinical respects except for the lack of definite cataplexy.
III. *Narcolepsy due to medical condition:* Narcolepsy with and without cataplexy is found in a number of medical and neurologic conditions (e.g., type C Niemann-Pick disease, Prader-Willi syndrome, structural lesions in the hypothalamic region including tumors, sarcoidosis, and multiple sclerosis).
IV. *Narcolepsy, unspecified:* Narcolepsy, unspecified, is defined by the ICSD-2 as a temporary classification for patients who meet clinical and laboratory criteria for narcolepsy but require additional evaluation for more precise classification.

BOX 10.1-2. ICSD-2 CLASSIFICATION OF HYPERSOMNIAS OF CENTRAL NERVOUS SYSTEM ORIGIN

Narcolepsy with cataplexy
Narcolepsy without cataplexy
Narcolepsy due to medical condition
Narcolepsy, unspecified
Recurrent hypersomnia
Kleine-Levin syndrome
Menstrual-related hypersomnia
Idiopathic hypersomnia with long sleep time
Idiopathic hypersomnia without long sleep time
Behaviorally induced insufficient sleep syndrome
Hypersomnia due to medical condition
Hypersomnia due to drug or substance
Hypersomnia not due to substance or known physiologic condition
Physiologic (organic) hypersomnia, unspecified

V. *Recurrent hypersomnia:* The recurrent hypersomnias are rare conditions in which prolonged episodes of excessive sleepiness are separated by periods of normal alertness and function.
   a. In Kleine-Levin syndrome (KLS), which typically affects teenage males, patients may sleep for all but a few hours daily for periods lasting days to several weeks. The syndrome may be accompanied by variable disturbances of mood, cognition, and temperament, often including increased appetite and significantly aggressive or hypersexual behavior. Episodes may occur up to 10 times yearly, often with gradual improvement over time.
   b. Menstrual-associated hypersomnia is a poorly characterized condition in which episodic sleepiness coincides with the menstrual cycle, and is believed to be related to hormonal influences.

VI. *Idiopathic hypersomnia with long sleep time:* Idiopathic hypersomnia with long sleep time is characterized by pervasive daytime sleepiness despite longer-than-average nighttime sleep (i.e., 10 or more hours).

VII. *Idiopathic hypersomnia without long sleep time:* Whereas earlier classifications allowed diagnosis of idiopathic hypersomnia only in the context of a prolonged nighttime sleep period, this classification refers to patients with comparable daytime sleepiness but normal to only slightly prolonged nighttime sleep of usually less than 10 hours.

VIII. *Behaviorally induced insufficient sleep syndrome:* Habitually insufficient total nighttime sleep results in excessive daytime sleepiness. Review of a sleep diary or sleep history of affected patients usually reveals a chronically limited and shortened nighttime sleep period that is reduced compared with the patient's premorbid baseline.

IX. *Hypersomnia due to medical condition:* Hypersomnia due to medical condition may be diagnosed when sleepiness is thought to be the direct result of a medical or neurologic condition, but the patient does not meet clinical or laboratory criteria for a diagnosis of narcolepsy.

X. *Hypersomnia due to drug or substance:* Hypersomnia due to drug or substance is characterized by excessive nighttime sleep, daytime somnolence, or excessive napping related either to use of drugs or alcohol or to their discontinuation.

XI. *Hypersomnia not due to substance or known physiologic condition (nonorganic hypersomnia, not otherwise specified):* Daytime somnolence is associated with an identifiable psychiatric diagnosis, which may become apparent after further detailed evaluation. Associated psychiatric conditions may include mood disorders, somatoform disorders, conversion disorders, and other psychiatric disturbances.

XII. *Physiologic (organic) hypersomnia, unspecified (organic hypersomnia, not otherwise specified):* Chronic sleepiness for at least 3 months' time with multiple sleep latency test (MSLT) evidence of excessive sleepiness may be classified as physiologic (organic) hypersomnia, unspecified, provided that the symptoms are believed to be physiologic and do not meet criteria for other disorders of excessive somnolence.

Pathophysiology

Recent evidence suggests that loss of hypocretin-1 secreting cells in the hypothalamus, possibly on an autoimmune basis, plays a pathogenetic role in the majority of cases of narcolepsy (Figs. 10.1-7 and 10.1-8). Cerebrospinal fluid (CSF) hypocretin-1 levels are most often normal in narcolepsy without cataplexy, whereas they are substantially decreased or undetectable when cataplexy is present (see Fig. 10.1-7).

The pathophysiology and pathogenesis of narcolepsy are remarkable for the tendency of REM sleep to occur within minutes of falling asleep. This is the "electrophysiologic signature" of narcolepsy. Narcolepsy is believed to represent a possible aberrant monoaminergic regulation of cholinergic REM sleep mechanisms (Fig. 10.1-9).

Data from Animal Studies

The hypocretin neuropeptides (hypocretin-1 and -2) (also called orexins) are located in a subregion of the dorsolateral hypothalamus. Hypocretin neurons project widely throughout the brain, most notably onto monoaminergic and cholinergic neurons, which are also involved in the regulation of sleep (see Fig. 10.1-8). These peptides are excitatory in almost all cases. In human narcolepsy brains, most cells producing hypocretin have been destroyed or cannot be detected (see damage to the lateral nucleus in Fig. 10.1-9).

The role of hypocretin in narcolepsy is further supported by the finding that hypocretin levels are abnormally low or undetectable in the CSF of most narcoleptic patients. Values below 110 pg/mL, or one third of mean normal control values, are highly diagnostic for narcolepsy in the absence of a severe brain pathology. Neurochemical abnormalities have been observed in the brains of both animals and humans with narcolepsy. The most consistent abnormalities were observed in the amygdala, where increased dopamine and metabolite levels were found. An increase in M2 receptors in the pontine reticular formation, a region associated with REM sleep, was also found. The pathophysiology of cataplexy includes inappropriate REM sleep motor atonia during periods of wakefulness and probably reflects an underlying deficit of hypocretin and an imbalance between excitatory and inhibitory motor systems.

Genetics of Narcolepsy

Narcolepsy is associated with both human leukocyte antigen (HLA) DR2 and DQ1. DQB1*0602 is a more sensitive marker for narcolepsy and appears to be correlated with both the frequency and severity of cataplexy. The DR2 appears to occur almost as frequently in narcolepsy without cataplexy as it does in the narcolepsy-cataplexy syndrome.

Cerebrospinal fluid

(pg/mL)

600

400

200

0

Narcolepsy (n = 38)

Neurologic controls (n = 19)

Control (n = 15)

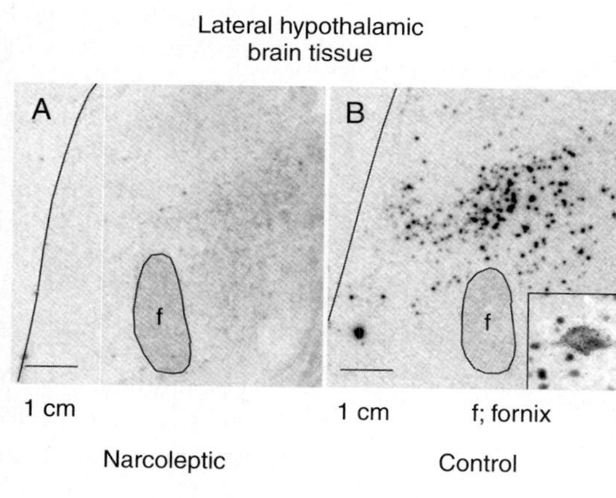

Figure 10.1-7.
Hypocretin deficiency in human narcolepsy. Cerebrospinal fluid (CSF) hypocretin is shown on the left panel comparing patients with narcolepsy with those with other neurologic conditions and with control patients. The right panel demonstrates lateral hypothalamic brain tissue staining in narcoleptic (A) versus control (B) patients. The studies show consistent reduction of CSF levels and brain tissue staining for hypocretin. (From Nishino S, Ripley B, Overeem S, et al: Hypocretin (orexin) deficiency in human narcolepsy. The Lancet 355(9197):39–40, 2000; Peyron C, Faraco J, Rogers W, et al: A mutation in a case of early onset narcolepsy and a generalized absence of hypocretin peptides in human narcoleptic brains. Nat Med 6:991–997, 2000. Courtesy Stanford Center for Narcolepsy.)

Figure 10.1-8.
Hypocretin deficiency in human narcolepsy. The number of hypocretin neurons is severely depleted in patients with narcolepsy and cataplexy. (Adapted from Thannickal T, Moore R, Nienhuis R, et al: Reduced number of hypocretin neurons in human narcolepsy. Neuron 27(3): 469–474, 2000.)

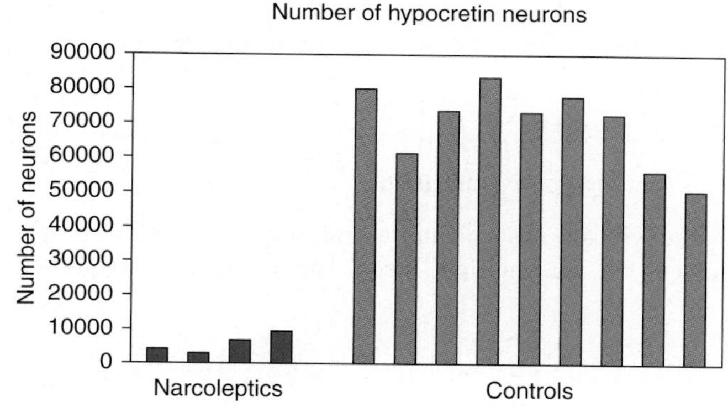

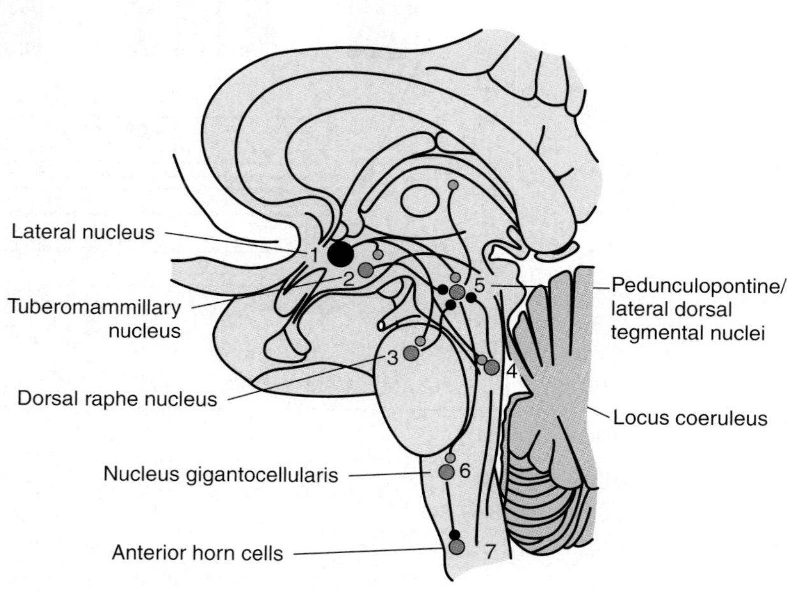

Figure 10.1-9.
Pathophysiologic representation of the brainstem in the proposed mechanism and structures involved in the generation of REM-related muscle atonia in narcolepsy. The paucity of hypocretin (orexin) cells in the lesioned lateral nucleus of the hypothalamus (1) results in a loss of what otherwise would have been wake-promoting effects on the tuberomammillary nucleus (2), the dorsal pontine raphe nucleus (3), the locus coeruleus (4), and the pedunculopontine/lateral dorsal tegmental nuclei (PPN/LDTN) (5). This leaves cholinergic "REM sleep – on" cells in the PPN/LDTN (5) uninhibited, allowing some of them to polysynaptically stimulate the nucleus gigantocellularis (6) (one of the medial groups of reticular nuclei in the medulla oblongata), which then causes a glycine-mediated hyperpolarization of anterior horn cells (7) in the spinal cord, resulting in atonia. (tan circles, facilitatory; blue circles, inhibitory.) (Adapted from Dyken ME, Yamada T: Narcolepsy and disorders of excessive somnolence. Prim Care Clin Office Pract 32:389–413, 2005.)

Diagnosis

Confirmation of diagnosis is aided by a number of objective and subjective tests.

SUBJECTIVE ASSESSMENT

Epworth Sleepiness Scale

The Epworth Sleepiness Scale (ESS) is an important instrument for assessing the degree of daytime sleepiness among patients with sleep complaints. This eight-item questionnaire is reviewed in Chapter 7.

The Fatigue Severity Scale

The Fatigue Severity Scale (FSS) is a self-rated test that assesses the degree of fatigue intensity on various functional and behavioral aspects of life. The FSS provides a subjective measurement of daytime fatigue that is largely independent of daytime sleepiness and depression. Each item is rated from 1 (strongly disagree) to 7 (strongly agree). Scoring involves calculating the mean score for all statements, with the range of possible scores being from 1 to 7, with higher scores reflecting greater fatigue.

SLEEP STUDIES

The nocturnal polysomnogram

Most typically, the nocturnal polysomnogram (PSG), followed by the multiple sleep latency test, is required. Polysomnographic features of narcolepsy include sleep disruption, repetitive awakenings, and decreased REM sleep latency. REM sleep onset (typically within less than 20 minutes of sleep onset) during the PSG occurs in approximately 50% of patients with narcolepsy and cataplexy, and is very rare in control subjects. A sleep-onset REM period (SOREMP) at night is highly predictive of narcolepsy (Fig. 10.1-10).

The Multiple Sleep Latency Test

The multiple sleep latency test (MSLT) is performed during the main period of wakefulness and is designed to determine a patient's propensity to fall asleep (Figs. 10.1-11, 10.1-12, 10.1-13). To be valid, the MSLT is usually performed the day after the nocturnal PSG. Current criteria for narcolepsy include a mean sleep latency (MSL) equal to or under 8 minutes and equal to or greater than two SOREMPs. Recent large studies have shown, however, that between 4% and 9% of the general population may have multiple SOREMPs on routine clinical MSLTs, and that of these patients 2% to 4% report daytime sleepiness that meets MSLT criteria for narcolepsy. Sleep-onset REM periods can also occur with depression, sleep-wake schedule disorders, drug and alcohol withdrawal, and REM sleep deprivation from sleep apnea. However, the absence of sleep-onset REM periods on an MSLT does not exclude narcolepsy, and their presence does not by itself confirm the diagnosis. The sleep-onset REM periods must be interpreted cautiously, particularly when sleep apnea is present.

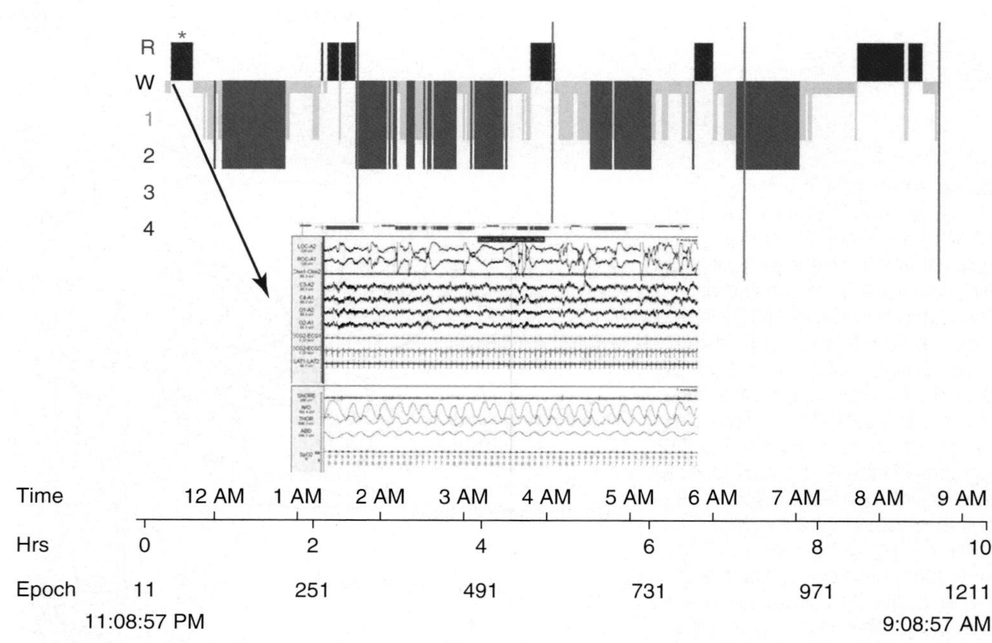

Figure 10.1-10.
Diagnostic polysomnogram in a patient with narcolepsy demonstrating REM sleep onset as soon as lights are out *(red star).*

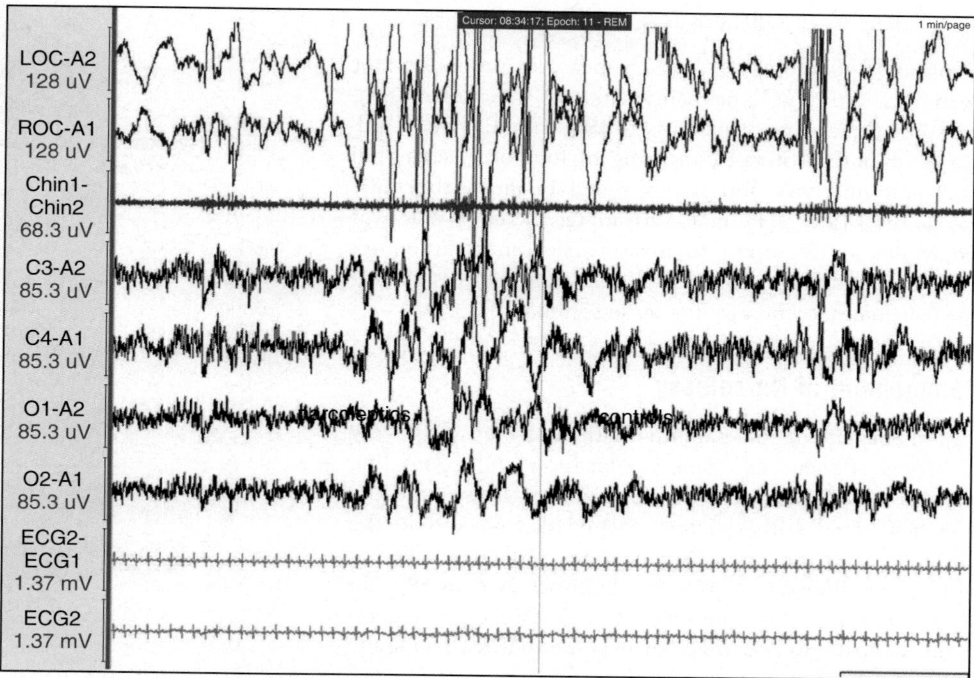

Figure 10.1-11. Multiple sleep latency tests (MSLTs) from the same patient shown in Figure 10.1-10. Following his polysomnogram the patient had a MSLT consisting of four naps. He went into REM sleep (shown here) in every single nap and had a severely reduced mean sleep latency of 2.8 minutes.

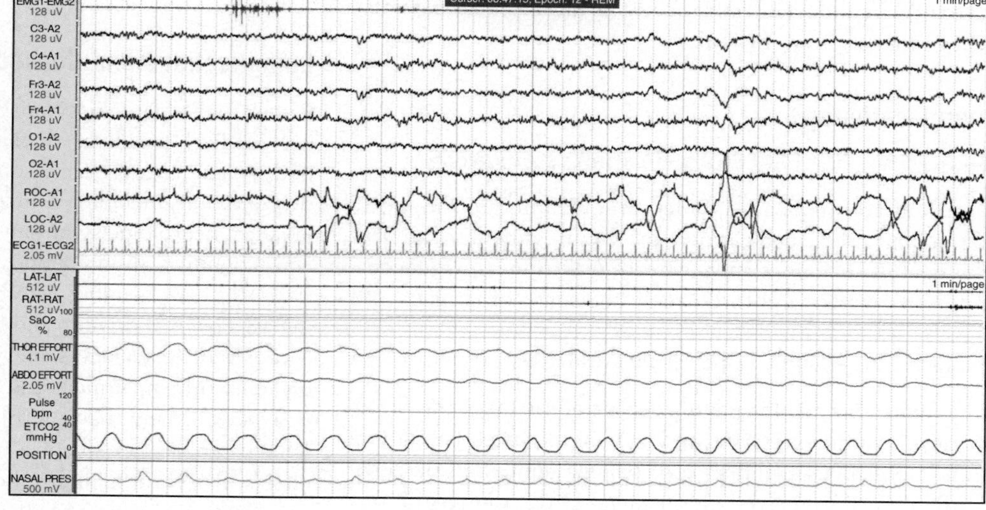

Figure 10.1-12. This is the first nap of a patient with narcolepsy showing the early onset of REM. The red vertical line is about 6 minutes into the recording. The epoch length shown here is 1 minute.

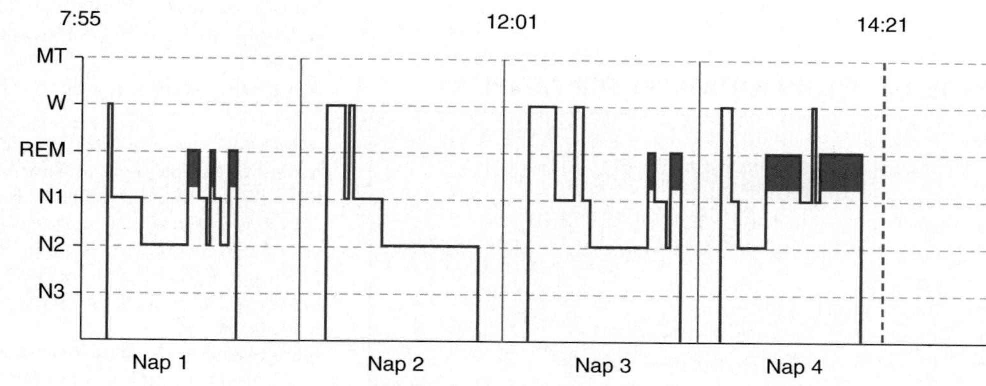

Figure 10.1-13. This is a histogram of four naps of a multiple sleep latency test (MSLT) showing early sleep onset in each of the naps and REM in all but the second nap. Each nap opportunity was 20 minutes. This is a classic finding for narcolepsy.

Maintenance of Wakefulness Test

As opposed to the MSLT, which measures propensity for sleepiness, the MWT, or maintenance of wakefulness test, measures the ability of patients to stay awake. The MWT is a 40-minute protocol consisting of four trials separated by 2-hour intervals and is performed in much the same way as the MSLT. The major advantage of the MWT over the MSLT is its ability to measure sleepiness at higher levels of somnolence. It is usually performed to assess efficacy of pharmacotherapy for hypersomnia.

Management of Narcolepsy

The management of patients with narcolepsy is very rewarding. Patient and family education and counseling are key, as is good sleep hygiene. Other factors are the risks associated with sleepiness while driving and in the workplace and the role of medications. Adequate sleep at night is also important, as sleep deprivation or insufficient sleep can aggravate symptoms. It is customary to recommend that patients take power naps. One to three 20-minute naps daily can lead to improvement in alertness and psychomotor performance without exacerbating nocturnal sleep disruption. Few studies on the effects of naps in narcolepsy have been conducted; still, many clinicians and patients believe that naps are helpful.

Pharmacotherapy

TREATMENT FOR EXCESSIVE DAYTIME SLEEPINESS

Modafinil and its R-enantiomer, armodafinil, are the most commonly used medications in the treatment of EDS. The goal of treatment is to increase wakefulness, vigilance, and performance, and to decrease the sense of fatigue.

Treatment for Abnormal REM Sleep Intrusions

Treatment for cataplexy and sleep paralysis takes the form of tricyclic antidepressants and sodium oxybate. The latter is an endogenous metabolite of gamma-aminobutyric acid (GABA). GABA received U.S. Federal Drug Administration (FDA) approval for the treatment of cataplexy in 2002 (Box 10.1-3).

BOX 10.1-3. PHARMACOTHERAPY FOR CATAPLEXY

Discontinuation of drugs may precipitate marked increase in number or severity of attacks, termed *rebound cataplexy* (status cataplecticus).

- Sodium oxybate (only FDA-approved medication)
- Variety of REM-sleep–suppressing medications widely used off-label
- Tricyclic antidepressants
- Serotonin-selective reuptake inhibitors
- Norepinephrine-selective reuptake inhibitors

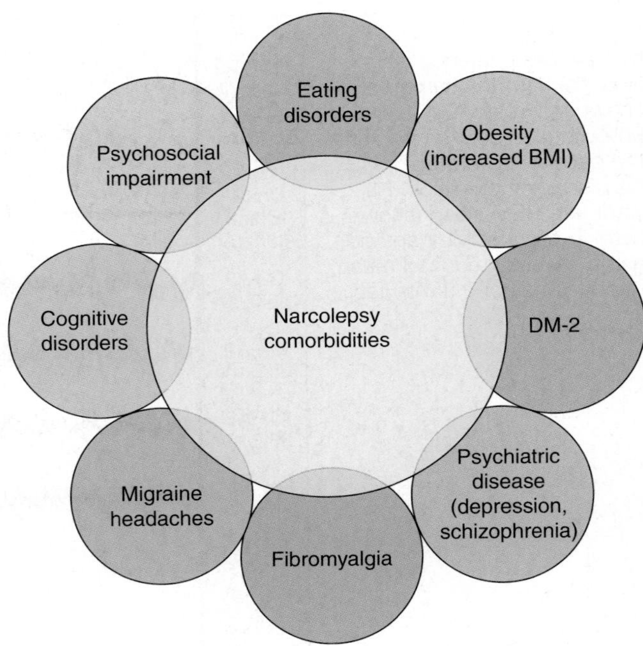

Figure 10.1-14.
Narcolepsy comorbidities. There are several medical and psychiatric comorbidities that can result in a reduced quality of life. BMI, body mass index; DM, diabetes mellitus.

Complications and Consequences of Narcolepsy

Patients with narcolepsy are at risk for a number of comorbid medical problems, including eating disorders, higher body mass index (obesity), diabetes types 1 and 2, psychiatric conditions including schizophrenia and depression, fibromyalgia, neurologic symptoms including migraine headaches and cognitive dysfunction, and psychosocial impairment (Fig. 10.1-14). Roughly two thirds of narcoleptics report falling asleep while driving, and 80% have fallen asleep at work. Motor vehicle accidents are common, and narcoleptics have greater work impairment and poorer driving records than do epileptics. Many have a high prevalence of depression, which probably reflects a psychosocial problem or the effects of a chronic illness, but there is little to suggest that narcolepsy is associated with specific psychopathology. Narcolepsy impacts a person's psychological and social functioning, especially at times of increasing responsibility at school or work. Patients often experience social isolation to avoid potentially embarrassing situations.

SELECTED REFERENCES

Aldrich MS: Sleep Medicine. Oxford, Oxford University Press, 1999.
Bassetti C: Narcolepsy. Curr Treat Options Neurol 1(4):291–298, 1999.
Black JE, Brooks SN, Nishino S: Narcolepsy and syndromes of primary excessive daytime somnolence. Semin Neurol 24(3):271–282, 2004.
Fry JM: Sleep disorders. Med Clin North Am 71(1):95–110, 1987.
International Classification of Sleep Disorders: Diagnostic and Coding Manual, 2nd ed (ICSD-2). Westchester, Ill, American Academy of Sleep Medicine, 2005.
Johns MW: A new method for measuring daytime sleepiness: The Epworth Sleepiness Scale. Sleep 14(6):540–545, 1991.

Korner Y, Meindorfner C, Moller JC, et al: Predictors of sudden onset of sleep in Parkinson's disease. Move Disord 19(11):1298–1305, 2004.
Mignot E: Narcolepsy: Pharmacology, pathophysiology and genetics. In Kryger M, Roth T, Dement W (eds): Principles and Practice of Sleep Medicine, 4th ed. Philadelphia, Elsevier Saunders, 2005, pp. 761–779.
Mignot E, Lammers GJ, Ripley B, et al: The role of cerebrospinal fluid hypocretin measurement in the diagnosis of narcolepsy and other hypersomnias. Arch Neurol 59(10):1553–1562, 2002.
Mitler MM, Hajdukovic R, Erman M, Koziol JA: Narcolepsy. J Clin Neurophysiol 7(1):93–118, 1990.
Silber MH: Sleep disorders. Neurol Clin 19(1):173–186, 2001.
Thorpy MJ: Cataplexy associated with narcolepsy: Epidemiology, pathophysiology and management. CNS Drugs 20(1):43–50, 2006.

Alon Y. Avidan

10.2 Restless Legs Syndrome and Periodic Limb Movements in Sleep

Restless legs syndrome (RLS) is a common disease that frequently presents with difficulty falling asleep and staying asleep.

Clinical Manifestations

The four essential criteria for the diagnosis of RLS are summarized in Fig. 10.2-1. Diagnostic criteria developed by the International RLS Study Group in collaboration with the National Institutes of Health are shown in Table 10.2-1.

RLS is characterized by a tetrad of leg discomfort, which usually occurs in the evening (see chapter 19, Patient Interview Videos). The most prominent symptom is the irresistible need to move the limbs. There is improvement of the discomfort with leg movement, with a return of the symptoms upon cessation of limb movements, described as quiesogenic (i.e., arising from rest). The disorder may cause sleep-onset insomnia.

RLS symptoms, which usually last for a few minutes to as long as several hours, are often bilateral and rarely unilateral. Although they can occur at any time of day, they typically occur in the evening, or when the patient is experiencing prolonged immobilization, such as when driving long distances, sitting in a movie theater, or flying on an airplane. RLS symptoms are most severe in the evening, increasing in intensity before bedtime, with a relatively free RLS zone between 6 A.M. and 10 A.M.

RLS has two forms, early and late onset. These may have different etiologies and different ages of onset, as seen in Table 10.2-2. Early-onset RLS typically begins before age 45, has a slower progression, and a female-to-male ratio of 2 to1. Late-onset RLS begins later in life, after age 45, has an equal male-to-female ratio, a faster progression, and no genetic etiology. It may be more severe with more frequent daily symptoms, and may be associated with medical, neurologic, and sleep disturbances as comorbidities, including neuropathies, radiculopathies, renal disease, and Parkinson's disease (Fig. 10.2-2). RLS may also be associated with iron deficiency anemia, uremia, renal failure,

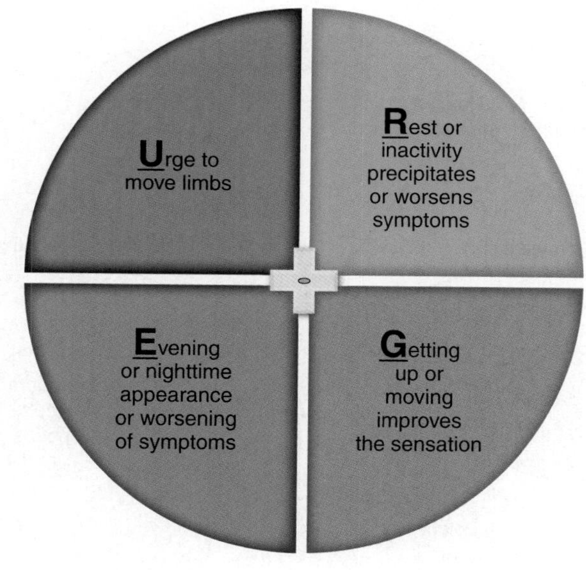

Figure 10.2-1. Essential criteria and core symptoms: "URGE." (Adapted from Allen RP, Picchietti D, Hening WA, et al: Restless legs syndrome: Diagnostic criteria, special considerations, and epidemiology. A report from the restless legs syndrome diagnosis and epidemiology workshop at the National Institutes of Health. Sleep Med 4[2]:101–119, 2003; Walters AS: Toward a better definition of the restless legs syndrome. Move Disord 10:634–642, 1995.)

Table 10.2-1. Key Diagnostic Criteria for RLS

Diagnostic criteria developed by the International RLS Study Group in collaboration with the National Institutes of Health.

KEY RLS DIAGNOSTIC CRITERIA	SUPPORTIVE FEATURES
Urge to move the legs or arms usually accompanied or caused by uncomfortable leg sensations	Sleep disturbances
Temporary relief with movement and partial or total relief from discomfort by walking or stretching	Involuntary leg movements
Onset or worsening of symptoms at rest or inactivity, such as when lying or sitting	Positive family history of RLS
	Positive response to dopaminergic therapy

ASSOCIATED FEATURES

Natural clinical course of the disorder

Can begin at any age, but most patients seen in clinical practice are middle-aged or older. Most patients seen in the clinic have a progressive clinical course, but a static clinical course is sometimes seen. Remissions of a month or more are sometimes reported.

Sleep disturbance

The leg discomfort and the need to move result in insomnia.

Medical investigation/neurologic examination

A neurologic examination is usual in idiopathic and familial forms of the syndrome.

Peripheral neuropathy or radiculopathy is sometimes experienced in the nonfamilial form of the syndrome. A low serum ferritin (50 g/L) may be associated with the syndrome.

Data from Allen RP, Picchietti D, Hening WA, et al: Restless legs syndrome: Diagnostic criteria, special considerations, and epidemiology: A report from the restless legs syndrome diagnosis and epidemiology workshop at the National Institutes of Health. Sleep Med 4(2):101–119, 2003; Walters AS: Toward a better definition of the restless legs syndrome. Move Disord 10:634–642, 1995.

Table 10.2-2. Difference Between Early- and Late-Onset RLS

EARLY-ONSET RLS	LATE-ONSET RLS
Age $\leq$ 45	Age $>$ 45
Slowly progressive	Rapidly progressive
Familial	Sporadic
Primary	Secondary/Primary

and neurologic conditions such as Parkinson's disease (Fig. 10.2-3). Certain medications may worsen RLS as well as periodic leg movements of sleep (PLMS). These include dopamine antagonists (particularly the antinausea agents), antihistamines (H1 antagonists), and antidepressants (tricyclics, selective serotonin reuptake inhibitors).

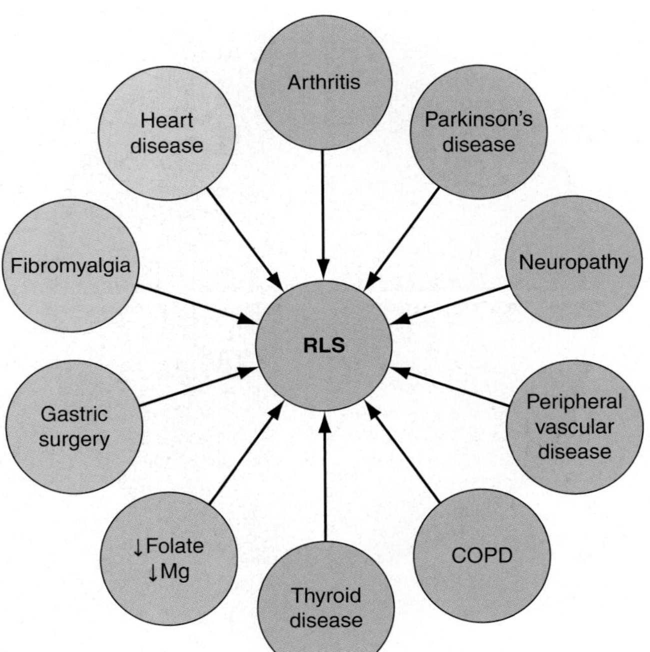

Figure 10.2-2.
Comorbid conditions associated with late-onset, secondary RLS. COPD, chronic obstructive pulmonary disease; Mg, magnesium.

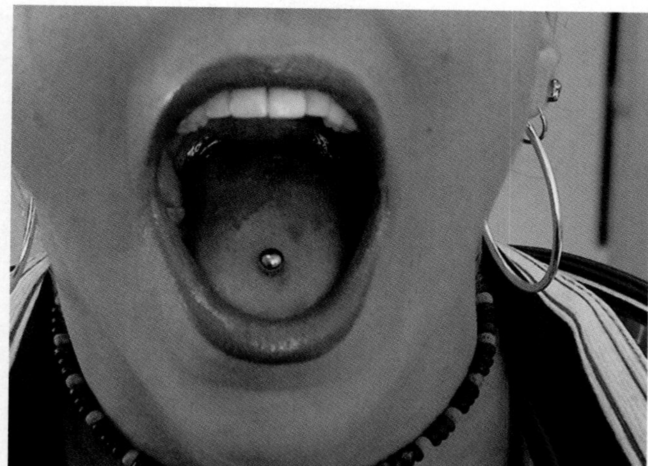

Figure 10.2-3.
RLS in iron deficiency. This young woman with RLS was a vegetarian on a poor diet and had severe, chronic iron deficiency. Her tongue had evidence of glossitis manifested as reddened atrophic mucosa. Burning of the tongue is a common symptom when this is present.

Epidemiology

RLS affects approximately 10% of U.S. adults. The prevalence of the disease increases with advanced age and tends to peak above age 50 (Figs. 10.2-4 and 10.2-5). Although the age of onset varies widely, most patients begin to experience symptoms after 40. RLS is present in both men and women, with greater prevalence in women (see Fig. 10.2-4). Symptoms of RLS occur in 5% to 15% of normal subjects. The prevalence of the disease increases in pregnancy (11%) and in patients with medical comorbidities. Fifteen percent to 20% of uremic patients and up to 30% of patients with rheumatoid arthritis experience RLS. The highest prevalence is in Western European nations, where rates range as high as 10%. South Asia and Turkey have reported lower prevalence rates.

RLS and Quality of Life

RLS has a significant impact on daytime function, according to a National Sleep Foundation survey conducted in

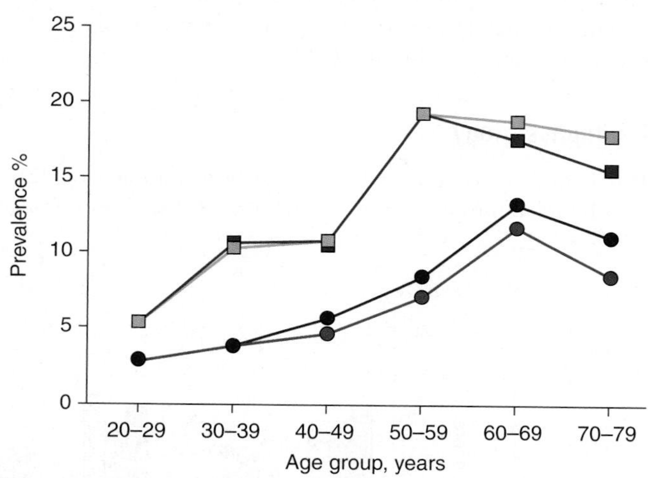

Figure 10.2-4.
Prevalence of RLS symptoms increases with age: Health of Pomerania Study in Germany ($n = 4310$). (Data from Berger K, Luedemann J, Trenkwalder C, et al: Sex and the risk of restless legs syndrome in the general population. Arch Intern Med 164:196–202, 2004.)

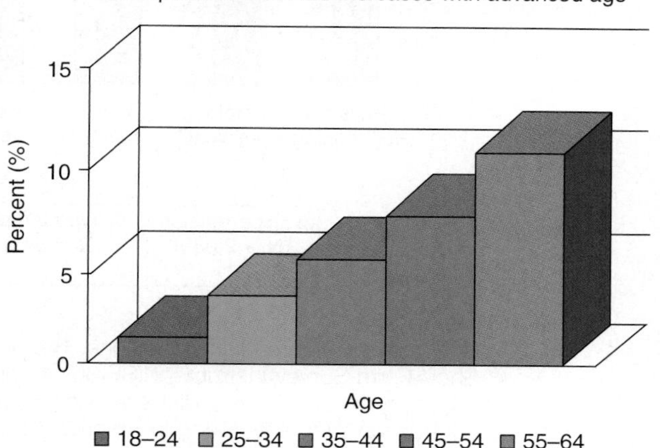

Figure 10.2-5.
RLS increases in older age. (Data from Ulfber J, Nystrom B, Carter N, Edling C: Prevalence of restless legs syndrome among men aged 18 to 64 years: An association with somatic disease and neuropsychiatric symptoms. Move Disord 16[6]:1159–1163, 2001.)

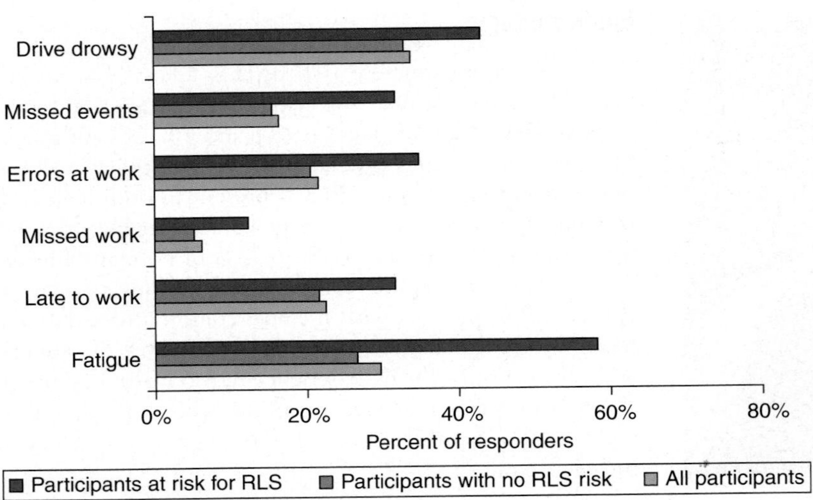

Figure 10.2-6.
Impact of RLS on daytime function. (Data from National Sleep Foundation Web site, Sleep in America Poll, 2005.)

2005 (Fig. 10.2-6), and on quality of life as measured by the Short Form Survey Instrument (SF 36). These are comparable to several domains reported by patients with serious conditions such as hypertension, type 2 diabetes, and acute myocardial infarction (Fig. 10.2-7).

Pathophysiology

It is believed that the underlying pathophysiology of RLS may be related to dopamine dysfunction. Other hypotheses concern brain iron storage deficiency and metabolism fueled by reduced cerebrospinal fluid iron content in RLS patients as compared with normal controls. Figures 10.2-8 and 10.2-9 highlight brain iron insufficiency in RLS patients on both postmortem tissue pathology (Fig. 10.2-8) and brain magnetic resonance imaging (MRI) (Fig. 10.2-9). Evidence shows reduced levels of iron in key areas subserving motor control, including the red nucleus and substantia nigra. The theory implicating iron deficiency and dopamine dysfunction can be appreciated in Figure 10.2-10. Iron is a

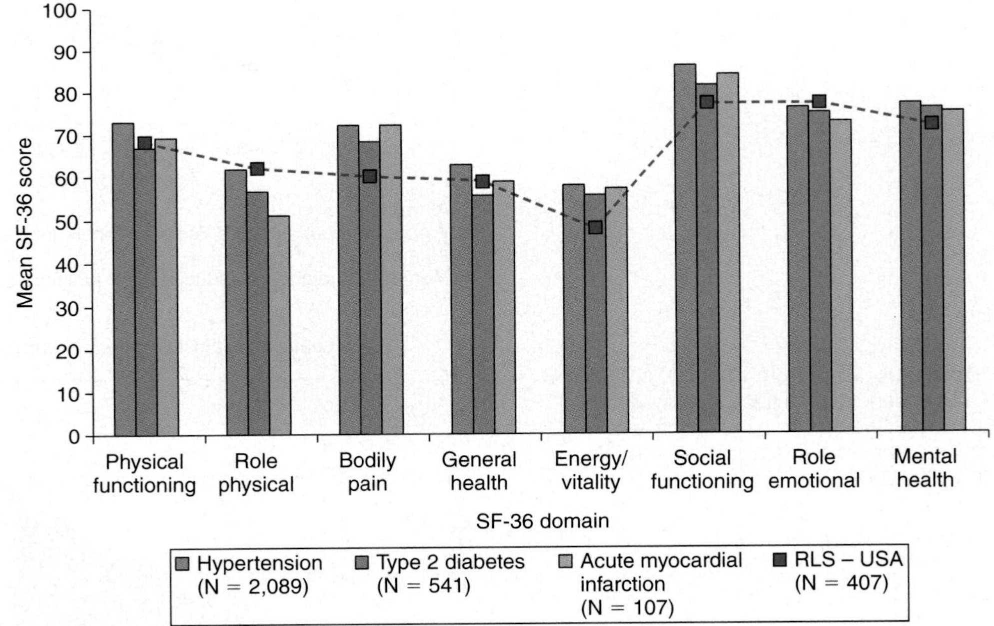

Figure 10.2-7.
RLS versus other medical conditions. The quality of life in patients with RLS as measured by the Short Form Survey Instrument (SF-36) is comparable to several domains reported by patients with hypertension, type 2 diabetes, and acute myocardial infarction. (Data from National Sleep Foundation Web site. Sleep in America Poll, 2005.)

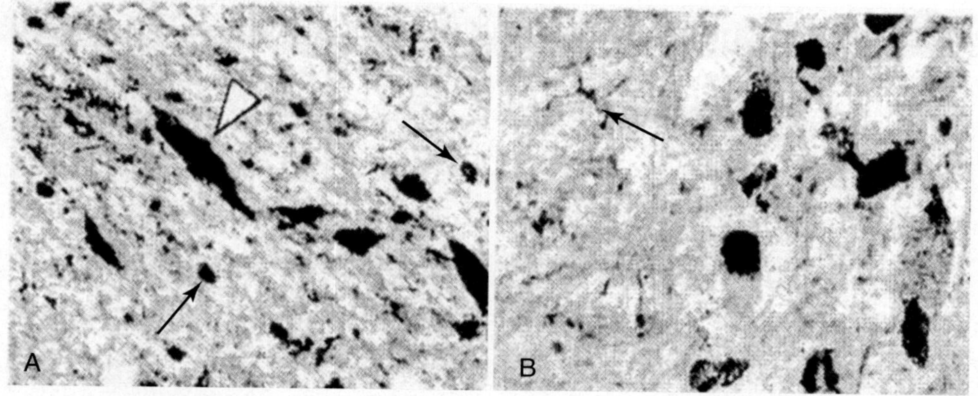

Figure 10.2-8.
RLS pathophysiology. Brain iron insufficiency neuropathological exam using iron stain for RLS controls (**A**) and patients (**B**). (From Connor JR, Boyer PJ, Menzies SL, et al: Neuropathological examination suggests impaired brain iron acquisition in restless legs syndrome. Neurology 6:301–309, 2003.)

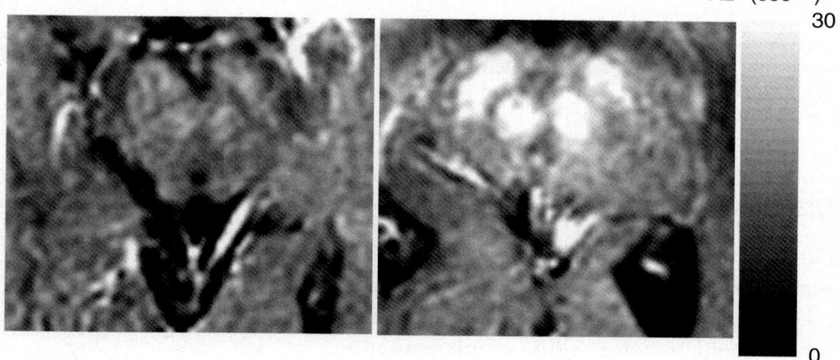

Figure 10.2-9.
Low brain iron tissue concentrations on MRI. R2* images in a 70-year-old RLS patient (*left*) and a 71-year-old control (*right*). Much lower R2* relaxation rates are apparent in the RLS case in both red nucleus and substantia nigra. (From Earley CJ, Barker PB, Horská A, Allen RP: MRI-determined regional brain iron concentrations in early- and late-onset restless legs syndrome. Sleep Med 7[5]:458–461, 2006.)

cofactor for dopamine synthesis and acts as a modulator in the dopamine transport across the blood-brain barrier. Its deficiency, therefore, is critical in contributing to dopamine dysfunction in many but not all patients with RLS.

RLS pathophysiology: iron-dopamine model of RLS

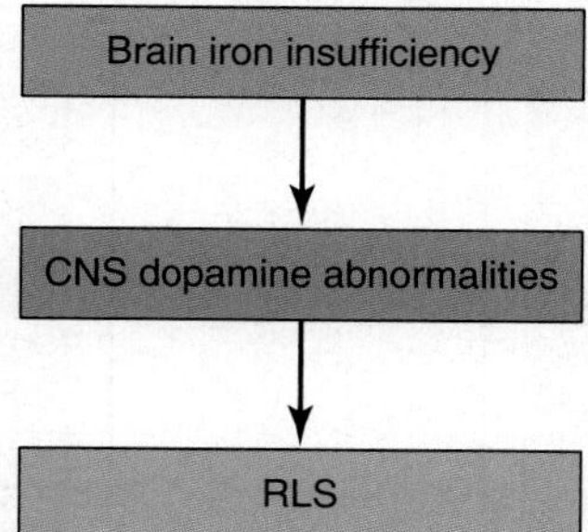

Figure 10.2-10.
Iron model of RLS. Iron deficiency may lead to dopamine abnormality leading to RLS. It is hypothesized that dysfunction of the iron–dopamine connection is central to the pathophysiology of RLS. (Adapted from Allen RP, Barker PB, Wehrl F, et al: MRI measurement of brain iron in patients with restless legs syndrome. Neurology 56[2]:263–265, 2001.)

Genetics

Several genes have recently been implicated in RLS. They include:

- Chromosome 2q (Tyrol)—having primarily autosomal dominant inheritance pattern
- Chromosome 9 (U.S. and Germany)—labeled as RLS3—having primarily autosomal dominant inheritance pattern
- Chromosome 12 (Quebec, Germany, and Iceland)—labeled as RLS1—having primarily autosomal recessive or no inheritance pattern defined
- Chromosome 14 (Tyrol)—labeled as RLS2—having primarily autosomal dominant inheritance pattern
- Chromosome 20p (Quebec)—having primarily autosomal dominant inheritance pattern

Differential Diagnosis

Table 10.2-3 lists the clinical conditions to consider in the differential diagnosis of RLS. Many of these disorders may be further evaluated and could be ruled out by history and clinical examination.

Table 10.2-3. Differential Diagnosis of RLS According to Clinical Features and Circadian Timing

DIAGNOSIS	CLINICAL FEATURES	CIRCADIAN TIMING
RLS	Clinical symptoms of uncomfortable sensation brought on at time of inactivity or rest, with relief once movement commences.	Night
PLMS	PSG findings characterized by periodic episodes of repetitive and stereotyped limb movements that occur during sleep. Lack sensory symptoms of RLS.	Night
Nocturnal leg cramps ("Charlie horse cramps")	Painful and palpable muscular contractions. Relieved with stretching.	Night
Painful peripheral neuropathy	Sensory symptoms described as numbness, burning, and pain. Typically not relieved while walking or during sustained movement.	Diurnal, increased at night
Neuroleptic-induced akathisia	Described as a "whole body sensation" rather than centered only in limbs. Does not improve with movement. Positive history of specific medication exposure.	None
Arthritis in lower limb	Discomfort is centered in the joints.	None
Volitional movements, foot tapping, leg rocking	Occurs in fidgety patients, during times of anxiety or boredom. Typically lack sensory symptoms, discomfort, or the urge to move.	None
Positional discomfort	Associated with prolonged sitting or lying in the same position, relieved by changing position.	None
Burning or painful feet and moving toes	Described as continuous slow writhing or repetitive movements of toes. Primary involvement of the feet.	None

Data from Lesage S, Hening WA: The restless legs syndrome and periodic limb movement disorder: A review of management. Semin Neurol 24(3):249–259, 2004.

Diagnostic Evaluation

Patients with clinical symptoms of RLS need to have their serum ferritin levels measured. Those with levels under 45 µg/L are at higher risk of having the disease and therefore should receive iron supplementation, as well as undergo an evaluation for iron deficiency anemia. Polysomnography (PSG) may be helpful, especially in children, when diagnosis is difficult to make clinically, and in adults to exclude other underlying primary sleep disorders such as sleep-disordered breathing. Sleep studies may also be helpful in RLS patients who do not respond to conventional therapy.

Treatment

Treatment for RLS may be divided into nonpharmacologic (conservative) therapy and pharmacotherapy (Figs. 10.2-11 and 10.2-12; Table 10.2-4). Patients with RLS will notice an improvement when they engage in mentally challenging activities. Patients with ferritin levels less than 45 µg/L should begin supplementation with iron sulfate (along with vitamin C to improve gastrointestinal absorption). Currently two dopamine agonists, ropinirole and pramipexole, have U.S. FDA (Food and Drug Administration) approval for RLS (see Fig. 10.2-12). Dopamine agonists are preferred as first-line therapy as they have substantial data to demonstrate their efficacy by objective verifiable indicators. If symptoms persist despite dopamine agonists, other medications such as levodopa/carbidopa and antiepileptic drugs such as gabapentin may be used. One significant drawback of dopamine precursor therapy is the potential for augmentation (onset of increased symptom severity earlier in the day) and rebound (worsening of RLS symptoms later at night or in the early morning hours). When treatment is refractory to traditional therapy, opiates (such as methadone) may be utilized.

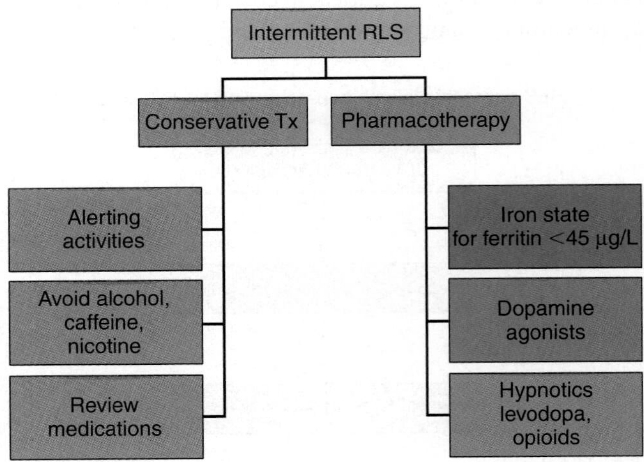

Figure 10.2-11.
Treatment algorithm for intermittent RLS divided according to conservative and pharmacologic therapies. (Adapted from Silber MH, Ehrenberg BL, Allen RP, et al: An algorithm for the management of restless legs syndrome. Mayo Clin Proc 79:916–922, 2004.)

Treatment for primary RLS

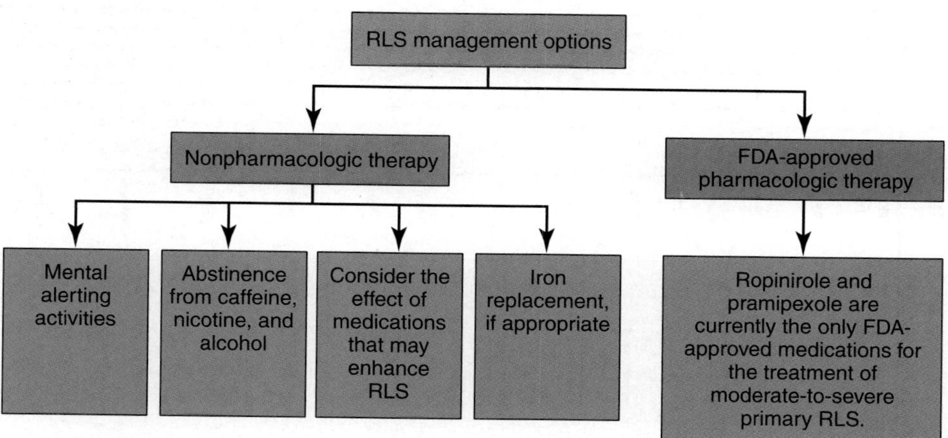

Figure 10.2-12.
Treatment algorithm for primary daily RLS. (Adapted from Silber MH, Ehrenberg BL, Allen RP, et al: An algorithm for the management of restless legs syndrome. Mayo Clin Proc 79:916–922, 2004.)

Periodic Limb Movements in Sleep

EPIDEMIOLOGY

The prevalence of periodic limb movements in sleep (PLMS) increases with advancing age. PLMS may be found in up to 34% of patients over 60 years of age and can be observed in a variety of sleep disorders including RLS, REM sleep behavior disorder, and narcolepsy.

CLINICAL MANIFESTATIONS

PLMS is an electromyographic finding observed during polysomnography. It is described as periodic episodes of repetitive and stereotyped limb (leg or arm) movements that occur during sleep (Figs. 10.2-13 and 10.2-14). The movements are often associated with a partial electroencephalographic arousal or awakening, often unrecognizable by the patient. When PLMS is severe and sleep fragmenta-

Table 10.2-4. Pharmacotherapy for RLS

GENERIC/BRAND	DOSE	RISKS
Iron: Ferrous sulfate	325 mg bid/tid Recommended for Ferritin < 50 mcg	Gastrointestinal side effects: constipation. Role in treatment under current investigation
Dopamine agonists: Pramipexole (Mirapex)* Ropinirole (Requip)*	0.125 to 0.5 mg, 1 hr before bedtime Start low and increase slowly 0.25 to 2 mg, 1 hr before bedime	Severe sleepiness; nausea reported in some cases. Nausea, vomiting, sleep attacks, (rare) compulsive gambling
Dopaminergic agents: Levodopa/Carbidopa (Sinemet)	25/200 mg: ½ to 3 tabs 30 min before bedtime	Nausea, sleepiness, augmentation of daytime symptoms, insomnia, gastrointestinal disturbances
Anticonvulsants: Gabapentin (Neurontin)	300 to 2700 mg/day divided tid	Daytime sleepiness, nausea
Benzodiazepines: Clonazepam (Klonopin)	0.125 to 0.5 mg ½ hr before bedtime	Nausea, sedation, dizziness
Clonidine: Catapres	0.1 mg bid May be helpful in patients with hypertension	Dry mouth, drowsiness, constipation, sedation, weakness, depression (1%), hypotension
Opioids: Darvocet (Darvoset-N) Darvon (Propoxyphene) Codeine	300 mg/day 65 to 135 mg at bedtime 30 mg	Nausea, vomiting, restlessness, constipation. Addiction; tolerance may be possible

**Only FDA-approved drug for RLS (as of November 2008).*
Reviewed from Earley CJ: N Engl J Med 348:2103–2109, 2003; Stiasny K, Oertel WH, Trenkwalder C: Clinical symptomatology and treatment of RLS and PLMD. Sleep Med Rev 6:253–265, 2002.

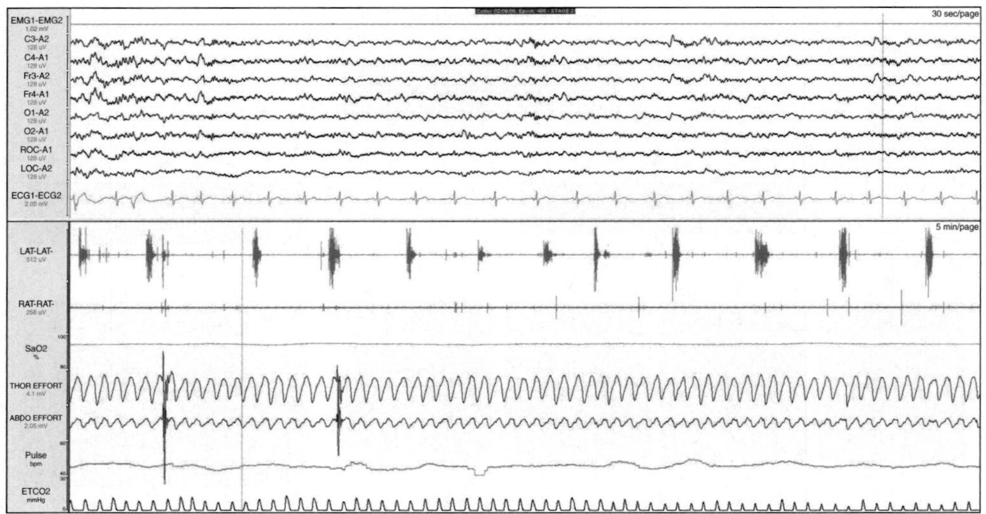

Figure 10.2-13.
The bottom 5-min window shows periodic limb movements that were present almost the entire night. They were seldom associated with EEG arousal, but often were associated with increases in heart rate, the latter perhaps reflecting subcortical arousals.

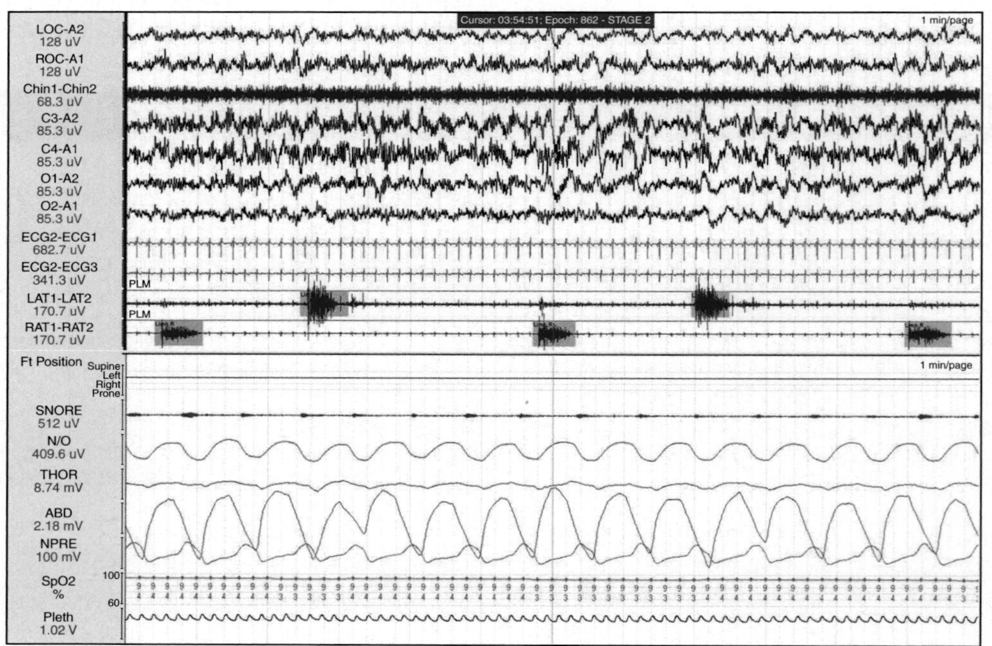

Figure 10.2-14.
This figure shows a 60-second sleep epoch from a diagnostic PSG of a 66-year-old woman with RLS and sleep initiation and maintenance insomnia. The figure illustrates successions of five periodic limb movements occurring in the right and left anterior tibialis (RAT/LAT) muscles. Channels are as follows: electro-oculogram (LOC-A2 *[left]*, ROC-A1 *[right]*), chin EMG (Chin-Chin), EEG (C3-A2 *[left central]*, C4-A1 *[right central]*, O1-A2 *[left occipital]*, O2-A1 *[right occipital]*), ECG, limb EMG (left leg [LAT], right leg [RAT]), patient position, snoring (SNORE), nasal-oral airflow (N/O), respiratory effort (thoracic [THOR], abdominal [ABD]), nasal pressure (NPRE), oxygen saturation (SpO_2), and plethysmography (Pleth).

Table 10.2-5. RLS and PLM in Sleep Are Very Different Clinical Entities

RESTLESS LEGS SYNDROME	PERIODIC LEG MOVEMENTS
Clinical diagnosis	Electromyographic finding seen during a sleep study
Confirmed by history and physical examination	Confirmed during a sleep study
About 80% have periodic leg movements	About 30% have restless legs syndrome

Allen RP, Picchietti D, Hening WA, et al: Restless legs syndrome: Diagnostic criteria, special considerations, and epidemiology: A report from the restless legs syndrome diagnosis and epidemiology workshop at the National Institutes of Health. Sleep Med 4(2): 101–119, 2003.

tion frequent, patients may experience excessive sleepiness. Table 10.2-5 distinguishes between RLS and PLMS. Whereas RLS is a clinical diagnosis, PLMS may be suspected but must be confirmed polysomnographically.

DIAGNOSTIC EVALUATION

Polysomnography reveals repetitive electromyogram (EMG) contractions of the anterior tibialis lasting 0.5 to 5 seconds (mean duration, 1.5 to 2.5 seconds). PLMS is diagnosed when over five leg movements occur per hour of sleep. Four or more consecutive movements are required, and the interval between movements is typically 20 to 40 seconds (see Fig. 10.2-14). To be categorized PLMS, movements that are separated by an interval less than 5 or greater than 90 seconds are not counted when determining the total number of movements, or movement indexes. PLMS may appear as early as sleep onset, may decrease in frequency in slow-wave sleep, and are usually absent during REM sleep. Figure 10.2-15 demonstrates polysomnography in a patient with RLS. As can be appreciated, there is a lack of periodicity to the motor activity and there is evidence of elevation of EMG tone during the awake state, representing a muscle artifact. Figure 10.2-16, on the other hand, shows the periodicity of PLMS in a sleeping patient.

Video monitoring can confirm the vigorous movements these patients may have (see chapter 18).

Management

The treatments for PLMS and RLS are somewhat similar, in that many patients respond to agents such as low-dose dopamine-agonist and benzodiazepines such as clonazepam. Clinicians should also be on the lookout for medications that may worsen PLMS, such as antidepressants, as shown in Figure 10.2-17.

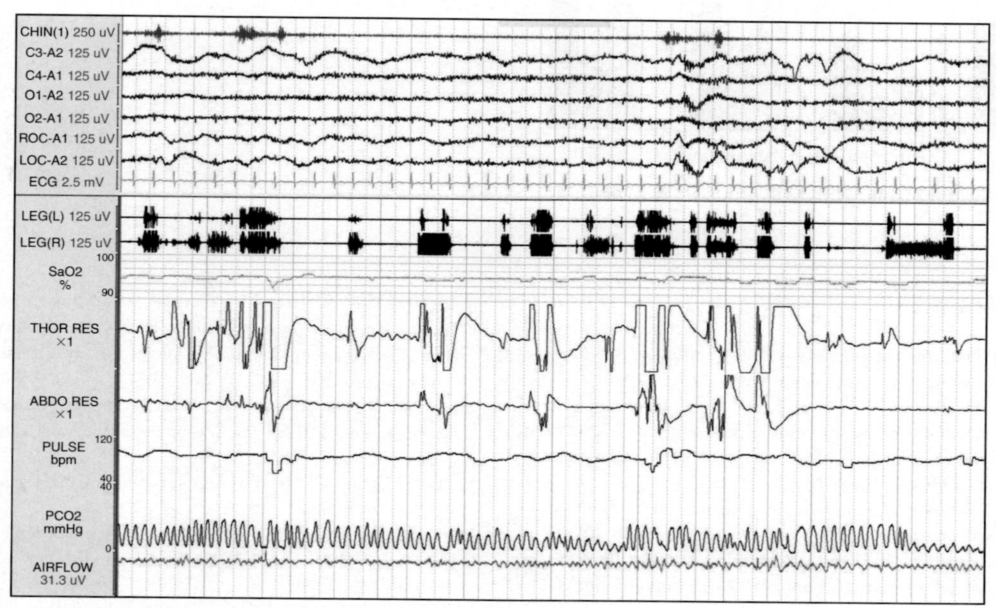

Figure 10.2-15.
PSG in RLS. This woman with RLS had severe sleep-onset insomnia. Her legs showed a great deal of activity while she was trying to fall asleep. The leg movements and body movements result in artifacts in the respiratory channels. She complained that her feet became very hot at night and she has to keep moving them. Her husband mentioned that she moves a great deal when she sleeps. There is a previous history of severe iron deficiency. Ferritin level is 12 µg/L.

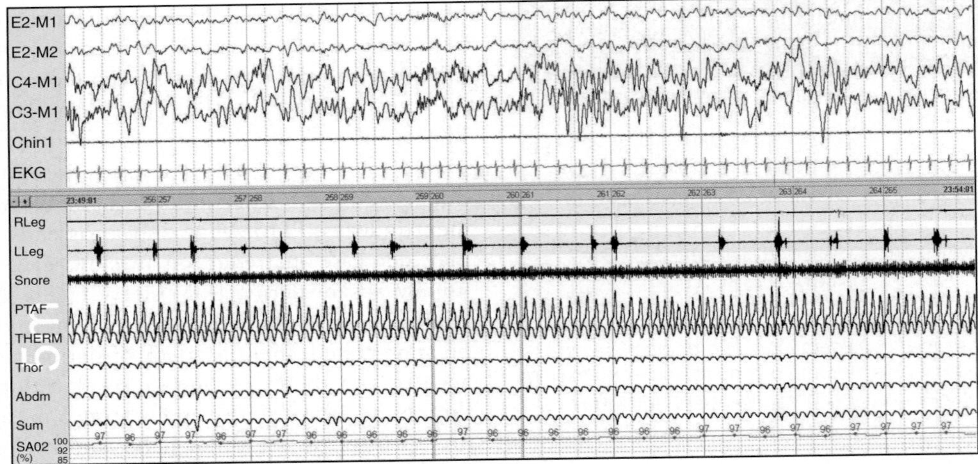

Figure 10.2-16.
PSG in a 6-year-old. As the findings here show, children can have PLMS. Such children may be referred with sleepiness and may have been diagnosed with attention deficit hyperactivity disorder. In this example inadequate gain resulted in the right leg not showing the movements.

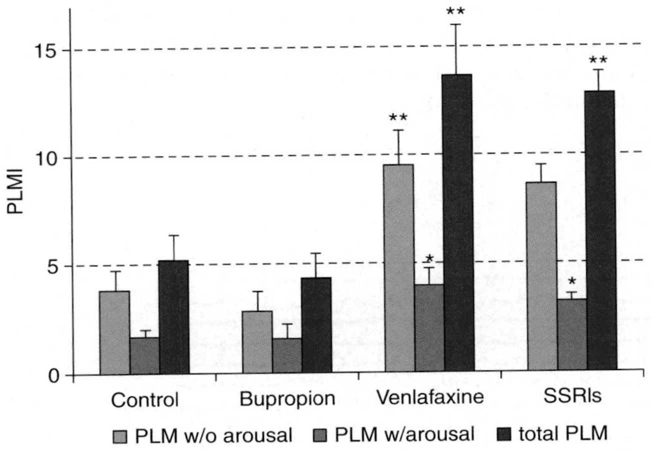

Figure 10.2-17.
Certain antidepressants can worsen RLS. In this example, the serotonin norepinephrine reuptake inhibitor (SNRI) venlafaxine (Effexor) is a risk factor for inducing periodic leg movements with and without arousals compared with control patients, those using selective serotonin reuptake inhibitors (SSRIs), and those on buproprion (Wellbutrin). (Adapted from Yang C, White DP, Winkelmann JW: Antidepressants and periodic leg movements of sleep. Biol Psychiatry 58:510–514, 2005.)

SELECTED REFERENCES

Allen RP, Earley CJ: Defining the phenotype of the restless legs syndrome (RLS) using age-of-symptom-onset. Sleep Med 1:11–19, 2000.

Allen RP, Picchietti D, Hening WA, et al: Restless legs syndrome: Diagnostic criteria, special considerations, and epidemiology: A report from the restless legs syndrome diagnosis and epidemiology workshop at the National Institutes of Health. Sleep Med 4(2):101–119, 2003.

Earley CJ, Allen RP, Beard JL, Connor JR: Insight into the pathophysiology of restless legs syndrome. J Neurosci Res 62(5):623–628, 2000.

Earley CJ, Connor JR, Allen RP: RLS patients have abnormally reduced CSF ferritin compared to normal controls. Neurology 52(Suppl 2): A111–A112, 1999.

Hening WA, Allen RP, Earley CJ, et al: An update on the dopaminergic treatment of restless legs syndrome and periodic limb movement disorder: An American Academy of Sleep Medicine interim review. Sleep 27(3):560–583, 2004.

Hening WA, Walters AS, Allen RP, et al: Impact, diagnosis and treatment of restless legs syndrome (RLS) in a primary care population: The REST (RLS epidemiology, symptoms, and treatment) primary care study. Sleep Med 5(3):237–246, 2004.

International Classification of Sleep Disorders: Diagnostic and Coding Manual, 2nd ed (ICSD-2). Westchester, Ill: American Academy of Sleep Medicine, 2005.

Lesage S, Earley CJ: Restless legs syndrome. Curr Treat Options Neurol 6 (3):209–219, 2004.

Lesage S, Hening WA: The restless legs syndrome and periodic limb movement disorder: A review of management. Semin Neurol 24 (3):249–259, 2004.

Sun ER, Chen CA, Ho G, et al: Iron and the restless legs syndrome. Sleep 21(4):371–377, 1998.

Winkelmann J, Provini F, Nevsimalova S, et al: Genetics of restless legs syndrome (RLS): State-of-the-art and future directions. Move Disord 22(Suppl 18):S449–S458, 2007.

Alon Y. Avidan

Sleep in Epilepsy 10.3

Epidemiology of Epilepsy and Comorbidities in Sleep Disorders

About 1% to 2% of the population has epilepsy, and 1 out of 10 people will have a seizure during their lifetime. Approximately 20% of patients with epilepsy will have seizures solely while asleep.

Nocturnal seizures should be distinguished from other nocturnal events such as parasomnias (see chapter 12), including those that occur during wakefulness, wake-sleep transition, and rapid eye movement (REM) and non-REM (NREM) sleep. The most difficult problem is to distinguish between frontal lobe seizures and parasomnias (Table 10.3-1). Sleep disorders such as sleep deprivation and sleep apnea may exacerbate seizures, and, conversely, seizures may affect sleep, as many of the current antiepileptic drugs produce undesirable side effects to sleep architecture and may predispose the patient to primary sleep disorders.

Table 10.3-1. Characteristics of Nocturnal Frontal Lobe Epilepsy (NFLE) vs. Parasomnias

CLINICAL FEATURE	NFLE	PARASOMNIAS
Age at onset (years)	11.8 ± 6.3	Usually<10
Attacks/month (n)	36 ± 12	1–4
Clinical course	Increasing or stable	Decreasing/ disappearing
Movement semiology	Stereotypic	Polymorphic
Attack onset	Any time during the night	First third of the night
Attack distribution	2-NREM (65%)	3-4 NREM
Motor pattern	2-3 repetitive types of attacks	Absence of motor pattern
Duration of the attacks	Less than 1 min (excl. prolonged episodes)	Some minutes

The Effects of Seizure Drugs on Sleep Organization and Architecture

Antiepileptic drugs have a variable effect on sleep. Table 10.3-2 summarizes their effects on sleep architecture and other secondary sleep disorders. For example, benzodiazepines decrease slow-wave sleep, phenytoin shortens sleep latency, and lamotrigine may induce insomnia.

Sleep State as a Facilitator of Epilepsy

REM sleep: The increased brainstem cholinergic input, which occurs during REM sleep, induces a state of cortical activation (Fig. 10.3-1).

NREM sleep: NREM sleep is a physiologic state of relative neuronal synchronization and predisposes to neuronal hyperpolarization.

Figure 10.3-2 demonstrates epileptogenicity as relating to the sleep states. REM sleep is least epileptogenetic, followed by wake. NREM sleep is most epileptogenetic owing to the relative synchrony of thalamocortical synaptic activity and the greater ease of propagation of epileptiform discharges.

Table 10.3-2. Effects of Antiepileptic Drugs on Sleep

DRUG	EDS	INSOMNIA	SL	REM	SLOW WAVE	AWAKENINGS	OTHER
Gabapentin	++			▲		▼	▲Weight
Lamotrigine		+		▲	▲	▲	
Levetiracetam	+						
Oxycarbazepine	+						
Tiagabine	+++				▲		
Topiramate	++						▼Weight
Zonisamide	+	+					
Carbamazepine	+			▼			▲PLMs
Phenytoin	+	+	▼			▲	
Valproate	+		▲				▲Weight
Phenobarbital	+++					▼	▲OSA
Ethosuximide		+			▼		
Felbamate		++					▲Weight

Key: + Mild effect, ++ Moderate effect, +++ Severe effect, ▼ Decrease/Reduce, ▲ Increase
EDS, excessive daytime sleepiness; SL, sleep latency.
Antiepileptic drugs have variable effects on sleep variables.

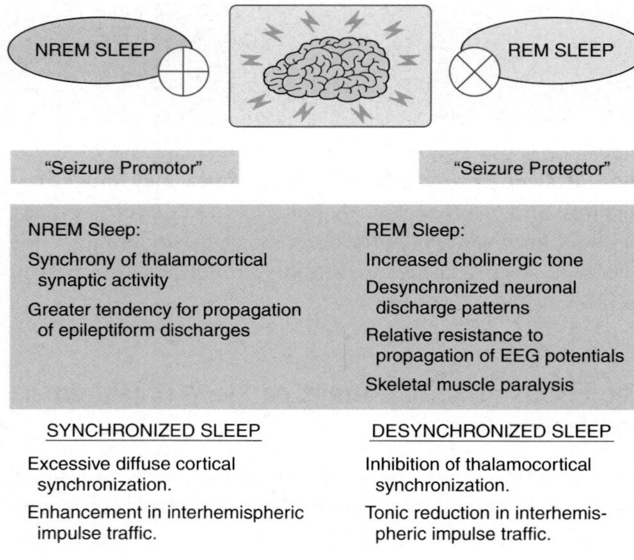

Figure 10.3-1.
Sleep state as a facilitator of epilepsy: NREM versus REM sleep.

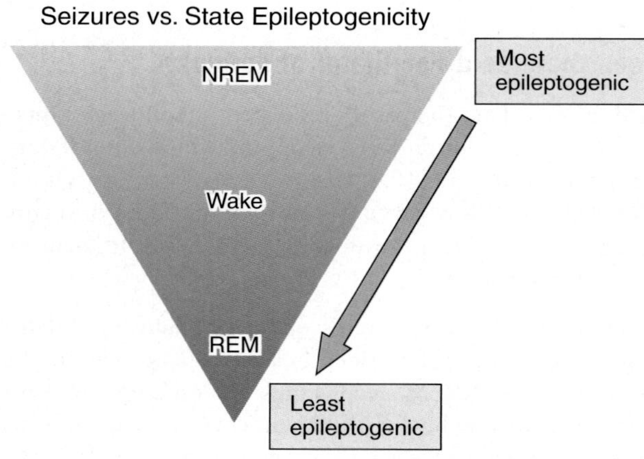

Figure 10.3-2.
Sleep state as a facilitator of epilepsy.

Regional Anatomy in Epilepsy Facilitation

Patients with frontal lobe epilepsy experience most of their seizures during sleep, whereas those with temporal lobe epilepsy experience most of their seizures while awake. The frontal lobe receives significant ascending input from the thalamus and has rich interconnections, demonstrating its propensity as a region to facilitate seizures during sleep.

Epilepsy Syndromes Associated with Sleep

Nocturnal seizures are bizarre, difficult to diagnose and evaluate, but usually have a consistent stereotypy, which remains a key factor in distinguishing them from other parasomnias. Stereotypical semiology is a major component of the clinical presentation and is often the one element in the history that directs the clinician toward the diagnosis of nocturnal seizures.

Nocturnal seizures have strange clinical manifestations, but as a rule there is preservation of consciousness during the spells with rapid recovery of the patient. Their evolution may be complicated by the lack of reliable characterization; the observer may be asleep, or may miss the beginning of a spell. The result is that the description of the spells is sometimes lacking or ambiguous. Furthermore, nocturnal epileptic spells have auras and postictal periods that tend to be masked by sleep. Behavioral manifestations are demonstrated in Figure 10.3-3.

Diagnosis of sleep-related seizures may be considered if the following elements are present:

- The patient has a history of epilepsy, even if the epilepsy is well controlled.
- The patient experiences stereotyped events that are repetitive and disruptive to the sleep of the patient and the patient's bedpartner.
- Episodes occur at any time of night (more commonly during NREM sleep than during REM sleep).
- Similar events may occur during the day.
- A trial of antiepileptic drugs produces a favorable response.

Figure 10.3-3.
Characteristics of frontal lobe epilepsy.

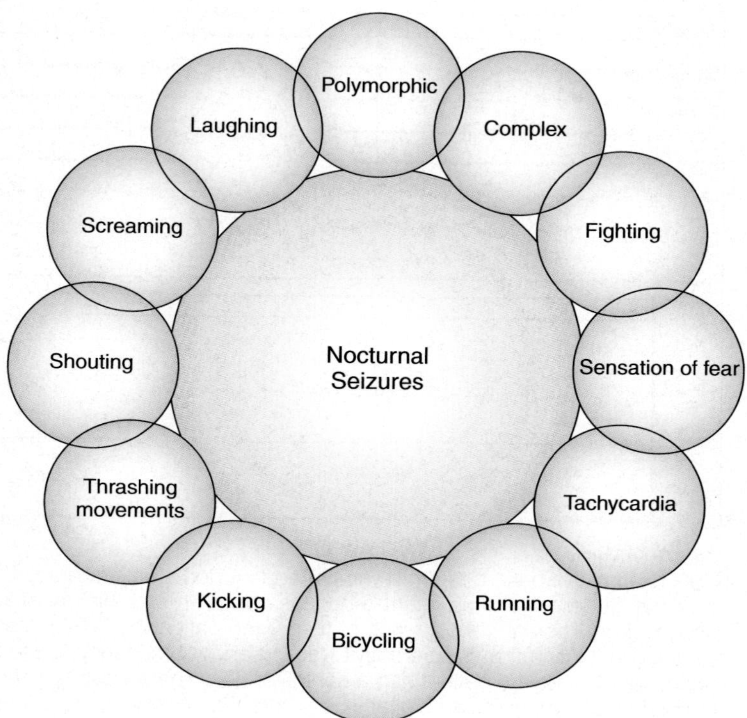

Nocturnal polysomnography (PSG) using a montage normally used for evaluating sleep breathing disorders may detect seizure activity (Figs. 10.3-4 and 10.3-5). More often a "seizure montage" is used in suspected cases in order to record many more electrode pairs and thereby allow for a more detailed evaluation (Fig. 10.3-6).

Sleep-related Epilepsy Syndromes

NOCTURNAL TEMPORAL LOBE EPILEPSY

Temporal lobe epilepsy is the most common type of partial epilepsy in adults (Fig. 10.3-7). Patients may lack an aura or may not recall the event. Spells consist of experiential,

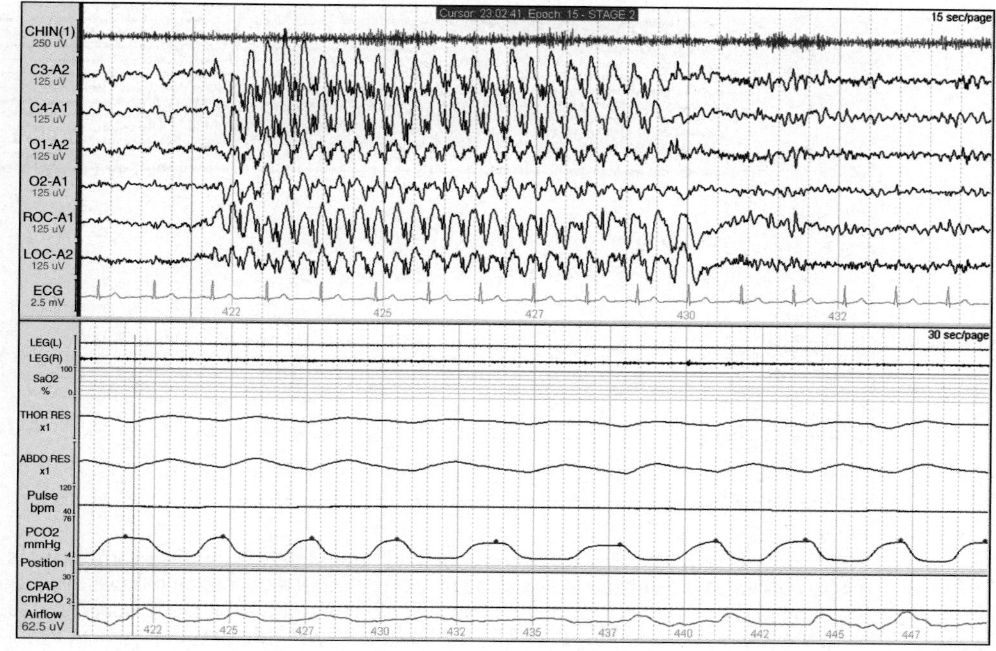

Figure 10.3-4.
PSG example of nocturnal frontal lobe epilepsy. This is a representative PSG sample from a 35-year-old woman with a history of bizarre nocturnal spells in the middle of the night. The episodes are usually brief, less than a minute. This PSG shows spike and slow-wave complexes more prominent centrally during stage N2 sleep. (PSG courtesy M. H. Kryger.)

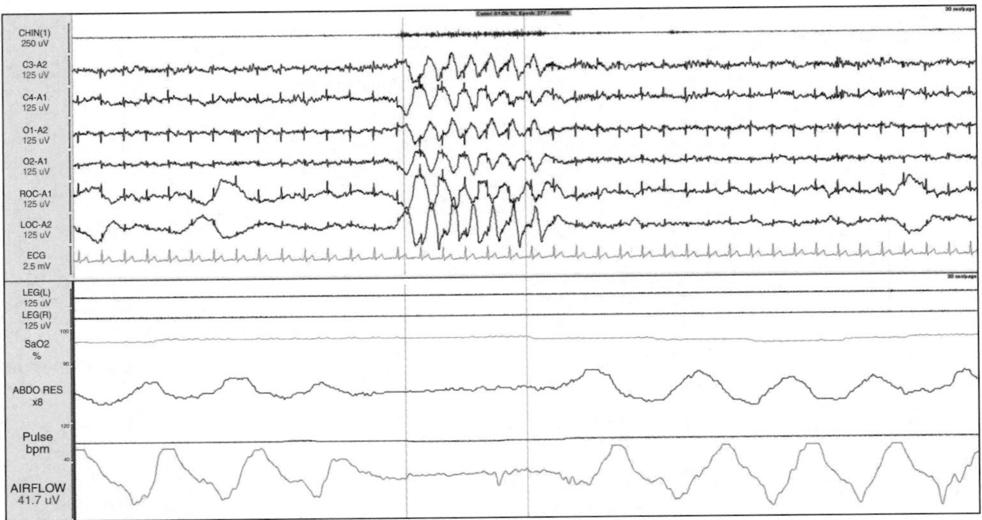

Figure 10.3-5.
PSG example of patient referred with infrequent nocturnal seizures. This example is from a 20-year-old student who was referred because of a 5-month history of infrequent seizures that occurred only at night. As a result of these, the patient had dislocated his shoulder and bitten his tongue. Notice the seizure activity lasting about 5 seconds in the middle of the epoch, during which time the patient had a central apnea. There were only three similar findings during the night. On synchronized digital video there was absolutely no movement visible. The sleep study may be entirely normal in patients with infrequent seizures. (PSG courtesy M. H. Kryger.)

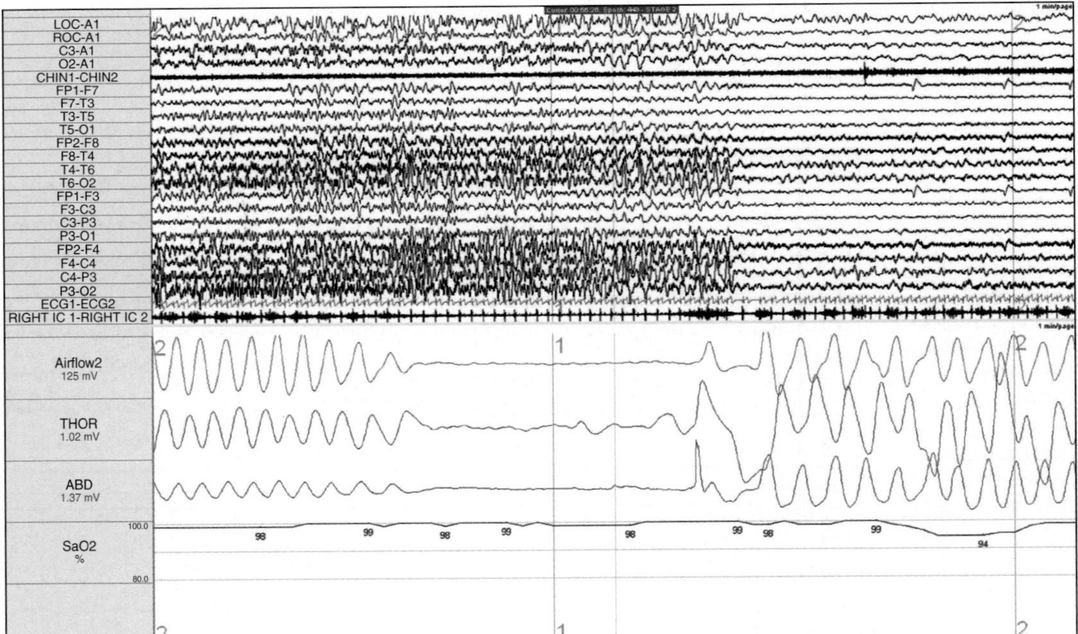

Figure 10.3-6.
PSG example of right-sided seizure resulting in central apnea. In this example the seizure was originally missed because the seizure activity was only on the right side (notice the even-numbered electrodes) and the scoring montage did not include them. Such a seizure montage is useful in cases of unexplained central apneas *(black, right; blue, left)*. (PSG courtesy M. Mahowald.)

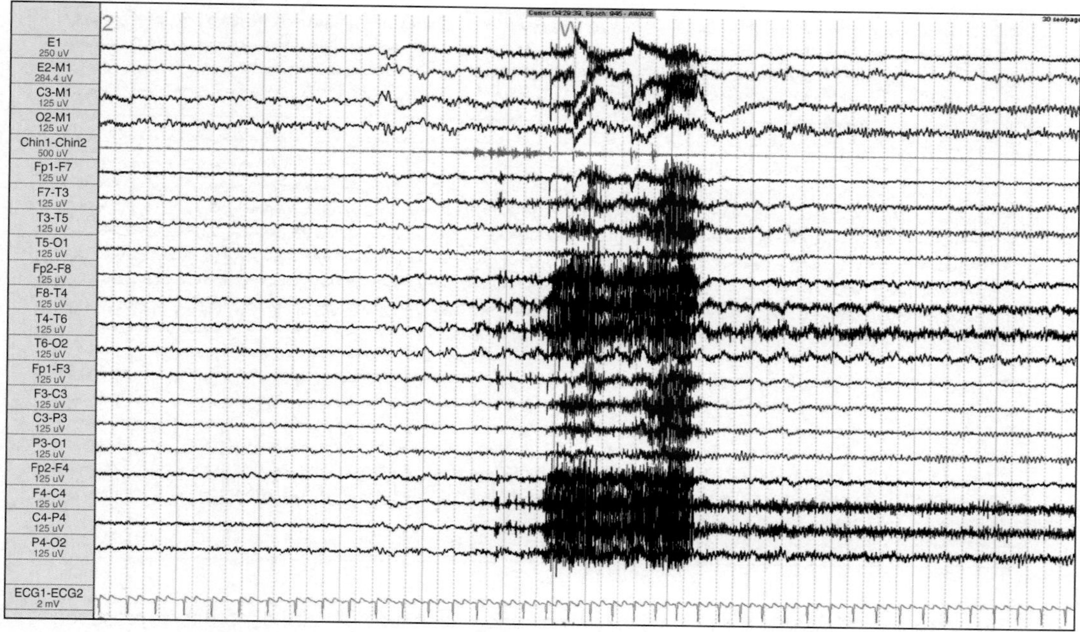

Figure 10.3-7.
PSG example of temporal seizure. In this example there are brief spikes in the right temporal region (note the abnormalities in T4-T6 and T6-O2) that begin just before the increased activity in the chin electrodes. This is followed by arousal. On the conventional sleep scoring montage, this would appear to be a simple, nonspecific arousal. The EEG montage reveals periodic spikes from the right mid-temporal region culminating in an arousal followed by residual postictal slowing over the same region. This "arousal" was actually the sole clinical manifestation of a focal temporal lobe epileptic discharge. (These may occur hundreds of times a night, resulting in frequent arousals [sleep fragmentation] presenting as excessive daytime sleepiness.) For this reason, it is prudent to employ a full seizure montage in all patients with a history of seizures and the complaint of excessive daytime sleepiness. If these arousals are associated with extremity movements, an erroneous diagnosis of periodic leg movements could be made *(black, right; blue, left)*. (PSG courtesy M. Mahowald.)

autonomic, or special sensory components associated with brief periods of impaired consciousness with motionless staring or automatisms.

BENIGN EPILEPSY OF CHILDHOOD WITH CENTROTEMPORAL SPIKES

Benign epilepsy with centrotemporal, or Rolandic, spikes is the most common form of partial epilepsy in children. In 70% to 80% of cases, seizures are confined to sleep. Spells are characterized by paresthesias in one half of the face, sometimes involving the tongue and lips, followed by clonic jerks involving the face, tongue, lips, larynx, and pharynx. The electroencephalogram (EEG) reveals characteristic high-amplitude interictal spikes followed by slow waves in the mid-temporal and central spikes, or sharp waves particularly during sleep (Fig. 10.3-8). The EEG pattern is inherited as an autosomal dominant trait.

NOCTURNAL PAROXYSMAL DYSTONIA

Nocturnal paroxysmal dystonia is a form of frontal lobe epilepsy that consists of a sudden arousal associated with a complex sequence of movements, repeated dystonia, or a dyskinetic (ballistic or choreoathetotic) pattern. Patients may also move their legs and arms with cycling or kicking movements, rock their trunks, and show tonic asymmetric or dystonic posture of the limbs. A few cases are characterized by a violent ballistic pattern with flaying of the limbs. Consciousness is often preserved. Carbamazepine is the agent of choice and provides an excellent response.

SUPPLEMENTARY SENSORIMOTOR SEIZURES

Supplementary sensorimotor seizures are associated with bilateral, contralateral, and ipsilateral somatosensory sensations of numbness or tingling. Nocturnal frontal lobe epilepsy (NFLE) includes spells with predominant motor manifestations and nocturnal preponderance. Frequent seizures often occur in clusters with many per day. These are brief seizures (less than a minute) that occur suddenly and present with little or no ictal confusion. There is often vocalization of variable complexity, and the attacks appear to be bizarre in nature.

AUTOSOMAL DOMINANT NOCTURNAL FRONTAL LOBE EPILEPSY

The clinical manifestations of autosomal dominant nocturnal frontal lobe epilepsy (ADNFLE) include clusters of brief nocturnal motor seizures with hyperkinetic or tonic

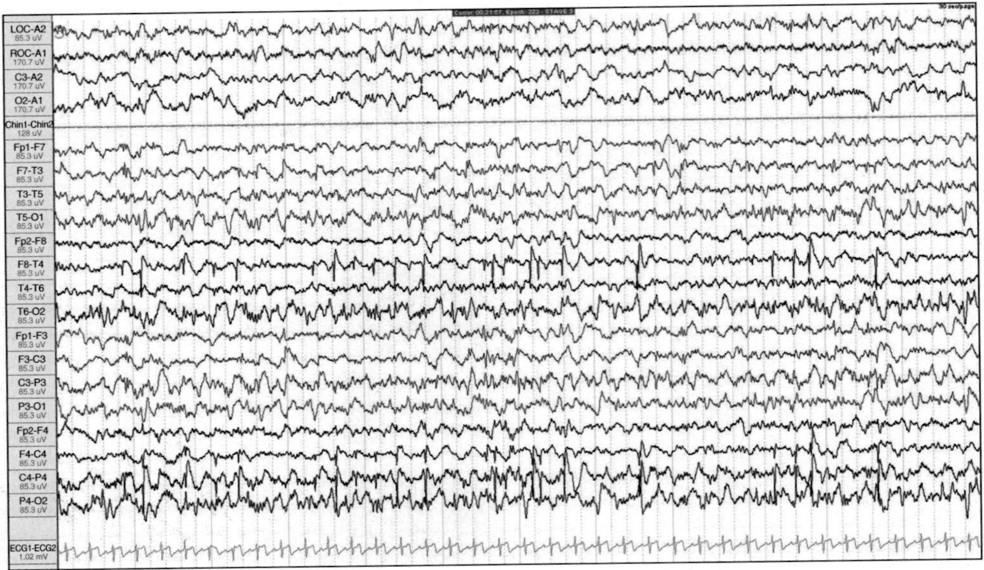

Figure 10.3-8.
PSG example of Rolandic spikes. In this example the spikes are right sided (note their presence primarily in even-numbered electrode pairs). These spikes are characteristic of Rolandic spikes (seen in benign Rolandic epilepsy). They are most prominent over the central and mid-temporal region and are often present only during NREM sleep, when they may become very active. Clinically, there may be twitching of the mouth on the contralateral side with or without drooling. Occasionally these usually trivial seizures will generalize. The prognosis is generally very good, with the natural history of spontaneous resolution over time, hence the term *benign Rolandic epilepsy (black, right; blue, left)*. (PSG courtesy M. Mahowald.)

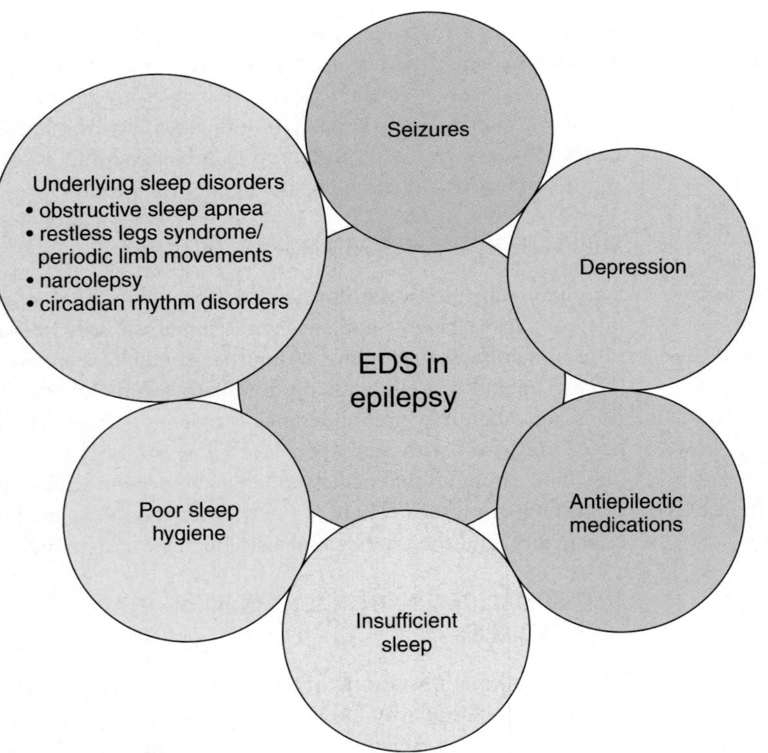

Figure 10.3-9.
Causes of excessive daytime sleepiness (EDS) in epilepsy.

manifestations. ADNFLE is a genetically heterogeneous disorder consisting of four known genetic loci. Genes encode various nicotinic acetylcholine receptor α and β subunits CHRNA-4, CHRNB-2, and CHRNA-2.

Epilepsy with Continuous-Spike–Slow-Wave Activity during Sleep

JUVENILE MYOCLONIC EPILEPSY

Epilepsy with continuous spike waves during slow-wave sleep (CSWS) has a heterogeneous clinical presentation. The defining feature of CSWS is an EEG pattern consisting of generalized slow spike-wave discharges, which are present during 85% to 90% of slow-wave sleep and relatively suppressed during REM sleep and wakefulness.

GENERALIZED TONIC-CLONIC SEIZURES UPON AWAKENING

Juvenile myoclonic epilepsy is one of the most common forms of idiopathic generalized epilepsy, consisting of a triad of three seizure types: myoclonic jerks, generalized tonic-clonic seizures, and absence seizures. A gene locus linked to the human leukocyte antigen (HLA) region on the short arm of chromosome 6 has been identified.

Hypersomnia in Epilepsy Patients

Common causes of hypersomnia in epilepsy patients are shown in Figure 10.3-9.

Obstructive Sleep Apnea and Epilepsy

Sleep apnea may coexist with epilepsy. Several potential mechanisms of action have been proposed as to the etiology of seizure facilitation in obstructive sleep apnea (OSA). Prolonged asystole, which may occur in OSA, may be associated with seizures. Some have proposed that sleep deprivation resulting from frequent arousals increases neuronal excitability. Frequent arousals or stage shifts into and out of sleep therefore facilitate sleep-related seizures. The treatment of OSA may improve seizure control, daytime sleepiness, or both.

SELECTED REFERENCES

Bazil CW: Sleep-related epilepsy. Curr Neurol Neurosci Rep 3:167–172, 2003.

Beran RG, Plunkett MJ, Holland GJ: Interface of epilepsy and sleep disorders. Seizure 8:97–102, 1999.

Foldvary-Schaefer N: Sleep complaints and epilepsy: The role of seizures, antiepileptic drugs and sleep disorders. J Clin Neurophysiol 19(6): 514–521, 2002.

Foldvary-Schaefer N, Grigg-Damberger M: Sleep and epilepsy: What we know, don't know, and need to know. J Clin Neurophysiol 23(1): 4–20, 2006.

Malow BA: Sleep and epilepsy. Neurol Clin 23(4):1127–1147, 2005.

Alon Y. Avidan

Sleep In Parkinson's Disease 10.4

Introduction

The most commonly seen neurodegenerative disorder seen in a sleep disorders center is Parkinson's disease (PD). The patients have a loss of neurons that results in the motor symptoms of resting tremor, rigidity, and akinesias. Sleep complaints are extremely common in PD.

Epidemiology of PD

Except for familial forms, which may begin before age 30, this is a disease of older people. The prevalence is about 1% in people in their late 60s and 5% in patients in their early 80s.

Pathophysiology of PD

The main abnormalities are in the substantia nigra. These result in a reduced content of dopamine in the basal ganglia that leads to the motor abnormalities. Other areas of the brain and neurotransmitter systems are affected. The biological basis of sleep disruption in PD may be due to the alteration of dopaminergic, noradrenergic, serotonergic, and cholinergic neurons in the brainstem.

Sleep Symptoms

The majority of patients with Parkinson's disease have sleep disorders that adversely affect their quality of life. These sleep disturbances include excessive daytime sleepiness, insomnia, motor disorders (related to restless legs syndrome and periodic limb movements), and parasomnias such as rapid eye movement (REM) sleep behavior disorder and nightmares (Fig. 10.4-1). Severe sleepiness and fatigue are common in PD patients and are two of the most disabling of their many symptoms (Fig. 10.4-2). Sleep complaints in PD patients increase with the increased severity of their

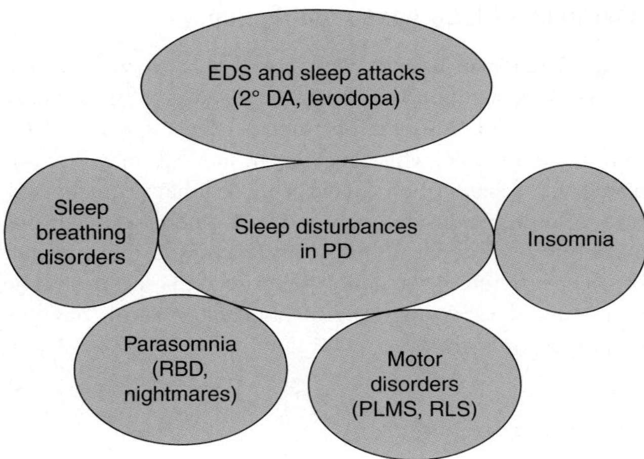

Figure 10.4-1.
The spectrum of sleep disorders in patients with PD, 2° DA, secondary to dopamine agonists; EDS, excessive daytime sleepiness; PLMS, periodic leg movements in sleep; RBD, REM sleep behavior disorder; RLS, restless legs syndrome.

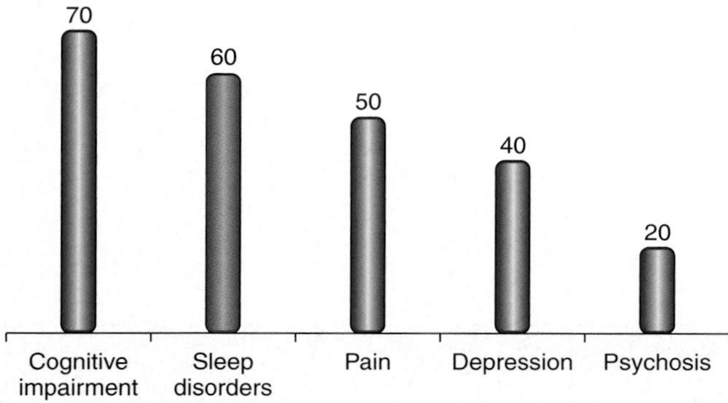

Figure 10.4-2.
The clinical symptoms of Parkinson's disease. Sleep disturbances are often more common than underlying psychiatric disorders and pain. (Data from Parkinson's Disease and Movement Disorders: Diagnosis and Treatment Guidelines for the Practicing Physician. Mayo Foundation for Medical Education and Research, 2002.)

disease. In severe PD, nocturia can disturb sleep and may be related to the development of dysautonomia in PD.

Sleep complaints occur in 60% to 90% of PD patients, and many other disease-related or secondary factors may play a role, including the medications used for PD treatment. The most common causes of excessive daytime sleepiness in PD are related to a variety of factors, as summarized in Figure 10.4-3.

Patients often have difficulty or inability turning over and getting out of bed. This is most likely secondary to bradykinesia. There are several prominent symptoms involving the limbs, including leg cramps and leg jerks

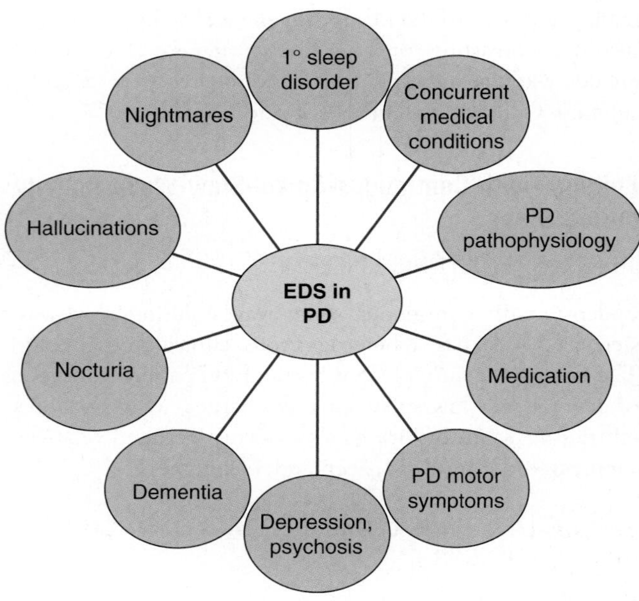

Figure 10.4-3.
Causes of excessive daytime sleepiness (EDS) in PD.

and dystonic spasms. Such spasms may also affect the face and back.

Laboratory Findings

The common sleep laboratory findings include fragmented sleep with an increased number of arousals and awakenings, motor phenomena such as nocturnal immobility, rest tremor, eye-blinking, dyskinesias, and other abnormalities (including periodic leg movements and restless legs syndrome), fragmentary myoclonus, and sleep breathing disorders. Sleep maintenance problems and difficulties with sleep initiation are the earliest and most frequent sleep disorders observed in these patients (Figs. 10.4-4 to 10.4-6).

Polysomnographic recordings confirm reduced sleep efficiency, increased wake after sleep onset, marked sleep fragmentation, reduced slow-wave sleep and REM sleep, disruption of the NREM-to-REM cycle, loss of muscle atonia, and increased EMG activity in REM sleep, which is the basis for REM sleep behavior disorder (see chapter 10.5). The latter, which is very common in PD, may also precede by years the onset of PD.

PD-specific motor abnormalities during sleep include the Parkinsonism tremor and REM-onset blepharospasm, which disappears in REM sleep. Patients have rapid blinking at sleep onset and REM intrusion into NREM sleep. Patients with PD who have posture reflex abnormalities and autonomic nervous system impairment are at an increased risk for sleep-related breathing disorders, including central sleep apnea, obstructive sleep apnea, and the alveolar hypoventilation syndrome. Parkinson's disease may lead to extrapulmonary lung restriction (Fig. 10.4-7).

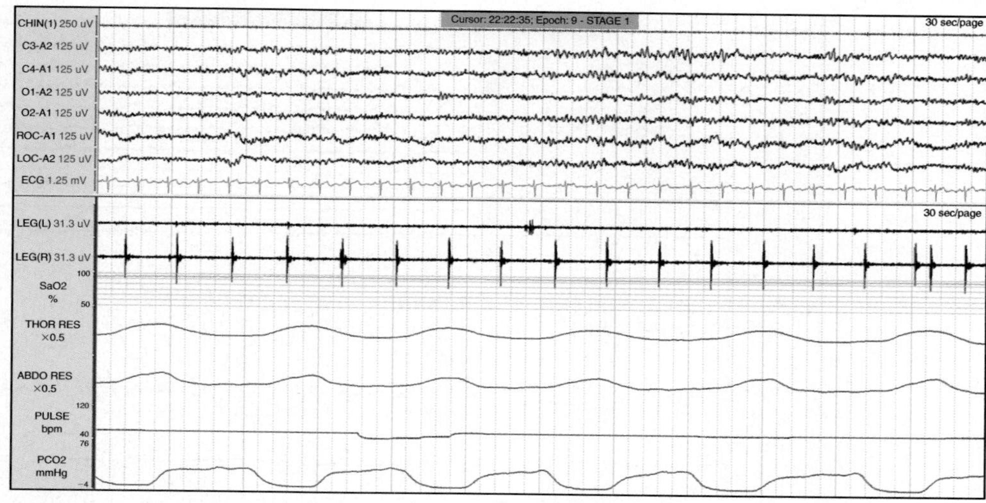

Figure 10.4-4. Polysomnographic recording of a patient with Parkinson's disease and rest tremor of the right leg during wakefulness. There is a regular unilateral rest tremor. The tremor continued during NREM sleep in this patient.

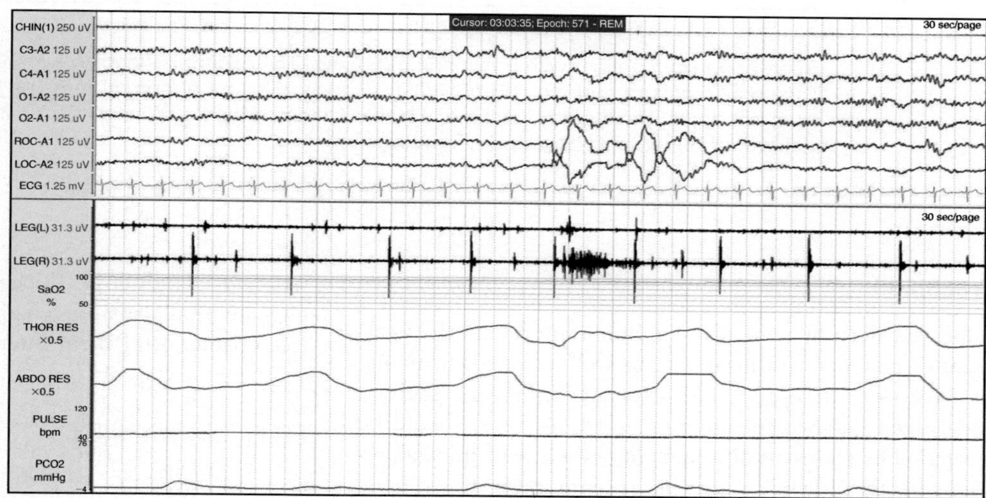

Figure 10.4-5. Polysomnographic recording of the patient with Parkinson's disease in Figure 10.4-4 during REM sleep. There is still unilateral tremor, but the frequency at which the tremors occurred decreased by about half, and there was much less regularity noted. There is increased activity in the right leg synchronous with REM. This patient also had REM sleep behavior disorder.

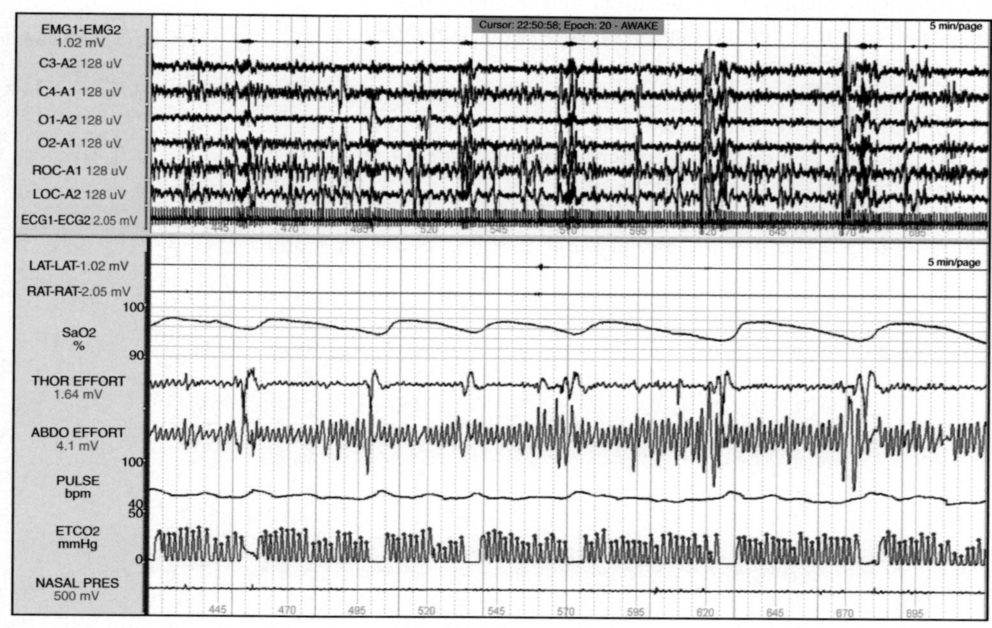

Figure 10.4-6. Oxygen desaturations and yawning during wakefulness in Parkinson's disease. This patient had sleep-onset insomnia and demonstrated progressive drops in SaO_2 terminating in a yawn during wakefulness. The findings mimic sleep apnea.

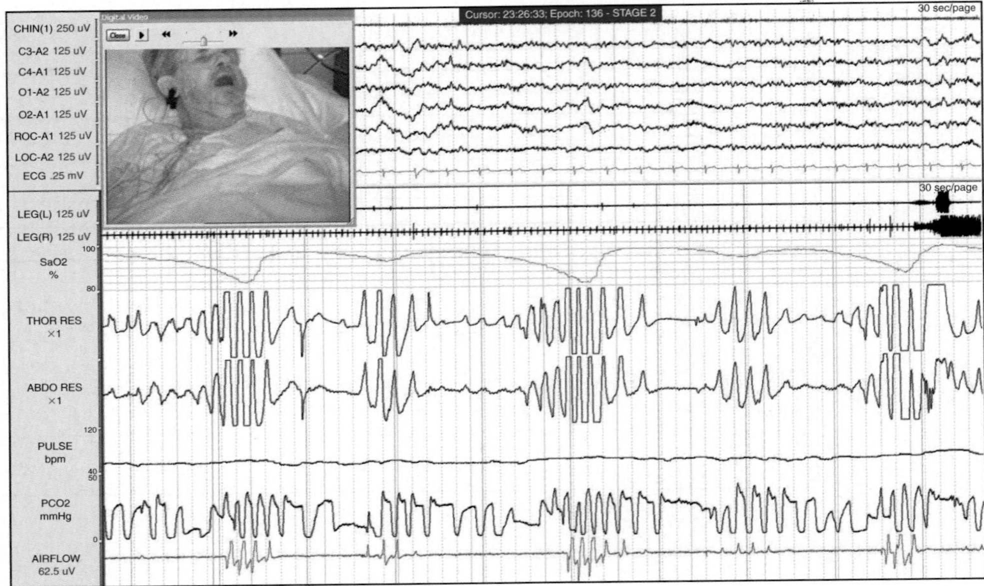

Figure 10.4-7.
Sleep apnea in a patient with Parkinson's disease. The patient is sleeping with his mouth open. The nasal pressure and the end-tidal CO_2 suggest different abnormalities. The nasal pressure does not detect the mouth breathing, which is detected by the oronasal CO_2 catheter. This has features of both obstructive and central apnea.

Treatment

Improved sleep hygiene plays an important role in the treatment of patients with insomnia. As well, any accompanying primary sleep disorders and associated problems such as REM sleep behavior disorder (see chapter 10.5) should be treated. The mainstay of treatment is the use of dopaminergic agonists. Sodium oxybate has recently been shown to be effective in improving sleep quality and daytime alertness in PD. Problems related to bradykinesia and nocturia may be improved by providing patients with a bedside commode. For patients with symptoms of restless legs syndrome, an evening and nighttime dose of dopaminergic D_3 agonist is useful. Patients in treatment may have additional sleep difficulties because low-dose dopaminergic agonists are often sedating. High-dose dopaminergic agonists may cause increased hallucinations, nightmares, and increased arousals (see chapter 19, Patient Interview Videos).

SELECTED READINGS

Dhawan V, Healy DG, Pal S, Chaudhuri KR: Sleep-related problems of Parkinson's disease. Age Ageing 35(3):220–228, 2006.

Frucht SJ, Greene PE, Fahn S: Sleep episodes in Parkinson's disease: A wake-up call. Move Disord 15:601–603, 2000.

Larsen JP, Tandberg E: Sleep disorders in patients with Parkinson's disease: Epidemiology and management. CNS Drugs 15(4):267–275, 2001.

Trenkwalder C: Parkinsonism. In Kryger M, Roth T, Dement WC (eds): Principles and Practice of Sleep Medicine, 4th ed. Philadelphia, Elsevier, 2005.

Alon Y. Avidan

REM Sleep Behavior Disorder 10.5

Introduction

Normally, during rapid eye movement (REM) sleep there is a loss of skeletal muscle tone throughout most of the body. REM sleep behavior disorder (RBD) is characterized by pathologic augmentation of skeletal muscle tone during REM sleep (Fig. 10.5-1). Patients present with unusual, complex, sometimes quite vigorous, sometimes violent motor activity during a dream. Motor activity ranges from simple limb movements to very complex apparent responses to dream content. The potential for patients to harm themselves and their bed partner is high (see chapter 12).

Epidemiology of RBD

The majority of cases are older people. In approximately 60% of older people the condition is idiopathic; the remaining 40% may have an underlying neurologic disease. RBD often presents in people in their 60s and 70s. It has increasingly been described in children and adolescents.

RBD is commonly seen in Parkinson's disease (PD). Many patients with PD but without sleep complaints may have subclinical or clinical RBD. RBD may precede the manifestation of Parkinsonism and other diseases by decades.

In addition to RBD being more common in PD (see chapter 10.4), RBD is more likely to occur in synucleinopathies

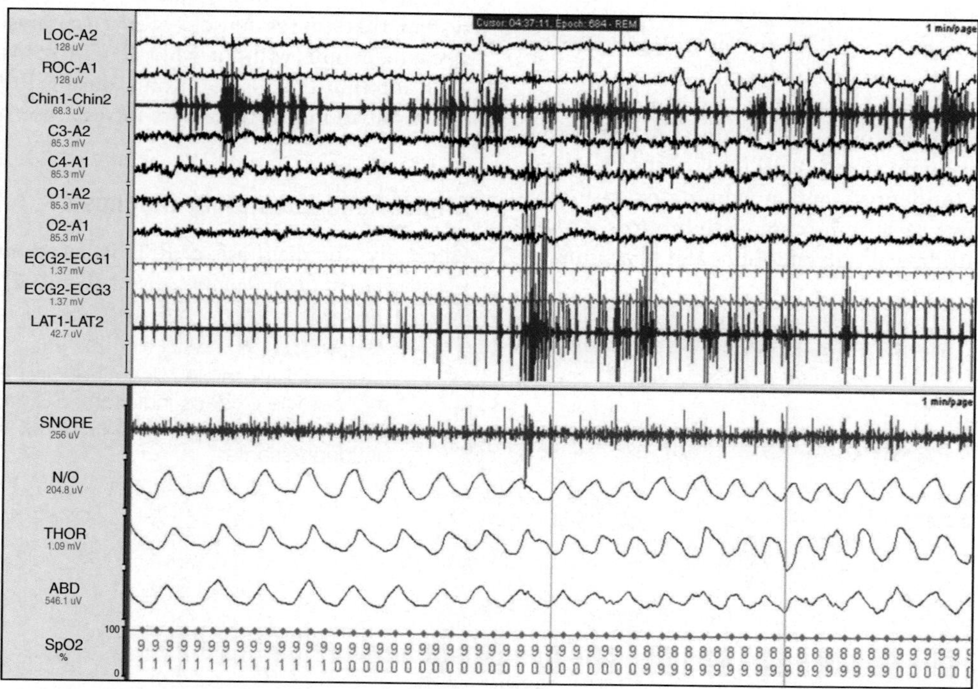

Figure 10.5-1.
A 1-minute epoch from the PSG of an 80-year-old man referred for evaluation of recurrent violent nighttime awakenings. Illustrated here is a typical event that this patient was experiencing. He was noted to yell, jump from bed, and have complex body movements. Although there is a great deal of intermittent muscle activity in the chin and leg, there is underlying REM-associated muscle atonia in the chin EMG and the left anterior tibialis muscle. The twitches in the latter are actually an EKG artifact (notice the synchrony with EKG). Channels are as follows: Electro-oculogram (LOC-A2, left; ROC-A1, right), chin electromyogram (EMG), electroencephalogram (left central, right central, left occipital, right occipital), two ECG channels, limb EMG (lateral), snore channel, nasal-oral airflow, respiratory effort (thoracic, abdominal), and oxygen saturation (SpO_2).

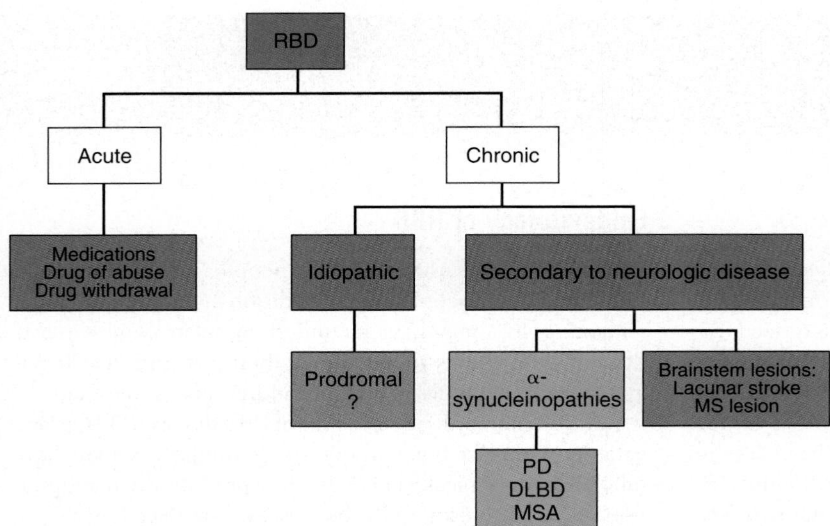

Figure 10.5-2.
RBD classification: Acute forms could be caused by underlying medications and drugs of abuse. The chronic form is most likely prodromal and related to alpha-synucleinopathies. DLBD, diffuse Lewy body disease; MS, multiple sclerosis; MSA, multiple system atrophy; PD, Parkinson's disease.

and other neurodegenerative disorders, including diffuse Lewy body disease, olivopontocerebellar degeneration, Shy-Drager syndrome, and multiple system atrophy.

In the secondary forms of RBD the neurologic diseases disrupt the brainstem centers involved in the muscle atonia of REM. These diseases include multiple sclerosis, cerebral vascular accidents, and brainstem neoplasms (Fig. 10.5-2). The acute onset of RBD is related to drugs such as tricyclic antidepressants, monamine oxidase inhibitors, and selective serotonin-reuptake inhibitors, as well as to acute withdrawal of alcohol and barbiturates (Fig. 10.5-3).

Pathophysiology of RBD

The pontine tegmentum appears to be the location of the system that causes muscle atonia (paralysis) during REM sleep in people without RBD (Fig. 10.5-4). In RBD there is an intermittent loss of atonia during REM sleep, which can result in motor behaviors in response to dreams.

Clinical and Laboratory Diagnosis

Clinically, the diagnosis of RBD is based on the *International Classification of Sleep Disorders, revised* (ICSD-2). In many cases,

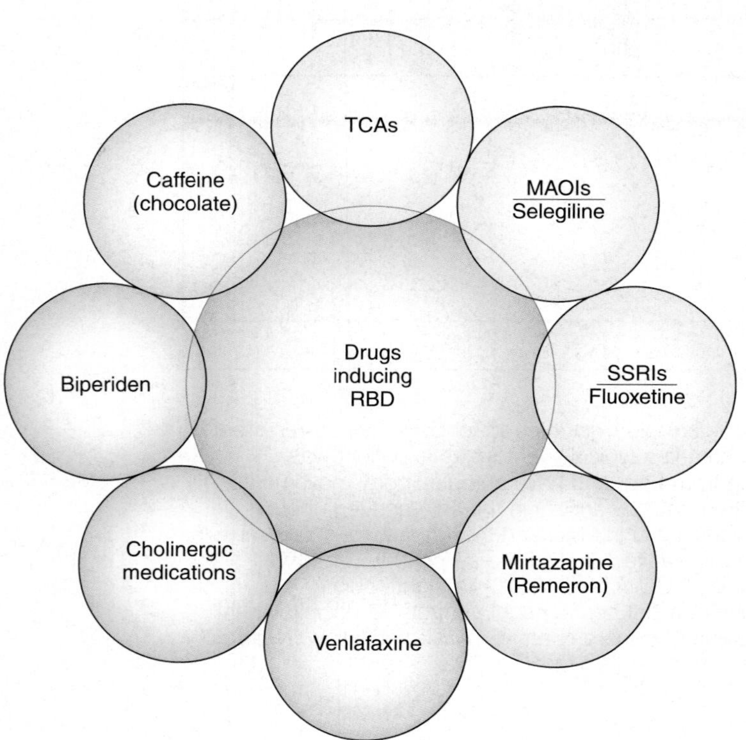

Figure 10.5-3.
Drugs with possible role in inducing RBD. MAOIs, monoamine oxidase inhibitors; SSRIs, selective serotonin reuptake inhibitors; TCAs, tricyclic antidepressants.

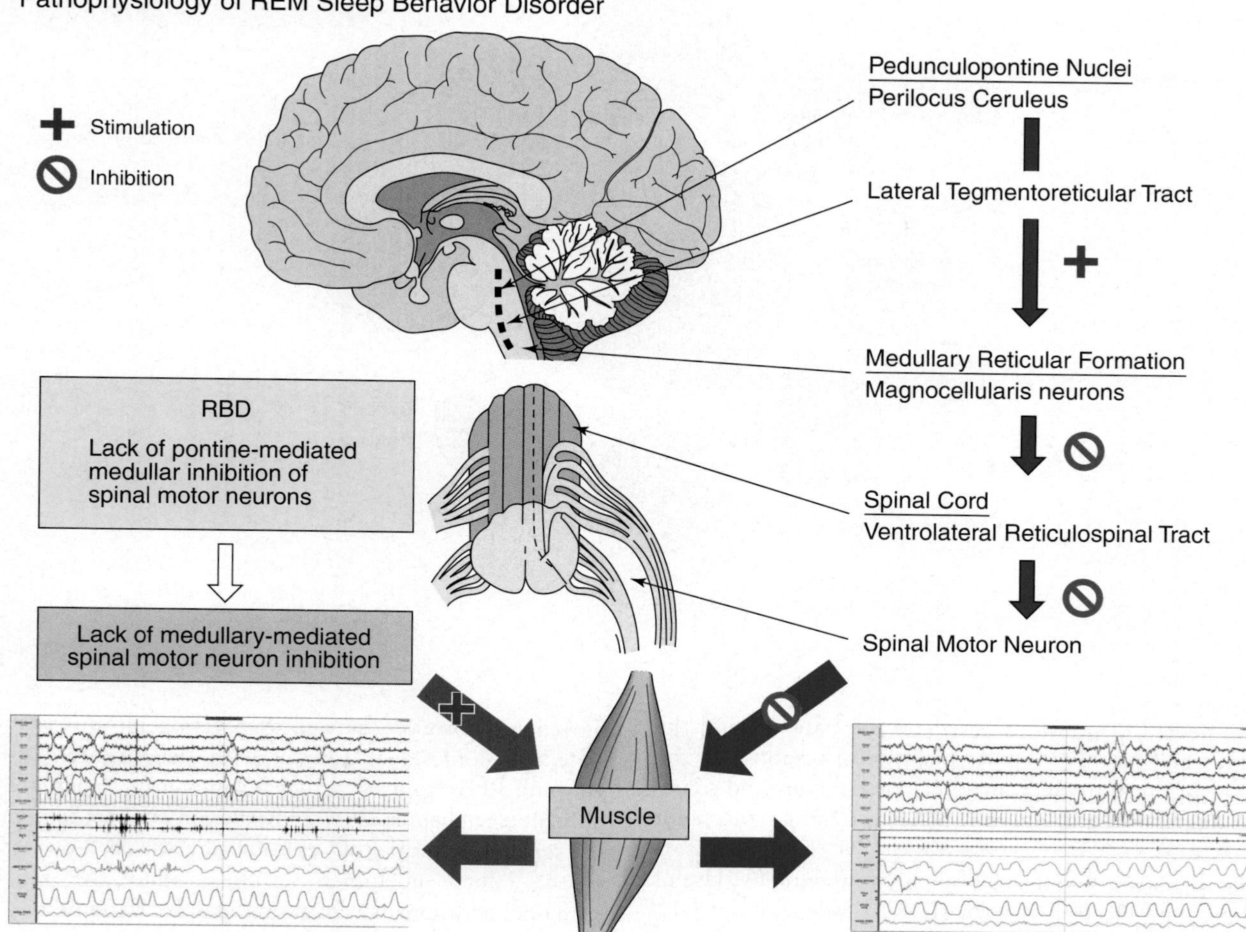

Figure 10.5-4.
Pathophysiology of RBD. Generalized muscle atonia during REM sleep results from pontine-mediated perilocus ceruleus inhibition of motor activity. This pontine activity exerts an excitatory influence on medullary reticular formation (magnocellularis neurons) through the lateral tegmentoreticular tract. These neuronal groups in turn hyperpolarize the spinal motor neuron postsynaptic membranes through the ventrolateral reticulospinal tract. In RBD, the brainstem mechanisms generating the muscle atonia normally seen in REM sleep may be disrupted. The pathophysiology of RBD in humans has been studied in a cat model, where bilateral pontine lesions result in a persistent absence of REM sleep atonia associated with prominent motor activity, similar to that observed in human RBD. The pathophysiology of the idiopathic form of RBD in humans may arise from reduction of central dopaminergic innervation. (Adapted from Primary care: Clinics in office practice. Special issue: Sleep disorders in the older patient. Sleep Med 32:563–586, 2005.)

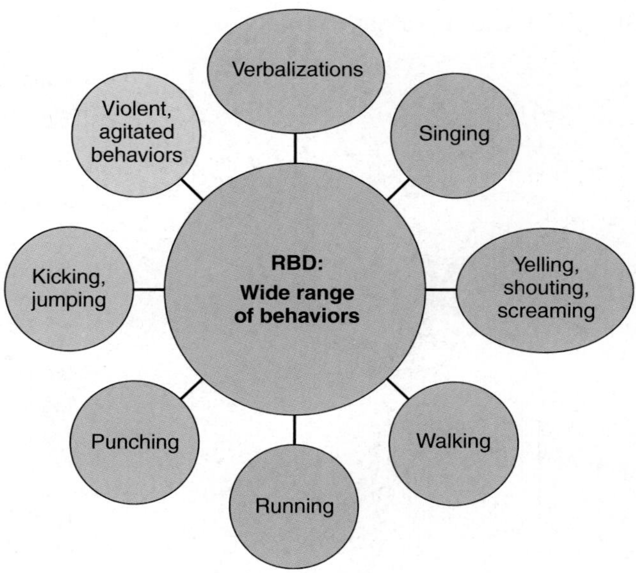

Figure 10.5-5.
Behavioral spectrum of RBD.

the suspected diagnosis is based on the patient's and the patient's bed partner's reports of physical response to the content of dreams, which may include complex and sometimes aggressive and vigorous behaviors during the night (Fig. 10.5-5).

The diagnosis is confirmed by polysomnography. Use of multiple-limb electromyogram (EMG) leads (Box 10.5-1), along with synchronized digital video monitoring demonstrating evidence of increased electromyographic bursts of chin EMG or limb electrodes during REM sleep, has some intrinsic limitations based on the patient's report or on ambiguous terminology, whereas polysomnography has a better reliability.

The differential diagnosis of RBD includes sleepwalking, nocturnal seizures, post-traumatic stress disorder, sleep terrors, nocturnal panic disorders, delirium, and periodic limb movements disorder, as well as psychogenic dissociative-state and confusional arousals with sleep apnea. Distinguishing RBD from nocturnal seizures may sometimes be difficult (see chapter 10.3). However, in contrast to nocturnal seizures, typical RBD episodes are usually not stereotyped. When nocturnal seizures cannot be reliably excluded, additional sleep testing may be warranted.

Treatment for RBD

Safety for the patient's bed partner as well as for the patient is crucial in every case of RBD. The sleeping environment may have to be modified by, for example, removing dangerous objects and padding the bed area.

Suggested treatment for RBD includes clonazepam (0.25 mg to 1 mg po, qhs), which is effective in 90% of

BOX 10.5-1. ICSD-2 CRITERIA FOR REM SLEEP BEHAVIOR DISORDER

DIAGNOSIS

Suspected clinically, confirmed by PSG.

DIAGNOSTIC CRITERIA

- PSG abnormality: elevated EMG tone during REM sleep in either submental or limb leads.
- Either a history of dream enactment behavior or observation of abnormal REM sleep behavior during the PSG.
- Absence of EEG epileptiform activity during REM sleep.
- The disorder is not better explained by another sleep, medical, neurologic, or psychiatric disorder; medication use; or substance abuse.

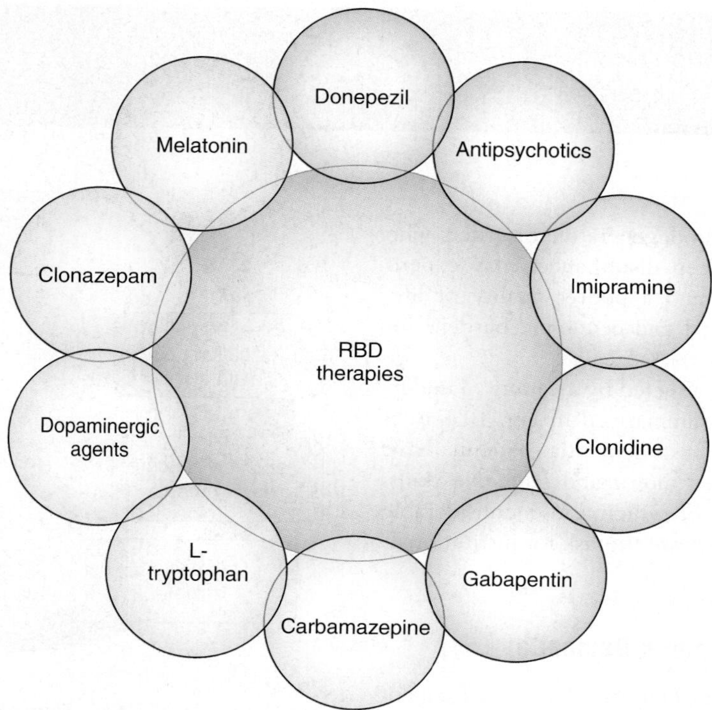

Figure 10.5-6.
Treatment options for RBD.

cases (Fig. 10.5-6). There is little evidence of tolerance or abuse with this. Abrupt discontinuation of treatment can precipitate withdrawal symptoms. Other agents that can be helpful include imipramine (25 mg po, qhs), carbamazepine (100 mg po, tid), and levodopa, in cases where RBD is associated with Parkinson's disease. There may be improvement with melatonin, which is believed to exert its effect by restoring REM sleep atonia. Two studies reported that melatonin was effective in 87% of patients taking 3 to 9 mg at bedtime, whereas a later study reported resolution in those taking 6 to 12 mg at bedtime. Tacrine, donepezil, and nefazodone, drugs used in Alzheimer's disease and other neurodegenerative disorders, may exacerbate RBD. Some antidepressants that potentially may increase total REM sleep may also worsen RBD.

SELECTED REFERENCES

Boeve BF, Silber MH, Ferman TJ: REM sleep behavior disorder in Parkinsons disease and dementia with Lewy bodies. J Geriatr Psychiatry Neurol 17(3):146–157, 2004.

Gugger JJ, Wagner ML: Rapid eye movement sleep behavior disorder. Ann Pharmacother 41(11):1833–1841, 2007.

Schenck CH, Bundlie SR, Mahowald MW: Delayed emergence of a Parkinsonian disorder in 38% of 29 older men initially diagnosed with idiopathic rapid eye movement sleep behavior disorder. Neurology 46:388–393, 1996.

Schenck CH, Bundlie SR, Patterson AL, Mahowald MW: Rapid eye movement sleep behavior disorder: A treatable parasomnia affecting older adults. JAMA 257(13):1786–1789, 1987.

Schenck CH, Mahowald MW: REM parasomnias. Neurology Clin 14:697–720, 1996.

Stores G: Rapid eye movement sleep behavior disorder in children and adolescents. Dev Med Child Neurol 50(10):728–732, 2008.

10.6 Sleep in Alzheimer's Disease

Alon Y. Avidan

Introduction

Patients with underlying neurodegenerative disorders who are affected by comorbid sleep disturbances may experience higher rates of injury and a poorer quality of life, and may impose greater social and economic burdens for caregivers and society.

Patients with dementia are affected by a variety of underlying sleep disturbances, as summarized in Fig. 10.6-1. In addition to these disturbances, dementia patients have increased irritability, impaired motor and cognitive skills, depression, and fatigue, all of which cause considerable caregiver burden and may increase the risk for institutionalization (Fig. 10.6-2).

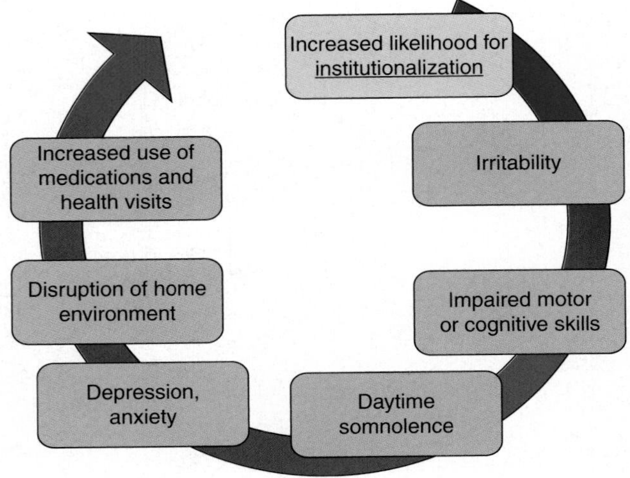

Figure 10.6-2.
Consequences of sleep disorders in dementia. Dementia patients with underlying sleep disorders experience significant irritability, impaired motor and cognitive skills, excessive daytime sleepiness, and depression and anxiety resulting in disruption of the home environment. Their increased use of medications and higher rates of health visits result in increased societal costs, finally culminating in increased likelihood for institutionalization.

Sleep Disorders in Alzheimer's Dementia

Sleep disorders in Alzheimer's dementia (AD) are frequent and correlated with the severity of the disease progression. The disturbances may be divided into internal (direct) and external (indirect) mechanisms, as shown in Table 10.6-1. Direct mechanisms, depicted in Figure 10.6-3, may be further related to the degeneration of specific nuclei in the brain: the cholinergic neurons in the nucleus basalis of Meynert, the pedunculopontine tegmental nuclei, the laterodorsal tegmental nuclei, and the noradrenergic neurons of the brainstem may be responsible for decreased rapid eye movement (REM) sleep in AD patients. It is thought that degeneration of the suprachiasmatic nucleus (SCN) may be primarily responsible for the underlying circadian rhythm disturbances seen in AD. Polysomnographic disturbances in AD consist of decreased sleep efficiency and reversal of circadian rhythmicity.

Indirect mechanisms of sleep disruption in AD include environmental factors such as reduced environmental light during the day, underlying medical, sleep, and psychiatric illnesses, medication-related side effects, and predictable age-related alterations in sleep (as described in chapter 4). Patients with AD have significant sleep architecture abnormalities. The hallmarks include reduction in sleep

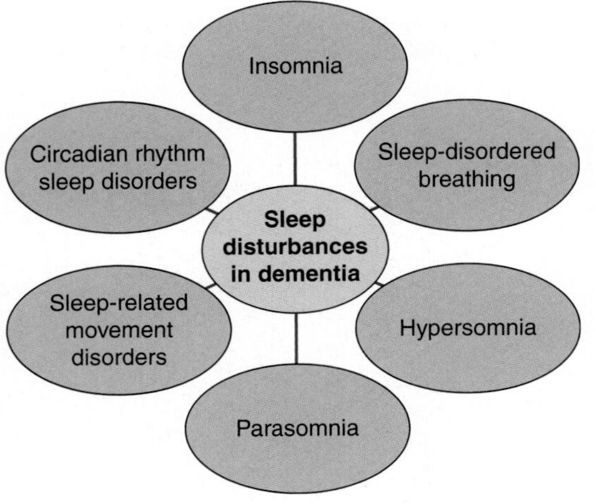

Figure 10.6-1.
The spectrum of sleep disorders in patients with dementia.

Table 10.6-1. Sleep Disruption in Dementia

EXTERNAL FACTORS	INTERNAL FACTORS	
Decreased periodic environmental stimuli (i.e., light exposure) Environmental factors: excessive noise and light	**Illness:**	Dementia Depression Medical illness Medications Inactivity
	Increased age:	Age-related changes in sleep Changes in the internal circadian clock Increased prevalence of 1° sleep disorders

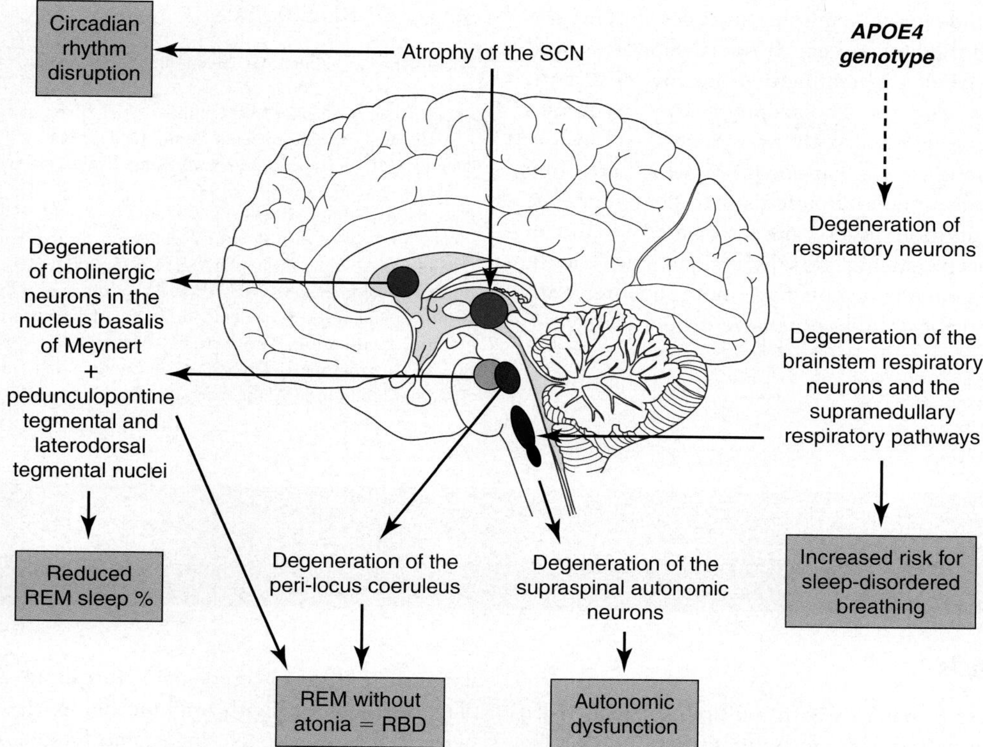

Figure 10.6-3.
Pathophysiology of sleep disruption in patients with Alzheimer's dementia: potential environmental and intrinsic factors. (Adapted from Avidan A: Sleep disturbances in dementia and other neurodegenerative disorders. In Culebras A [ed]: Sleep Disorders and Neurologic Diseases, 2nd ed. New York, Taylor & Francis Group, 2007, pp. 315–336.)

efficiency, increase in non-REM (NREM) stage N1 sleep, increase in arousal and awakening frequency, decrease in total sleep time, and reduction in sleep spindles and K complexes. A profound disruption in sleep-wake rhythmicity occurs primarily early in the onset of the disease. Sleep fragmentation subsequently leads to increased daytime sleepiness, nocturnal insomnia, nocturnal wandering, increase in cognitive decline, increase in the number of daytime naps, increase in time in bed and time spent awake in bed, and increase in the frequency of nocturnal wandering, disorientation, and confusion. Later, as the disease progresses, patients with AD manifest more dramatic reduction of REM sleep, increased REM sleep latency, and a marked alteration of the circadian rhythm resulting in sleepiness. In fact, sleep and cognitive dysfunction are positively correlated in AD.

Sundowning Syndrome

Sundowning refers to agitation in dementia patients that has specific temporal exacerbation during the early evening or nocturnal hours. Patients with sundowning syndrome experience nocturnal confusion, hyperactivity, delirium, disorganized thinking, wandering, restlessness, impaired attention, agitation, insomnia, hypersomnia, hallucinations, anger, delusions, anxiety, and illusions. Patients with AD have increased susceptibility to sundowning, which is a frequent cause of institutionalization. The term *sundowning* is often used too loosely and ambiguously, describing nocturnal agitation without specifically connoting a precise pathophysiologic mechanism or diagnosis. Specific therapy for sundowning is targeted at uncovering the underlying causes. Figure 10.6-4 summarizes the contributing factors to sundowning syndrome.

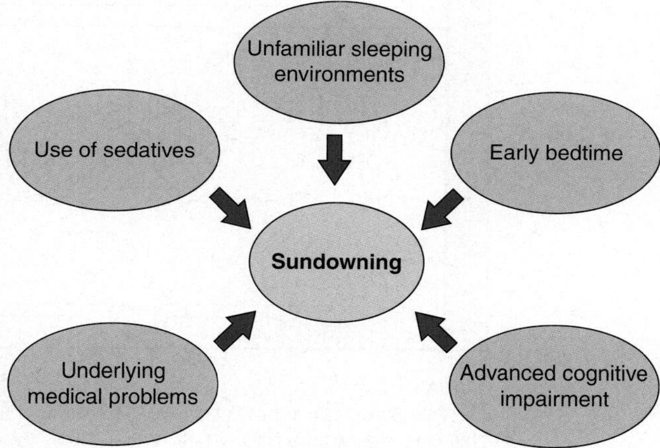

Figure 10.6-4.
Etiology of sundowning syndrome. Several factors may play a role in sundowning.

Therapy for sundowning syndrome includes the integration of behavioral therapy and psychosocial support as well as specific pharmacologic treatment using low-dose antipsychotic agents and benzodiazepines. Antipsychotics often have adverse effects, such as sedation, confusion, orthostatic hypotension, and Parkinsonism, which are often clinically significant in elderly patients with dementia. The "high-potency" antipsychotics are associated with an increased risk of producing extrapyramidal side effects, whereas the "low-potency" agents have more sedating, anticholinergic, and orthostatic hypotensive properties.

SELECTED REFERENCES

Ancoli-Israel S, Alessi C: Sleep and aging. Am J Geriatr Psychiatry 13(5):341–343, 2005.

Ancoli-Israel S, Klauber MR, Gillin JC, et al: Sleep in non-institutionalized Alzheimer's disease patients. Aging (Milan) 6(6):451–458, 1994.

Bachman DL: Sleep disorders with aging: Evaluation and treatment. Geriatrics 47(9):53–56, 59–61, 1992.

Blass JP: Alzheimer's disease. Dis Mon 31(4):1–69, 1985.

Bliwise DL: Sleep disorders in Alzheimer's disease and other dementias. Clin Cornerstone 6(Suppl 1A):S16–S28, 2004.

Bliwise DL, Hughes M, McMahon PM, Kutner N: Observed sleep/wakefulness and severity of dementia in an Alzheimer's disease special care unit. J Gerontology 50A(6):M303–M306, 1995.

Bliwise D, Yesavage J, Tinklenberg J: Sundowning and rate of decline in mental function in Alzheimer's disease. Dementia 3:335–341, 1992.

10.7 Sleep in Other Neurologic Disorders

Alon Y. Avidan

Multiple Sclerosis

Sleep disturbances in patients with multiple sclerosis (MS) are related to underlying comorbidities that include leg spasms, pain, immobility, nocturia, and immune-modulating therapies. Common sleep disorders in patients with MS include sleep apnea (Fig. 10.7-1; see chapter 19, Patient Interview Videos), insomnia, restless legs syndrome, narcolepsy, and rapid eye movement (REM) sleep behavior disorder typically resulting in hypersomnolence, increased fatigue, and a lowered pain threshold (Table 10.7-1). Treatment of MS with immunotherapy is often associated with hypersomnolence, increasing fatigue, depression, and insomnia. MS plaques affecting the diencephalon (hypothalamic region) have also been shown to cause hypersomnia and narcoleptic symptoms in the context of low cerebrospinal fluid (CSF) hypocretin-1 (orexin-1) levels. An increased clinical awareness of sleep-related problems is warranted in this patient population because these

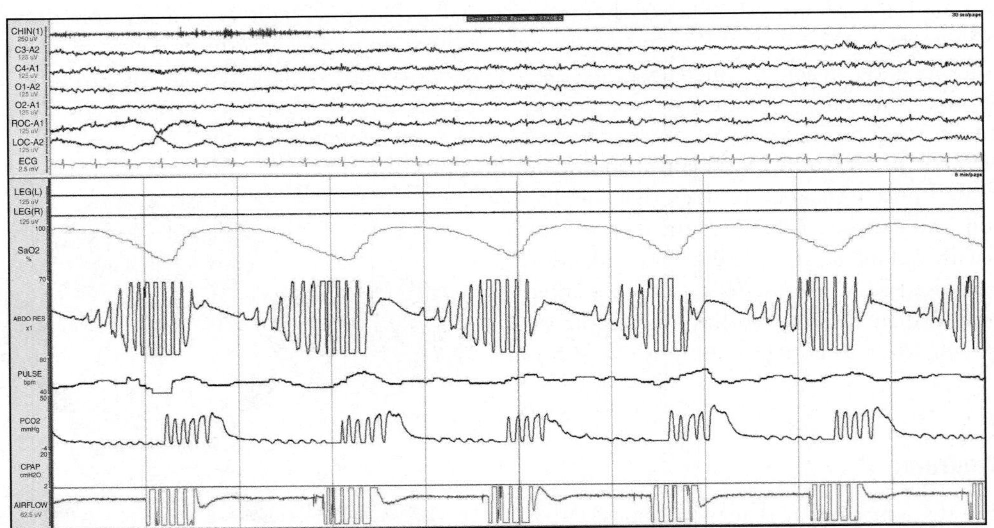

Figure 10.7-1.
Central sleep apnea in a 56-year-old male patient with multiple sclerosis, snoring, obesity, and daytime sleepiness. He was found to have a periodic breathing pattern with few breaths in each cycle alternating with mixed apnea (respiratory effort at the end of the cycles but without airflow). Continuous positive airway pressure was not successful, and the patient required bilevel pressure.

Table 10.7-1. Summary of the Etiology of Sleep Problems in Multiple Sclerosis Based on Direct and Indirect Causes

DIRECT	INDIRECT
• Sleep apnea	• Leg spasm
• Insomnia	• Immobility
• Restless legs syndrome	• Pain
• Narcolepsy	• Nocturia
• REM sleep behavior disorder	

problems are extremely common and have the potential to negatively impact overall health and quality of life.

Chronic Pain and Fibromyalgia

Sleep and pain have a bidirectional interaction, which ultimately impacts the biological and behavioral capacity of the individual. Sleep studies of patients experiencing acute pain during postoperative recovery demonstrate shortened and fragmented sleep with reduced amounts of slow-wave sleep and REM sleep. Recovery is accompanied by normalization of sleep architecture. Chronic pain disturbances such as arthritis frequently coexist with insomnia. Chronic pain can also produce a vicious cycle of inactivity and hypersomnia during the day, as well as insomnia at night. Patients with chronic pain disorders, including fibromyalgia, report significantly more sleepiness, more fatigue, and less refreshing sleep. Successful management of chronic pain requires treatment of the pain and the associated comorbid mood disorders. Treatment of pain with opiates, however, can lead to the development of severe central apnea (Fig. 10.7-2).

Fibromyalgia is commonly associated with sleep disturbances characterized by nonrestorative sleep and increased nocturnal awakenings (Fig. 10.7-3). The sleep disturbances and chronic stress related to fibromyalgia may be

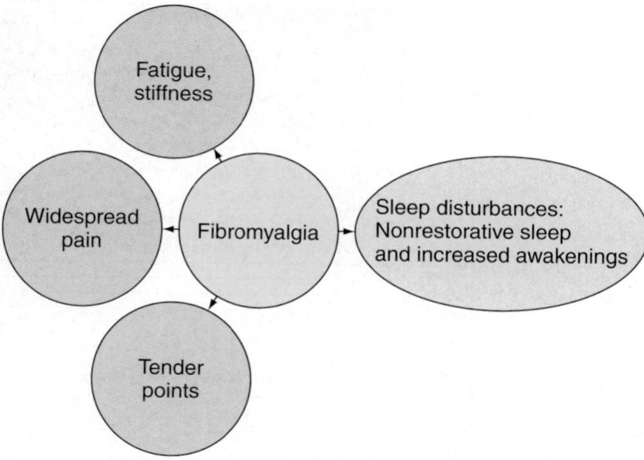

Figure 10.7-3.
Clinical features of fibromyalgia. Chronic widespread pain is the defining feature of fibromyalgia. Frequent sleep disturbances, fatigue, morning stiffness, and tenderness are also key features. The key sleep disturbances include nonrestorative sleep and increased awakenings.

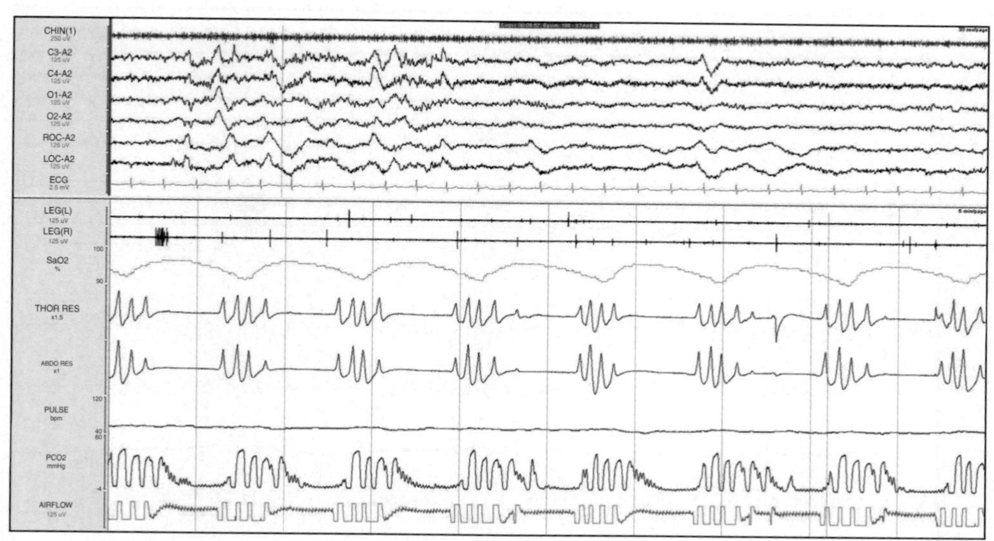

Figure 10.7-2.
Central sleep apnea in a 62-year-old male patient with multiple sclerosis and daytime sleepiness. He had been taking OxyContin for severe pain in his extremities. There is no history of snoring. He was found to have a periodic breathing pattern with few breaths in each cycle alternating with central apnea. Note the cardiogenic oscillations in the CO_2 trace and the nasal pressure trace indicating that the upper airway was patent. There was no audible snoring. Surprisingly, the breathing pattern normalized entirely on oxygen treatment.

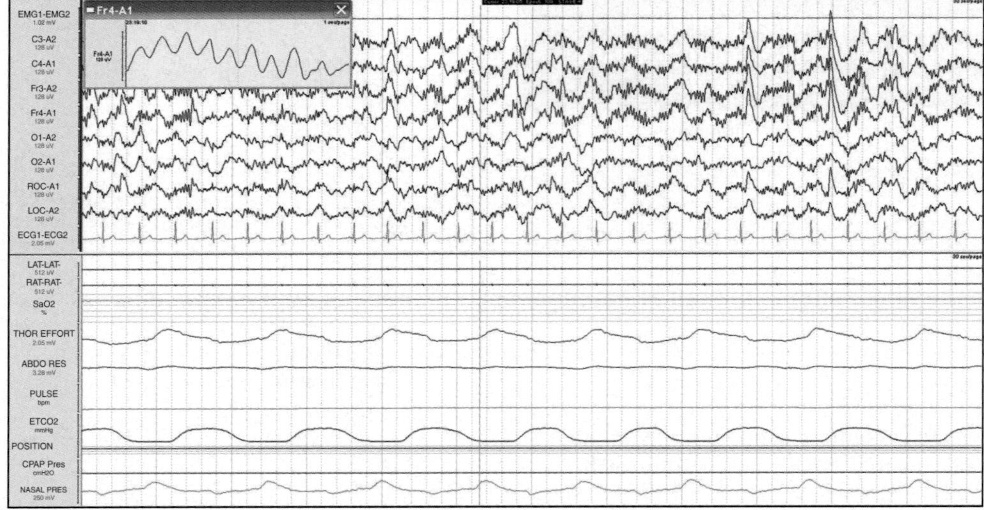

Figure 10.7-4.
Alpha-delta sleep in a 40-year-old woman with a history of sleepiness and tossing and turning. With modern systems one may drill into the PSG. The inset shows a 1-second window from one of the EEG channels showing 10 peaks in 1 second, typical of alpha activity (8 to 13 Hz) (see chapter 17, Table 17.2).

associated with fatigue, cognitive difficulties, and other stress-related symptoms. The hallmark signature of sleep studies in patients with fibromyalgia is alpha-delta sleep (Fig. 10.7-4).

Sleep and Cerebrovascular Accidents

Sleep and cerebrovascular accidents (CVAs) interact in a number of fascinating and complex ways. As high as 60%

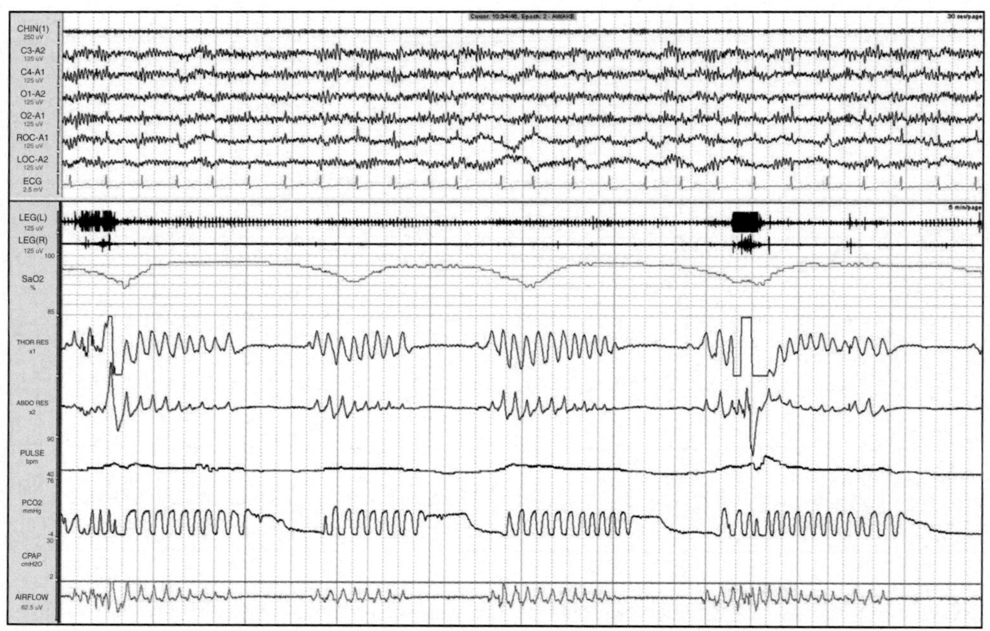

Figure 10.7-5.
Central apnea in a 81-year-old female with a 3-year history of severe insomnia that began immediately after a stroke. Note that the patient is awake. The patient had this breathing pattern the entire night and did not achieve persistent sleep.

of patients who present with stroke have obstructive sleep apnea (OSA), and, in fact, snoring alone is associated with a relative risk of 3.2 for stroke. OSA is the most common form of sleep-disordered breathing in CVA, but central sleep apnea (Fig. 10.7-5) and Cheyne Stokes breathing (Fig. 10.7-6) may predominate in 30% to 40% of patients. Brainstem and spinal CVA are infrequent causes of central hypoventilation, failure of automatic breathing (Ondine's curse), and other neurogenic breathing patterns (Table 10.7-2). Patients with deep hemispheric lesions may present with increased yawning and a constant urge for sleep, while patients with subcortical, thalamic, and pontine strokes are often likely to suffer from insomnia. Those with bilateral injury to the pontine tegmentum may theoretically develop REM sleep without atonia. Sleep apnea may be associated with a transient surge of morning blood pressure, which, over time, may lead to nocturnal then diurnal hypertension. Changes in cerebral autoregulation during apneic events and increased carbon dioxide reactivity may contribute to the increased morning stroke risk; indeed, several studies have shown that there is a significant increase in intracranial pressure and a decrease in cerebral perfusion during obstructive apneas.

Table 10.7-2. Neuroanatomic Breathing Centers and Resultant Breathing Pattern Disturbances

ANATOMIC LESION	RESPIRATORY PATHOLOGY
Afferents to medulla (spinal)	Central or obstructive apnea
Direct medulla	Ataxic breathing, failure of automatic breathing
Efferent respiratory control (anterior medulla)	Central or obstructive apnea
Supramedullary breathing control centers	Respiratory apraxia, failure of voluntary breathing
Pontomedullary centers	Irregular breathing

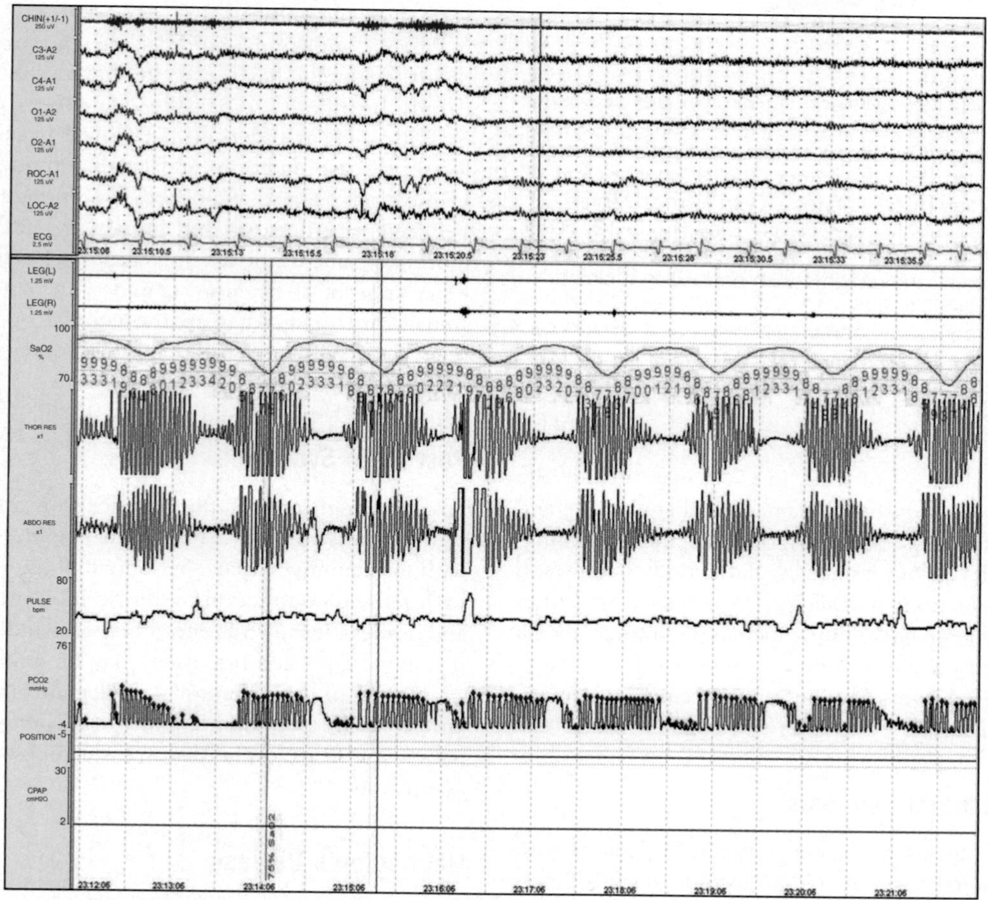

Figure 10.7-6.
Cheyne Stokes breathing in a patient with subacute left-hemispheric stroke. This breathing pattern is confirmed when the following is met: At least three consecutive cycles of cyclical crescendo and decrescendo change in breathing amplitude and at least one of the following: (1) five or more central apneas or hypopneas per hour of sleep; (2) the cyclic crescendo and decrescendo change in breathing amplitude has a duration of at least 10 consecutive minutes.

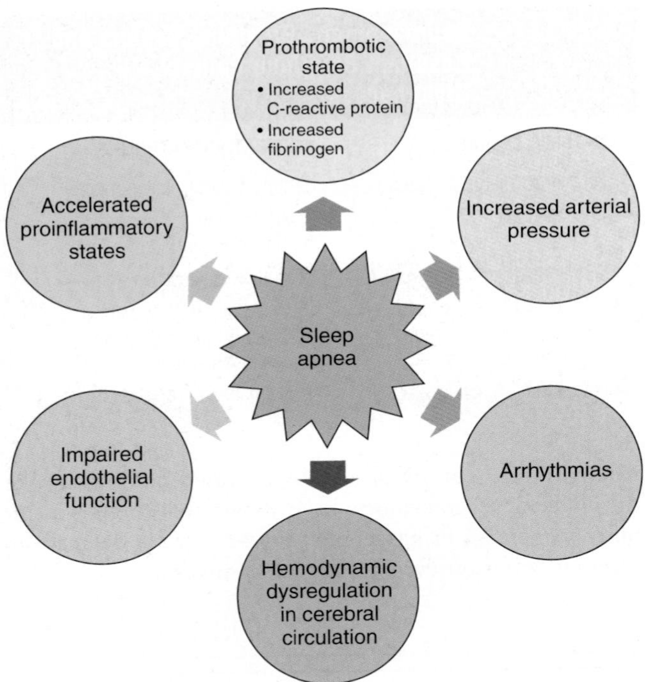

Figure 10.7-7.
Pathophysiology of sleep apnea in cerebrovascular accidents. OSA has been linked to cerebrovascular risk through various pathways, including reduction in cerebral blood flow, altered cerebral autoregulation, impaired endothelial function, and accelerated proinflammatory states. (Data from Culebras A: Sleep apnea and stroke. Rev Neurol Dis 2[1]:13–19, 2005; Dziewas R, Ritter M, Kruger L, et al: C-reactive protein and fibrinogen in acute stroke patients with and without sleep apnea. Cerebrovasc Dis 24[5]:412–417, 2007; Munoz R, Ramos C: Sleep apnea-hypopnea syndrome and stroke. An Sist Sanit Navar 30[Suppl 1]:97–106, 2007.)

The pathophysiology of OSA in CVA may include the following factors: endothelial damage, inflammation and atherosclerosis, arterial hypertension, systemic inflammation, increased levels of plasma vascular endothelial growth factor, and production of reactive oxygen species. Other factors are hypercoagulability, increased intima media thickness, increased aortic stiffness, reduced flow dilatation, and increased levels of adhesion molecules, as demonstrated in Figure 10.7-7.

Amyotrophic Lateral Sclerosis

The many sleep disturbances encountered in patients with amyotrophic lateral sclerosis (ALS) include severe hypersomnia, likely caused by underlying, sleep-related respiratory disturbances and insomnia. Proposed underlying mechanisms of respiratory disturbance in ALS include increased collapsibility and weakness of the upper airways (caused by bulbar weakness), diaphragmatic weakness or paralysis (due to a phrenic nerve lesion), and intercostal muscle weakness (due to the degeneration of intercostal nerve nuclei). Degeneration of the central respiratory neurons accounts for both central and obstructive sleep apnea. Polysomnographic findings in patients with ALS include central, obstructive, mixed apneas, frequent awakenings, increased sleep fragmentation, and reduced nocturnal oxygen saturation.

Spinal Cord Diseases

Patients with ALS and spinal cord injury (SCI) often present with sleep disturbances related to respiratory dysfunction. In SCI this is particularly critical when the lesion occurs in the upper cervical spinal cord within the vicinity of the phrenic nerve nuclei. Patients with SCI have a greater difficulty with sleep initiation, describe more frequent awakenings, are more likely to be prescribed hypnotics, sleep more hours, take more frequent and prolonged naps, and are more likely to snore when compared with controls. Patients with spinal cord disorders are at a higher risk for muscular spasms, pain, paraesthesia, and voiding difficulties, which subsequently have a higher association with sleep difficulties.

Patients with spinal cord disease who present with tetraplegia generally have a higher incidence of sleep-disordered breathing, especially if other conditions are present, such as older age, increased neck circumference, longer disease duration, and an underlying use of cardiac medications. These associated conditions implicate a link between sleep-disordered breathing and cardiovascular morbidity, one of the leading causes of death in tetraplegia. OSA appears to be more common in older patients with spinal cord injury than in the general population, and is related to ventilatory dysfunction secondary to spinal cord injury.

Post-Polio Syndrome

Besides a high predilection for sleep-disordered breathing, post-polio syndrome (PPS) often manifests itself in sleep with random myoclonus, periodic limb movements in sleep with muscle contractions, ballistic movements of the legs, and restless legs syndrome. Poliovirus-induced damage to the spinal cord and brainstem may be implicated as a possible cause of these abnormal movements in sleep. It is suggested that polysomnography be performed on PPS patients with excessive daytime sleepiness and respiratory complaints.

Huntington's Disease

Sleep disturbances are common in Huntington's disease (HD) and are summarized in Box 10.7-1. These abnormalities are correlated in part with duration of illness, severity of clinical symptoms, and degree of atrophy of the caudate nucleus. Based on actigraphy data, patients with HD demonstrate significant activity and spend more time making high-acceleration movements compared with age-matched

BOX 10.7-1. SLEEP DISORDERS IN HUNTINGTON'S DISEASE

Disturbed sleep pattern
Increased sleep-onset latency
Reduced sleep efficiency
Increased arousal frequency and sleep fragmentation
Frequent nocturnal awakenings
Decreased slow-wave sleep
Increased density of sleep spindles
Reduced sleep efficiency
Increased time spent awake

controls. These patients may have long episodes of obstructive apnea (Fig. 10.7-8). Circadian-rhythm sleep disturbances, however, are an important pathological feature of HD, and may arise from a disruption of the expression of the circadian clock genes mPer2 and mBmal1 in the suprachiasmatic nucleus, the principal circadian pacemaker in the brain.

Myotonic Dystrophy

Sleep abnormalities in patients with myotonic dystrophy (MD) include severe hypersomnia that correlates with the severity of muscular impairment. Sleep study characteristics of patients with MD are a short sleep latency and sleep-onset REM periods during the multiple sleep latency test, as seen in patients with narcolepsy. Corpus callosum atrophy might occur in MD patients, and the size of the corpus callosum anterior area might be associated with the hypersomnia. Patients with MD report a longer sleep period, a less restorative sleep, difficulties with sleep initiation, and hypersomnia comparable with those found in idiopathic hypersomnia.

Patients with MD are found to have an increased risk of OSA, central sleep apnea, and excessive daytime sleepiness. These patients are also thought to have centrally mediated impaired breathing, probably related to brainstem respiratory center disorder rather than respiratory muscle weakness. Neuropathologic findings in patients with MD consist of severe neuronal loss and gliosis in the midbrain and pontine raphe, particularly in the dorsal raphe nucleus and superior central nucleus, and the pontine and medullary reticular formation. Alveolar hypoventilation and the hypersomnia in MD may be attributed to these morphological abnormalities, and would appear to be central in nature.

Fatal Familial Insomnia

This is a very rare prion disease that leads to loss of neuroendocrine regulation and loss of vegetative circadian rhythmicity, and ultimately to the demise of the patient. Patients develop very severe progressive insomnia, loss of orthostatic stability, increased salivation, increased body temperature, and daytime stupor alternating with wakefulness. In

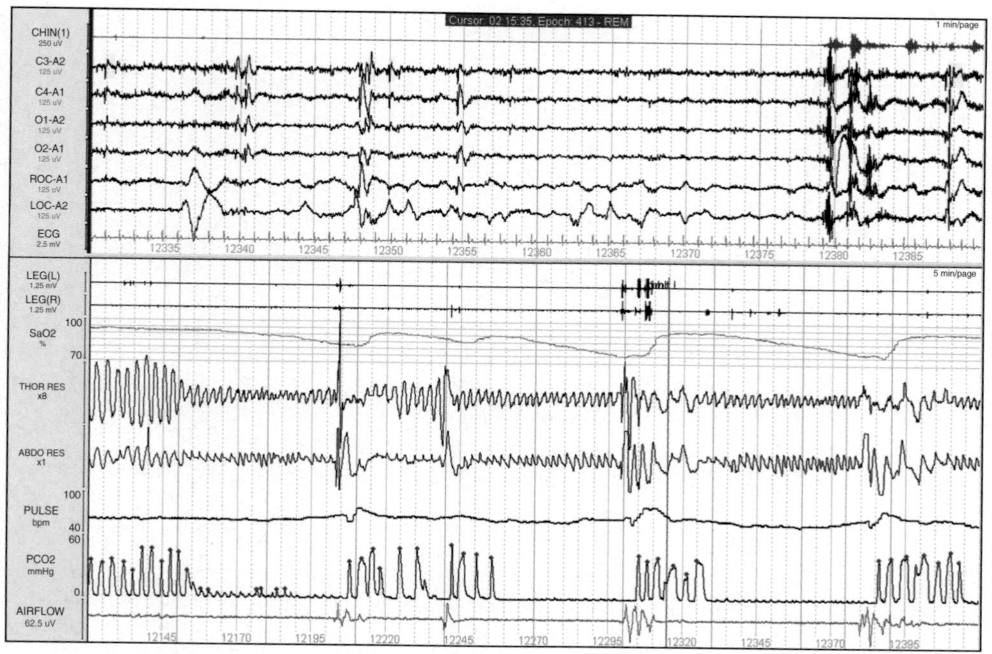

Figure 10.7-8.
This fragment is from a 60-year-old female with Huntington's disease. She had continuous choreoathetotic movements while awake that decreased when she fell asleep. During REM she had very long episodes of obstructive apnea.

the final stage of the disease, patients may become very agitated, confused, and disoriented. These patients eventually develop progressive stupor, then coma, and finally die.

SELECTED REFERENCES

Aboussouan LS, Lewis RA: Sleep, respiration and ALS. J Neurol Sci 164: 1–2, 1999.

Arnulf I, Similowski T, Salachas F, et al: Sleep disorders and diaphragmatic function in patients with amyotrophic lateral sclerosis. Am J Respir Crit Care Med 161:849–856, 2000.

Bollen EL, Den Heijer JC, Ponsioen C, et al: Respiration during sleep in Huntington's chorea. J Neurol Sci 84:63–68, 1988.

Butz M, Wollinsky KH, Wiedemuth-Catrinescu U, et al: Longitudinal effects of noninvasive positive-pressure ventilation in patients with amyotrophic lateral sclerosis. Am J Phys Med Rehabil 82:597–604, 2003.

Cote KA, Moldofsky H: Sleep, daytime symptoms, and cognitive performance in patients with fibromyalgia. J Rheumatol 24:2014–2023, 1997.

Culebras A: Sleep disorders and neuromuscular disease. Semin Neurol 25:33–38, 2005.

Ferguson KA, Strong MJ, Ahmad D, George CF: Sleep-disordered breathing in amyotrophic lateral sclerosis. Chest 110:664–669, 1996.

Fleming WE, Pollak CP: Sleep disorders in multiple sclerosis. Semin Neurol 25:64–68, 2005.

Hansotia P, Wall R, Berendes J: Sleep disturbances and severity of Huntington's disease. Neurology 35:1672–1674, 1985.

Laberge L, Begin P, Montplaisir J, Mathieu J: Sleep complaints in patients with myotonic dystrophy. J Sleep Res 13:95–100, 2004.

Leppavuori A, Pohjasvaara T, Vataja R, et al: Insomnia in ischemic stroke patients. Cerebrovasc Dis 14:90–97, 2002.

Mahowald ML, Mahowald MW: Nighttime sleep and daytime functioning (sleepiness and fatigue) in less well-defined chronic rheumatic diseases with particular reference to the "alpha-delta NREM sleep anomaly." Sleep Med 1:195–207, 2000.

Martinez-Rodriguez JE, Lin L, Iranzo A, et al: Decreased hypocretin-1 (Orexin-A) levels in the cerebrospinal fluid of patients with myotonic dystrophy and excessive daytime sleepiness. Sleep 26:287–290, 2003.

Roehrs T, Roth T: Sleep and pain: Interaction of two vital functions. Semin Neurol 25:106–116, 2005.

Steljes DG, Kryger MH, Kirk BW, Millar TW: Sleep in postpolio syndrome. Chest 98:133–140, 1990.

SLEEP BREATHING DISORDERS

CHAPTER 11

Meir Kryger

Examination of the Patient with Suspected Sleep Apnea

11.1

Because many patients with sleep apnea have anatomic abnormalities and obstruction of the upper airway, and because findings may lead to specific treatment decisions, examination of the face and all the structures of the upper airway is done in all patients suspected of having sleep apnea. In some patients abnormal findings may lead to a suspicion of sleep apnea. All the patients whose findings are shown in this chapter had documented sleep apnea.

Overall Inspection of the Patient

Sleep apnea can occur in any age group, in both genders, and in all ethnic groups. It often runs in families. Many patients do not fit the stereotype of the obese middle-aged male. The child shown in Figure 11.1-1 had sleep apnea caused by enlarged tonsils. The mother and her son in Figure 11.1-2 both had sleep apnea. She had hypothyroidism (see chapter 14.1) and her son was obese. The two brothers shown in Figure 11.1-3 had sleep apnea, as did both of their parents.

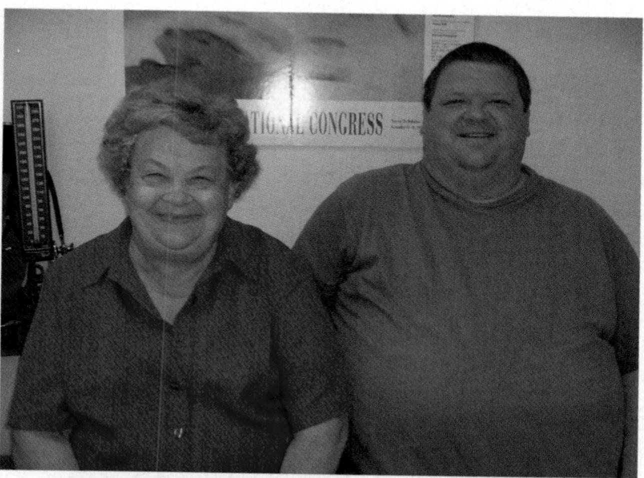

Figure 11.1-2.
Mother and son with sleep apnea.

Facial and Jaw Structures

Many anatomic abnormalities can lead to sleep apnea. For example, either an upper jaw (maxilla) or lower jaw (mandible) that is too far posterior can lead to sleep apnea by encroaching on the pharyngeal airway. This can occur not only directly but also indirectly since some structures (e.g., tongue) are attached to the mandible. The physical examination includes an intraoral exam and offers many clues as to the cause of sleep apnea.

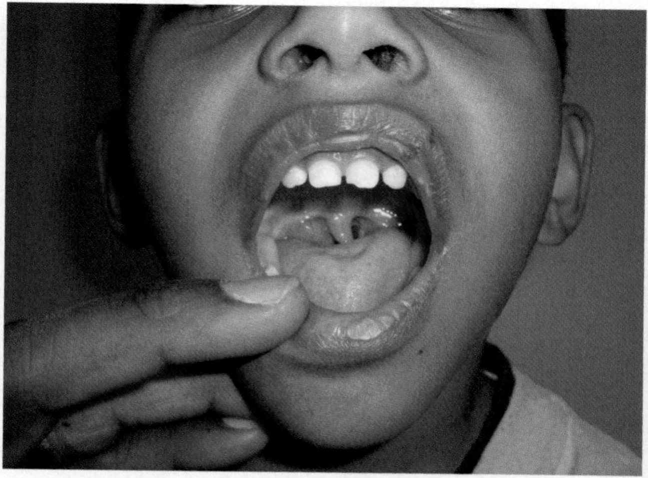

Figure 11.1-1.
Enlarged tonsils in a child.

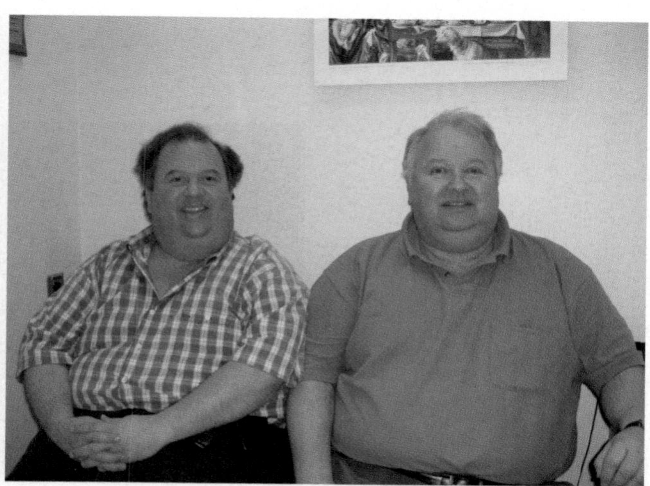

Figure 11.1-3.
Brothers with sleep apnea.

INSPECTION OF THE FACE

In some patients inspection of the face can reveal the disease—for example, thyroid disease (see chapter 14.1) or acromegaly (see chapter 14.2)—that may be causing sleep apnea. Inspection can also give insight into physiologic abnormalities.

In many instances sleep apnea is apparent at the first meeting with the patient. For example, drooping eyelids suggest sleepiness (Figs. 11.1-4 and 11.1-5).

The patient shown in Figure 11.1-6 is obese, cyanotic, and has bloodshot eyes. The latter finding was related to polycythemia. Obesity hypoventilation syndrome or overlap syndrome should be suspected when a patient has these findings. This patient has an overlap syndrome (see chapter 11.3).

All patients with Down syndrome should be suspected of having sleep apnea (Fig. 11.1-7).

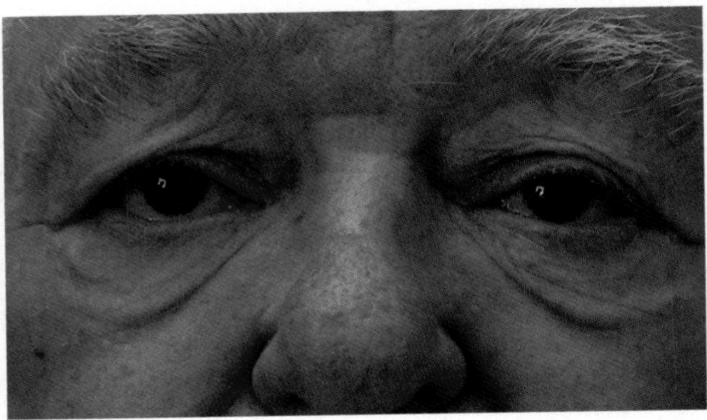

Figure 11.1-6.
Bloodshot eyes in man with overlap syndrome.

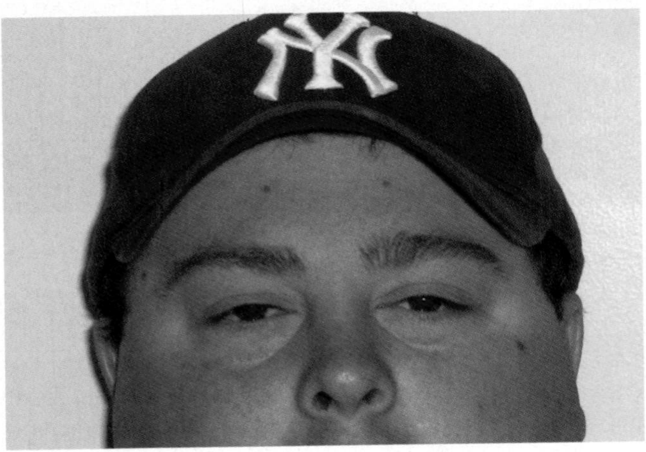

Figure 11.1-4.
Drooping eyelids in young man with sleep apnea.

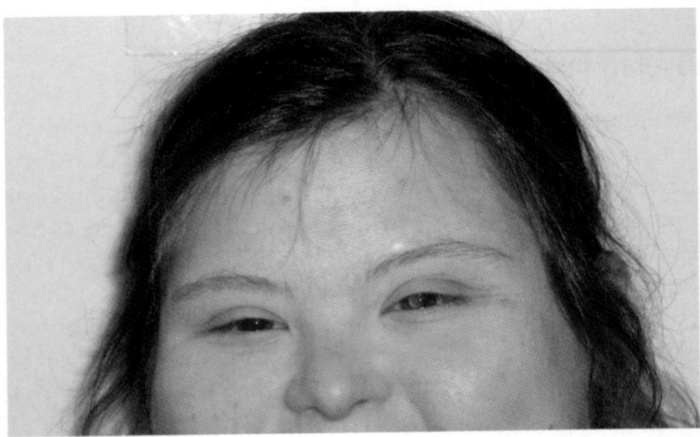

Figure 11.1-7.
Patient with Down syndrome.

BONY STRUCTURES

Abnormalities in the skeletal structures of the face can lead to an abnormal position of the attached soft tissues. This can obstruct the pharyngeal airway (Figs. 11.1-8 and 11.1-9).

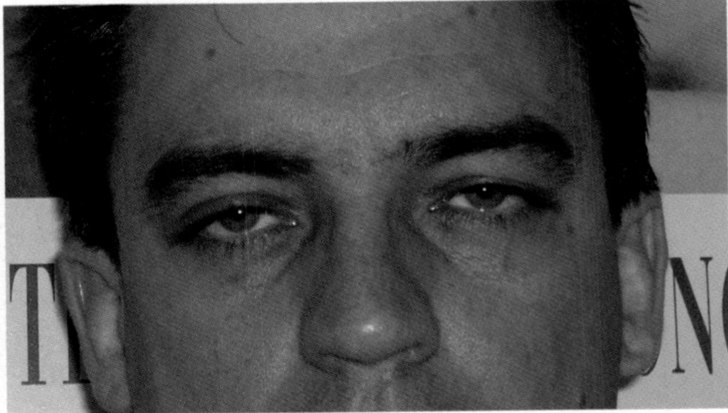

Figure 11.1-5.
Drooping eyelids in middle-aged male.

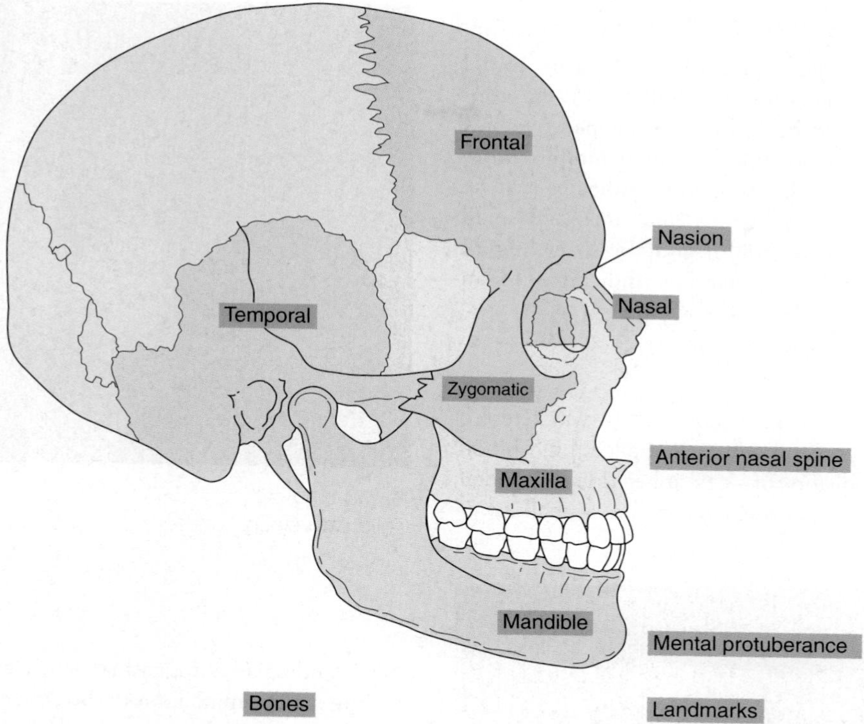

Figure 11.1-8.
Landmarks (*brown*) and bones (*blue*) of human skull.

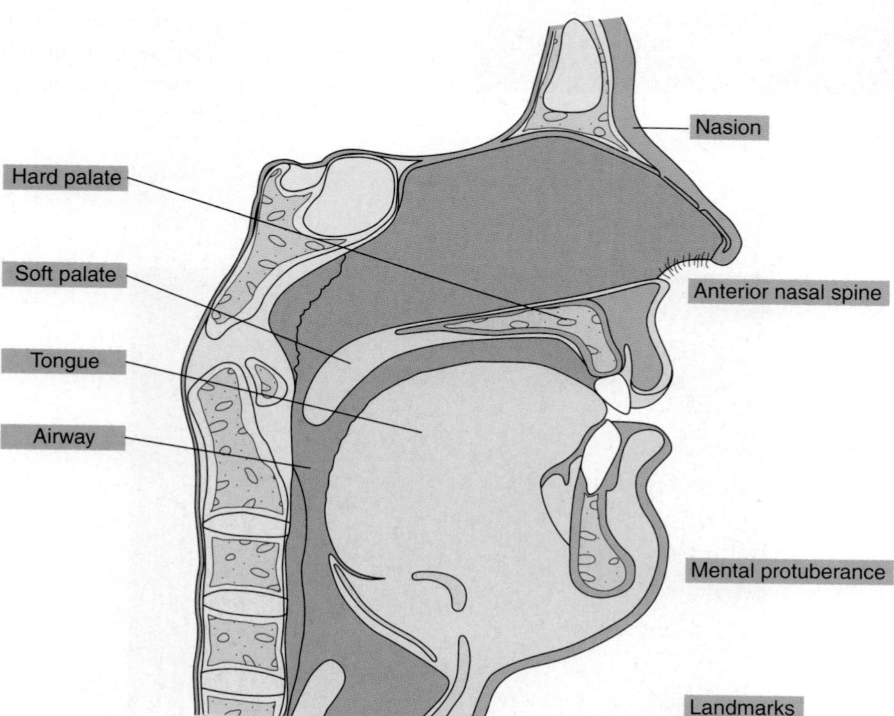

Figure 11.1-9.
Landmarks and anatomy of sagittal section.

MAXILLARY AND MANDIBULAR INSUFFICIENCY

The patient shown in Figure 11.1-10 appeared on initial inspection to have a prognathic mandible. Note the concave facial profile. In fact, he has a large fat pad over his chin giving the appearance of a prognathic mandible. More detailed examination of his facial features indicates that he has maxillary insufficiency (note his "flat" face and small "cheek bone," or zygomatic bone), and the crowding of the mandibular anterior teeth may be indicative of an undersized mandible (Fig. 11.1-11).

SMALL LOWER JAW

The 8-year-old child shown in Figure 11.1-12 was referred because of sleepiness, poor school performance, high blood pressure, and a family history of sleep apnea. He responded to continuous positive airway pressure. He has a small lower jaw (mandibular retrognathia) that was only apparent when his bite was examined. Note the convex facial profile, which is a feature of a child with an underdeveloped mandible. Retrognathia causes the patient's tongue to rest in a more posterior and superior position, thus impinging on the airway.

Thus, a receding chin is a sign of mandibular insufficiency. Such patients usually have an overjet with the mandibular anterior teeth excessively lingual (or posterior) to the maxillary anterior teeth. Figures 11.1-13 through 11.1-15 demonstrate the overjet during a lateral exam. Figures 11.1-16 through 11.1-18 show a patient with complete overlap of the maxillary over the mandibular anterior teeth (excessive overbite) when the patient is fully in occlusion on the posterior teeth.

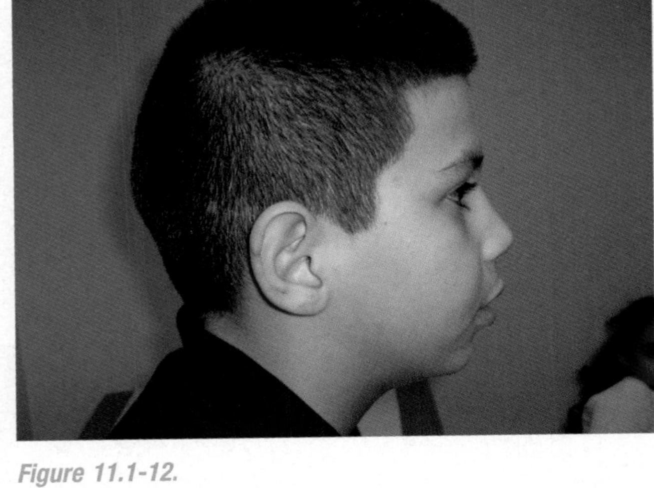

Figure 11.1-12.
Child with sleep apnea.

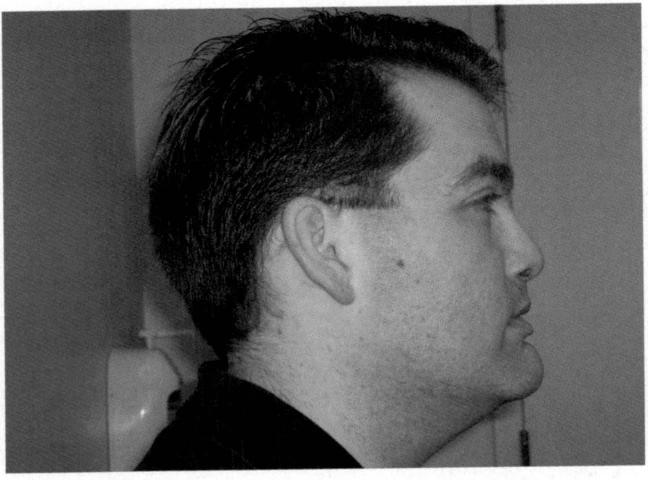

Figure 11.1-10.
Maxillary insufficiency.

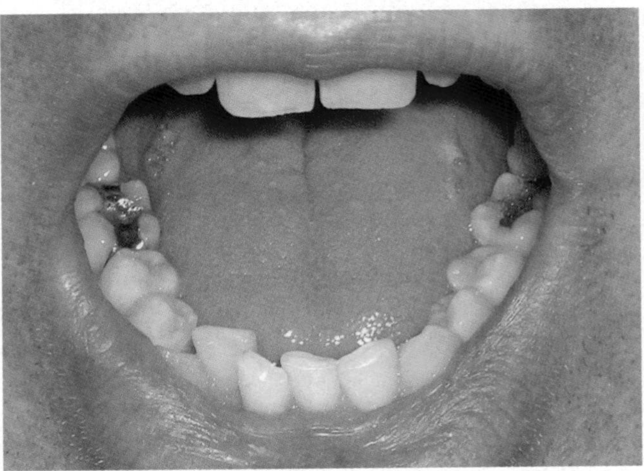

Figure 11.1-11.
Crowded teeth indicate a small mandible.

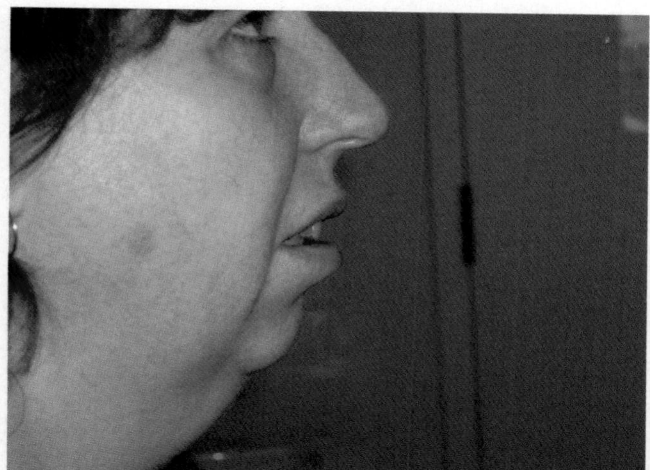

Figure 11.1-13.
Receding chin.

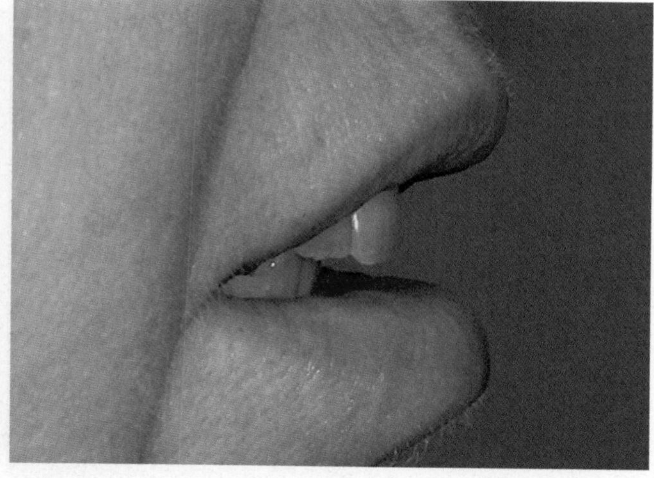

Figure 11.1-14.
Overjet. Patient from Figure 11.1-13.

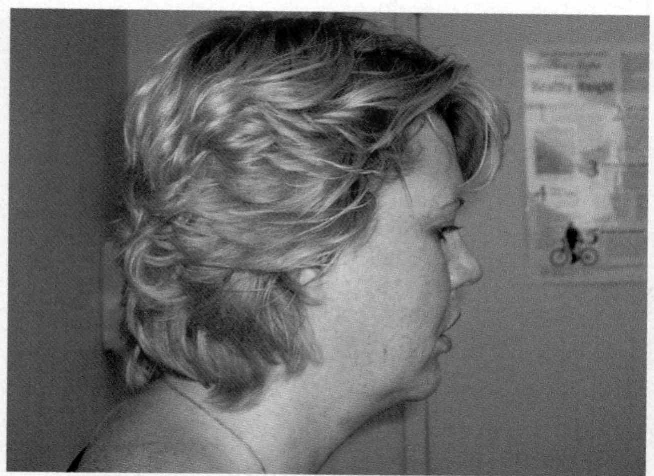

Figure 11.1-15.
Receding chin.

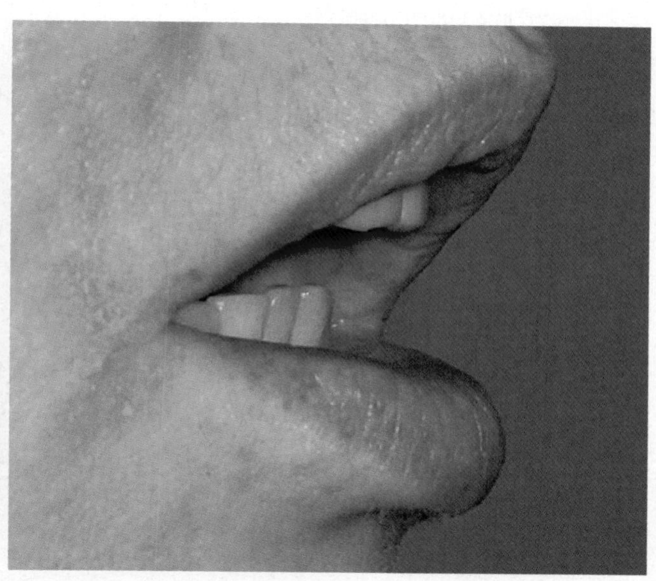

Figure 11.1-16.
Close-up of patient in Figure 11.1-15.

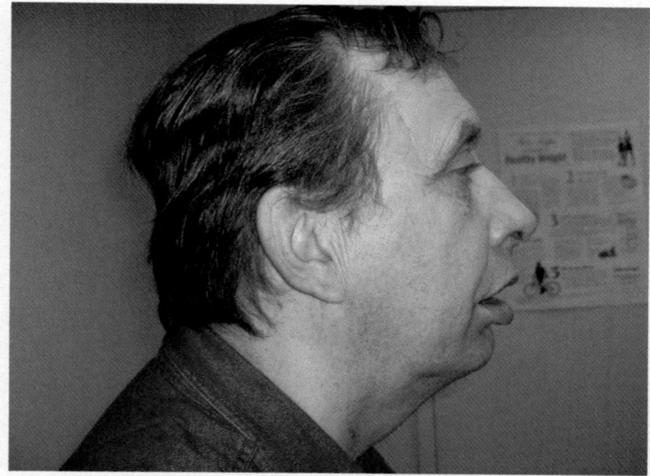

Figure 11.1-17.
Retrognathia.

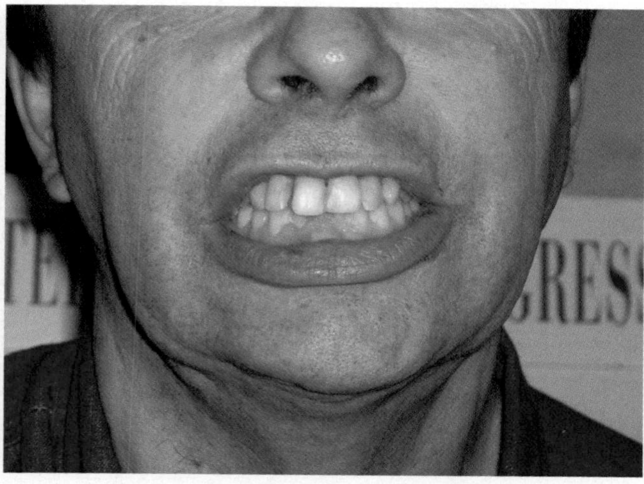

Figure 11.1-18.
The upper teeth overlap lower teeth.

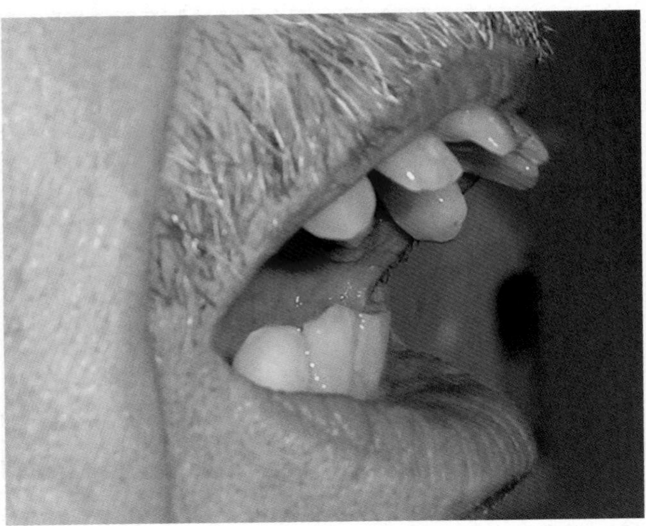

Figure 11.1-19.
"Buck teeth" in an older male.

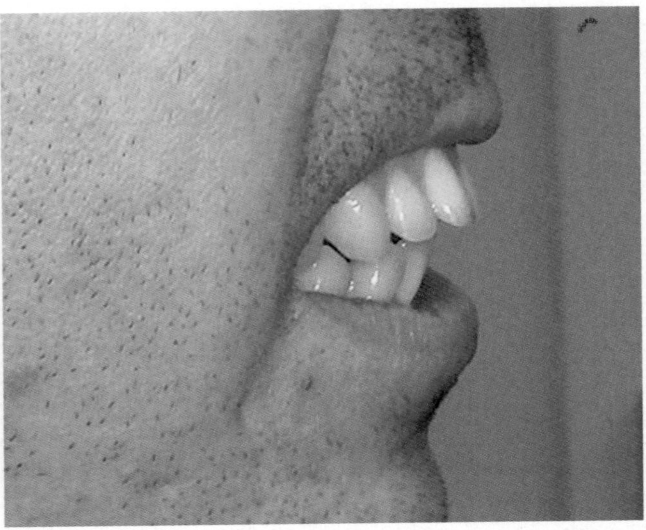

Figure 11.1-20.
"Buck teeth" in a younger male.

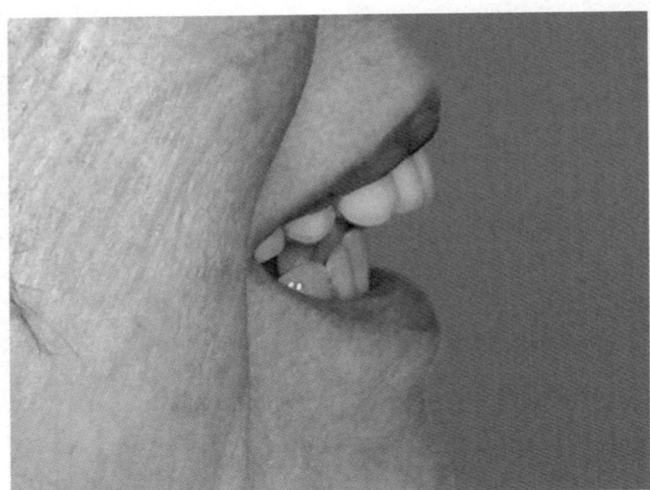

Figure 11.1-21.
"Buck teeth" in a middle-aged female.

Patients with protrusive maxillary anterior teeth ("buck teeth") frequently have retrognathic mandibles. Some patients present with an anterior open bite that may be the result of a severe tongue thrust or even a consequence of severe thumb sucking (Figs.11.1-19 to 11.1-21).

Patients with abnormal maxillary and mandibular arches and with asymmetry or crowding may have a micrognathic (small) mandible and be at risk for sleep apnea. The crowding of the lower arch causes inadequate space for the anterior portion of the tongue to move anteriorly. This in turn may cause the posterior part of the tongue to "bunch up." Such patients may develop a scalloped tongue from the tongue constantly pressing anteriorly (Figs. 11.1-22 to 11.1-25).

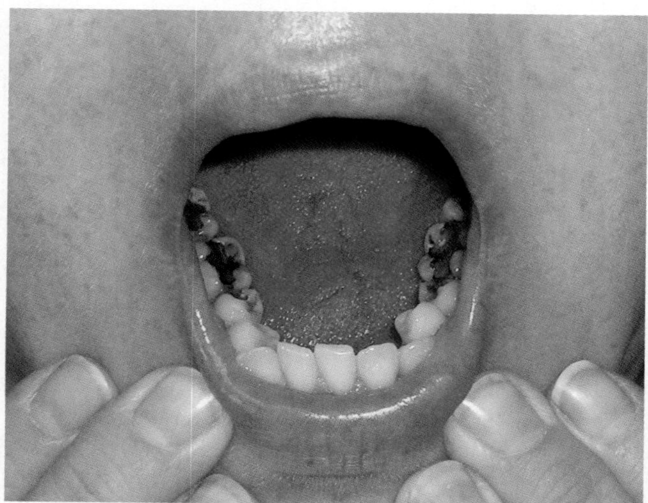

Figure 11.1-22.
Abnormal mandibular arch.

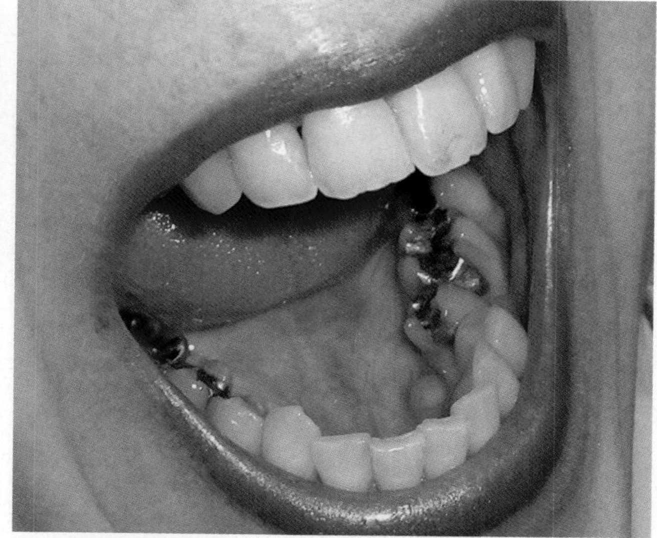

Figure 11.1-23.
Asymmetric mandibular arch.

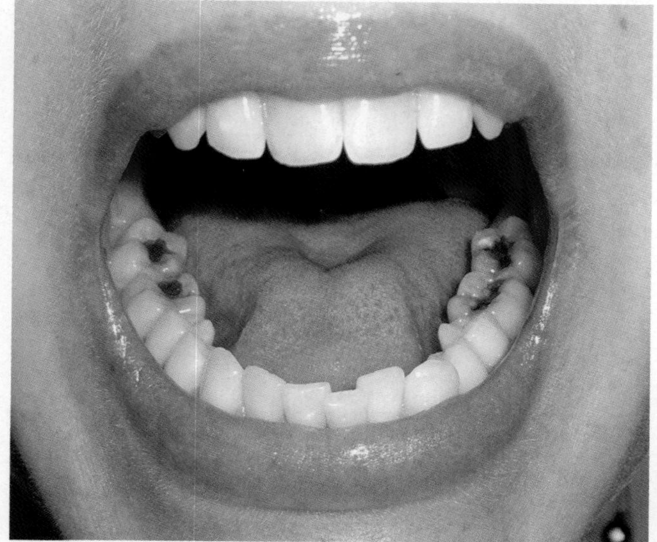

Figure 11.1-24.
Scalloped tongue.

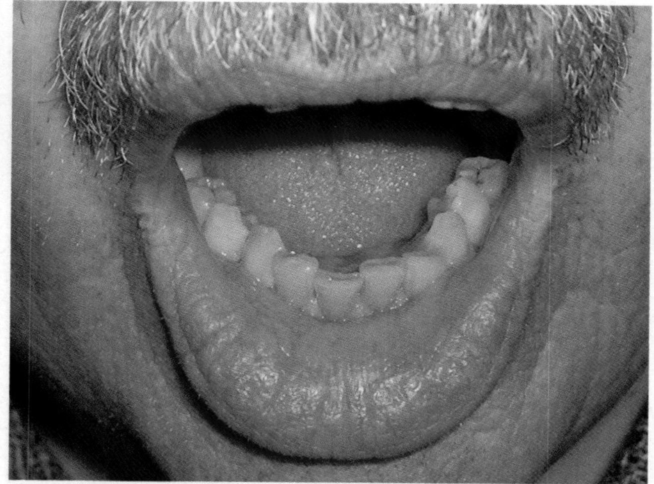

Figure 11.1-25.
Small mandible, crease in tongue, bruxism.

Nasal Airway

Examination of the nasal airway should include inspection of nasal symmetry and a search for anatomic abnormalities that might lead to nasal obstruction.

DISEASES AFFECTING NOSE AND NARES

The patient shown in Figures 11.1-26 through 11.1-29 has severe rosacea. This disease can lead to nasal obstruction and sleep apnea.

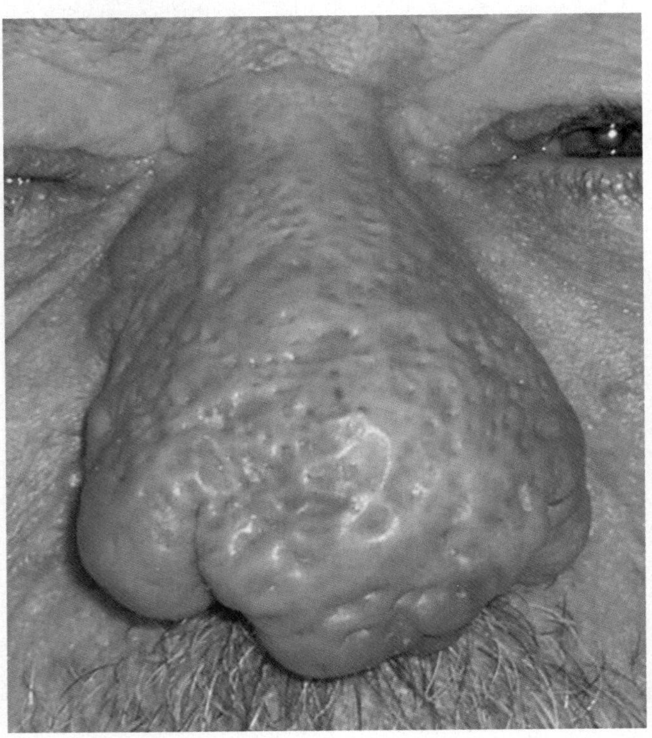

Figure 11.1-26.
Severe rosacea and rhinophyma.

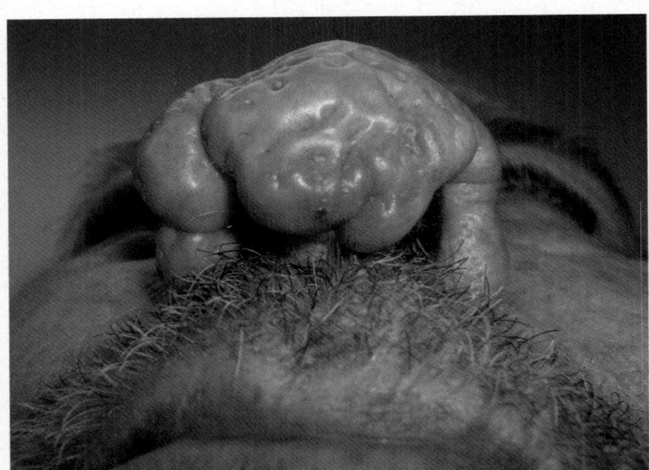

Figure 11.1-27.
Rhinophyma from below.

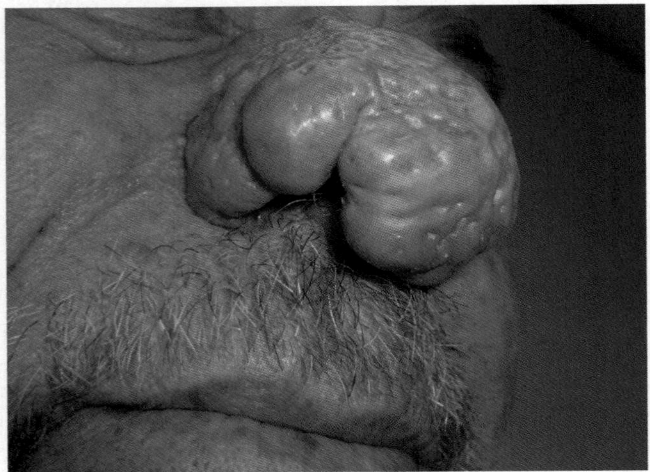

Figure 11.1-28.
Right nare is occluded.

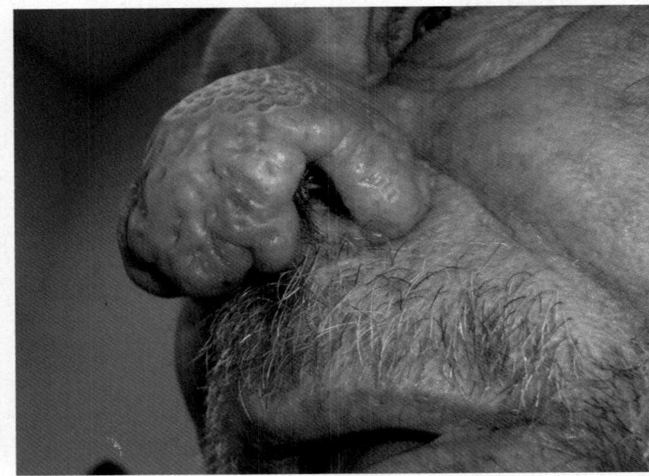

Figure 11.1-29.
View from left side.

TRAUMA AFFECTING NOSE AND NARES

The patient shown in Figures 11.1-30 and 11.1-31 had severe trauma from a gunshot wound to his face that required extensive reconstructive surgery. His remaining nose is entirely reconstructed. It does not have an airway leading to the nasopharyngeal airway, so he breathes exclusively via his oral airway, which also had reconstructive surgery.

TRAUMATIC INJURY TO THE NOSE

Inspection reveals asymmetry of the nose. These patients may have been told they now have a deviated septum. In these examples the patients are not overweight.

The patient shown in Figure 11.1-32 had a broken nose. Note the asymmetry of the nose. The patient shown in Figure 11.1-33 had been a boxer. The region below the

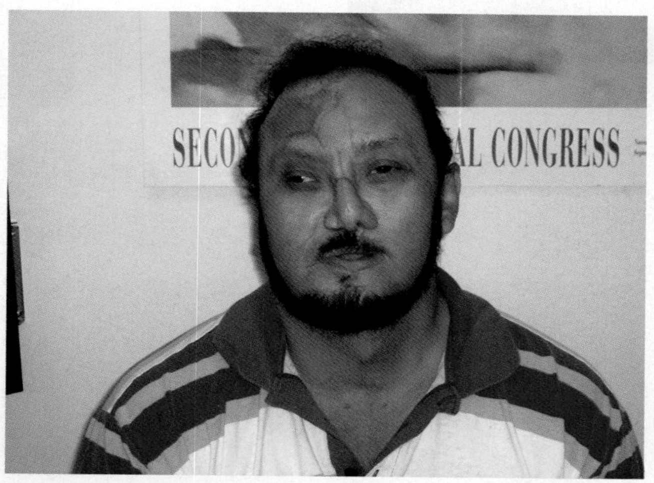

Figure 11.1-30.
Facial reconstruction after a gunshot wound.

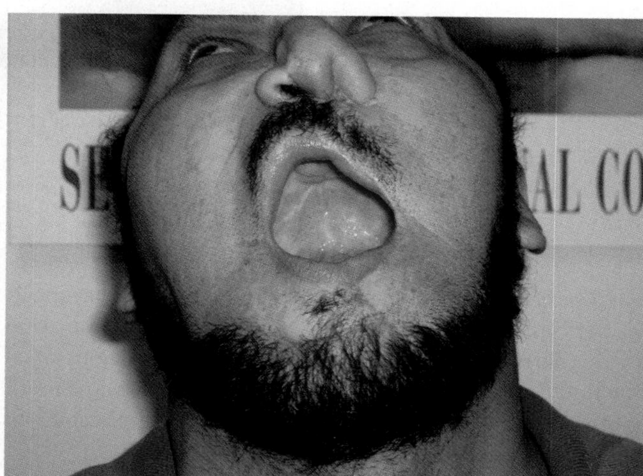

Figure 11.1-31.
Nasal reconstruction led to total obstruction.

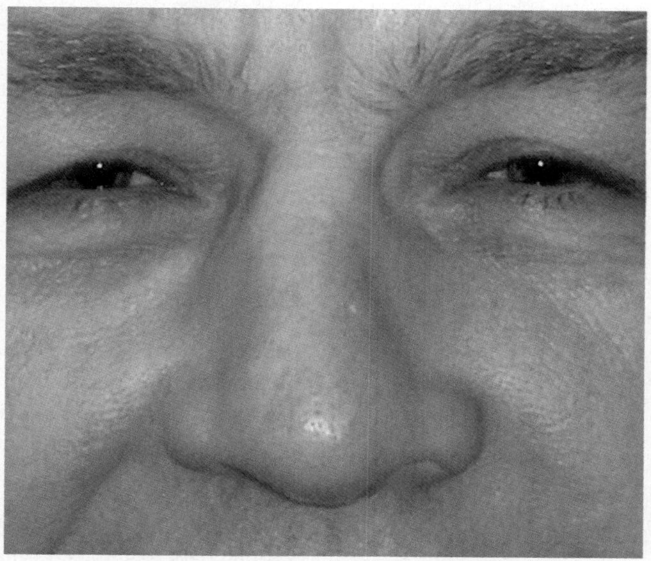

Figure 11.1-32.
Broken nose.

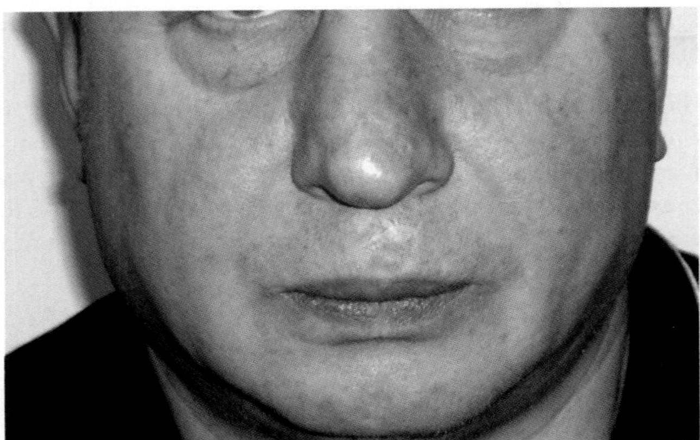

Figure 11.1-33.
Previously fractured nose.

nasal bone is wide and hard to palpation. Note the cyanosis of the lips. Figures 11.1-34 and 11.1-35 show examination of the nares from below in a patient with a previous nasal fracture. Bulging of the septum in left nostril is apparent. Note the size of the left nasal airway after application of an external nasal strip (see Fig. 11.1-35).

Examination of the Pharynx

MALLAMPATI CLASSIFICATION

The Mallampati classification describes the relationship between the tongue and the size of the pharynx. The patient, in the sitting position, is asked to open his or her mouth as far as possible and to protrude the tongue. This classification was first described as a method for anesthesiologists to predict difficult tracheal intubation.

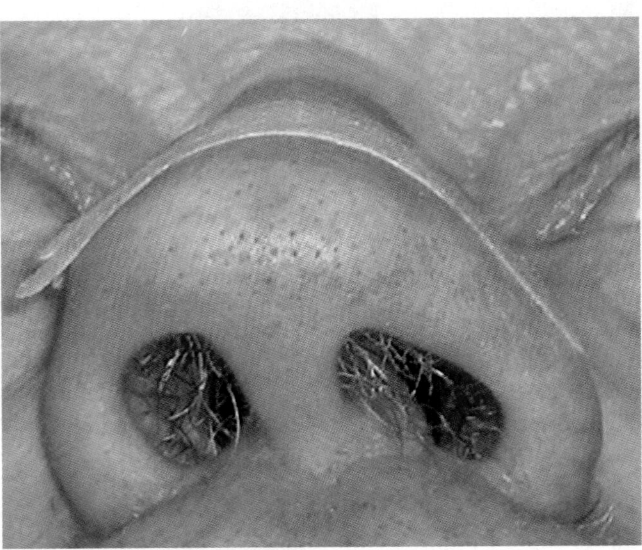

Figure 11.1-35.
Broken nose with nasal strip.

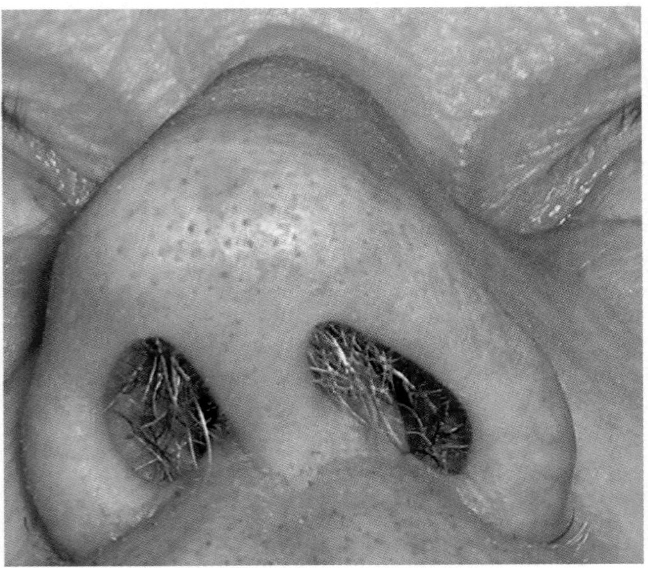

Figure 11.1-34.
Broken nose without nasal strip. Note bulge.

The Mallampati classification is as follows:

Class I: Soft palate, fauces, uvula, and posterior and anterior pillars are visible (Figs. 11.1-36 and 11.1-37).

Class II: Soft palate, fauces, and uvula are visible (Figs. 11.1-38 and 11.1-39).

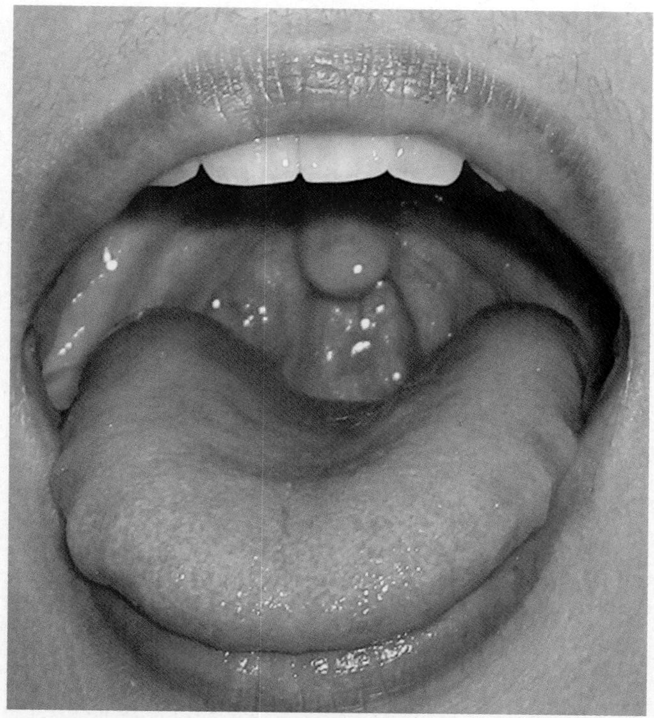

Figure 11.1-36.
Mallampati Class I. All structures visible.

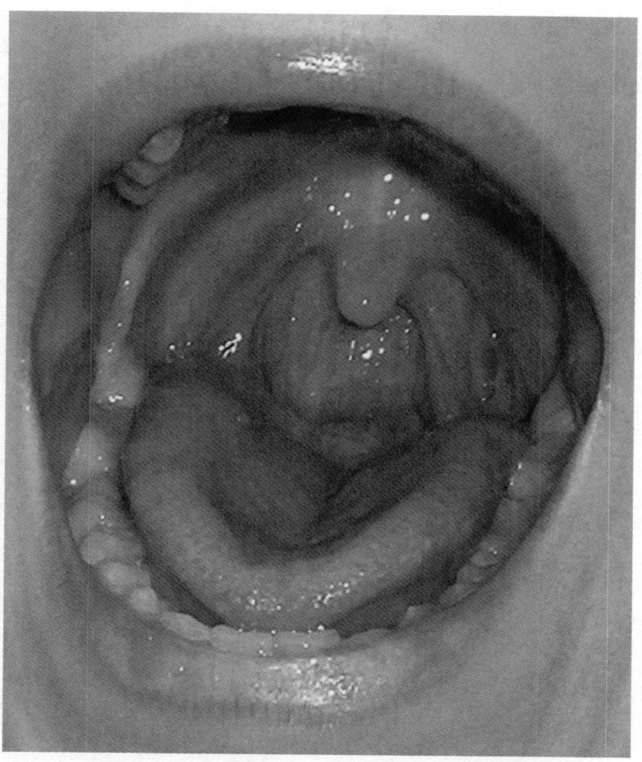

Figure 11.1-37.
Mallampati Class I. All structures visible.

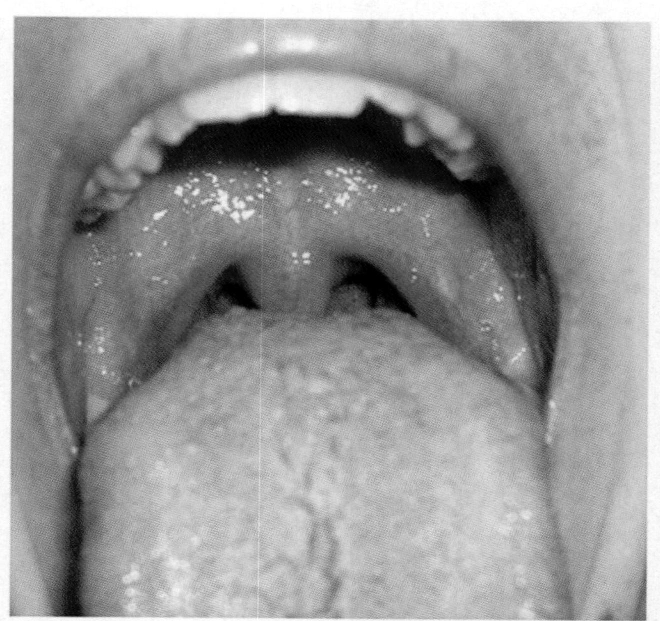

Figure 11.1-38.
Mallampati Class II. Posterior pillers and much of uvula not visible.

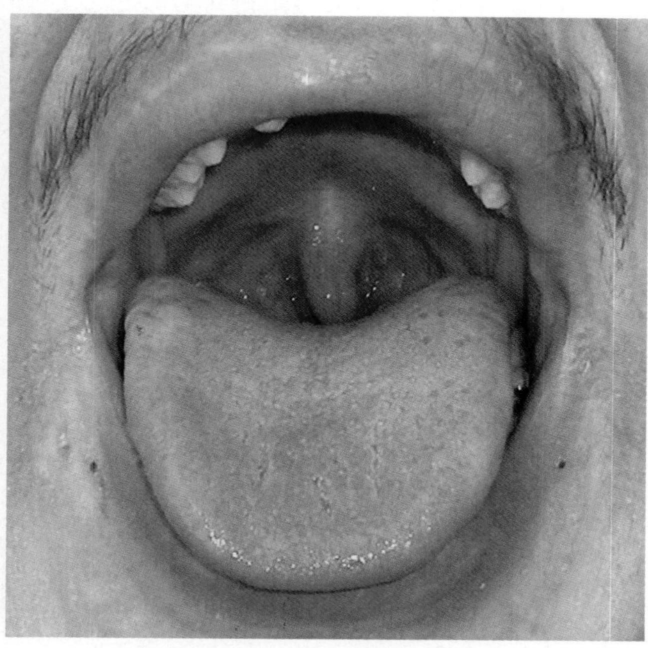

Figure 11.1-39.
Mallampati Class II. Tip of uvula not visible.

Class III: Soft palate, fauces, and only base of uvula are visible (Figs. 11.1-40 and 11.1-41).
Class IV: Soft palate is not visible (Fig. 11.1-42).

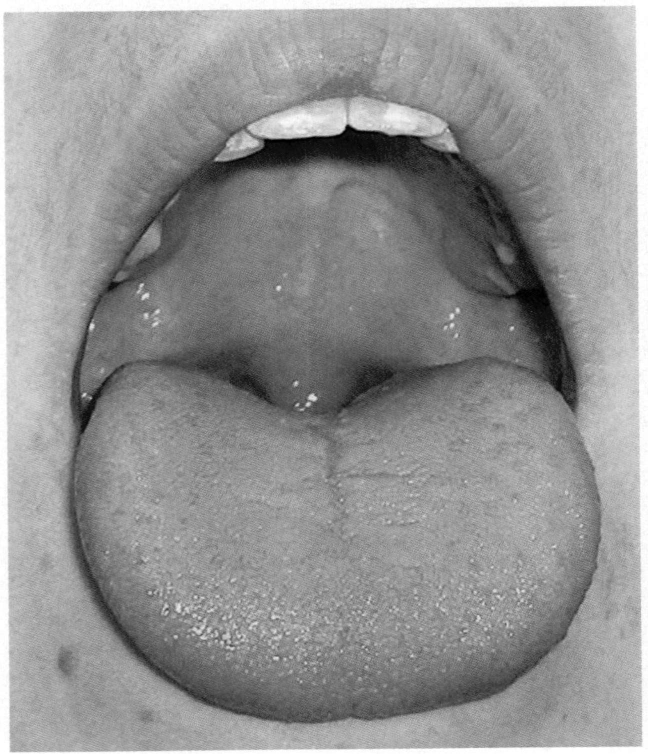

Figure 11.1-40.
Mallampati Class III. Only base of uvula seen.

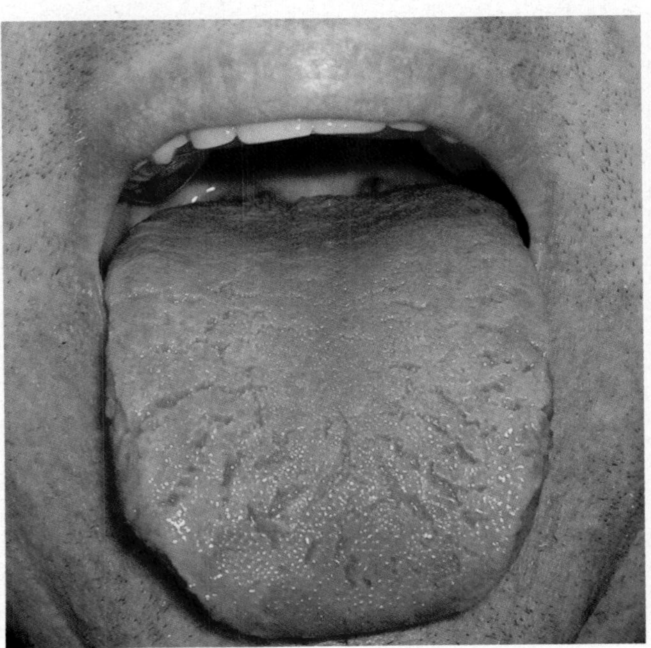

Figure 11.1-41.
Mallampati Class III. Base of uvula barely visible.

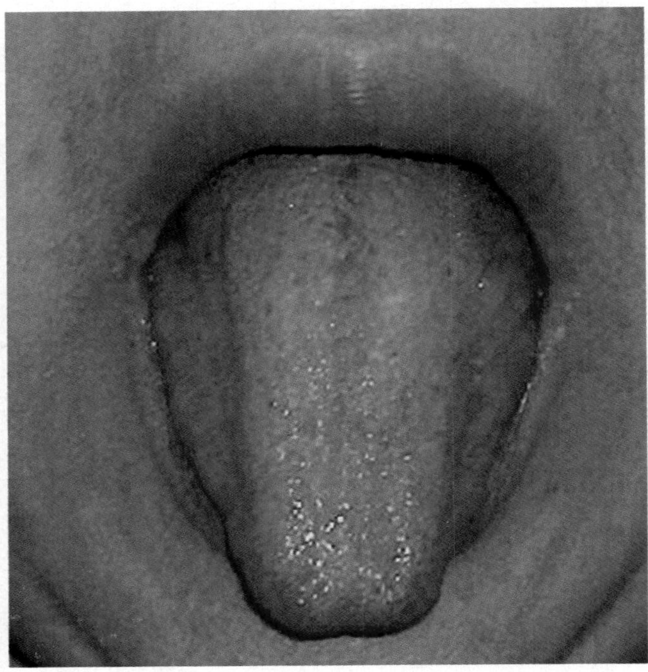

Figure 11.1-42.
Mallampati Class IV. Soft palate not visible.

Examination of the Tonsils

Enlarged tonsils and adenoids can lead to sleep apnea by obstructing the upper airway during sleep. Adenoids cannot be visualized in a routine physical examination. Enlarged tonsils and adenoids are the most common cause of sleep apnea in the pediatric population. Examination of the tonsils may or may not require using a tongue blade.

Tonsil size is graded on a scale from 0 (absent tonsils) to 4 ("kissing tonsils," touching at midline):

Grade 0. Absent tonsils. In this example the uvula is abnormally wide, and almost bifid. This is a variant of normal (Fig. 11.1-43).

Grade 1. Tonsils are hidden behind tonsillar pillars.

Grade 2. Tonsils extend to the pillars. In Figure 11.1-44, the right tonsil is Grade 1 and the left is Grade 2.

Grade 3. Tonsils are visible beyond the pillars (Fig. 11.1-45).

Grade 4. Tonsils are enlarged to midline (Figs. 11.1-46 to 11.1-48).

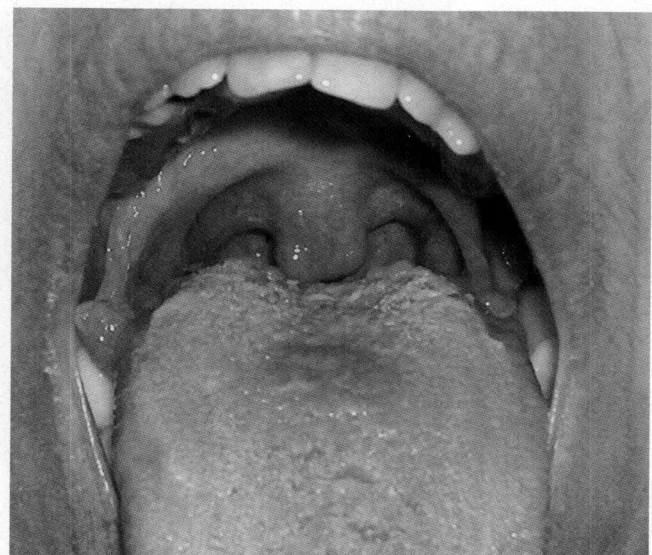

Figure 11.1-43. Grade 0 tonsils.

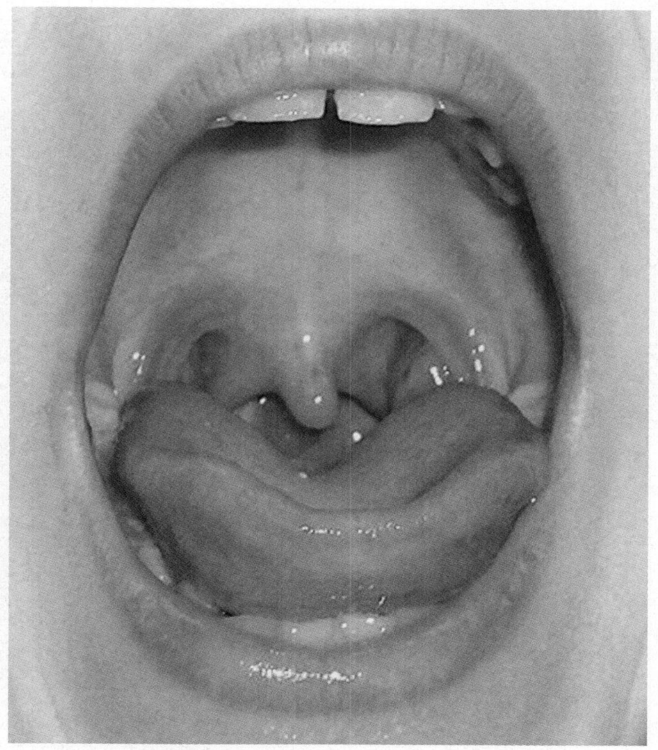

Figure 11.1-44. Grades 1 (right tonsil) and 2 (left tonsil).

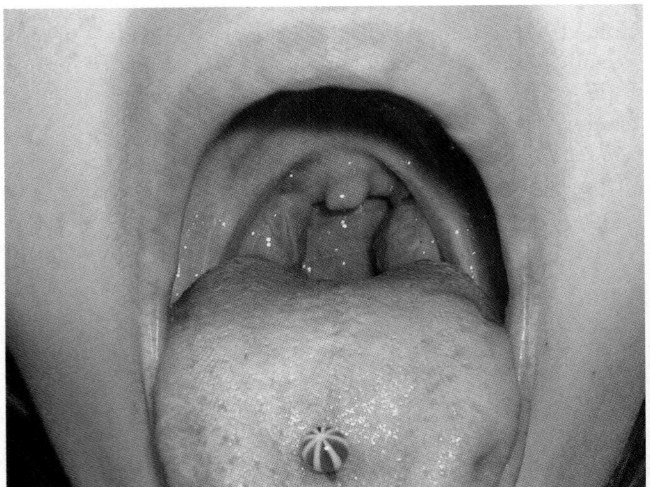

Figure 11.1-45.
Grade 3 tonsils.

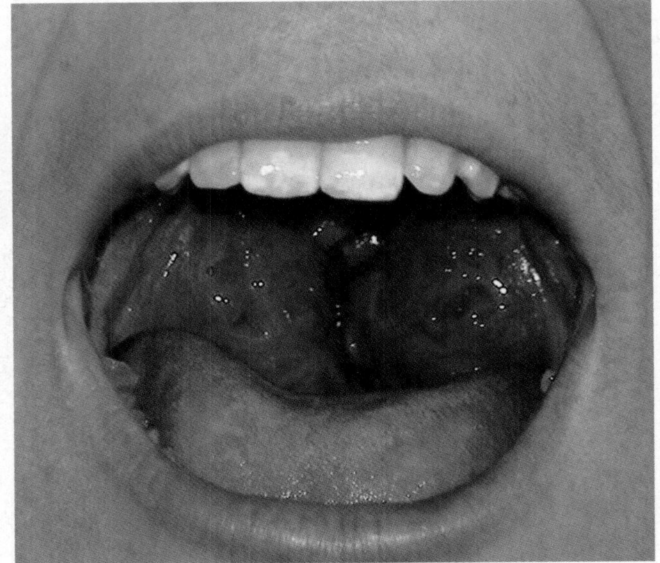

Figure 11.1-46.
Grade 4 tonsils.

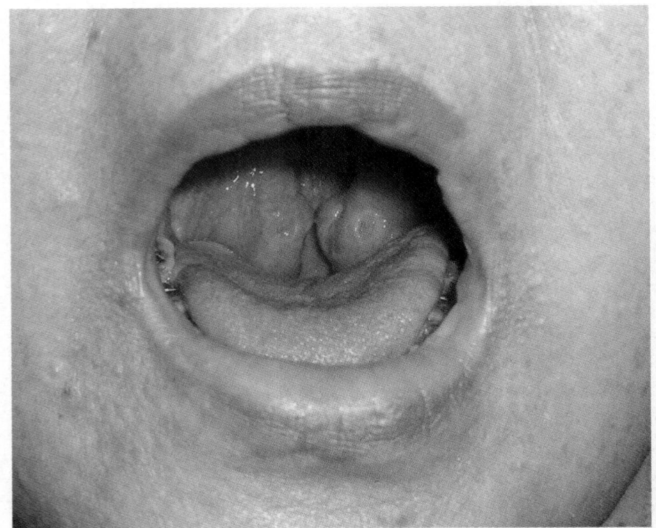

Figure 11.1-47.
Grade 4 tonsils.

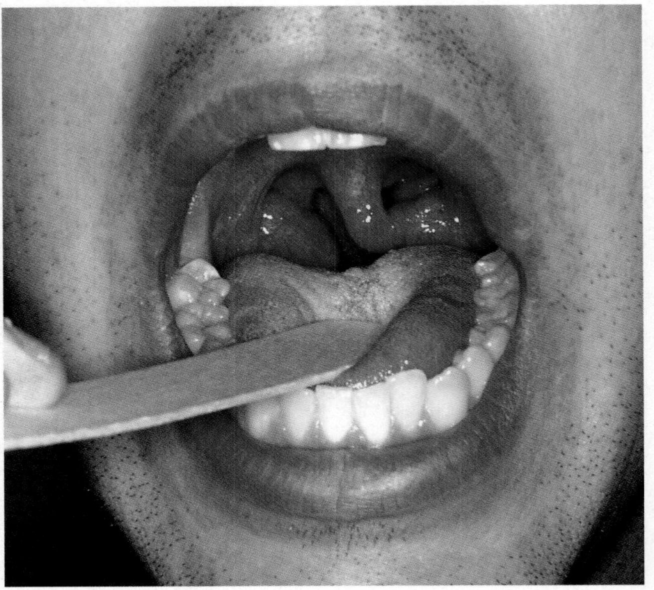

Figure 11.1-48.
Grade 4 tonsils.

VARIANTS AND ABNORMAL AIRWAY PHARYNGEAL FINDINGS

In Figure 11.1-49 the right tonsil is much larger than the left and extends beyond the midline. It was initially difficult to visualize because it extended behind the uvula. This would be classified as equivalent to Grade 4 enlarged tonsils.

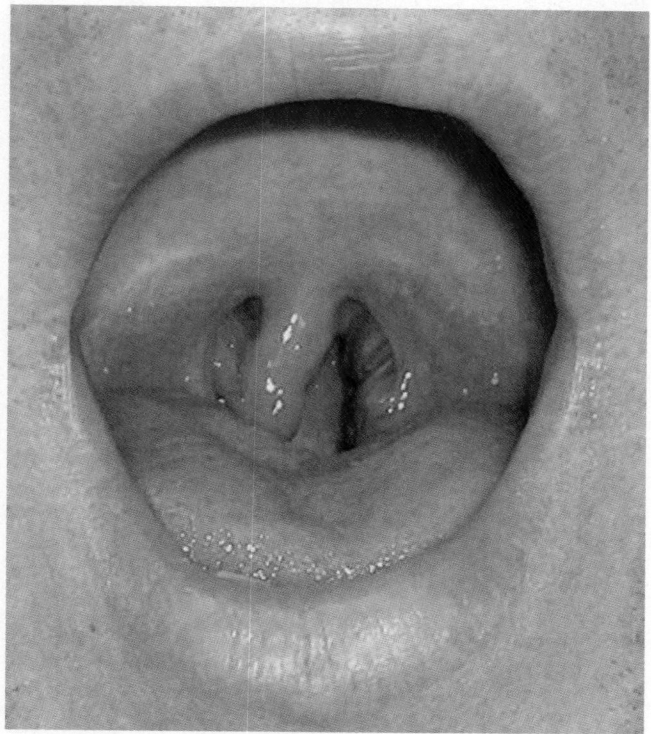

Figure 11.1-49.
Grade 4 enlarged tonsils. The right tonsil extends behind the uvula.

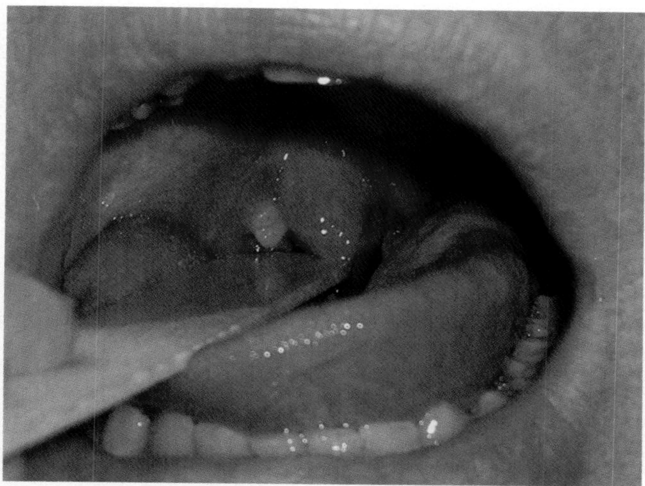

Figure 11.1-51.
Soft palate tumor.

In Figure 11.1-50, a nubbin of left tonsillar tissue can be seen. This patient frequently awakened with a sore throat, and the pharyngeal tissues show evidence of trauma (redness) due to snoring.

Figure 11.1-51 shows an unexpected finding in a sleep apnea patient, a tiny neoplastic lesion just to the right of the uvula. The most common surgical procedure involving the upper airway is uvulopalatopharyngoplasty (UPPP). UPPP usually involves removal of the uvula, variable amounts of the soft palate (depending on the surgeon), tonsils, adenoids, and redundant tissue in the pharynx. In the cases shown in Figures 11.1-52 through 11.1-55 UPPP was unsuccessful in treating the apnea. Note the differences in anatomic outcome in these examples.

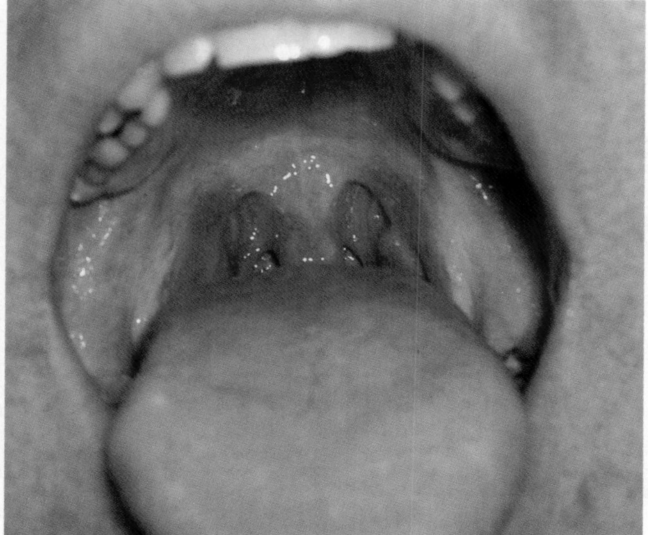

Figure 11.1-50.
Trauma (redness) due to snoring.

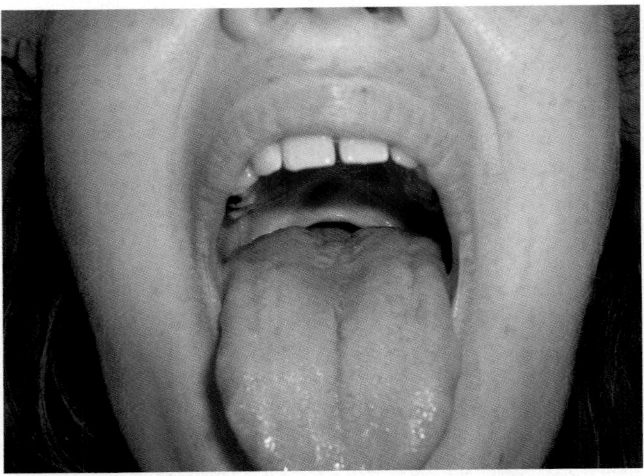

Figure 11.1-52.
Outcome of uvulopalatopharyngoplasty (UPPP).

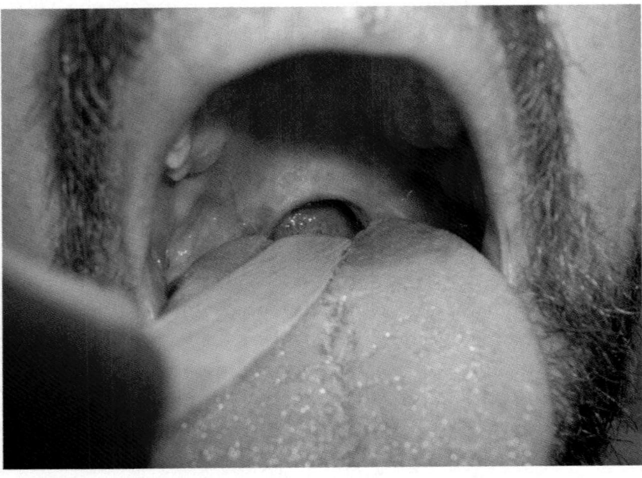

Figure 11.1-53.
UPPP with small pharyngeal opening.

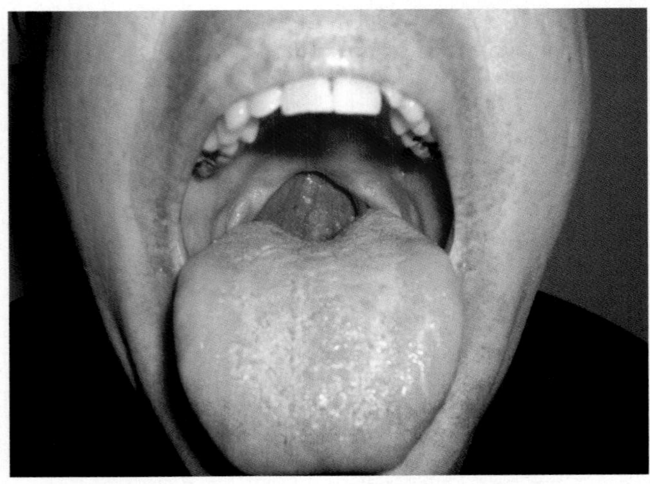

Figure 11.1-54.
UPPP with triangular pharyngeal opening.

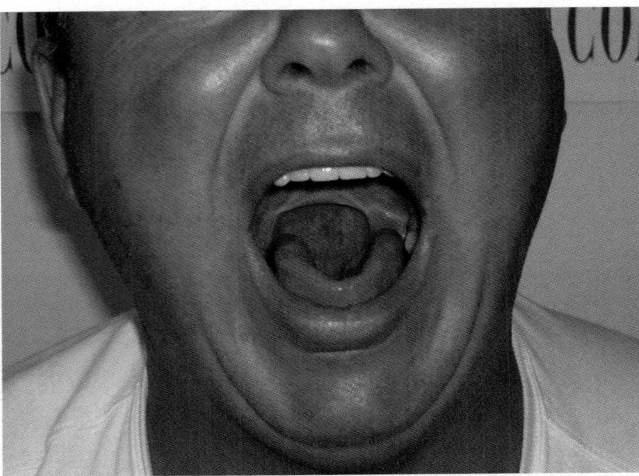

Figure 11.1-55.
UPPP with large pharyngeal opening.

Examination of the Neck

A large neck collar size is a robust statistical predictor of obstructive apnea, more so in men than women. The patient shown in Figures 11.1-56 and 11.1-57 has a neck collar size of 49 cm, or 19.3 inches. Most obese patients with apnea have a neck collar size of at least 43 cm, or 17 inches.

Congenital abnormalities involving the neck can also lead to sleep apnea. The patient shown in Figures 11.1-58 and 11.1-59 has severe sleep apnea due to Klippel-Feil syndrome. She also has polycystic ovarian syndrome (see chapter 15.1). Note the acne of the face. Findings in the neck are also seen in diseases of the thyroid gland (see chapter 14.1).

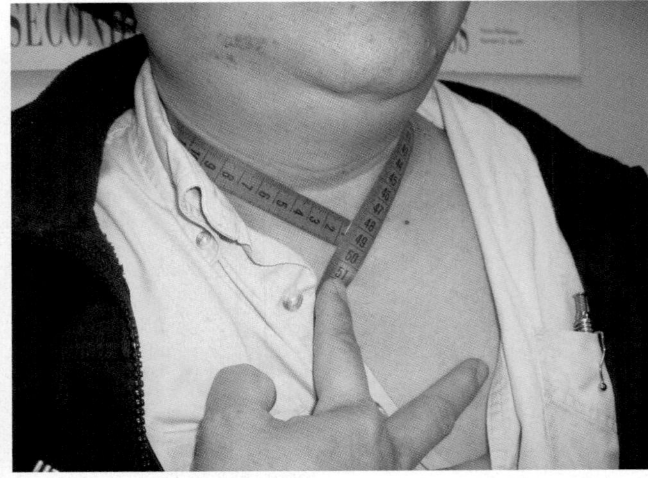

Figure 11.1-56.
Measuring neck collar size.

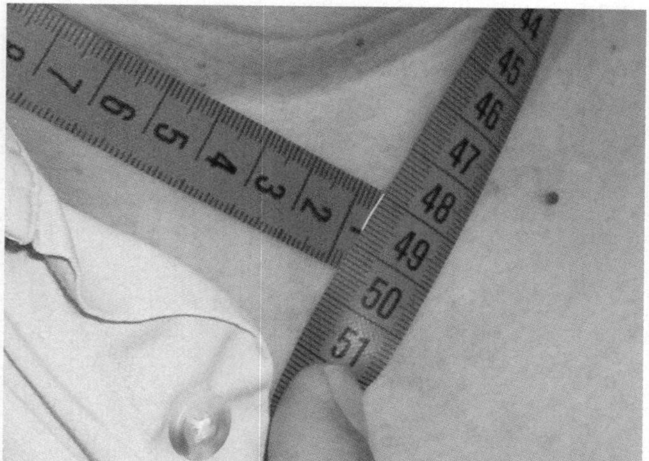

Figure 11.1-57.
Neck collar size exceeding 43 cm is associated with sleep apnea.

Examination of the Abdomen

Central obesity is a very common finding in sleep apnea patients. Note the striae in Figure 11.1-60.

Bariatric surgery is commonly done to treat morbid obesity and may result in resolution of sleep apnea. The patient shown in Figure 11.1-61 continued to have sleep apnea after having lost more than 100 kg. Note the abdominal scar and redundant tissue in this male patient.

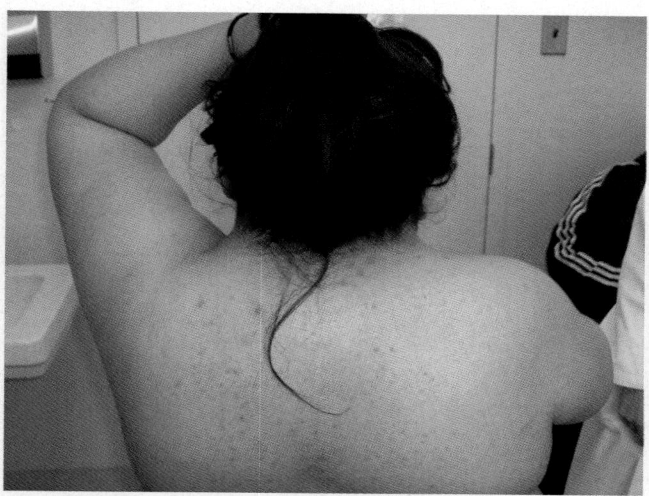

Figure 11.1-58.
Sleep apnea can be due to Klippel-Feil syndrome.

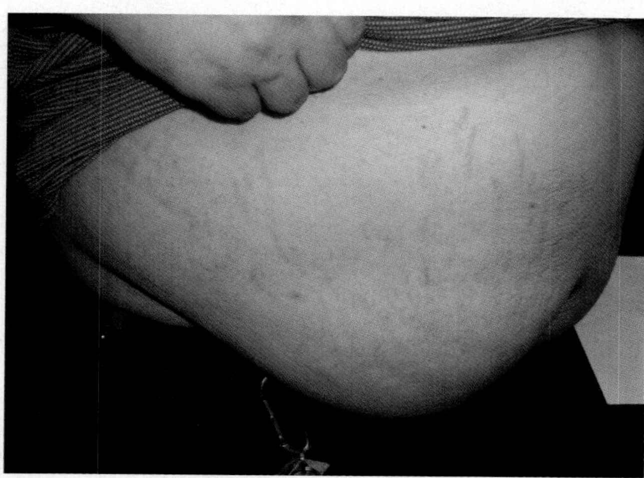

Figure 11.1-60.
Central obesity.

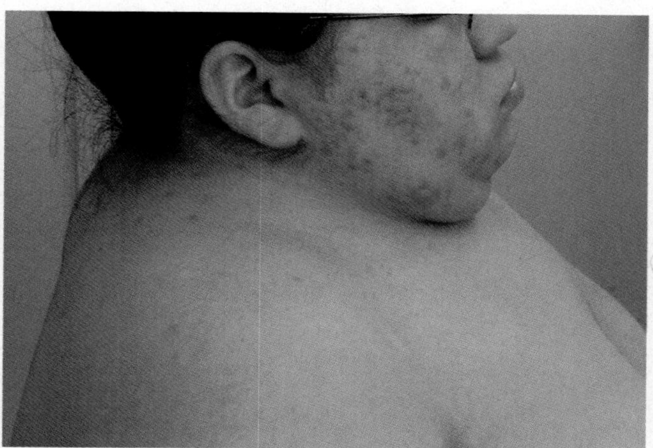

Figure 11.1-59.
Patients with Klippel-Feil syndrome have a low hairline and a short, webbed neck.

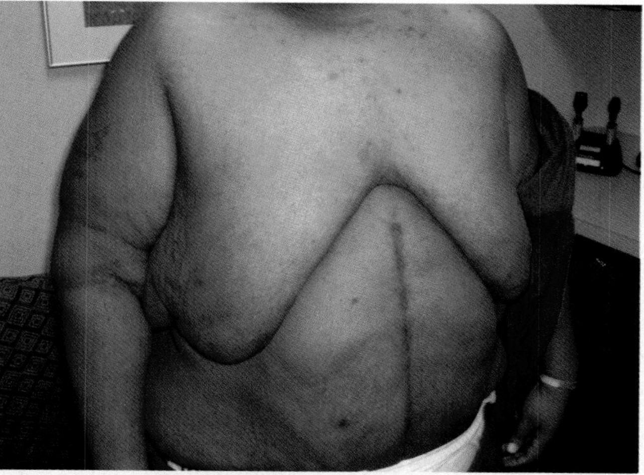

Figure 11.1-61.
Bariatric surgery results in weight loss, often leaving excess skin.

Examination of the Extremities

PERIPHERAL EDEMA

In very obese patients who spend most of their time in bed, edema might not always be maximal in the ankles and feet (Figs. 11.1-62 and 11.1-63). When edema is very severe in a patient with a sleep breathing disorder, it is almost always in the context of a hypoventilation syndrome (Fig. 11.1-64). Chronic edema results in discoloration and may result in infections that are difficult to treat (Figs. 11.1-65 and 11.1-66).

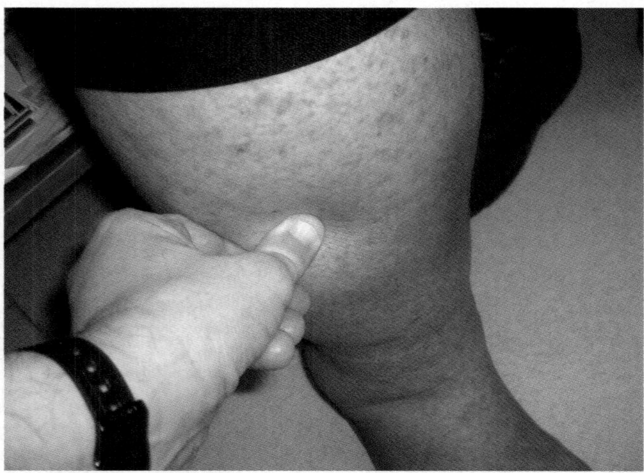

Figure 11.1-62.
Edema is not always present in ankles and feet.

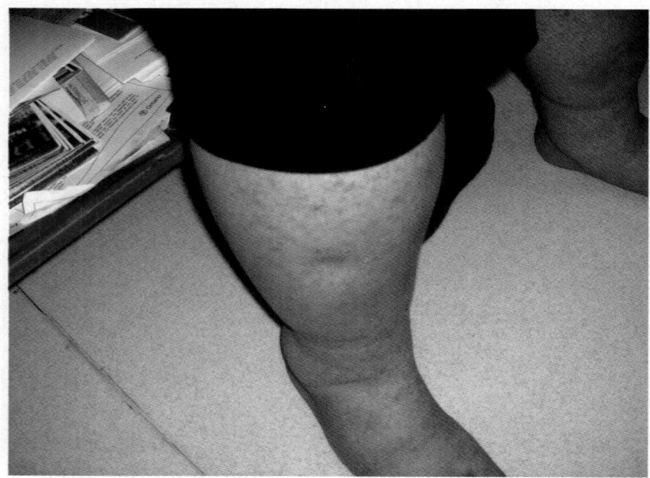

Figure 11.1-63.
Pitting edema.

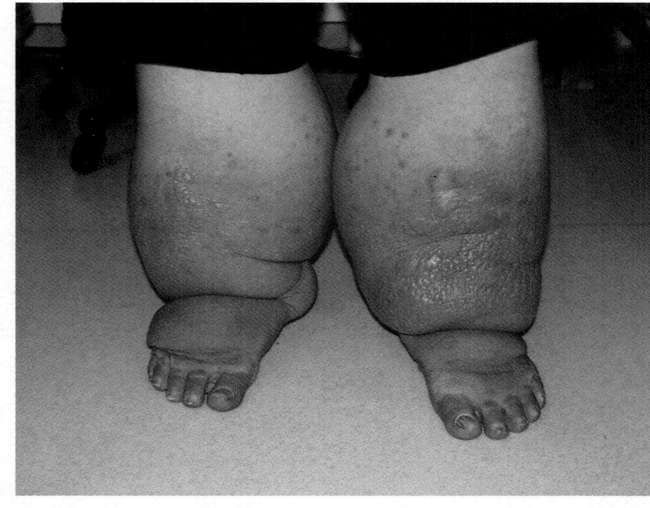

Figure 11.1-64.
Edema in patient with hypoventilation syndrome.

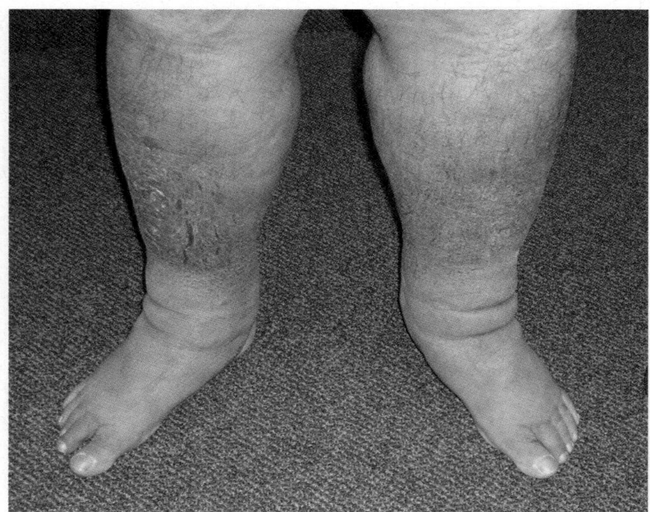

Figure 11.1-65.
Chronic edema, even when resolved, may result in discoloration.

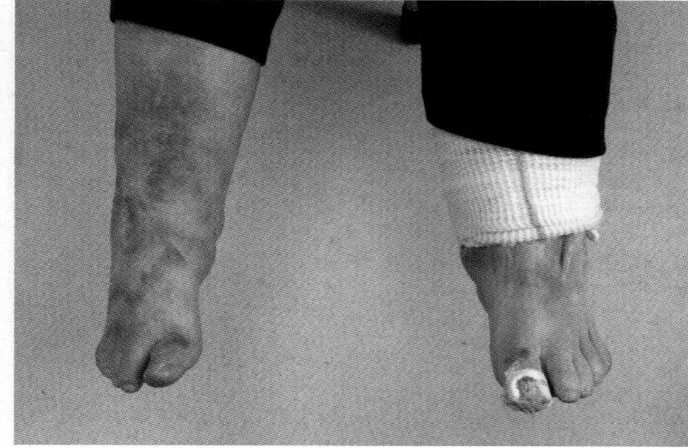

Figure 11.1-66.
Chronic edema may result in infections.

Don Hayes, Jr., and
Barbara Phillips

Sleep Apnea 11.2

Overview

Sleep breathing disorders encompass a wide variety of respiratory problems that appear exclusively in sleep, that affect sleep, or that are exacerbated by sleep. The classification schemes presented in the *International Classification of Sleep Disorders*, 2nd edition (ICSD-2), and in the *International Classification of Disease*, 9th edition (ICD-9) appear in Boxes 11.2-1 and 11.2-2.

BOX 11.2-1. SLEEP-RELATED BREATHING DISORDERS (ADAPTED FROM ICSD-2)

- Central sleep apnea syndromes
  - Primary central sleep apnea
  - Central sleep apnea due to Cheyne Stokes breathing pattern
  - Central sleep apnea due to high-altitude periodic breathing
  - Central sleep apnea due to medical condition not Cheyne Stokes
  - Central sleep apnea due to drug or substance
  - Primary sleep apnea of infancy
- Obstructive sleep apnea syndromes
  - Obstructive sleep apnea, adult
  - Obstructive sleep apnea, pediatric
- Sleep-related hypoventilation/hypoxemia syndromes
  - Sleep-related nonobstructive alveolar hypoventilation, idiopathic
  - Congenital central alveolar hypoventilation syndrome
- Sleep-related hypoventilation/hypoxemia due to medical condition
  - Sleep-related hypoventilation/hypoxemia due to pulmonary parenchyma or vascular pathology
  - Sleep-related hypoventilation/hypoxemia due to lower airways obstruction
  - Sleep-related hypoventilation/hypoxemia due to neuromuscular and chest wall disorders
- Other sleep-related breathing disorders

BOX 11.2-2. SLEEP-RELATED BREATHING DISORDERS (ADAPTED FROM ICD-9)

- Primary central sleep apnea (327.21)
- Central sleep apnea due to Cheyne Stokes breathing pattern (786.04)
- Central sleep apnea due to medical condition not Cheyne Stokes (327.27)
- Central sleep apnea due to drug or substance (327.29)
- Primary sleep apnea of infancy (770.81)
- Obstructive sleep apnea (327.23)
- Sleep-related nonobstructive alveolar hypoventilation, idiopathic (327.24)

Definitions

The term *sleep-disordered breathing* (SDB) refers to a spectrum of breathing disorders. Included are both obstructive events, in which airflow is limited despite respiratory effort, and central events, in which airflow ceases because of lack of respiratory effort.

The metric most commonly used to define and assess the severity of sleep apnea is the apnea plus hypopnea index, or AHI. Practically speaking, an individual is at risk for sleep apnea if the AHI is 5 or more. For this reason, measurement and definition of apneas and hypopneas are critical.

Among the obstructive sleep-disordered breathing disorders, the line between normal and pathologic is at times unclear (Box 11.2-3). The mildest form of an obstructed sleep-related breathing disorder is intermittent snoring, which may be a nuisance but is without significant health sequelae. (Evidence is accumulating, however, that chronic snoring may have consequences that are similar to those of frank obstructive sleep apnea.) The most severe form of sleep-disordered breathing is the obesity-hypoventilation syndrome (formerly called the Pickwickian syndrome), which is associated with severe morbidity and very high mortality. Between these two extremes are disorders of gradually increasing impact on morbidity and mortality: persistent snoring, upper airway resistance syndrome, and obstructive sleep apnea syndrome.

In contrast to obstructive sleep-disordered breathing, central sleep apnea typically occurs in the absence of respiratory effort and has very different risk factors and morbidities than has obstructive sleep apnea. The different pathophysiology of the two apnea types is reviewed in chapter 3.6.

Risk Factors

Obesity is the most important risk factor for obstructive SDB in Caucasians; the risk of significant SDB rises with body mass index. Obstructive sleep apnea (OSA) is about twice as common in men as in women before the age of 50, but may be equally prevalent in older men and women. Emerging data indicate that being Asian, African-American, or Hispanic is an independent risk factor for sleep apnea.

BOX 11.2-3. THE SPECTRUM OF SLEEP-DISORDERED BREATHING

- Obesity-hypoventilation syndrome (Pickwickian syndrome)
- Severe obstructive sleep apnea
- Moderate obstructive sleep apnea
- Mild obstructive sleep apnea
- Upper airways resistance syndrome
- Chronic, heavy snoring
- Intermittent snoring
- Quiet breathing

The prevalence of SDB also increases with age. In addition, there appear to be genetic risk factors for OSA. Other risk factors include hypothyroidism, nasal obstruction, and syndromes affecting airway caliber or craniofacial anatomy, such as trisomy 21, Pierre Robin, Alpert, Treacher Collins, and Marfan syndromes, to name a few. Behavioral factors, including alcohol consumption, use of sedative medication, and cigarette smoking, also contribute to an increased risk of SDB. Central sleep apnea, on the other hand, is associated with congestive heart failure, use of respiratory depressants such as opioids, and acute cerebrovascular injury (e.g., stroke).

Clinical Assessment

SYMPTOMS

Symptoms have generally been present for years before the diagnosis is made. The cardinal symptoms of OSA appear in Box 11.2-4 and in chapter 7. An interview of the patient (see chapter 19) will shed light on the symptoms and how they impact the patient's life.

BOX 11.2-4. SYMPTOMS OF OBSTRUCTIVE SLEEP-DISORDERED BREATHING

- Snoring
- Witnessed apnea
- Excessive daytime sleepiness
- Morning headache
- Dry throat in the morning
- Depressive symptoms
- Erectile dysfunction
- Insomnia
- Impaired vigilance and memory

EXAMINATION

The examination of the patient with sleep-disordered breathing is covered in detail in chapter 11.1. In OSA, the primary findings in adults are obesity, a crowded posterior airway, hypertension (especially difficult-to-control hypertension), and other abnormalities that may narrow the airway, such as retrognathia, an enlarged tongue, or a "birdlike face," as seen in Treacher Collins syndrome.

LABORATORY EVALUATION

The comprehensive overnight polysomnogram is currently the most widely used diagnostic test to document sleep apnea.

Data Obtained in a Sleep Study

The current American Academy of Sleep Medicine (AASM) scoring manual specifies the use of an oronasal thermal sensor to assess airflow for apnea and a pressure transducer to assess airflow for hypopnea. Information from a nasal pressure transducer may be misleading in a mouth breather, and the signal from a temperature sensor is not linear. Measuring end-tidal CO_2 adds an additional dimension of helpful information. The reader is encouraged not to slavishly follow the manual at all times, but to examine all the available data in order to assess and understand the physiologic abnormalities. Synchronized digital video is often invaluable in assessing the patient (see chapter 17).

Scoring of Respiratory Events

Both apneas and hypopneas must last at least 10 seconds, with the former occurring when inferred airflow is reduced by 90% or more from baseline, and the latter occurring

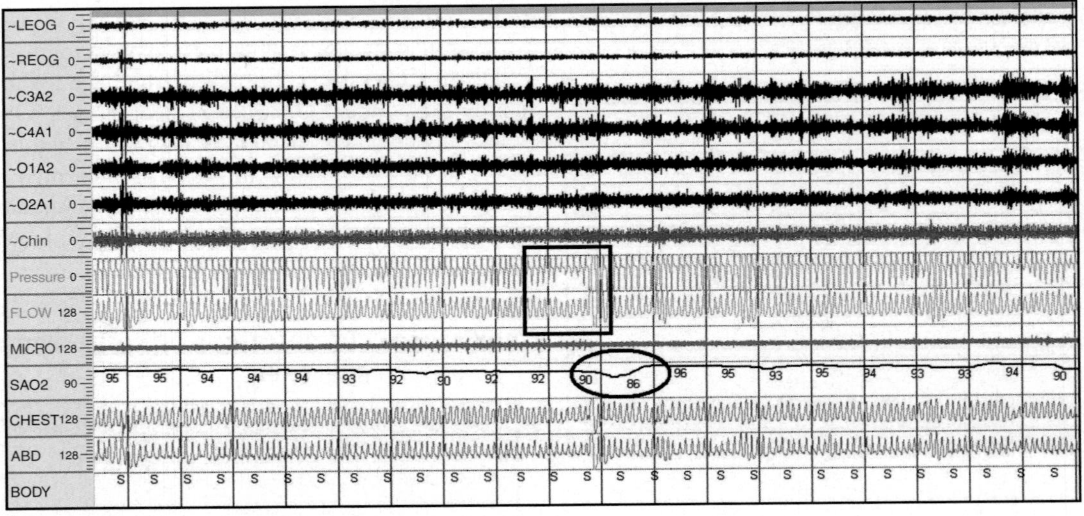

Figure 11.2-1.
Hypopnea. Shown here is a 10-minute, compressed epoch that demonstrates the features of a standard hypopnea, with reduction to about 30% of baseline of the pressure transducer signal and 4% oxygen desaturation. Also shown is the difference in the pressure transducer and thermal sensor (flow) signals, with noticeable change in the former, but little change in the latter.

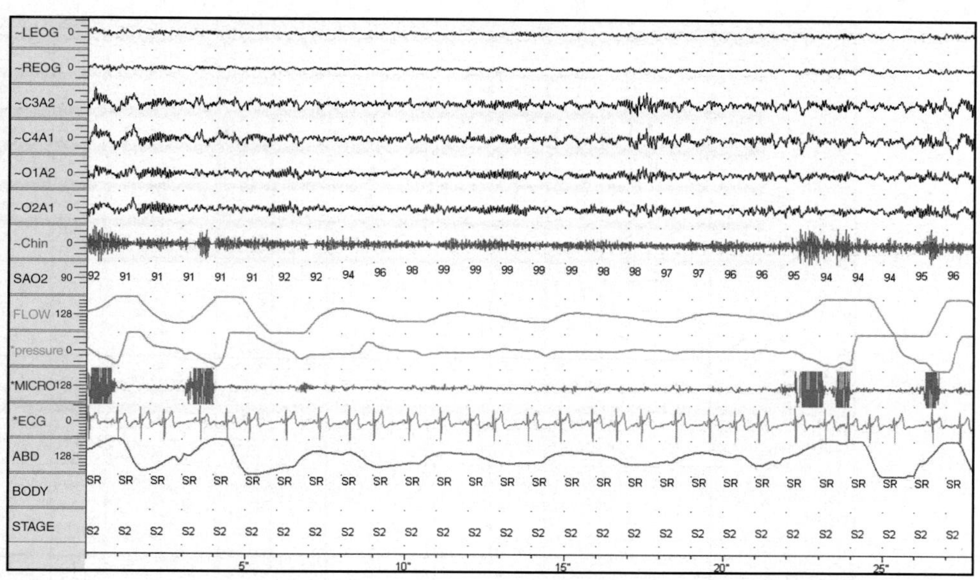

Figure 11.2-2.
Hypopnea. Shown here is a 30-second epoch that demonstrates a hypopnea with a fall in oxygen saturation from 99% to 94%. Flow measured by thermocouple is not quite reduced by 90%. The associated changes in heart rate and SaO_2 are similar to what would be seen in an apneic episode. Thus, the separation between apnea and hypopnea is often arbitrary, and the two events are combined to generate the apnea-hypopnea index (the number of events per hour of sleep).

when there is a reduction by 30% or more from baseline airflow with either a 4% or greater drop in SaO_2. An alternative rule for hypopnea requires a 50% or more reduction in flow with a 3% or greater drop in SaO_2 associated with an arousal. If respiratory effort is present during the event, it is classified as obstructive, and if not, it is classified as central. Figure 11.2-1 demonstrates a respiratory event that meets criteria for a hypopnea, with a marked reduction in the pressure transducer (but not the airflow or thermal sensor) signal and a drop in SaO_2 from 90% to 86%. Figure 11.2-2 demonstrates a hypopnea in which the SaO_2 never falls below 94%. In Figure 11.2-3, the somewhat arbitrary nature of these definitions, as well as the difference in thermal and pressure signals, is demonstrated. The term *respiratory effort-related arousal* (RERA) was coined to capture respiratory events that do not qualify as apneas or

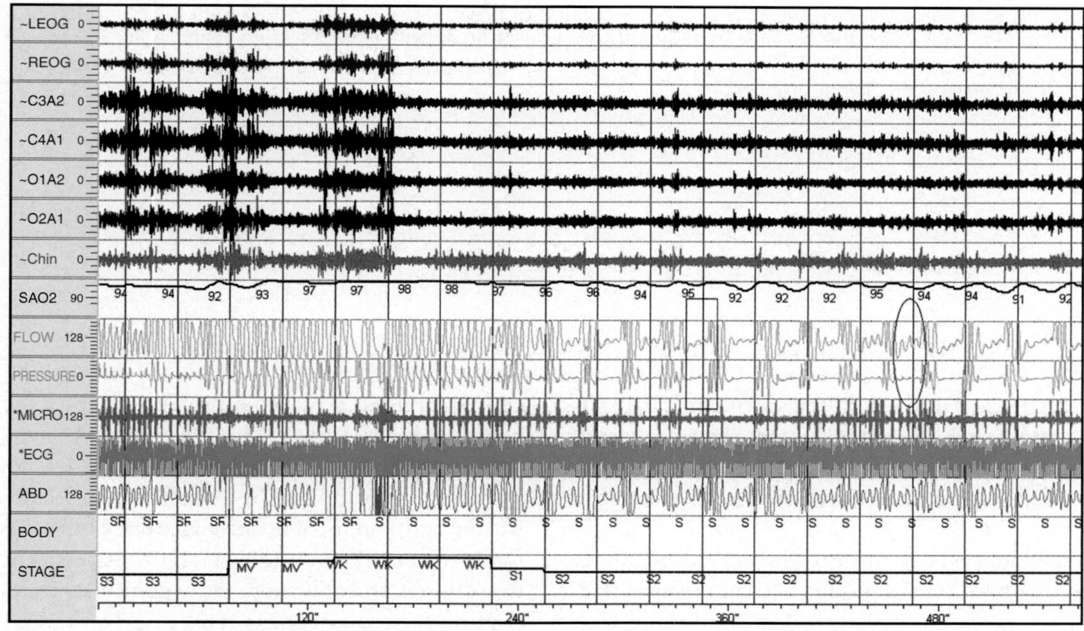

Figure 11.2-3.
Apneas and possible hypopnea. In this 10-minute compressed epoch, the "flow" channel represents the thermocouple signal and the "pressure" channel is nasal pressure. The event marked with the rectangle meets the criteria for an apnea, because the flow signal is reduced by more than 90% of baseline for more than 10 seconds (about 15 seconds). The oval marks an event that does not "qualify" as either an apnea or a hypopnea; the oxygen saturation only falls 1% (from 95 to 94), which precludes designating it as a hypopnea, and the thermocouple signal is reduced by about 80% of baseline (by standard criterion, a fall by 90% or more on the thermocouple [not flow transducer] channel is required for an apnea).

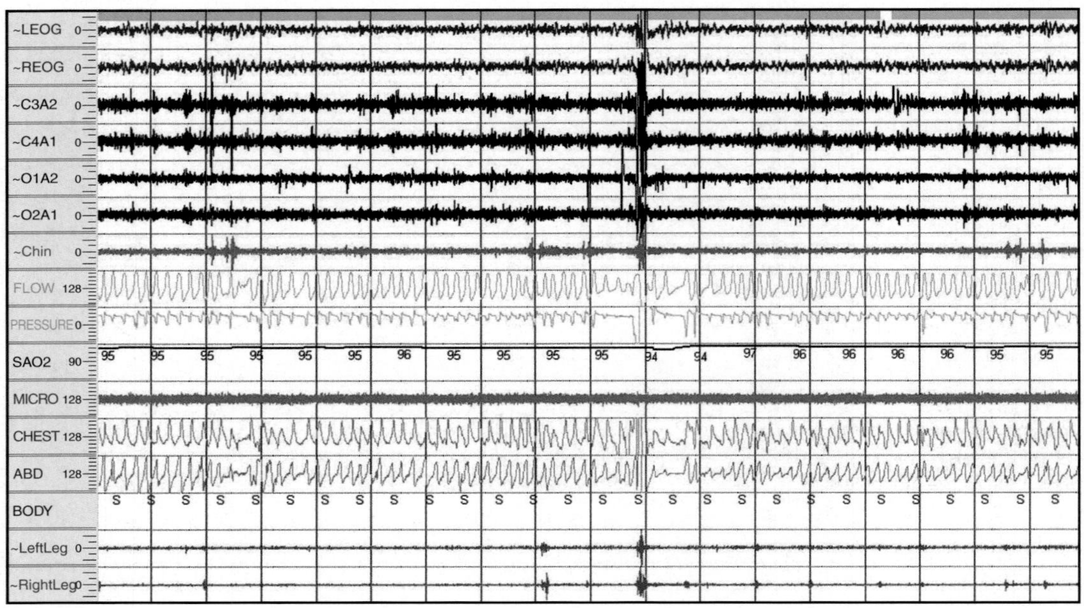

Figure 11.2-4.
Respiratory effort-related arousal. The difference in the sensitivity of pressure transducers ("pressure") and thermocouples ("flow") is demonstrated in this figure, in which a reduction of the pressure transducer signal to much less than 10% is evident, but the reduction in the flow channel is minimal. According to the scoring rules of the American Academy of Sleep Medicine, this event does not qualify as either an apnea or a hypopnea, since assessment of flow for apneas is supposed to be done by a thermal sensor. This cannot be a hypopnea by the scoring rules, because there is only a 1% oxygen desaturation. There is, however, an impressive arousal, including a leg jerk, and it is hard to argue that this event is not significant. This most likely represents a respiratory effort-related arousal (RERA), but does not meet scoring criteria for RERA, either. The current rules define RERA as "a sequence of breaths lasting at least 10 seconds characterized by increasing respiratory effort or flattening of the nasal pressure waveform leading to an arousal from sleep when the sequence of breaths does not meet criteria for an apnea or hypopnea." However, the scoring manual calls for use of an esophageal pressure manometer or respiratory inductance plethysmography in order to assess respiratory effort; these devices are not commonly used in clinical practice.

hypopneas (Fig. 11.2-4). However, the scoring manual calls for either an esophageal pressure manometer or respiratory inductance plethysmography in order to assess respiratory effort; these devices are almost never used in routine clinical practice.

The presence and severity of sleep-disordered breathing can be dependent both on sleep stage and on position (Fig. 11.2-5). Many patients, particularly women and those with milder disease, only experience events during rapid eye movement (REM) sleep and/or when supine.

By definition, central apneic events occur in the absence of respiratory effort. They are commonly seen in heart failure, in acute cerebrovascular events, and in the presence of respiratory depressants, but they also occur frequently in nonapneic individuals following arousal (Fig. 11.2-6). The central apneas may be linked to sleep stage and may decrease in REM (Figs. 11.2-7 to 11.2-9).

Cheyne Stokes respiration (also called Cheyne Stokes breathing), a pattern of at least three consecutive cycles of waxing and waning of breathing, is one of the most prevalent forms of central apnea (Fig. 11.2-10). Assessment of respiratory effort is probably more easily done in compressed epochs than in 30-second epochs (Fig. 11.2-11); there is markedly reduced movement in the chest and abdomen channels of this epoch during the apnea, more so than during airflow.

Both central and obstructive events can be seen in the same individual under a variety of circumstances (Fig. 11.2-12). Mixed sleep apneas share characteristics of both obstructive and central apneas, but typically respond well to treatment for obstructive apnea (Figs. 11.2-13 and 11.2-14).

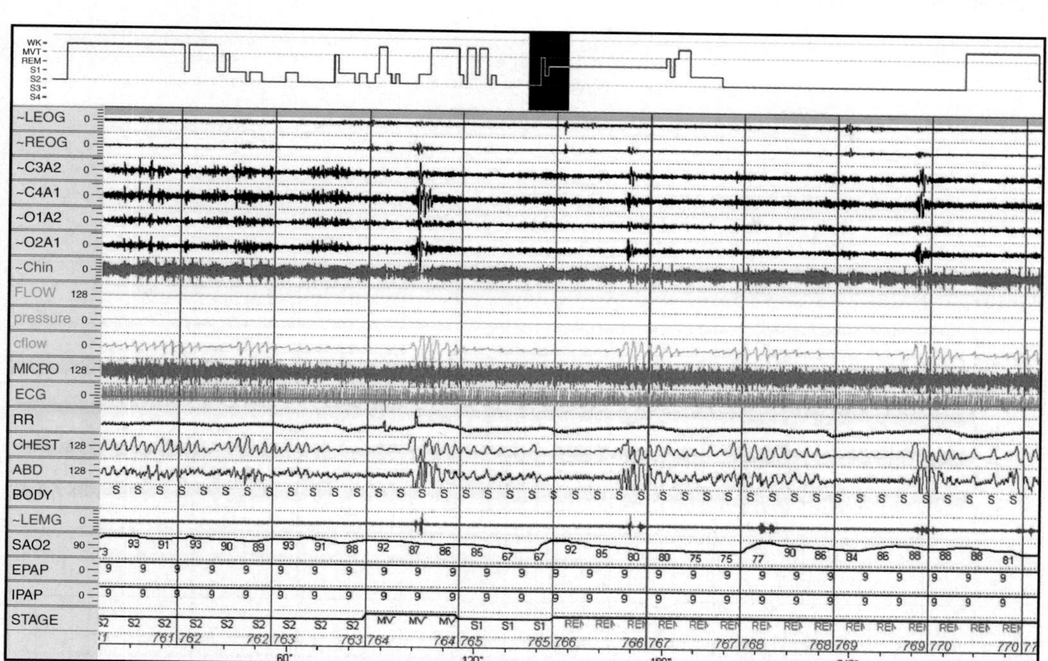

A

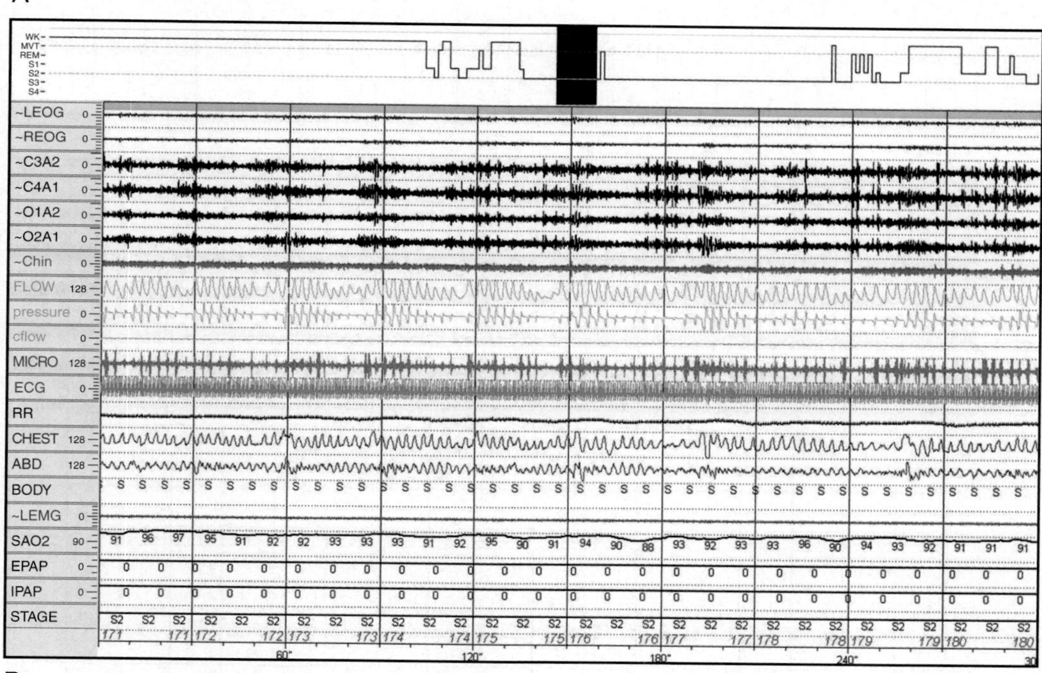

B

Figure 11.2-5.
Sleep stage effect on sleep-disordered breathing. The graphs illustrate epochs from a 38-year-old male patient diagnosed with obstructive sleep apnea based on an apnea-hypopnea index of 42 respiratory events per hour. **A,** The graph demonstrates worsening respiratory instability as the patient transitions from stage 2 to REM sleep. **B,** The graph illustrates his respiratory pattern soon after sleep onset. Physiologic changes in muscle tone occur phasically with the respiratory cycle and during sleep stage transitions. The REM sleep–specific phenomena are expressed not only in postural but also in respiratory muscles. This loss of muscle tone is greater than that seen during other phases of sleep, and the reduction in upper airway tone may be more profound than the depression of the main respiratory pump muscle activity, the diaphragm.

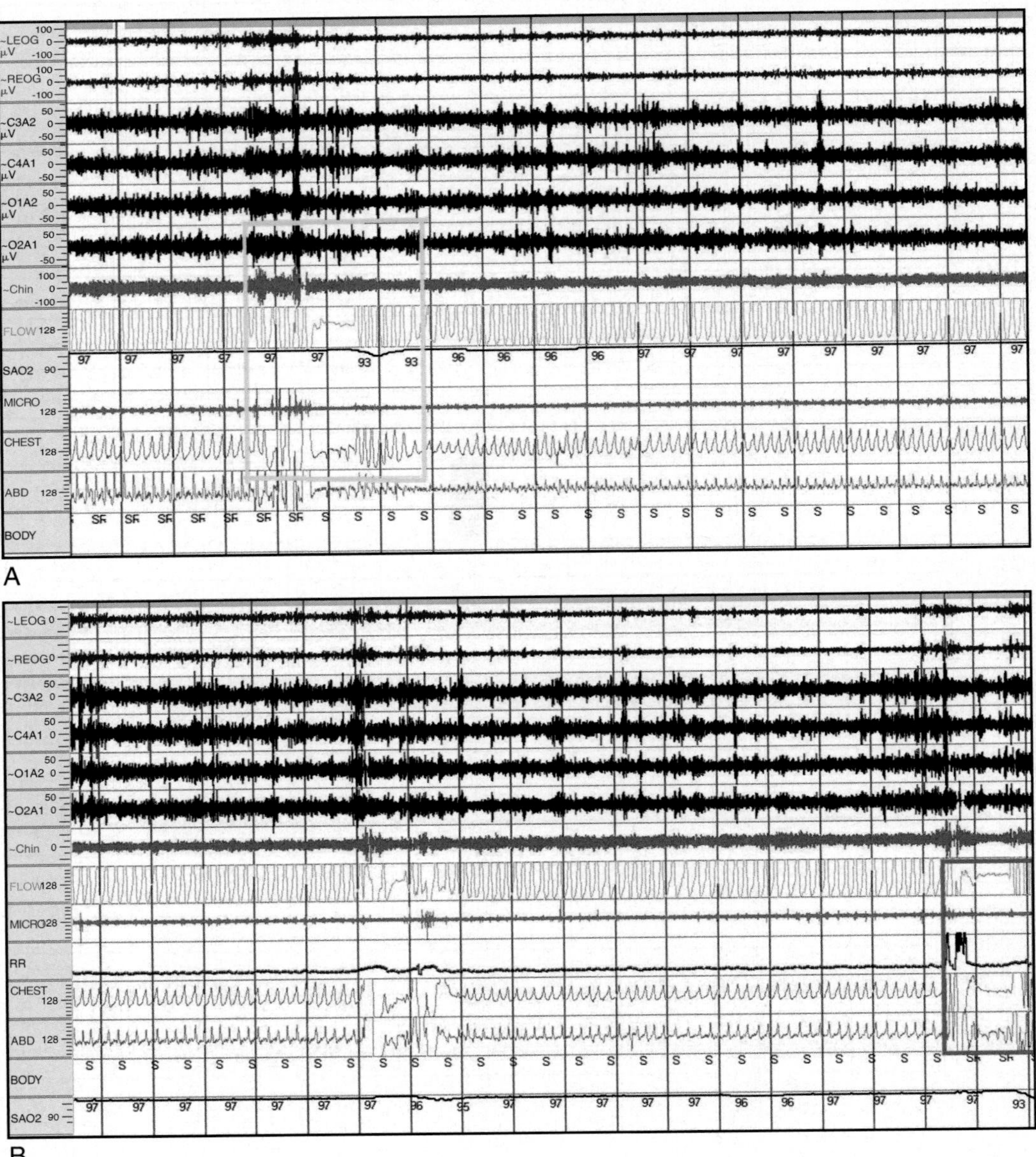

Figure 11.2-6.
Central apneas (A and B). These compressed 10-minute epochs demonstrate isolated central apneas following arousals. The lack of airflow in the pressure or flow channel, coupled with markedly reduced movement/effort in the abdomen/chest channel, marks these events as central.

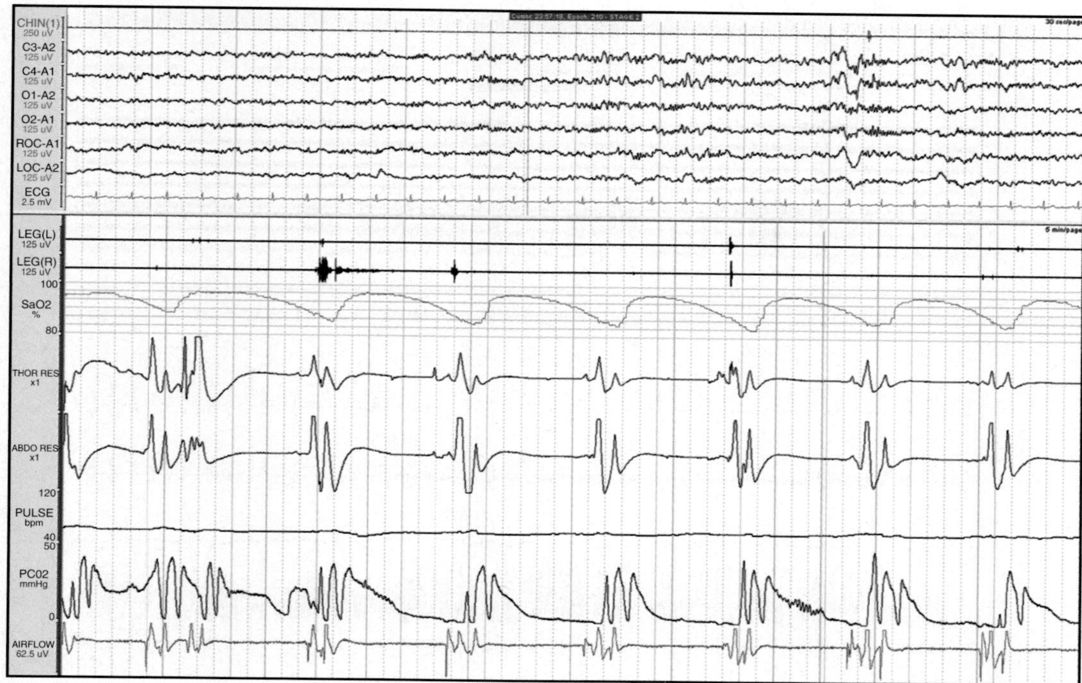

Figure 11.2-7.
In this illustration the top window has a 30-second epoch and the bottom window a 5-minute epoch. These are repetitive episodes of central apnea in a 44-year-old patient using opiates for pain in an injured ankle. Notice the small number of breaths in each cycle. There are cardiogenic oscillations in the CO_2 trace, best seen in the third apneic episode from the right.

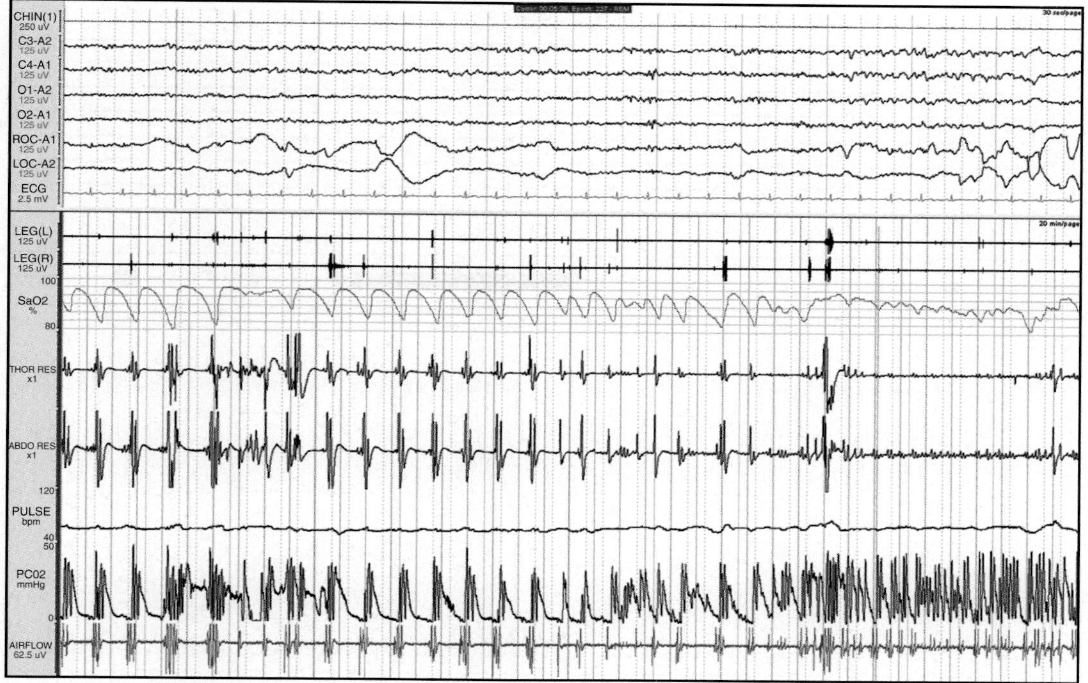

Figure 11.2-8.
This graph is from the same patient as seen in Figure 11.2-7. The bottom window is now a 20-minute epoch. The patient is going into REM sleep and the number of central apneas is decreased, but the patient is still hypoxic.

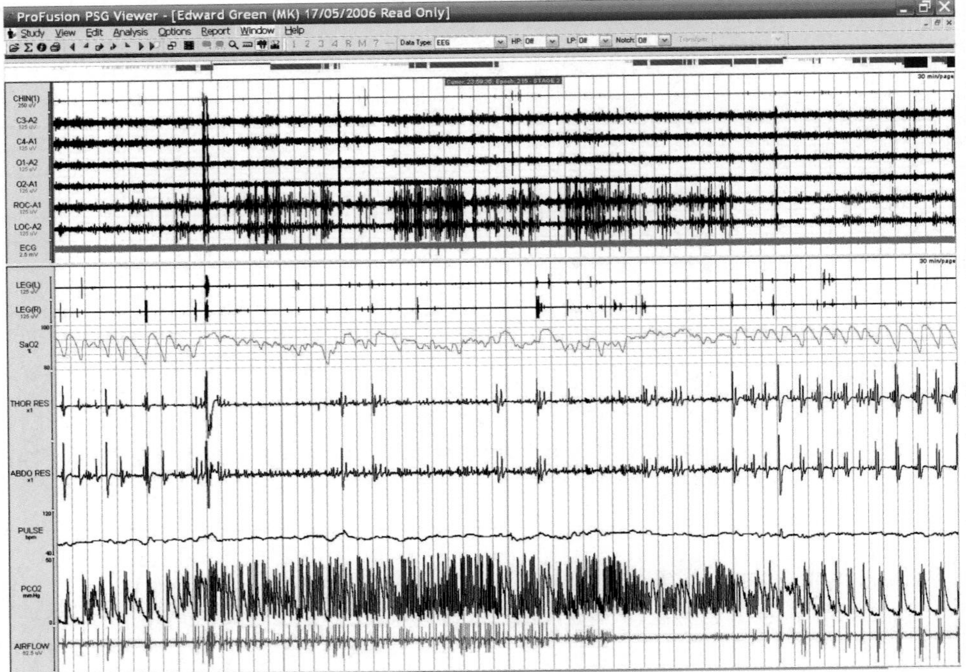

Figure 11.2-9.
This graph, from the same patient in Figure 11.2-8, shows a 30-minute compression in top and bottom windows. REMs can be seen where there are large deflections in the eye channels (ROC-A1 and LOC-A2). The periodic nature of the central apneas decreases when REM is entered and returns when NREM returns.

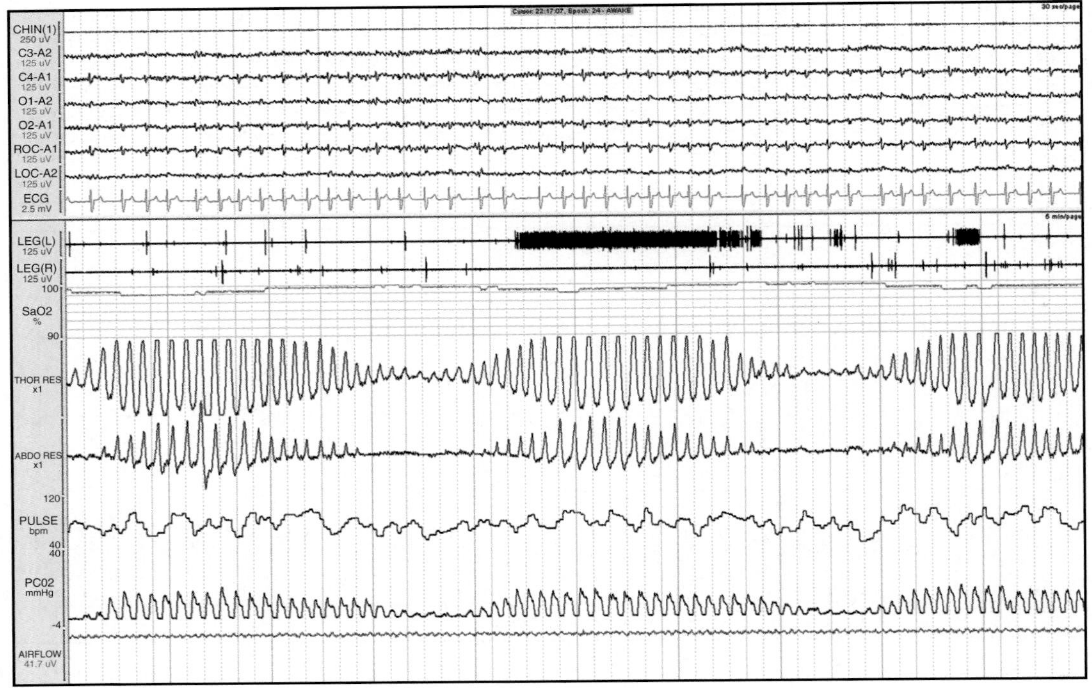

Figure 11.2-10.
See opposite page for legend.

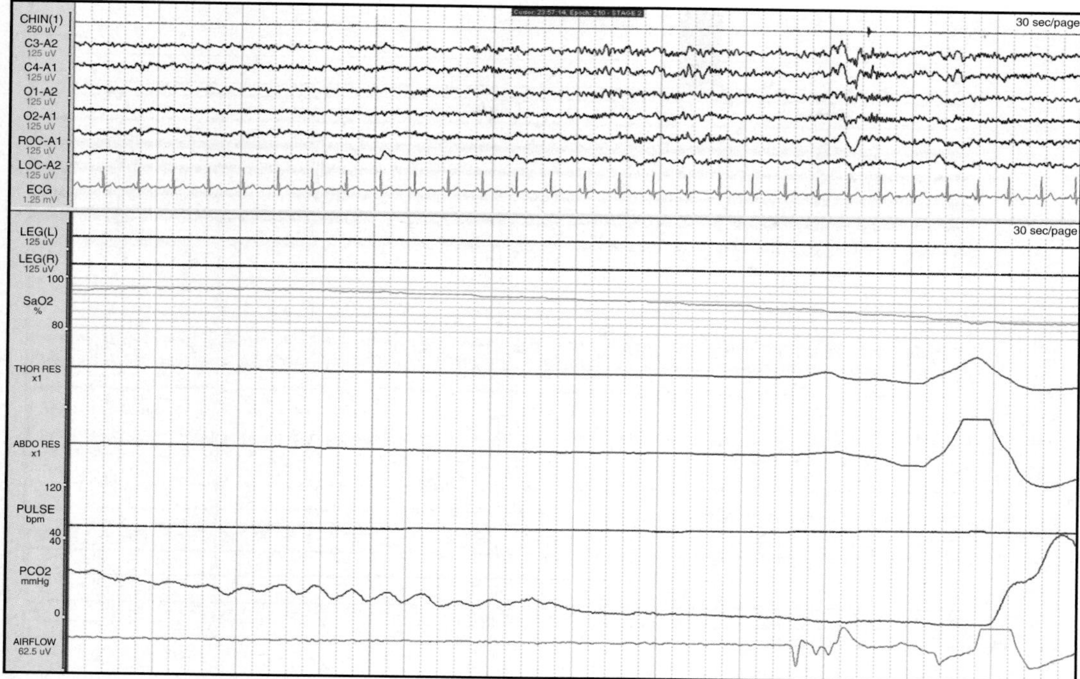

Figure 11.2-11.
Central apnea. The 30-second epoch seen here demonstrates the end of an apnea (no movement in the CO_2 or pressure channel during the apnea). Chest and abdominal signals are markedly reduced during the apnea. Note the cardiogenic oscillations in the CO_2 channel, adding evidence that this is a central apnea. Overall patterns in breathing are more easily appreciated in longer epoch lengths.

Figure 11.2-10.
Cheyne Stokes respirations (CSR). The compressed, 5-minute epoch in the bottom window is from a nocturnal polysomnogram of a patient with congestive heart failure and atrial fibrillation. It demonstrates classic central apneas separated by crescendo-decrescendo breathing, with absence or reduction of abdominal and chest movement during the apneas. Oronasal CO_2 is being recorded, and the nasal pressure (labeled "airflow") shows little activity because the patient is mouth breathing. CSR can be seen in patients with poorly controlled heart failure when they are awake (as in this example) and when they are sleeping; its presence is a negative prognostic sign. CSR can be predicted if the patient complains of paroxysmal nocturnal dyspnea.

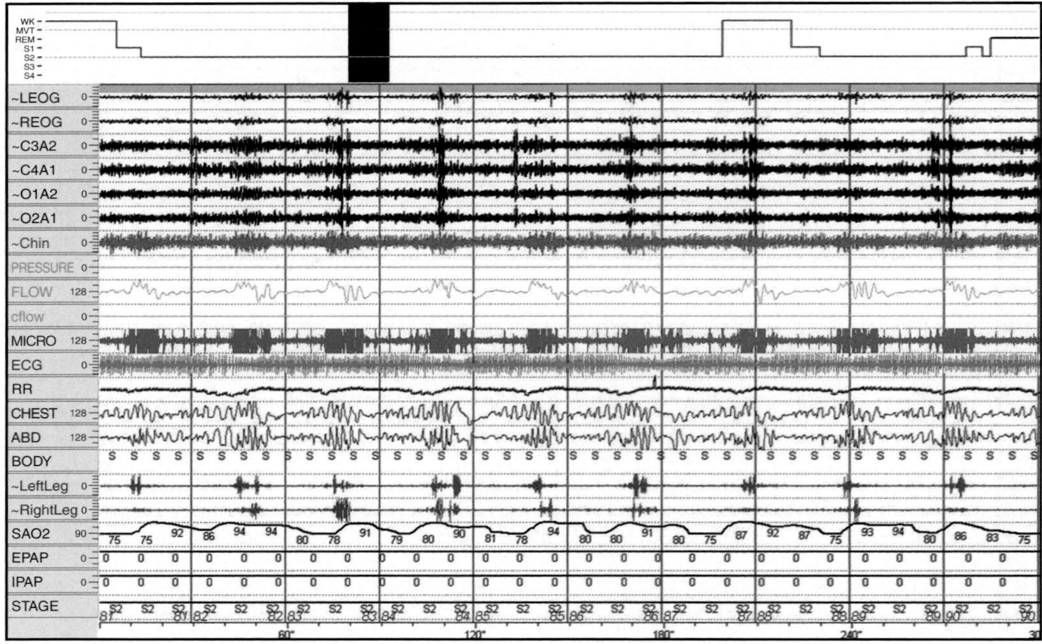

A

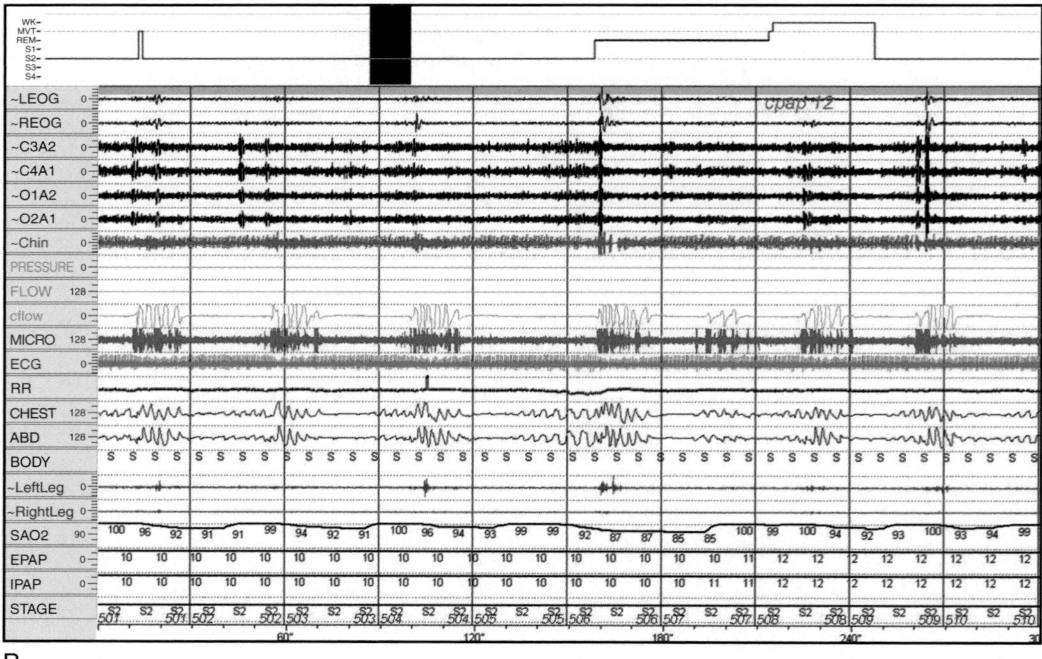

B

Figure 11.2-12.
Treatment-emergent central apneas ("complex" sleep apnea). These four graphs (**A–D**) illustrate epochs from a split-night nocturnal polysomnogram (NPSG) performed on a 37-year-old male who weighed 250 pounds with a body mass index of 36. The diagnostic component of the NPSG identified obstructive sleep apnea with an apnea-hypopnea index of 90.2 respiratory events per hour with lowest measured oxygen saturation of 72%. **A,** Seen here are obstructive apneas during the diagnostic component of the NPSG. During the therapeutic component of the study, the patient developed mixed apnea (**B** and **C**) with both continuous positive airway pressure (**B**) and bilevel continuous positive airway pressure (BiPAP) (**C**) treatment. The patient's upper airway obstruction was eventually resolved at a BiPAP pressure of 20/16.

(Continued)

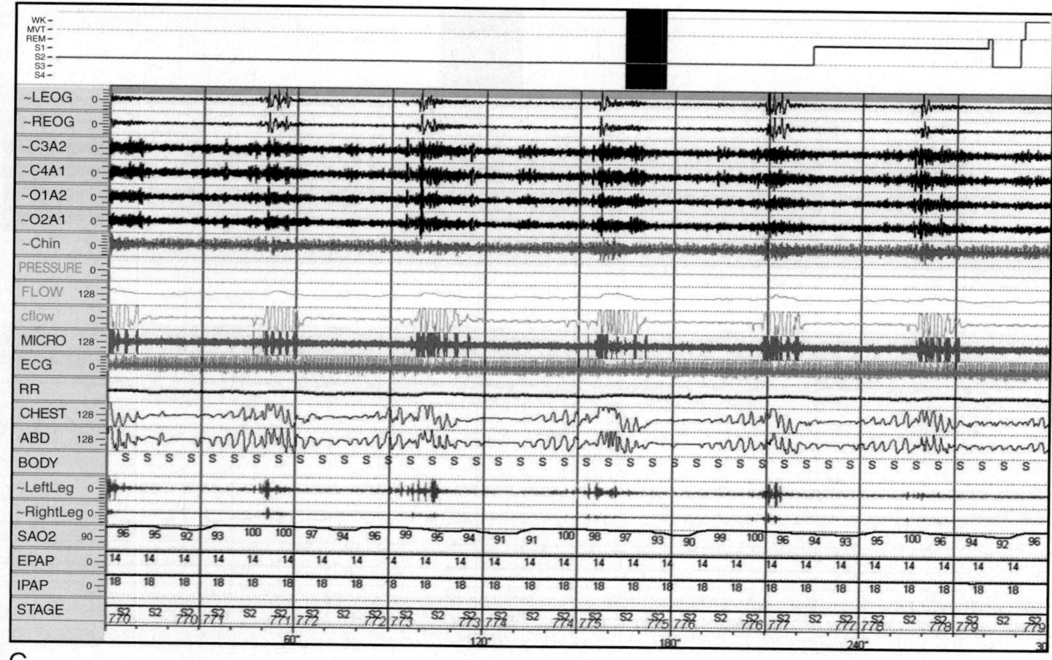

C

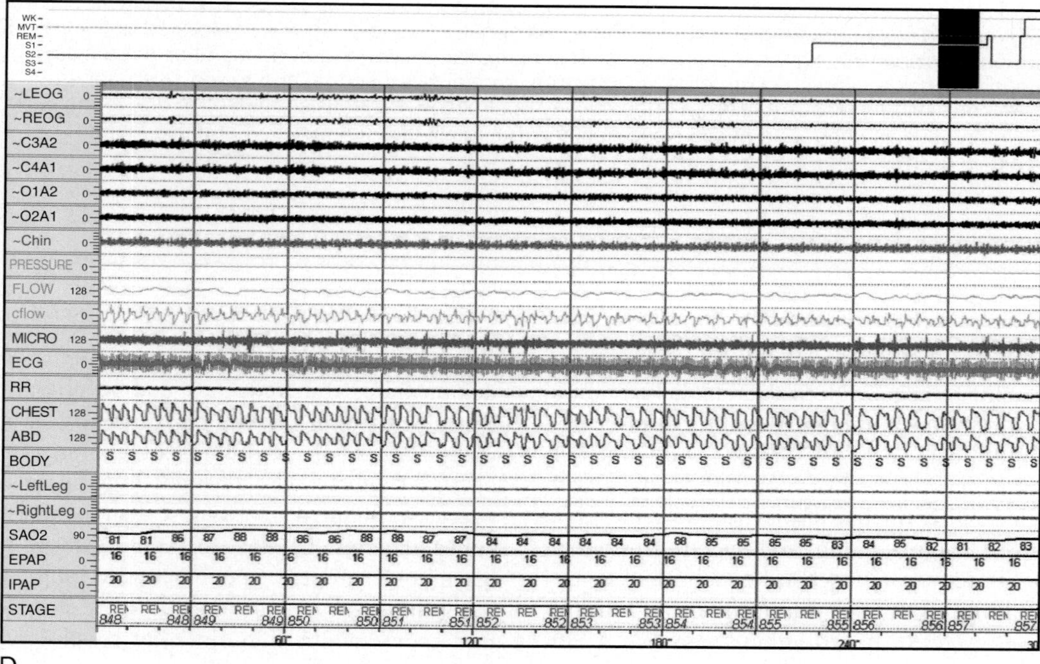

D

Figure 11.2-12. cont'd

D, The patient continued to have oxygen desaturations during REM sleep, so supplemental oxygen was started at 2 liters per minute with BiPAP therapy at 20/16 with complete resolution of his sleep-disordered breathing.

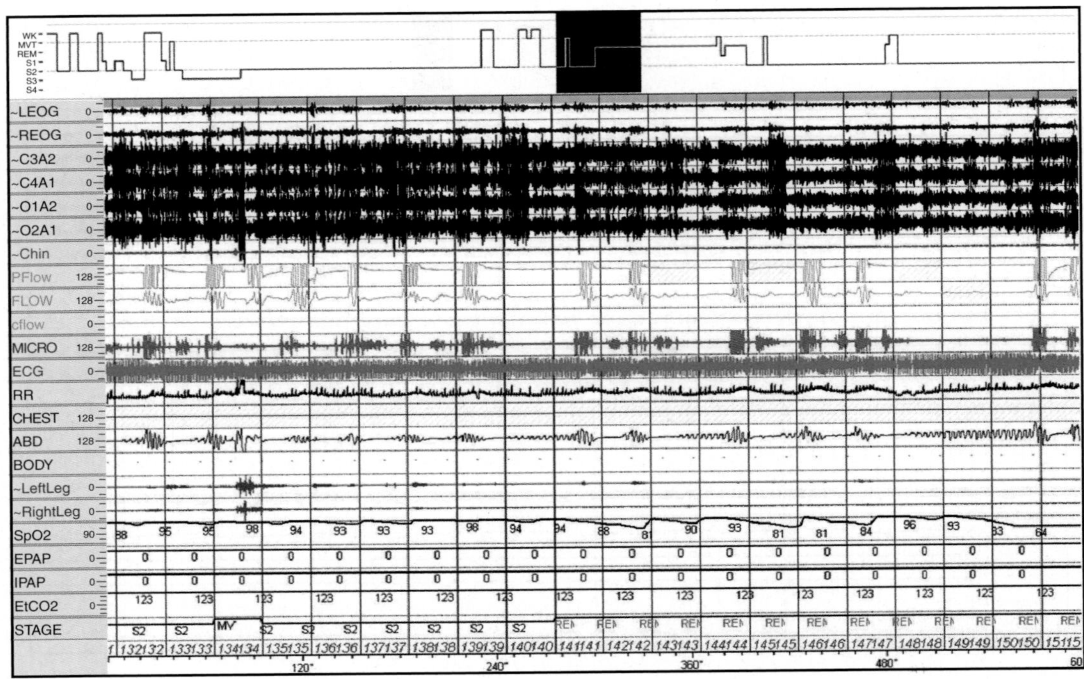

Figure 11.2-13.
Mixed sleep apnea. This figure demonstrates mixed sleep apnea in a compressed 10-minute epoch from a 50-year-old male with congestive heart failure. His apnea-hypopnea index was elevated at 92.1 events per hour of sleep with significant hypoxemia. This particular patient had evidence of all three main categories of sleep apnea: obstructive sleep apnea, central sleep apnea, and mixed sleep apnea. Obstructive sleep apnea results from upper airway obstruction, central sleep apnea is due to the lack of inspiratory muscle effort, and mixed sleep apnea is the result of a combination of these factors.

SCORING INTERVALS

Because almost all labs acquire sleep data digitally, and the data are displayed digitally on high-resolution displays, the polysomnographic data can be scored with different degrees of time compression. Data can be displayed with different epoch lengths on the display at the same time. In general, sleep stage scoring and electrocardiogram evaluation are best done in 30-second epochs, and assessment of respiratory events and leg movements is facilitated by compressed 5- or 10-minute epochs. A 30-second epoch demonstrating a hypopnea is seen in Figure 11.2-15; the compressed epoch seen in Figure 11.2-16 demonstrates the frequency and severity of sleep-disordered breathing much more clearly. Figure 11.2-17 demonstrates the usefulness of compressing the epoch up to 5 minutes. The all-night hypnogram gives a quick overview; Figure 11.2-18 most demonstrates REM-related apnea. Figures 11.2-19 to 11.2-22 show the utility of examining different epoch lengths using a split screen to examine the variables used to score sleep with a 30-second epoch, while using different epoch lengths to examine the respiratory variables.

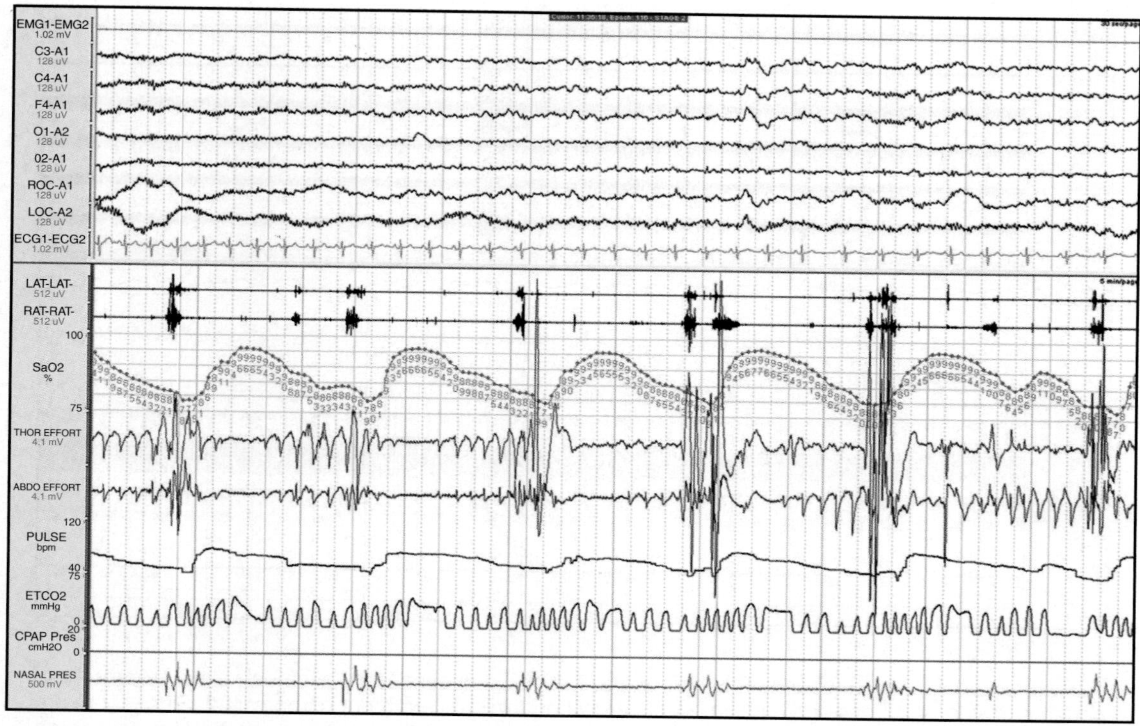

Figure 11.2-14.
Mixed apnea usually begins with central apnea and ends with obstructive apnea. In this example there are vigorous leg movements at the end of the apneic episodes. Continuous positive airway pressure abolished the apneas but the leg movements persisted.

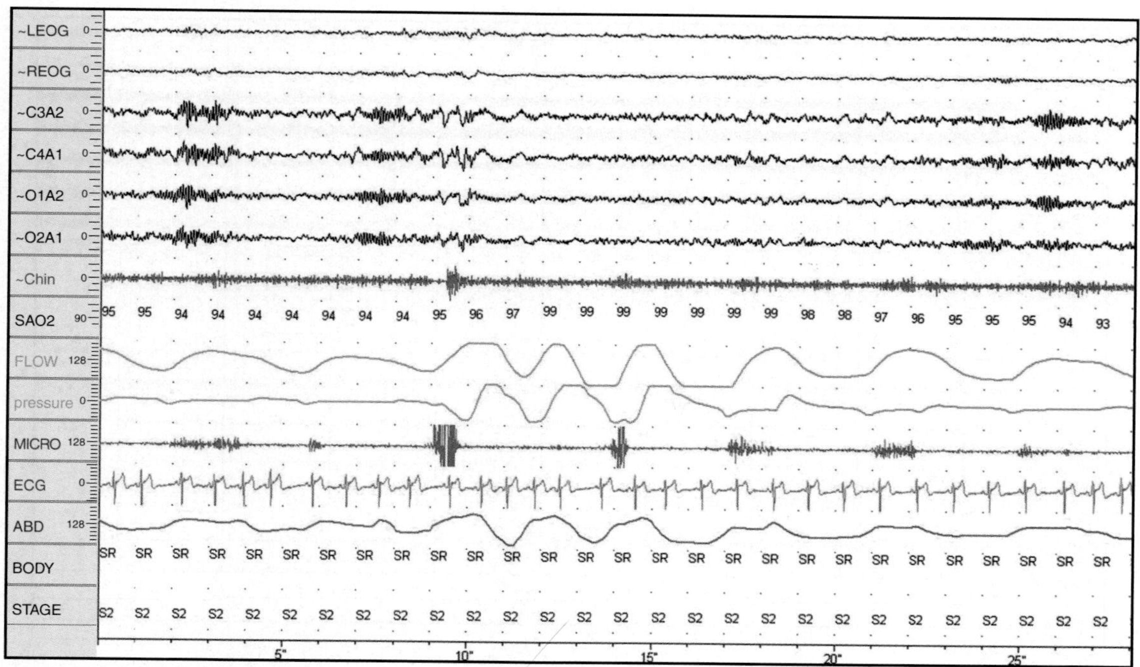

Figure 11.2-15.
A 30-second epoch. This 30-second epoch demonstrates stage 2 NREM sleep and the end of one hypopnea and the beginning of another.

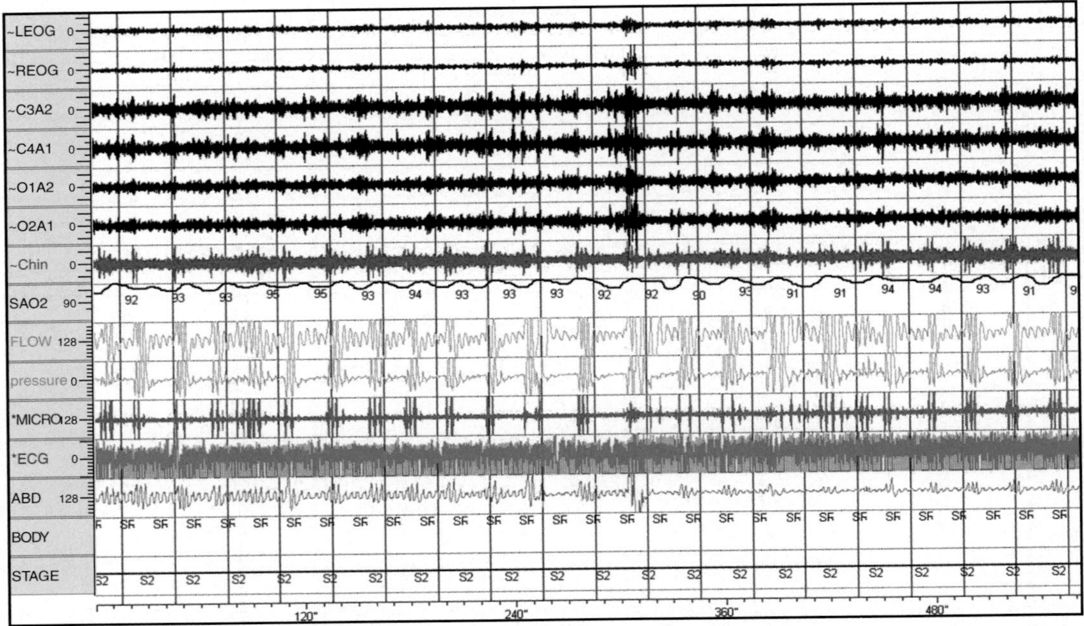

Figure 11.2-16.
A compressed 10-minute epoch. This compressed epoch demonstrates how much more evident the patterns of sleep-disordered breathing events are when the data are more compressed. Since there are no 3% falls in oxygen saturation here, no hypopneas can be scored by standard criteria. Very few of the falls in the flow (thermistry, not pressure, is recommended to identify apneas, according to the American Academy of Sleep Medicine scoring manual) actually meet the fall in flow to 10% of baseline. Yet, it would be difficult to argue that this patient is not having salvos of respiratory events, most of which are causing electroencephalogram (EEG) arousals.

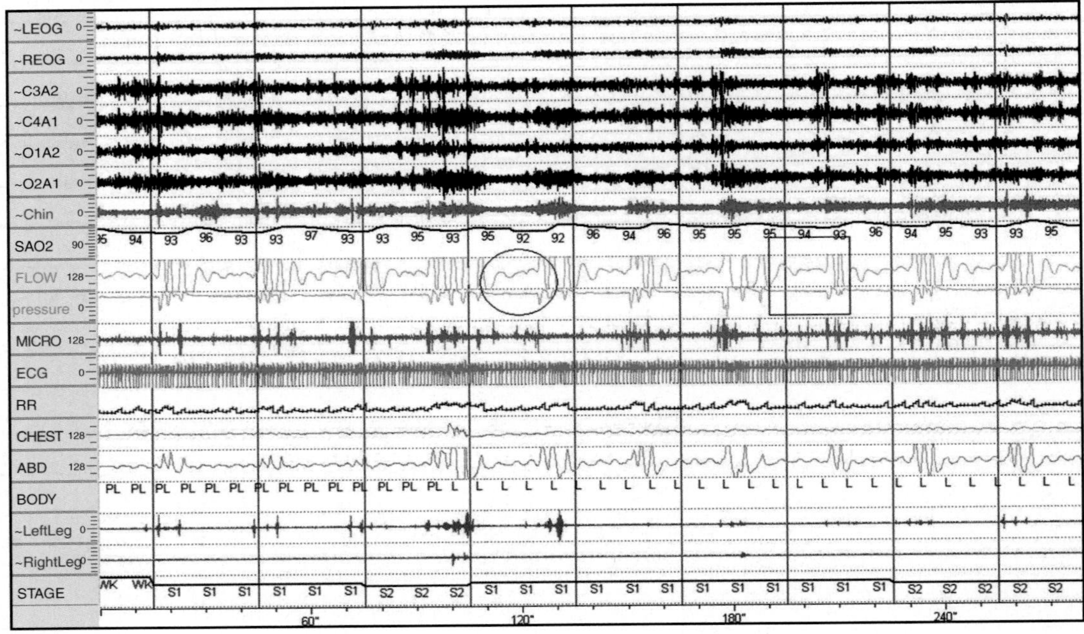

Figure 11.2-17.
A compressed 5-minute epoch. This compressed epoch (5 minutes, in contrast to the 10 minutes of data seen in Figure 11.2-16) demonstrates the usefulness of compressing data. The circle indicates an event that probably meets the criteria for an apnea, and can certainly be scored as a hypopnea if one is not convinced that the flow channel is decreased by 90% or more. The event indicated by the square is more ambiguous. It cannot be a hypopnea, since the oxygen saturation only falls from 95% to 93%, and many would score it as an apnea.

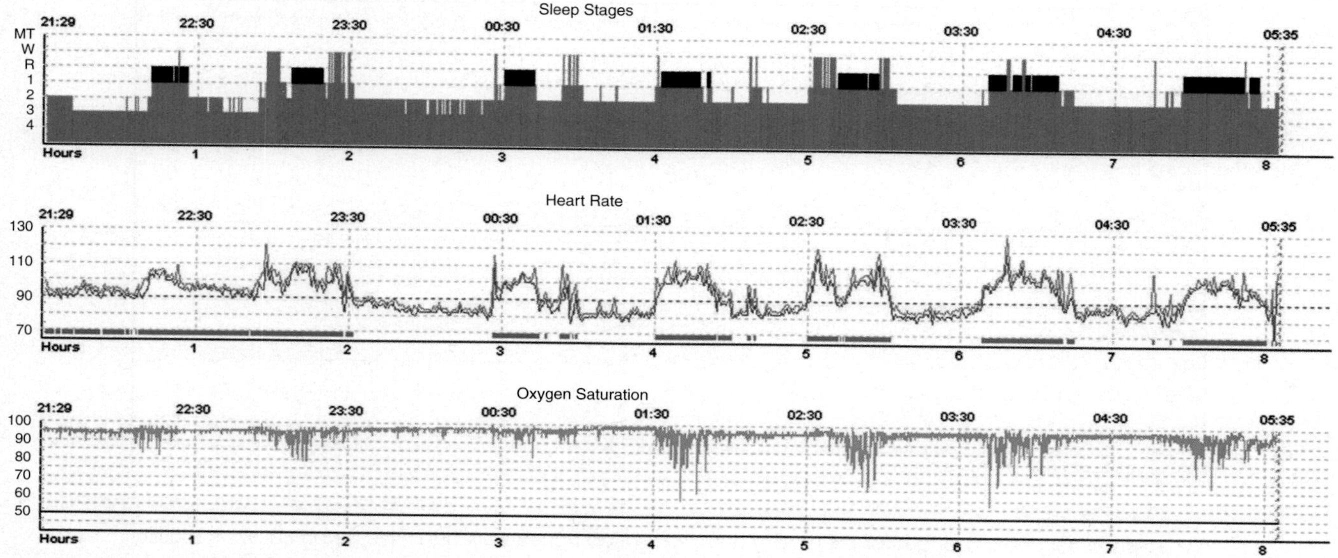

Figure 11.2-18.
Hypnogram with REM-related desaturation. This all-night hypnogram demonstrates profound oxygen desaturation during REM sleep. Notice the increases in heart rate that also occur during REM. These data are from a 2-year, 11-month-old child with loud snoring, witnessed apneas, and restless sleep. The patient had enlarged tonsils and a strong family history of apnea. Among adults, this phenomenon appears to be more common in women than in men.

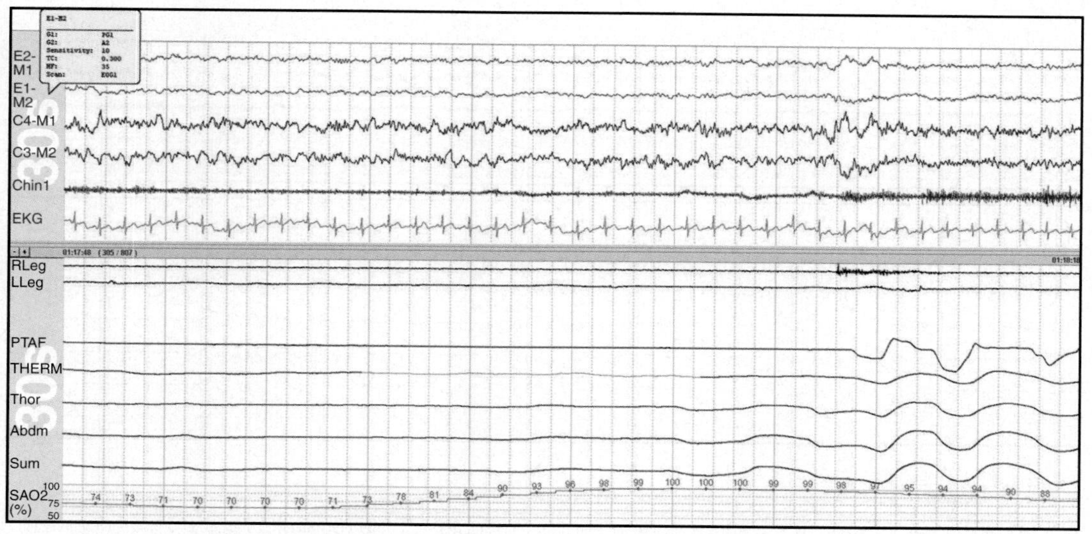

Figure 11.2-19.
What is the best epoch length for examining data from sleep apnea patients? Since 1969, an epoch length of 30 seconds has been considered "standard" based on a paper speed of 30 seconds per page. This is acceptable for optimal scoring of sleep stage, but often is not optimal for examining breathing. This figure shows a 30-second epoch. An entire abnormal breathing cycle cannot be seen. Figures 11.2-20 to 22 show that using different time compressions of the same data can be useful.

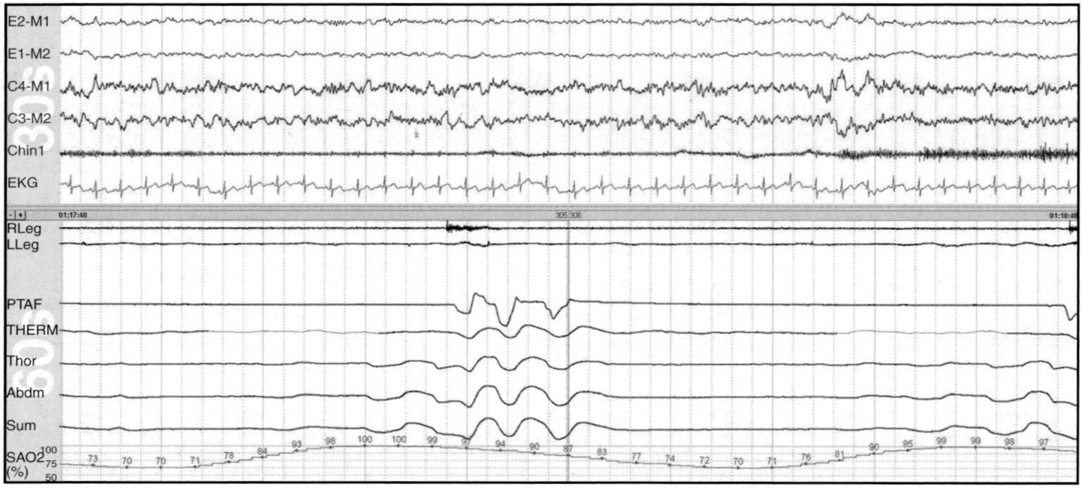

Figure 11.2-20.
What is the best epoch length for examining data from sleep apnea patients? This graph shows the utility of a split screen using different time compression. The top half of the split screen shows a 30-second epoch for the neurophysiologic variables and electrocardiogram (EKG). The bottom half shows 1 minute of the respiratory data. The longer-term pattern is still not clear from this.

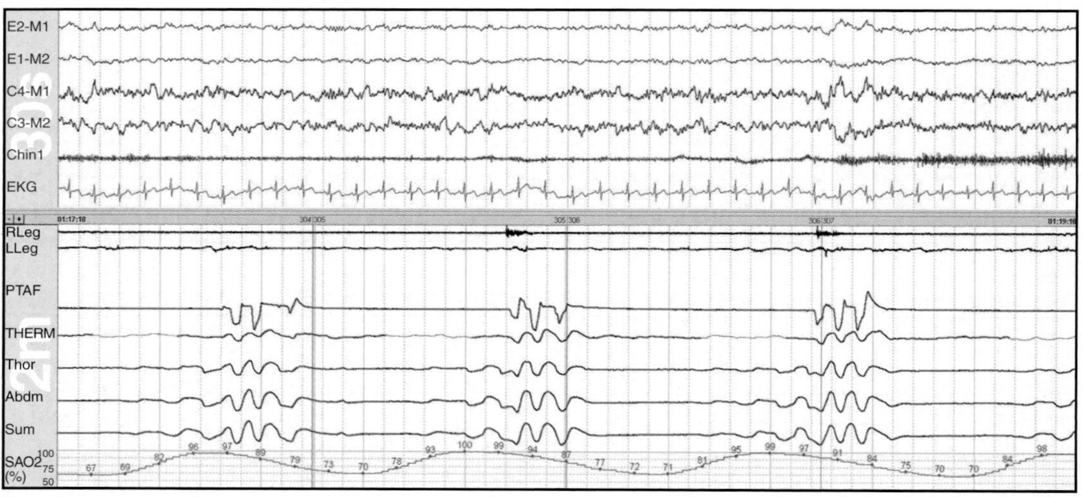

Figure 11.2-21.
The top portion of the split screen shows a 30-second epoch for the neurophysiologic variables and electrocardiogram (EKG). The bottom portion shows 2 minutes of the respiratory data. The longer-term pattern is now much clearer.

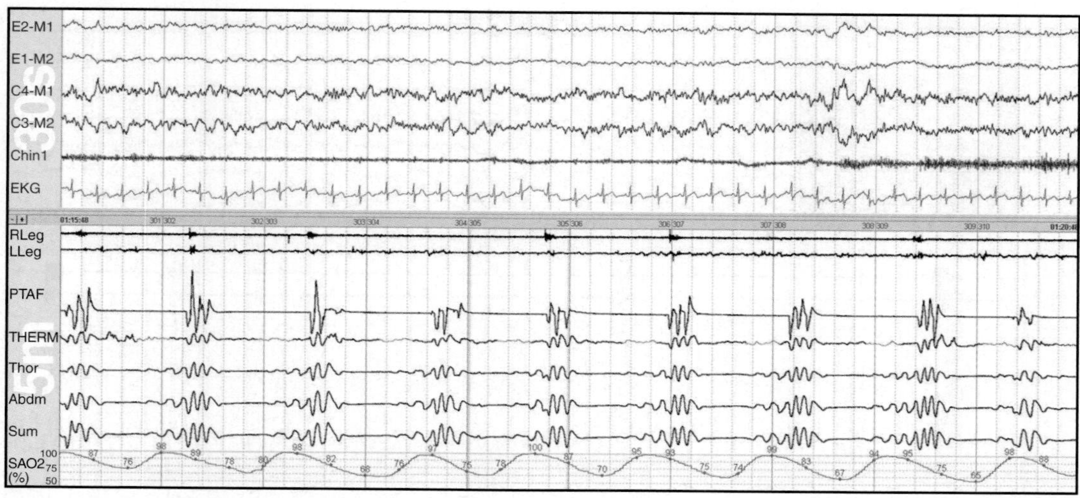

Figure 11.2-22.
The top portion of the split screen shows a 30-second epoch for the neurophysiologic variables and electrocardiogram (EKG). The bottom portion shows 5 minutes of the respiratory data. The monotonous regularity of the breathing suggests a Cheyne Stokes breathing pattern in this patient with heart failure and morbid obesity. Thus, this patient has features of obstruction caused by obesity and the Cheyne Stokes (central) component caused by heart failure. The leg movements noted in the leg channels are clearly linked to the breathing events and would not be scored as periodic limb movements.

Nonapneic Respiratory Events

Oxygen saturation falls during the night for humans, typically reaching a nadir in the early morning hours. For those with underlying lung diseases, this nocturnal desaturation can be exaggerated, as in the example shown in Figure 11.2-23. Oxygen saturation values hover in the mid-80s, even though airflow appears to be continually present. One may see such a pattern in patients with hypoventilation and in some cases of obesity.

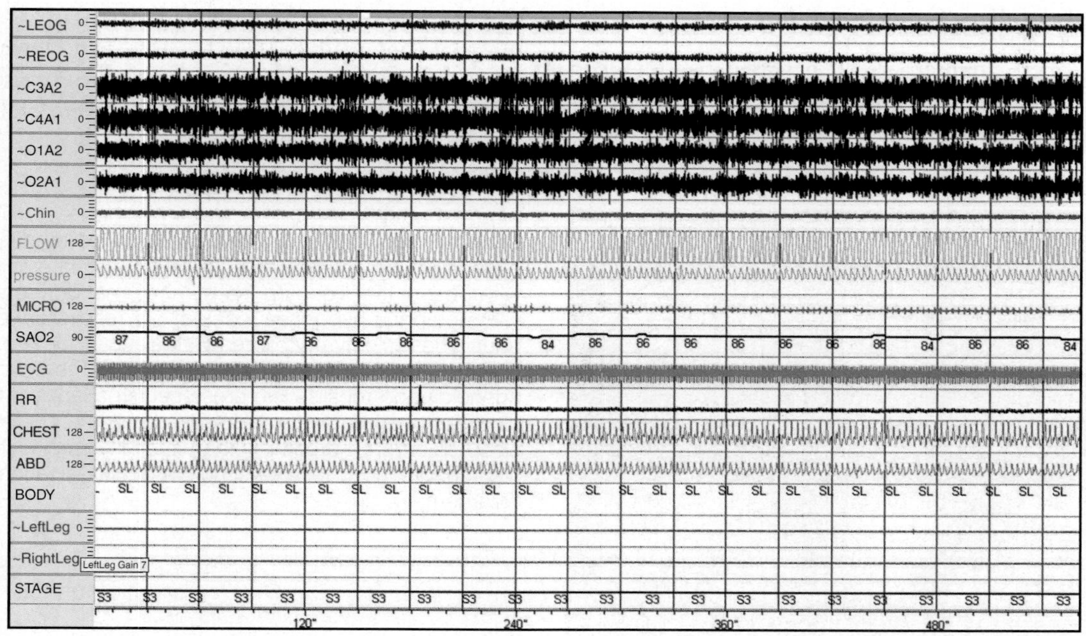

Figure 11.2-23.
Nonapneic hypoxemia. This 10-minute compressed epoch demonstrates oxygen saturations consistently in the mid-80s, despite excellent flow. This patient had chronic obstructive pulmonary disease with mild diurnal hypoxemia (see also Chapter 11.3).

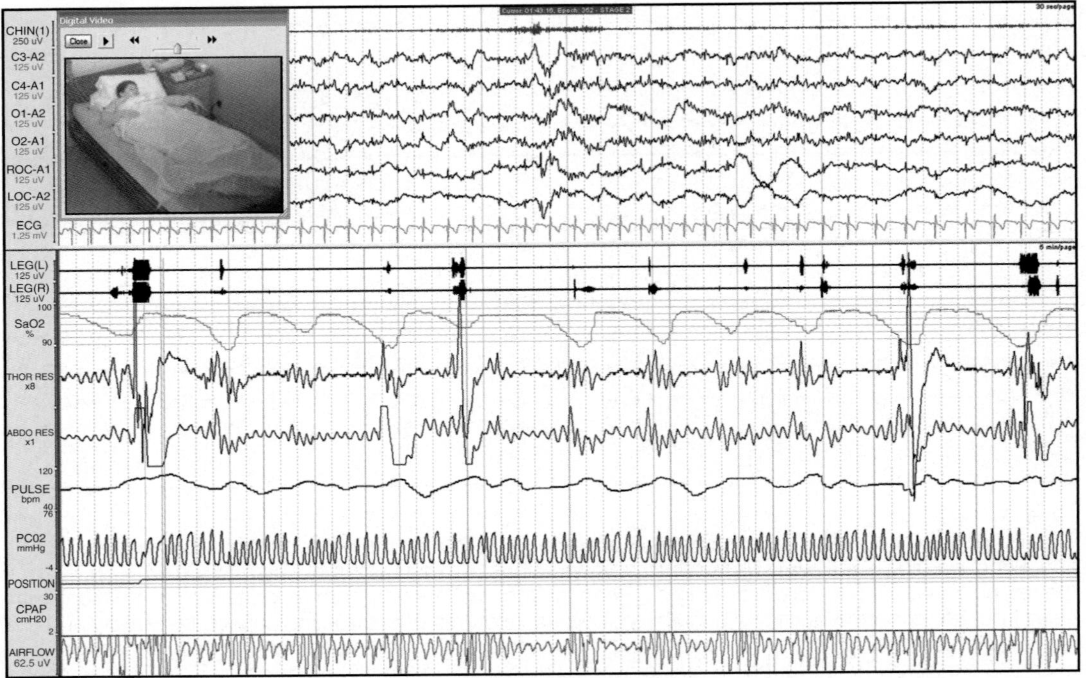

Figure 11.2-24.
Obstructive sleep apnea (OSA) in an obese child. This figure illustrates a 5-minute epoch of a 12-year-old who weighed 225 pounds and had tonsillar hypertrophy. At presentation, the patient complained of snoring and daytime hypersomnolence. His apnea-hypopnea index (AHI) was 42 respiratory events per hour with lowest measured oxygen saturation of 62%. Forgoing adenotonsillectomy for treatment, the patient underwent nasal continuous positive airway pressure titration with resolution of OSA. AHI scores are higher in obese compared with normal-weight children with OSA. Obese children are also less responsive to adenotonsillectomy as treatment for OSA, compared with normal-weight children.

Pediatric Sleep-disordered Breathing

Like adults, obese children are at increased risk for sleep apnea (Fig. 11.2-24). Other risk factors include tonsillar and adenoidal hypertrophy (Fig. 11.2-25), laryngomalacia (Fig. 11.2-26), pharyngolaryngomalacia (Fig. 11.2-27), craniofacial abnormalities (Fig. 11.2-28), and Down syndrome (Fig. 11.2-29). (See also chapter 11.1.) Neuromuscular disorders, such as spinal muscle atrophy and severe kyphoscoliosis,

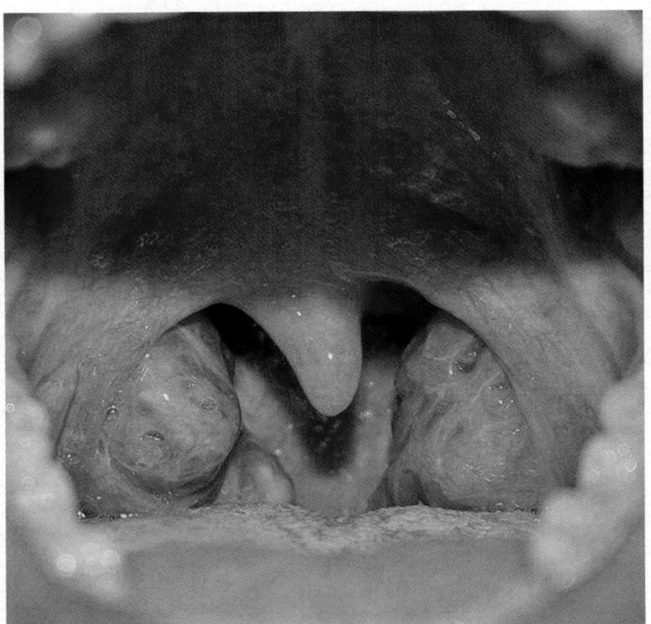

Figure 11.2-25.
Tonsillar hypertrophy. This image illustrates tonsillar hypertrophy in a 4-year-old child who was later diagnosed with obstructive sleep apnea by nocturnal polysomnogram with an apnea-hypopnea index of 6.5 respiratory events per hour. The majority of children with sleep-disordered breathing obstruct their upper airway at the level of the enlarged adenoids and tonsils. The cross-sectional area of the narrowest segment is significantly smaller in children with sleep-disordered breathing than it is in normal children. See also chapter 11.1 for a description of classification of tonsil enlargement.

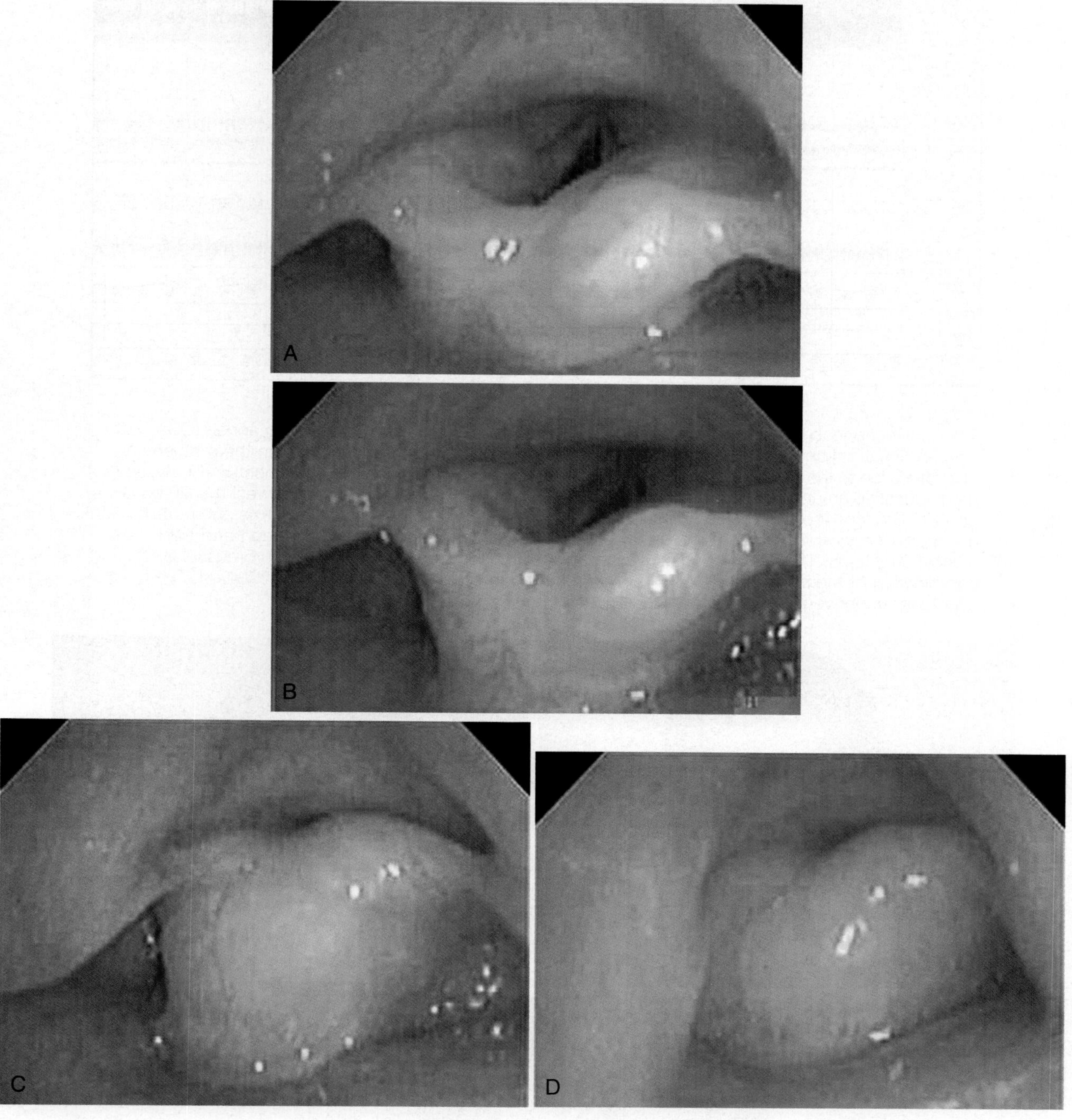

Figures 11.2-26.
Laryngomalacia in a child. These bronchoscopic images (A–D) demonstrate laryngomalacia at different points during inspiration, leading to airway closure in a 3-year-old. The child had persistent inspiratory stridor, snoring, gastroesophageal reflux, and suboptimal growth. The redundant tissue in the arytenoids region, which is more severe on the right, prolapses toward the glottic lumen. The patient was later diagnosed with obstructive sleep apnea (OSA) with an apnea-hypopnea index of 12 respiratory events per hour. The patient was referred to pediatric otolaryngology and underwent supraglottoplasty with resolution of OSA on repeat nocturnal polysomnogram after surgery.

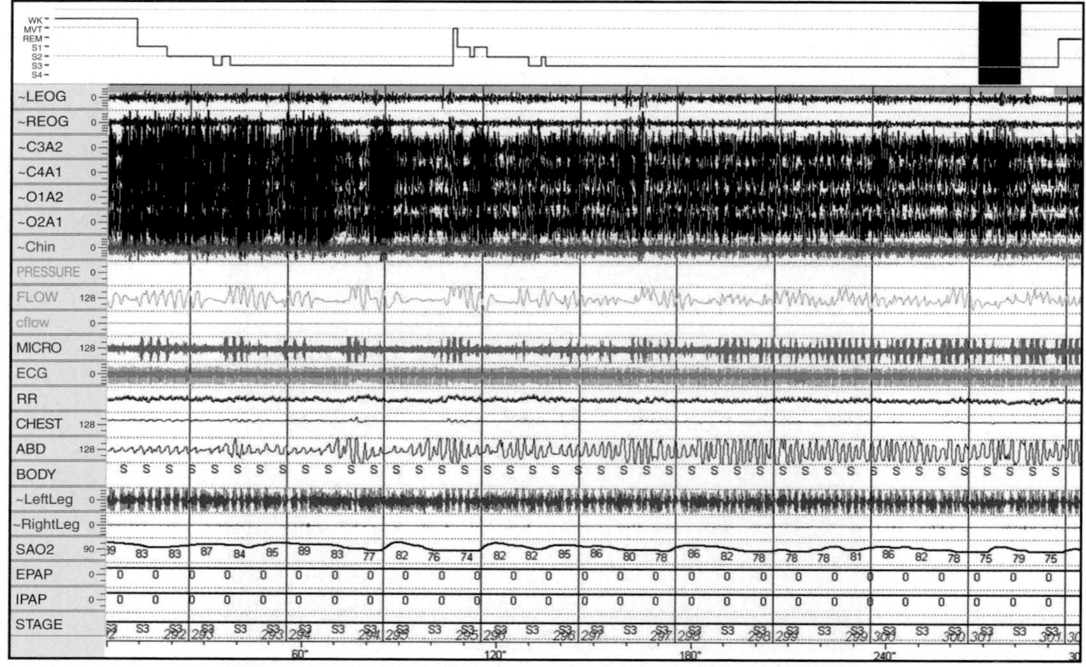

Figure 11.2-27.
Obstructive apneas in an underweight child. This graph illustrates obstructive sleep apnea (OSA) with oxygen desaturation in an 18-month-old child with delayed growth. On presentation the mother was frustrated due to the delay in referral for this long-standing problem since birth. The nocturnal polysomnogram identified an apnea-hypopnea index of 23.1 respiratory events per hour with lowest measured SaO_2 of 70%. Bronchoscopy revealed an infantile-shaped epiglottis that folds on its long axis and retracts with arytenoids having redundant mucosa that prolapsed over the laryngeal inlet with short and tight aryepiglottic folds. The final diagnosis was pharyngolaryngomalacia with loss of neuromuscular coordination of the entire pharynx and larynx, resulting in collapse of all structures involved. The child eventually underwent tracheostomy placement.

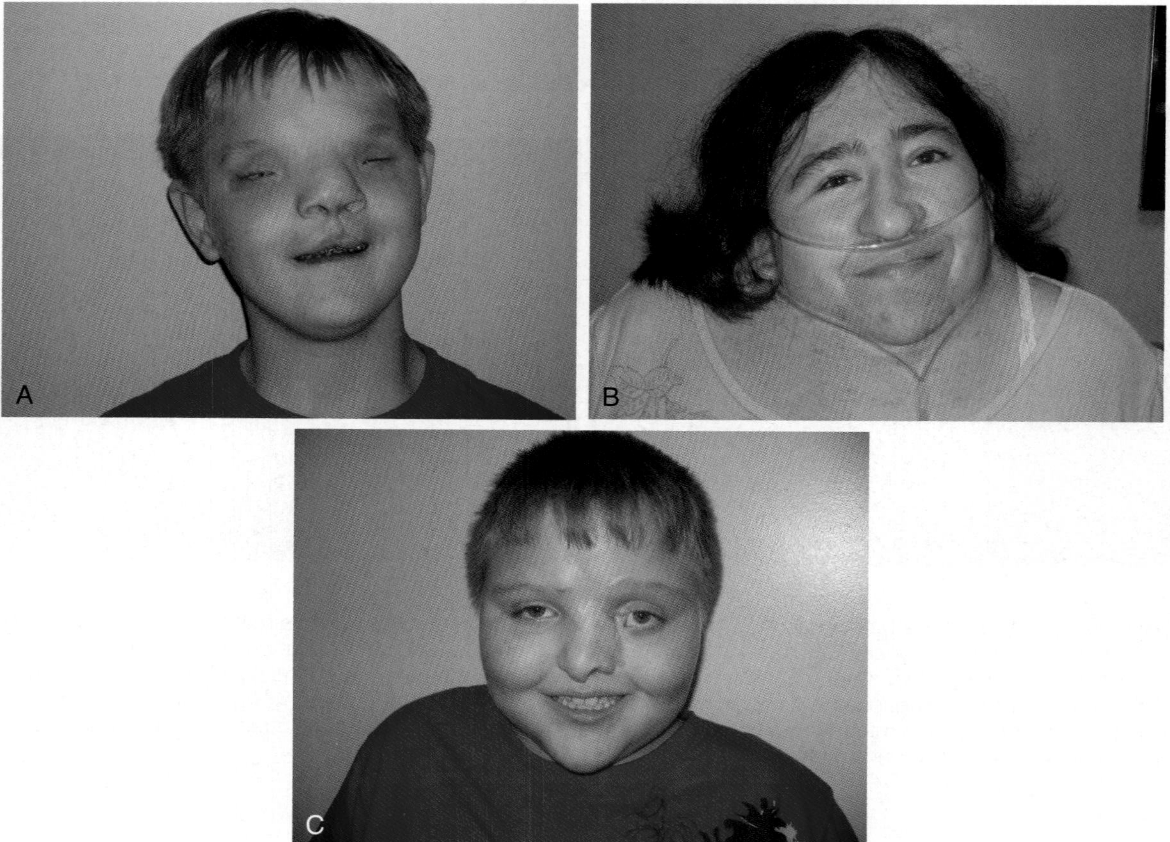

Figure 11.2-28.
See opposite page for legend.

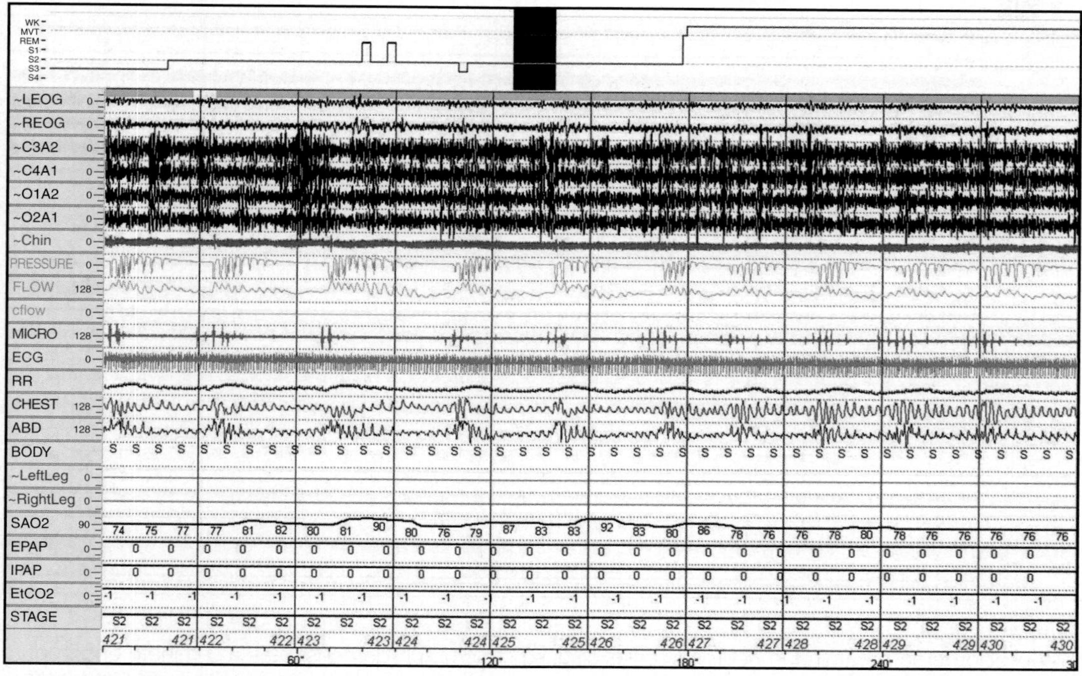

Figure 11.2-29.
Severe obstructive apnea in Down syndrome. This graph illustrates obstructive sleep apnea (OSA) in a 25-year-old male patient with Down syndrome who presented to the clinic with complaints of daytime hypersomnolence with snoring. Physical examination identified midface hypoplasia, macroglossia, and a body mass index of 32. The nocturnal polysomnogram identified an apnea-hypopnea index of 48.2 respiratory events per hour with lowest measured saturation of 65%. Facial dysmorphisms and upper airway abnormalities place patients with Down syndrome at risk for upper airway obstruction and OSA. The prevalence of sleep-disordered breathing in children with Down syndrome is very high. Obesity, adenoid hyperplasia, previous tonsillectomy or adenoidectomy, congenital heart disease, malocclusion, and macroglossia do not affect the prevalence. Nocturnal polysomnography should be a routine investigation for children with Down syndrome regardless of body habitus.

can also result in sleep-disordered breathing, particularly in children (Fig. 11.2-30). Prematurity is the most important risk factor for central apneas and periodic breathing in newborns (Figs. 11.2-31 and 11.2-32). In both children and adults, sleep apnea is not the only sleep disorder that may interfere with sleep or alertness (Fig. 11.2-33).

Figure 11.2-28.
A, This image is of a 16-year-old male patient with a history of multiple craniofacial anomalies due to an unidentifiable genetic disorder. To assess daytime hypersomnia and snoring, a nocturnal polysomnogram was performed. The polysomnogram identified mild obstructive sleep apnea with an apnea-hypopnea index of 7.5 respiratory events per hour. The family opted for nasal continuous positive airway pressure therapy with a custom-fitted nasal mask, which resulted in the resolution of his snoring and hypersomnia. **B** and **C**, These images are of relatives (aunt and nephew) with congenital craniofacial and musculoskeletal abnormalities of the head and neck and sleep-disordered breathing. This 26-year-old female (**B**) has Klippel-Feil syndrome (KFS) and severe scoliosis. (KFS is an autosomal dominant congenital disorder characterized by a defect in the formation or segmentation of the cervical vertebrae during the early weeks of fetal development, resulting in a fused appearance. The clinical triad for KFS consists of a short neck, low posterior hairline, and limited neck movement; less than 50% of patients demonstrate all three clinical features.) This 8-year-old male (**C**) has frontofacionasal dysostosis (FFND). (FFND is a congenital disorder that appears to be inherited as an autosomal recessive trait. Physical traits commonly seen include brachycephaly, cleft lip or palate, hypoplasia of the nose with malformation of the nostrils, narrowing of the palpebral fissures, blepharophimosis, ocular hypertelorism, coloboma, and lagophthalmos as well as other eye abnormalities.) This patient's complicated medical history also included surgical repair of tetralogy of Fallot and DiGeorge syndrome.

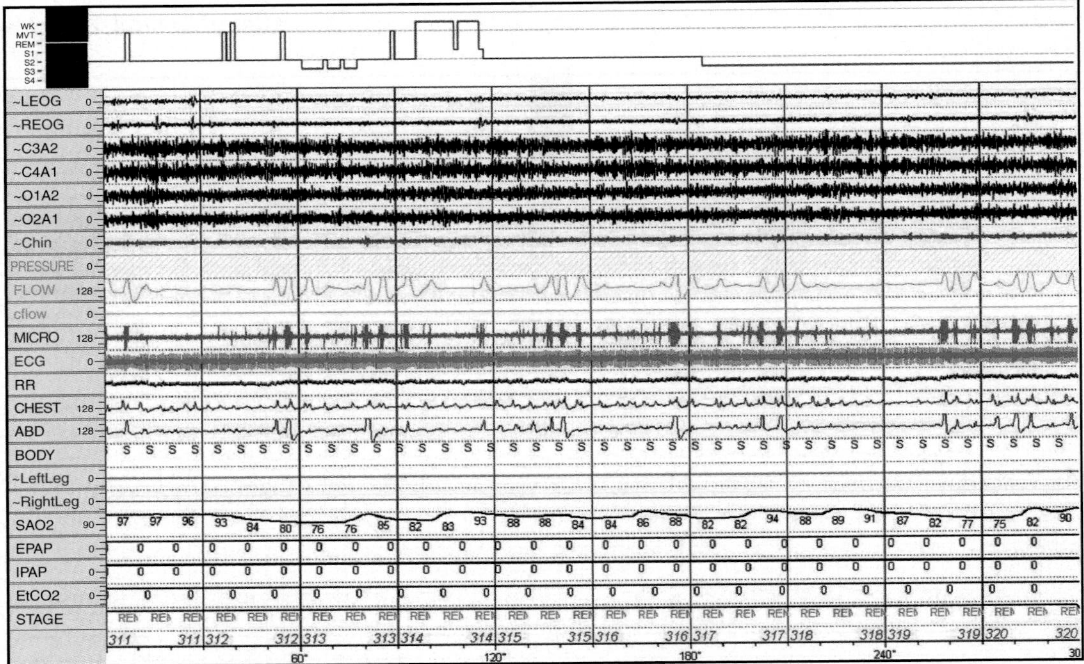

Figure 11.2-30.
Sleep-disordered breathing in neuromuscular disease. This graph demonstrates a 5-minute epoch of a 12-year-old female with type II spinal muscle atrophy and severe kyphoscoliosis. The family had been noncompliant, but eventually referred the child for a nocturnal polysomnogram. The apnea-hypopnea index was 30 events per hour of sleep with severe hypoxemia. This graph illustrates respiratory instability during REM sleep. The child underwent successful bilevel pressure titration. In children with spinal muscular atrophy, sleep-disordered breathing leads to relevant impairment of sleep and well-being. Improvement in both sleep and well-being is possible with nocturnal noninvasive ventilation.

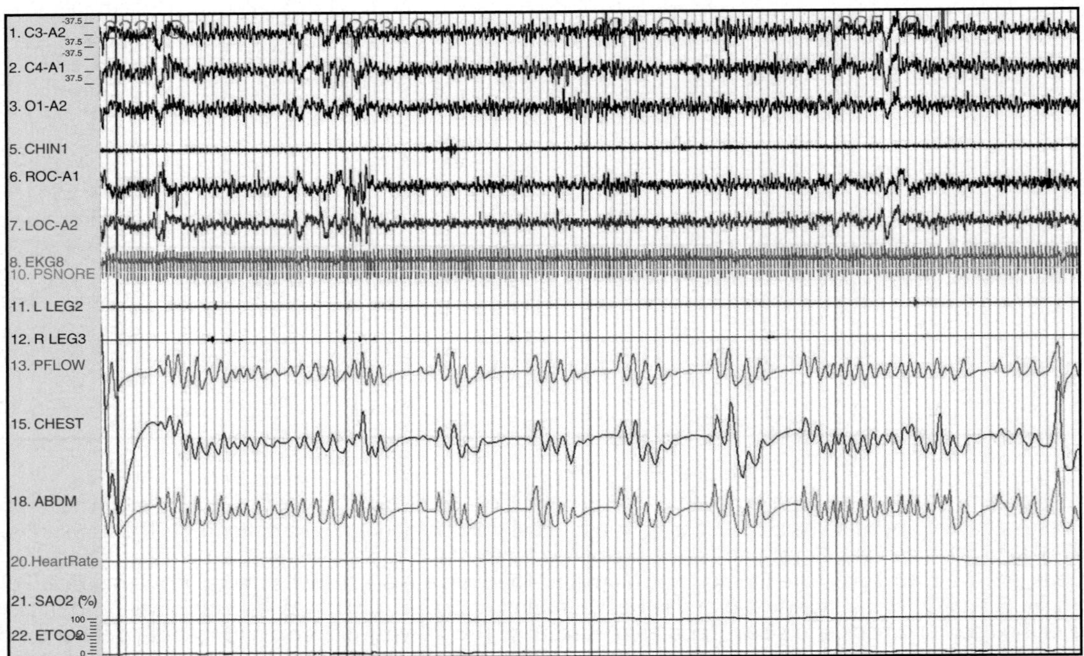

Figure 11.2-31.
Central apneas in an infant. The graph shown here illustrates central apneas during quiet sleep in a 4-month-old female infant who was born at 31 weeks gestation due to maternal preeclampsia. The infant had very mild bronchopulmonary dysplasia (BPD), requiring supplemental oxygen for the first month of life. Prematurely born infants with and without BPD sleep more efficiently in the prone position; however, central apneas are more prevalent while prone, thus emphasizing the importance of supine sleeping after neonatal unit discharge.

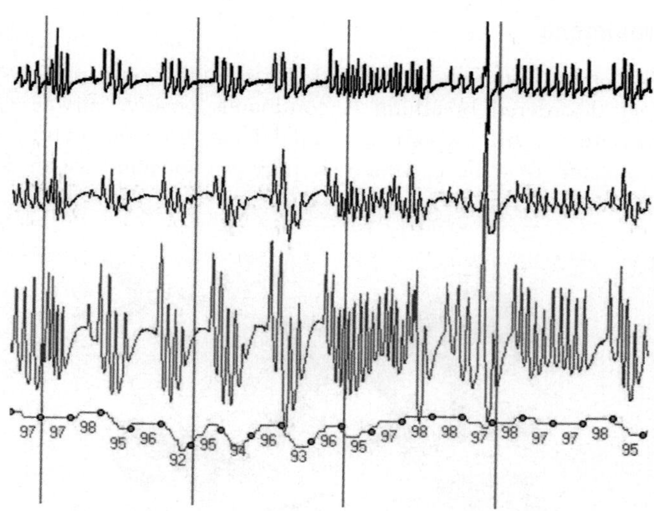

Figure 11.2-32.
Periodic respirations in an infant. This figure demonstrates periodic respirations with mild desaturations to 92% in a 2-month-old male infant, born 6 weeks premature, who presented for evaluation after an acute life-threatening event. Magnetic resonance imaging (MRI) of the brain was normal, without evidence of an abnormality or signs of an Arnold-Chiari malformation. The child was placed on apnea-bradycardia monitoring as a protective measure. Over the next 4 months the apneas slowly resolved while the child continued to grow normally.

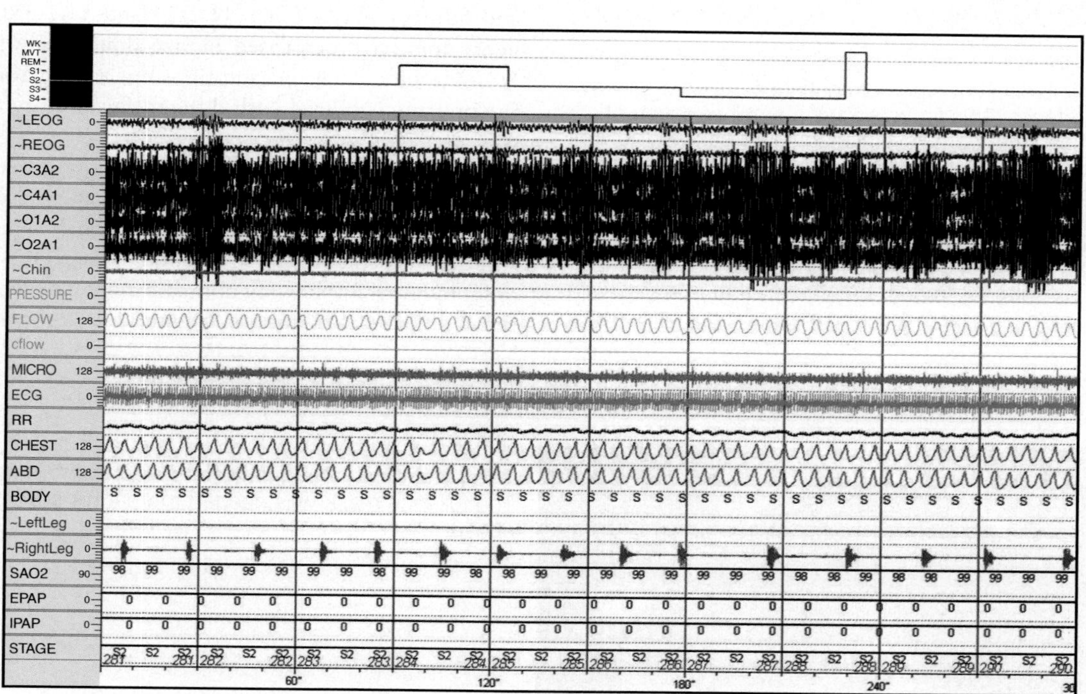

Figure 11.2-33.
Periodic limb movements in a child. A 10-year-old male child presented with concerns of sleep-disordered breathing based on a history of attention deficit hyperactivity disorder with aggressive behavior related to nonrestorative sleep. The parents reported no history of snoring or of witnessed apneas during sleep. Further history elicited long-standing growing pains that were more prevalent in the right leg and sporadic sleep-maintenance insomnia, along with the nonrestorative sleep. The patient occasionally had a morning headache. Family history identified two grandparents who may have had restless legs syndrome (RLS). A nocturnal polysomnogram does not identify sleep-disordered breathing but reveals periodic limb movements, primarily involving the right leg, as illustrated here. With a diagnosis of RLS and periodic limb movements disorder, laboratory analysis identified an iron deficiency anemia with a ferritin level of 5 ng/mL, so ferrous sulfate therapy was started. Follow-up 3 months later revealed resolution of growing pains along with more consolidated sleep. Further follow-up 6 months later revealed correction of anemia with a ferritin level of 50 ng/mL. Some children who are diagnosed with growing pains meet the diagnostic criteria for RLS. A positive family history is common for these children.

Treatment

The most commonly prescribed treatment for obstructive sleep-disordered breathing is continuous positive airway pressure (CPAP), which is created by a flow generator connected to a hose, which in turn is connected to an interface. There are many different CPAP masks, but they all fall under three general types: nasal masks, nasal pillows, and full-face masks (Figs. 11.2-34 and 11.2-35). The flow generators have decreased in size dramatically (Fig. 11.2-36). Machines may be autotitrating, and in some devices the pressure is bilevel with different inspiratory and expiratory pressures.

CPAP can be "titrated" in the sleep laboratory to determine the setting required to eliminate respiratory events. Figure 11.2-37 is a compressed, 20-minute epoch which demonstrates an acceptable CPAP titration. Figure 11.2-38 is an all-night hypnogram showing normalization of oxygenation over the night of a CPAP titration. Figure 11.2-39 shows the results

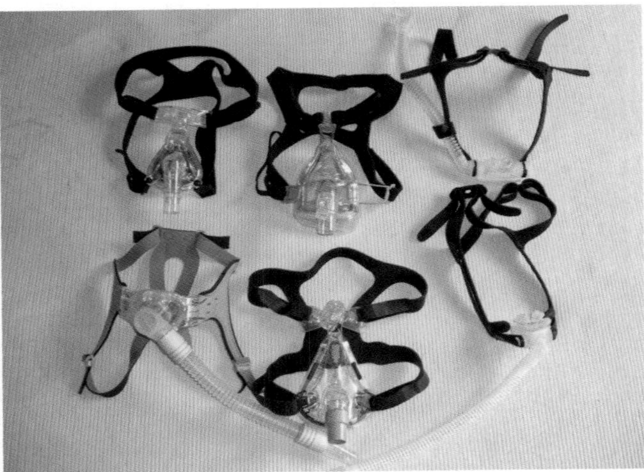

Figure 11.2-34.
There are many different types of continuous positive airway pressure interfaces. This figure shows a small selection of masks and headgear from several manufacturers. On the right are two nasal pillow-type masks, in the middle two full-face masks, and on the left two nasal masks. The bottom nasal mask is designed for a child. In the nasal pillow mask, prongs are inserted into the nostrils to deliver the positive airway pressure. The full-face mask fits over both the nose and the mouth and is useful for "mouth breathers," that is, those with nasal obstruction, and for those who have had palatal surgery.

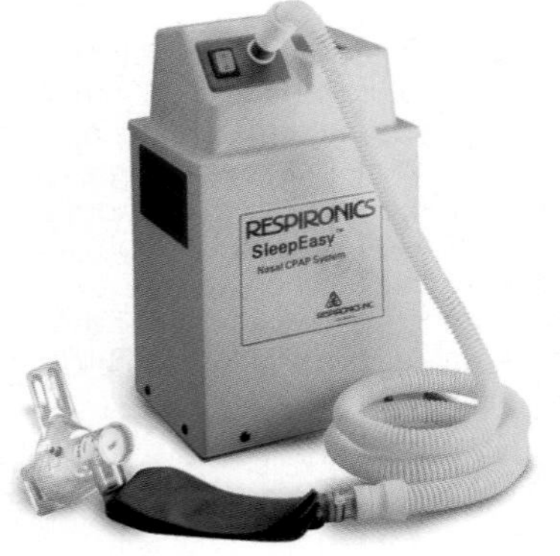

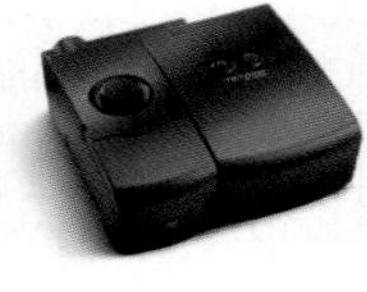

Figure 11.2-36.
Commercially available continuous positive airway pressure machines have decreased in size dramatically since their introduction in the mid-1980s. (Images courtesy Respironics Inc.)

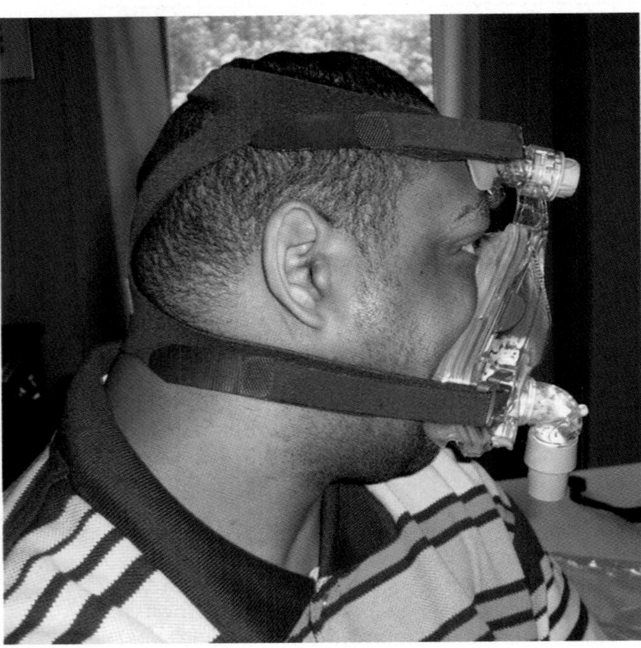

Figure 11.2-35.
This patient had retrognathia and slept with his mouth open. The full-face mask was needed to treat his severe sleep apnea.

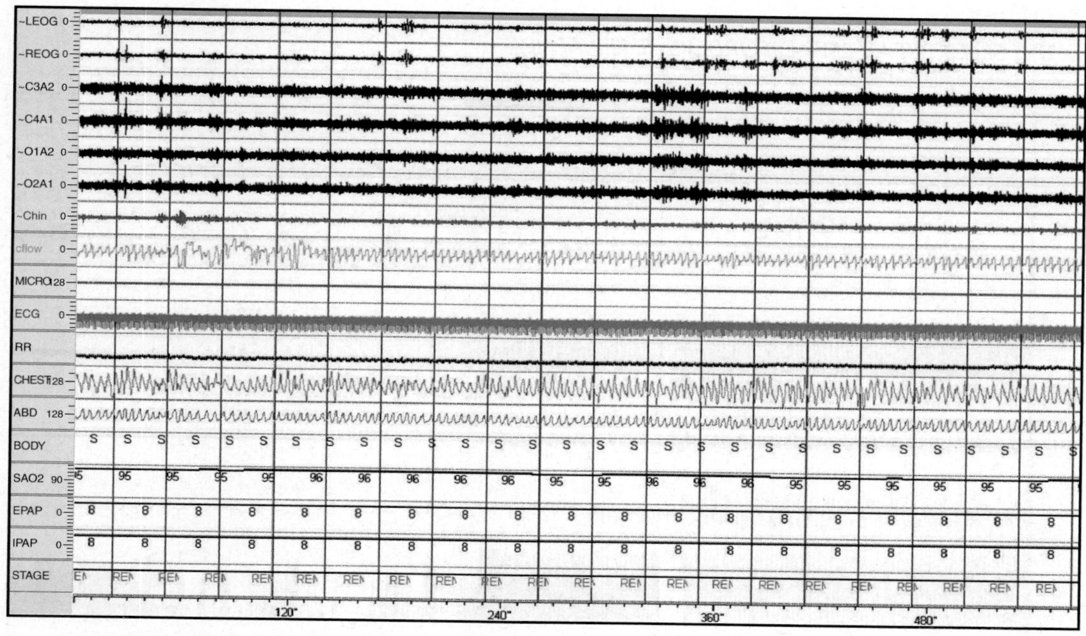

Figure 11.2-37.
Adequate continuous positive airway pressure (CPAP) titration. This 10-minute compressed epoch demonstrates a positive outcome of CPAP titration. The patient is in REM sleep (indicated by the stage scoring at the bottom of the montage, and also by the eye jerks in the electro-oculogram and low chin tone). The patient is also supine (indicated by the "S" in the "body" channel). The flow channel is stable, as is saturation (at 95% to 96%), and the microphone ("micro") is silent. This patient should do well on 8 cm H_2O CPAP.

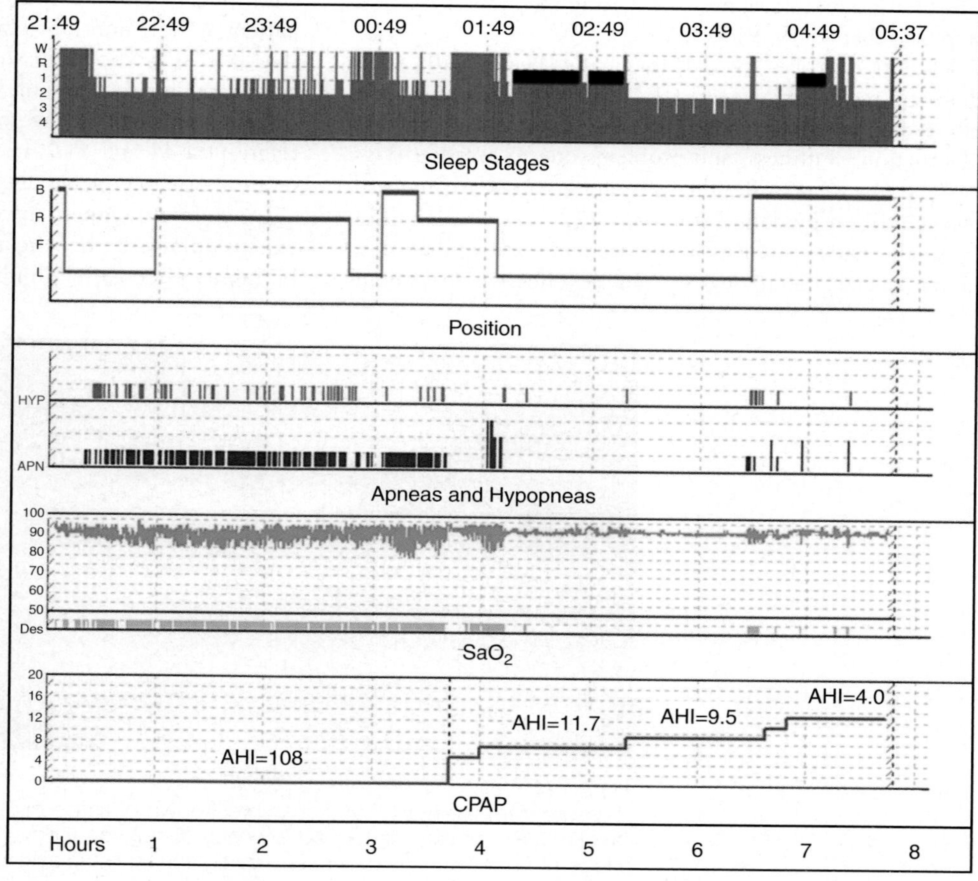

Figure 11.2-38.
Adequate continuous positive airway pressure (CPAP) titration. This all-night hypnogram consists of (from top to bottom) sleep stages, position, presence of apneas and hypopneas, SaO_2 desaturations, and CPAP pressure over almost 8 hours of a split-night study. Notice that before CPAP sleep is unstable, there is no REM, and there are many apneas and hypopneas with large oscillations in SaO_2. On the final CPAP pressure the apnea-hypopnea index is normal and the patient has REM sleep.

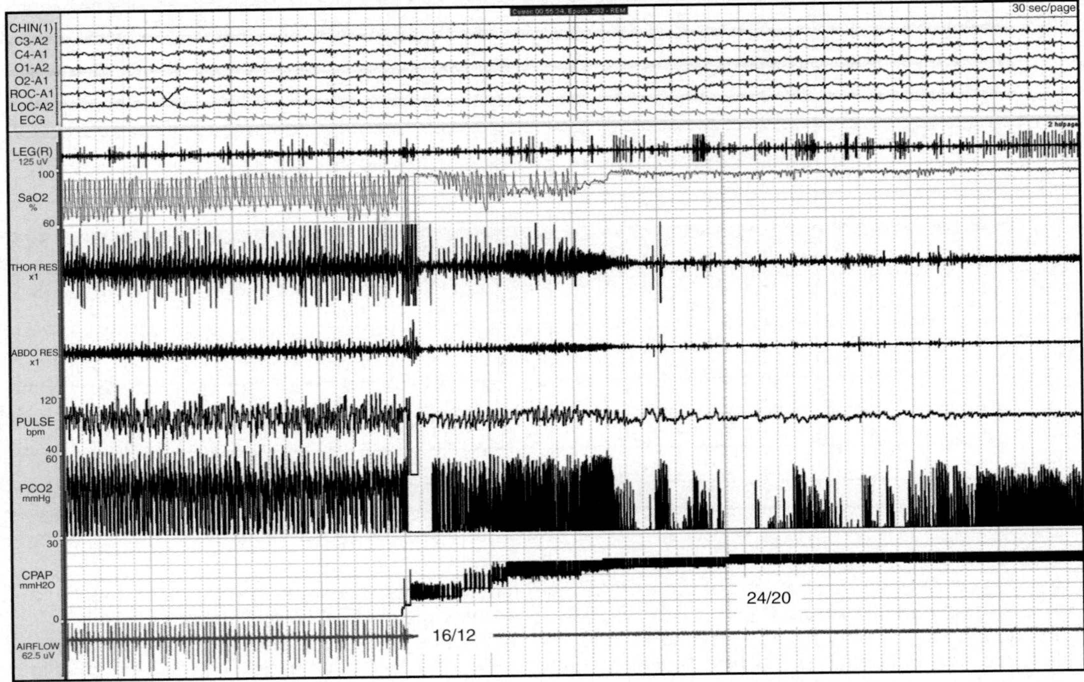

Figure 11.2-39.
The top window shows 30 seconds of data and the bottom 2 hours of data. The band in the CPAP channel represents the pressure swings with bilevel pressure. The patient was initially tried on 16 inspiratory pressure (cm H_2O) and 12 expiratory pressure and the pressures were increased in steps to 24/20. This corrected the very severe cyclic hypoxemia.

of a titration on bilevel pressure. Fitting the mask is a critical step (see chapter 19, Video 8).

Patients can be treated for many years, with often dramatic results. However, CPAP may result in unwanted effect. Patients may develop nasal symptoms such as nasal obstruction, stuffiness, and problems due to pressure (Figs. 11.2-40 to 11.2-42). Residual sleepiness can be treated with modafinil or armodafinil (see page 77).

An alternative to CPAP is the use of an oral appliance, or dental device. Such devices can be effective in patients with mild to moderate obstructive apnea, especially if the patient is not morbidly obese. Patients with retrognathia (Fig. 11.2-43) who sleep with their mouths open are good candidates for such treatment. The most widely used type of oral appliance is the mandibular advancement device (Figs. 11.2-44 and 11.2-45). There are dozens of different models available, generally through a dentist.

In children, upper airway surgery or rapid maxillary expansion may be beneficial (Fig. 11.2-46). CPAP can also be highly effective in children (Fig. 11.2-47).

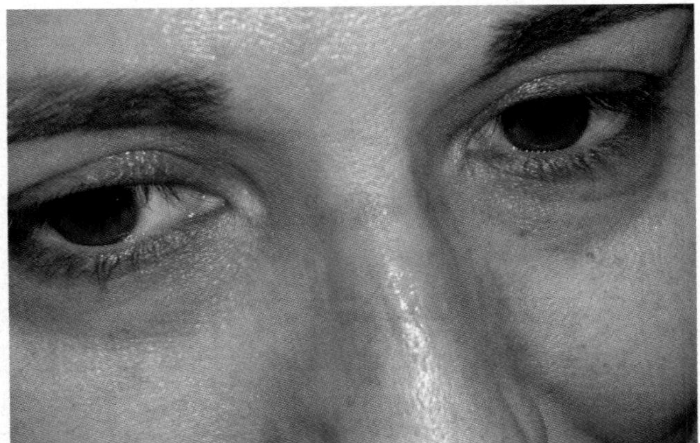

Figure 11.2-40.
Pressure from the mask can cause breakdown of tissue or infection. This patient developed a weepy pustule on the bridge of her nose. She had been overtightening her mask. Switching masks and education solved her problem.

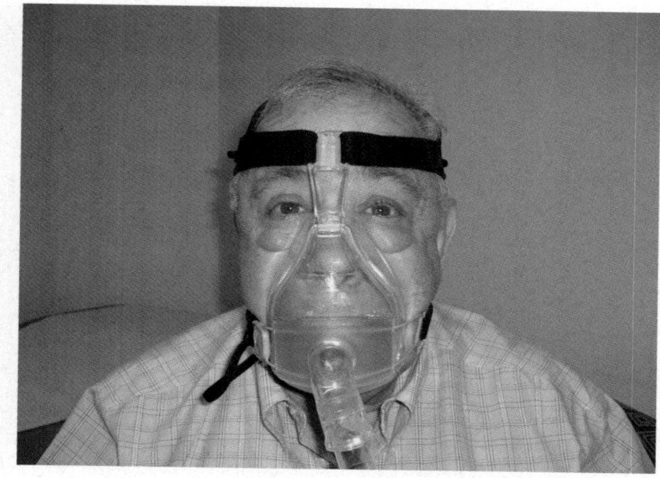

Figure 11.2-41.
This patient wore a full-face mask for several years. He was doing well on continuous positive airway pressure but developed "waterbags" under his eyes.

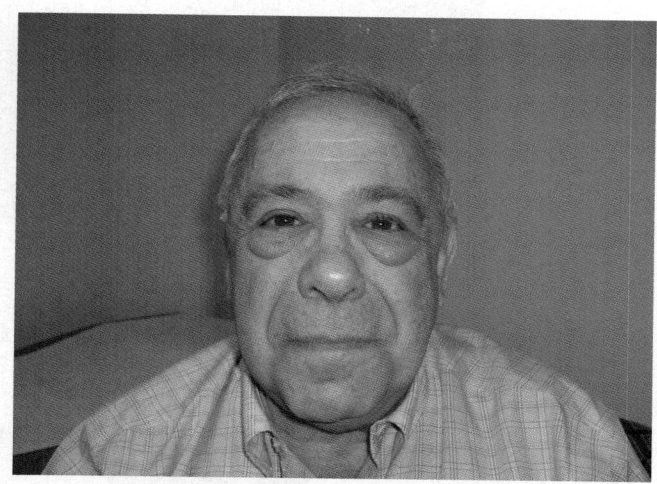

Figure 11.2-42.
Although this patient tried several interfaces, only the mask shown in Figure 11.2-41 was effective, and he elected to continue to use it. The "waterbags" under his eyes did not result in symptoms.

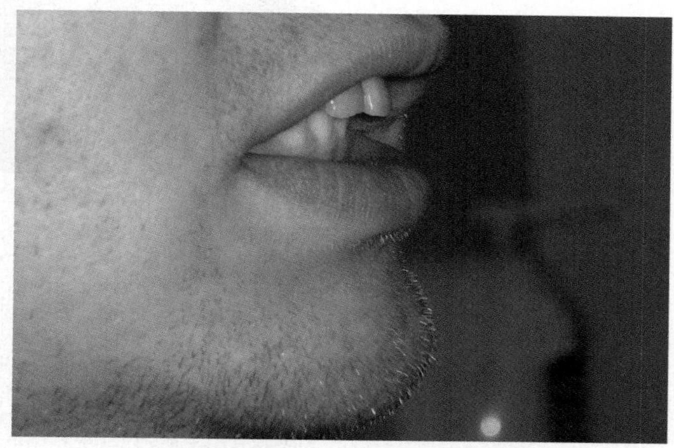

Figure 11.2-43.
A good candidate for an oral appliance is the patient with retrognathia. Note that in this patient, although the mandible is retrognathic as evidenced by the overjet, the lower jaw appears normal because of a pad of soft tissue on the chin. In fitting for an oral appliance, an impression of the maxilla and the mandible and a specific bite is taken with the mandible advanced to or beyond normal occlusion. When in place, oral devices then advance the lower jaw, which opens the posterior airway.

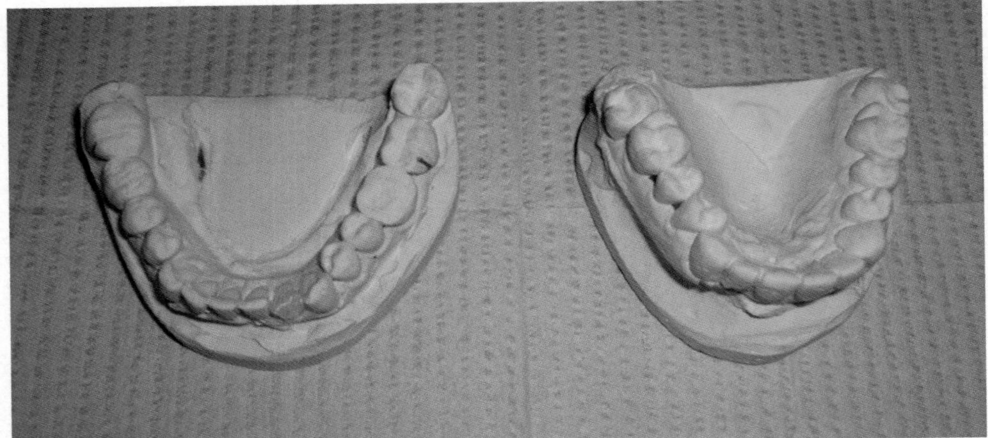

Figure 11.2-44.
A mandibular advancement device is custom-fabricated for each patient. The first step after determining that there are a sufficient number of teeth of adequate integrity and strength is to obtain separate impressions of the upper *(right)* and lower *(left)* teeth that will anchor the device. Note that the impression shows a narrow upper arch and a high arched palate.

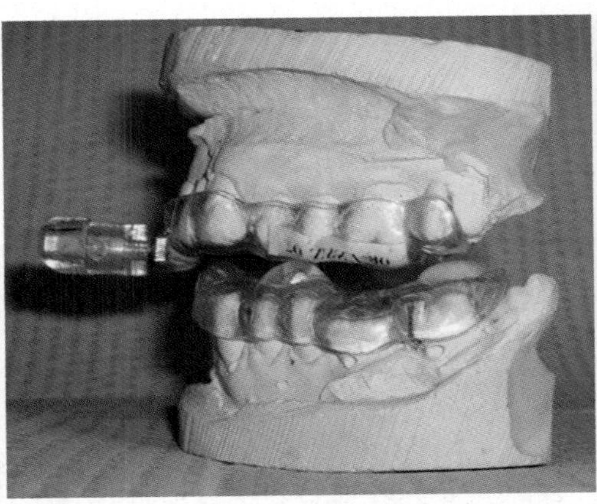

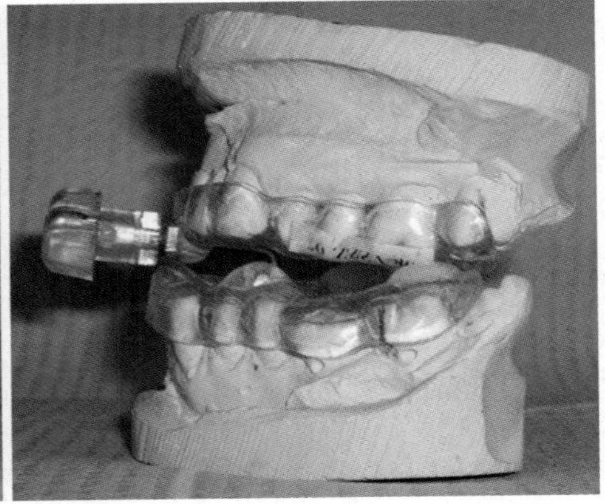

Figure 11.2-45.
These images show a mandibular advancement device on the dental impressions shown in Figure 11.2-44. The left image shows the natural position of the mandible, which is retrognathic. The right shows the anterior position of the mandible after the appliance has been adjusted. There has been substantial forward movement of the mandible.

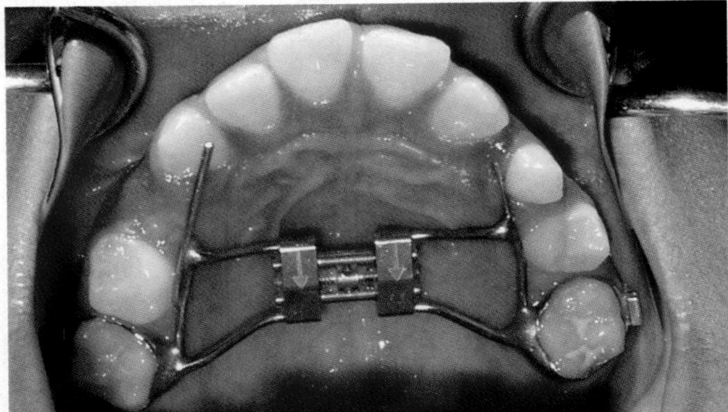

Figure 11.2-46.
Rapid maxillary expansion. This image illustrates a rapid maxillary palate expander in a 12-year-old child with a body mass index of 75% predicted. The young girl, who had a history of snoring and restless sleep, was referred to an orthodontist for dental occlusion at the same time she was referred for a nocturnal polysomnogram (NPSG). The NPSG identified obstructive sleep apnea syndrome with an apnea-hypopnea index (AHI) of 5.8 respiratory events per hour. The rapid maxillary expansion was placed, and a repeat NPSG 6 months after completion of maxillary expansion revealed an AHI of 0.6 respiratory events per hour.

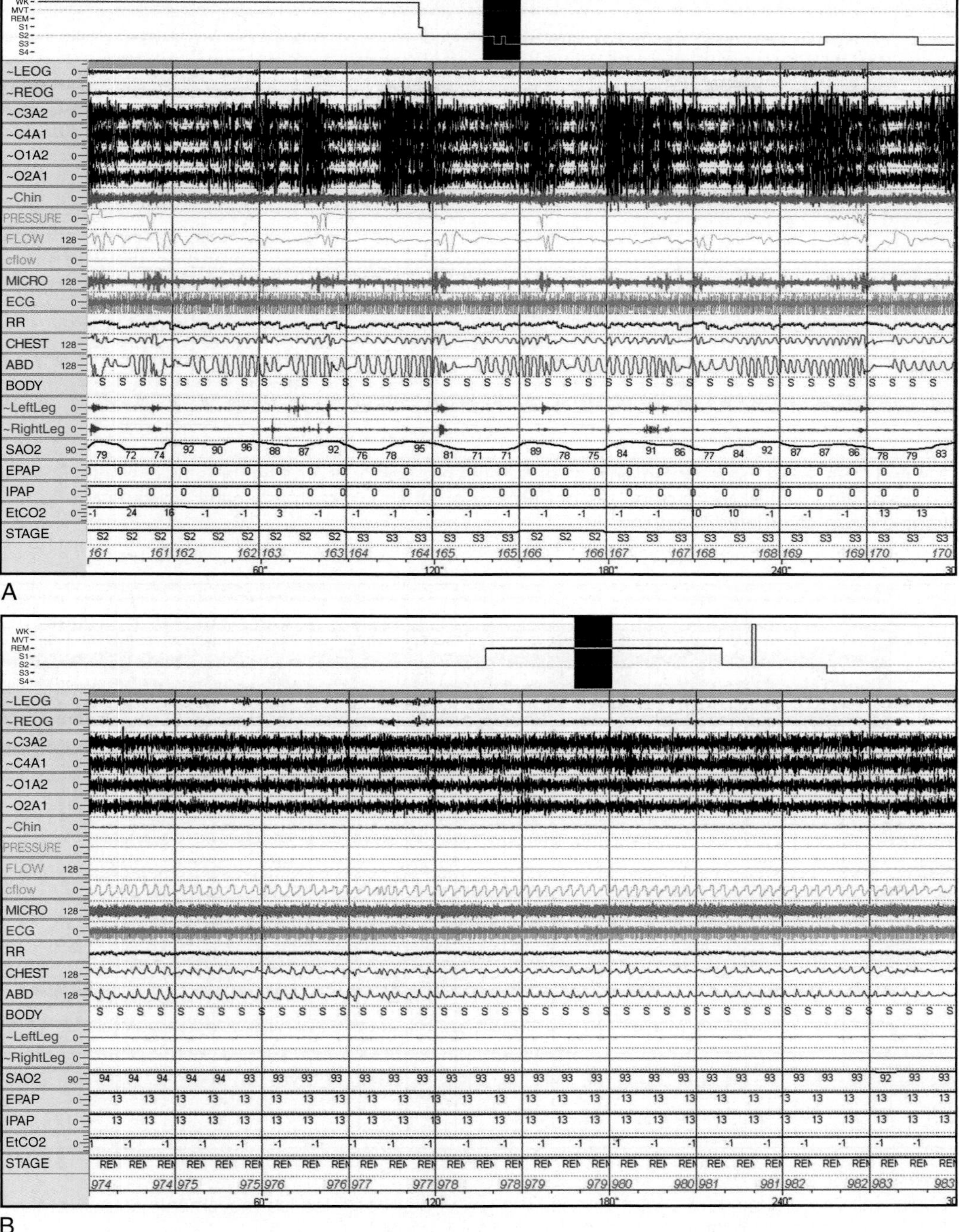

Figure 11.2-47.
Continuous positive airway pressure (CPAP) titration in a child. The two images illustrate epochs of a nocturnal polysomnogram (NPSG) in a 7-year-old child who weighed 152 pounds and had undergone adenotonsillectomy 3 years prior. **A,** The initial NPSG identified obstructive sleep apnea with an apnea-hypopnea index of 24 respiratory events per hour with lowest measured saturation of 71%. **B,** The patient underwent a CPAP titration with resolution of respiratory events occurring best at a CPAP pressure of 9 cm H_2O.

Leg Movement Artifacts

Sleep-disordered breathing has been demonstrated to be associated with periodic limb movements (PLMs). Often, the leg jerks are part of the arousal response to the sleep-disordered breathing event. Such leg jerks should not be scored in as PLMs, as they are simply electrophysiologic epiphenomena in this scenario. Figures 11.2-48 and 11.2-49 demonstrate this phenomenon in obstructive and central sleep apnea, respectively.

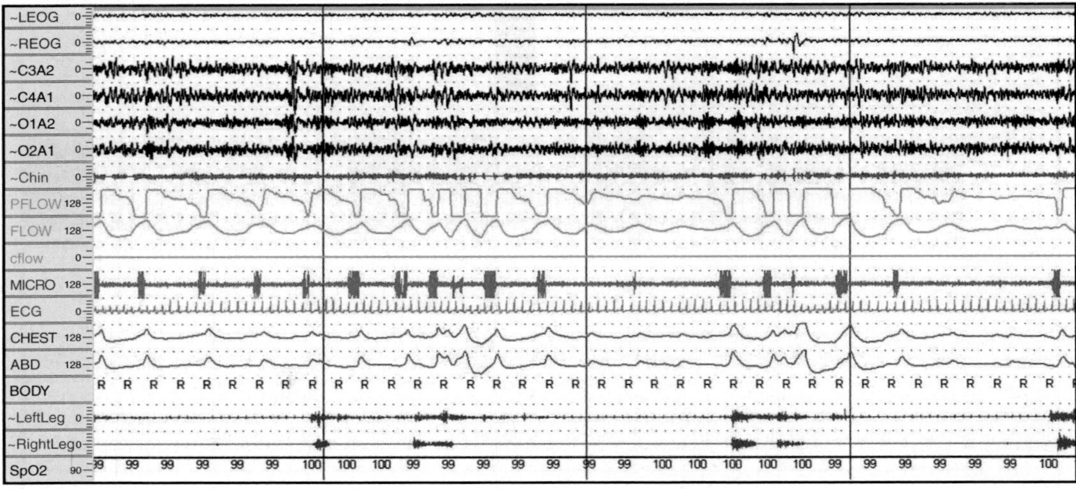

Figure 11.2-48.
PLMs and OSA. Here there are leg jerks as part of the arousal for obstructed breathing events. OSA has been associated with PLMs; a diagnosis of PLMs disorder should be made cautiously in those with untreated sleep-disordered breathing.

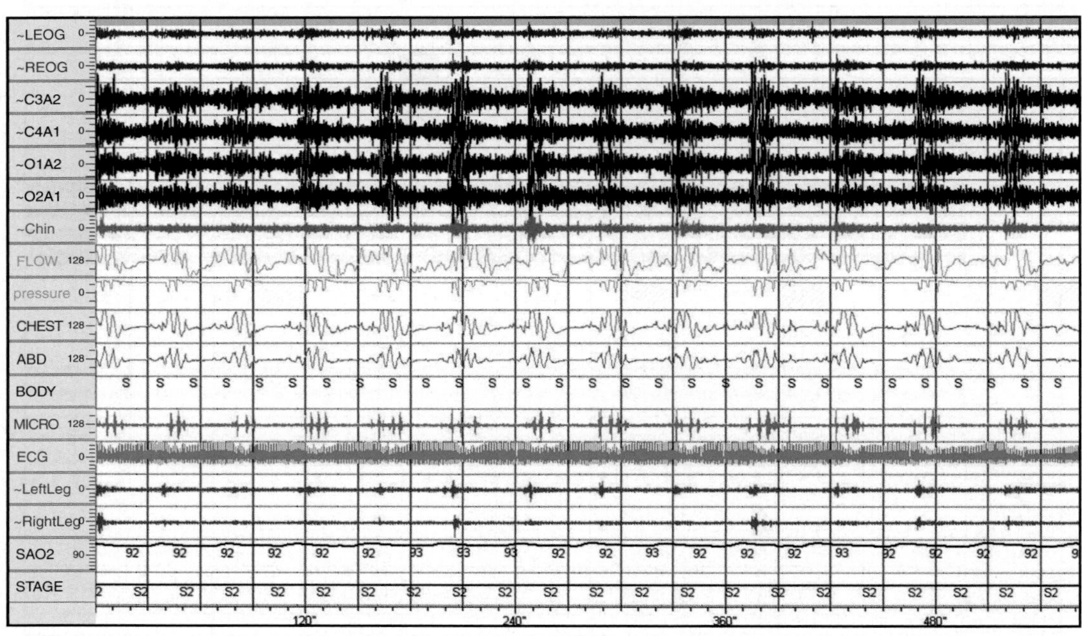

Figure 11.2-49.
Periodic limb movements and central apnea. The graph demonstrates leg movements as part of the arousal response to respiratory events that are primarily central.

SELECTED READINGS

Fitzgerald DA, Paul A, Richmond C: Severity of obstructive apnoea in children with Down syndrome who snore. Arch Dis Child 92(5):423–425, 2007.

Guilleminault C, Stoohs R, Clerk A, et al: A cause of excessive daytime sleepiness. Chest 104:781–787, 1993.

Iber C, Ancoli-Israel S, Chesson A, Quan SF: The AASM Manual for the Scoring of Sleep and Associated Events: Rules, Terminology and Technical Specifications. Westchester, Ill, American Academy of Sleep Medicine, 2007.

International Classification of Sleep Disorders, 2nd ed. Diagnostic and Coding Manual. Westchester, Ill, American Academy of Sleep Medicine, 2005.

Kushida CA, Morgenthaler TI, Littner MR, et al: Practice parameters for the treatment of snoring and obstructive sleep apnea with oral appliances: An update for 2005. Sleep 29(2):240–243, 2006.

Mitchell RB, Kelly J: Outcome of adenotonsillectomy for obstructive sleep apnea in obese and normal-weight children. Otolaryngol Head Neck Surg 137(1):43–48, 2007.

Mulgrew AT, Fox N, Ayas NT, Ryan CF: Diagnosis and initial management of obstructive sleep apnea without polysomnography: A randomized validation study. Ann Intern Med 146:157–166, 2007.

Tishler PV, Larkin EK, Schluchter MD, Redline S: Incidence of sleep-disordered breathing in an urban adult population. JAMA 289:2230–2237, 2003.

Young T, Peppard PE, Gottlieb DJ: Epidemiology of obstructive sleep apnea: A population health perspective. Am J Respir Crit Care Med 165:1217–1239, 2002.

Meir Kryger

Respiratory Diseases and the Overlap Syndromes 11.3

The term *overlap syndrome* was originally introduced to categorize those patients who had sleep apnea and chronic obstructive pulmonary disease (COPD). The notion is that such patients would demonstrate the clinical and laboratory features of their underlying respiratory disease and those of their sleep breathing disorder. In reality, in the sleep clinic one encounters patients who have features of several respiratory diseases and sleep disorders, not just COPD. Here we consider the respiratory overlap syndromes.

Obstructive Pulmonary Diseases

The common element in obstructive pulmonary diseases is that they all result in obstruction to airflow because they all affect the lungs and the airways in the lungs. These diseases include COPD, asthma, and cystic fibrosis. Although patients with asthma and cystic fibrosis frequently have nocturnal wheezing and/or cough, they are seldom referred to a sleep disorders center by their primary care physicians.

BOX 11.3-1. ABNORMAL SLEEP PHYSIOLOGY IN COPD

• Increased airway resistance	→	Dyspnea
• Pooling of secretions	→	Cough
• Accessory muscle atonia in REM sleep	→	Hypoxemia
• Ventilation/perfusion mismatch in lung	→	Hypoxemia
• Decreased ventilatory drive	→	Hypoxemia

BOX 11.3-2. SLEEP DISTURBANCE IN COPD

- More than 50% of patients have difficulty initiating and maintaining sleep
- Reduced sleep efficiency
- Increased awakenings, sometimes to smoke
- Multiple arousals and stage changes
- Daytime fatigue, frequent naps

COPD can be considered a spectrum of disorders ranging from chronic bronchitis, which can include the pathophysiologic abnormalities of lower airway inflammation and bronchial muscle constriction, to emphysema in which there is destruction of lung tissue. Many COPD patients have elements of both. The likeliest cause in most cases is cigarette smoking (Box 11.3-1).

Patients with COPD often have unstable sleep due to production of secretions, coughing, and dyspnea related to constriction of airways (see videos in chapter 20). Sleep is often fragmented in patients with severe findings. In COPD without sleep apnea, significant hypoxemia occurs, primarily during REM sleep due to hypoventilation most likely caused by the loss of muscle tone of the accessory muscles of respiration (Box 11.3-2).

In the typical sleep disorders clinic, one is less likely to encounter a patient with COPD and sleep disruption only related to COPD. More commonly encountered are referred patients with the overlap syndrome. In this syndrome there is the combination of sleep-disordered breathing and the findings related to COPD.

Although a formal designation does not exist for these overlap patients we recommend using a designation that describes their sleep breathing abnormality and their pulmonary disease, followed by an indication of whether the sleep breathing disorder is present throughout sleep or primarily in REM sleep. Furthermore, such cases can be further designated to indicate if hypoventilation and/or right heart failure is present. Following are examples of such patient groups.

The nonobese patient with COPD may present only with the typical sleep findings of COPD, mainly oxygen desaturation during REM sleep, which is believed to be related to REM atonia affecting the respiratory muscles (Fig. 11.3-1). There may be additional hypoxemia when snoring (without apnea) is present. Snoring that is causing the hypoxemia may respond to continuous positive airway pressure. In our experience, COPD patients frequently have a movement disorder (Figs. 11.3-2 to 11.3-4).

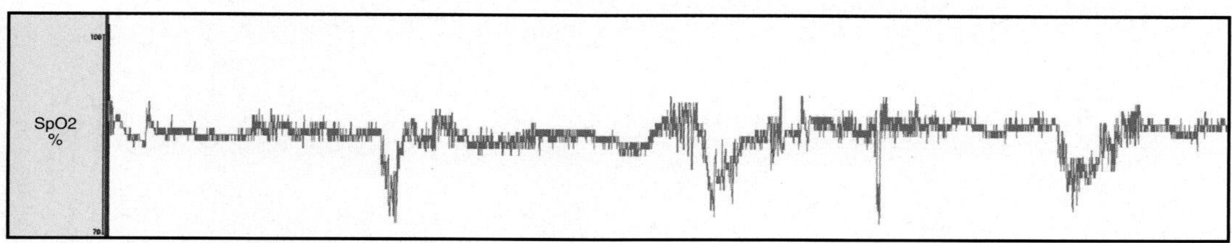

Figure 11.3-1.
This all-night oximetry trace shows three prolonged episodes of desaturations in a typical patient with COPD. The desaturations occurred in REM sleep.

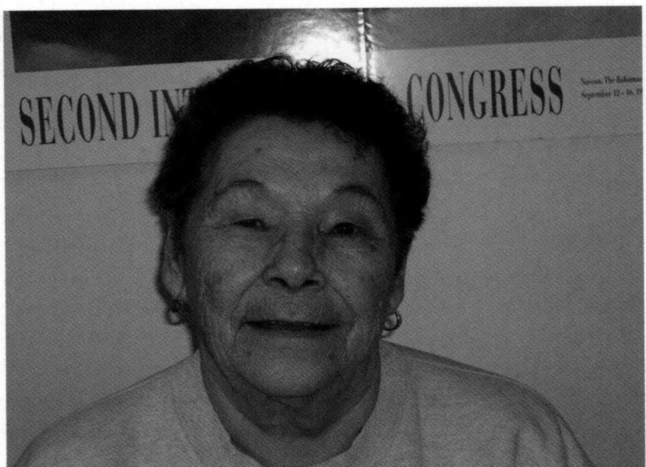

Figure 11.3-2.
This patient has severe COPD (note the smoking-induced wrinkles in her face). Fragments of her PSGs are in Figures 11.3-3 and 11.3-4.

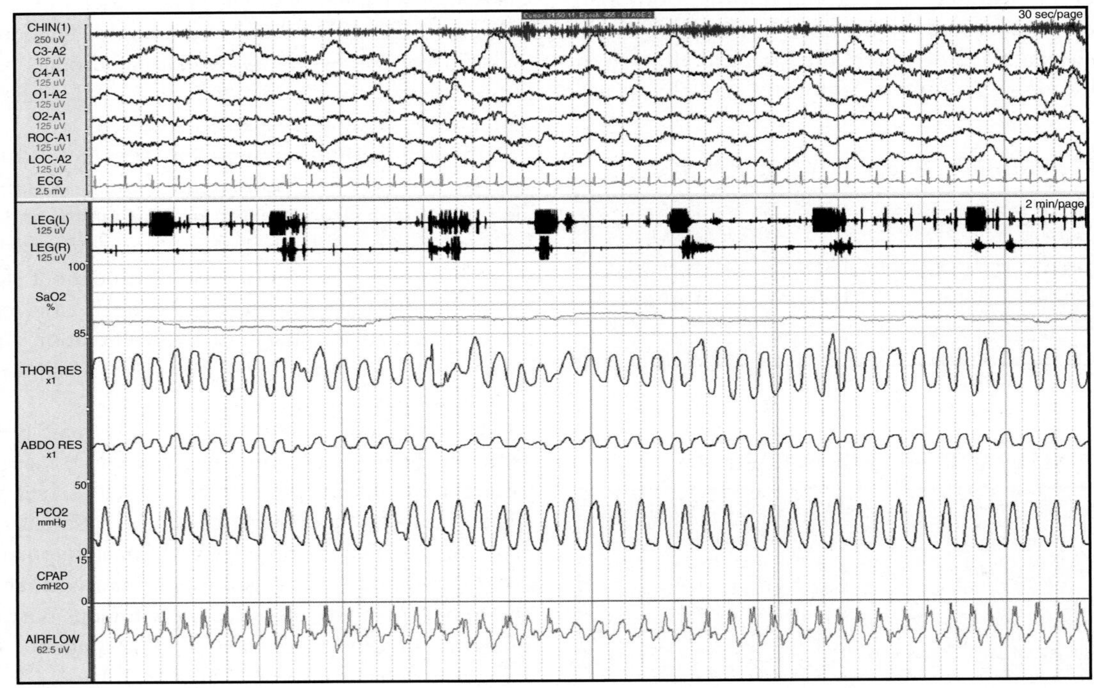

Figure 11.3-3.
At baseline there is hypoxemia and evidence of a significant movement disorder. This patient is noted to snore. (Note the respiratory artifact caused by lead A2.)

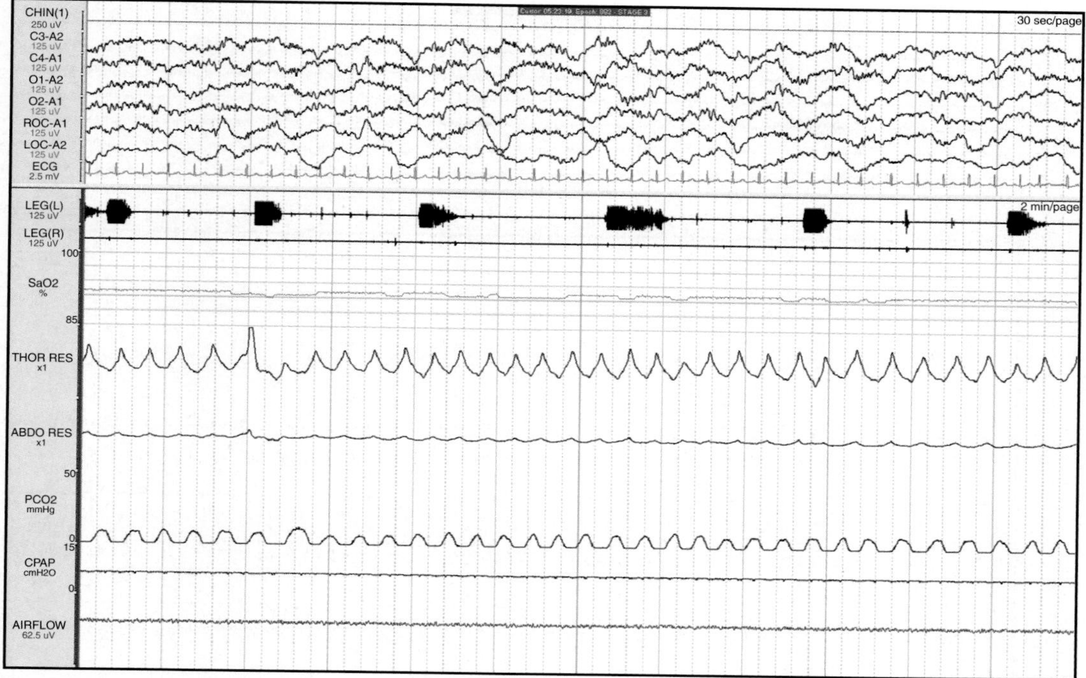

Figure 11.3-4.
Continuous positive airway pressure has corrected the hypoxemia in the patient shown in Figure 11.3-2. The periodic limb movements continue.

The obese COPD patient may have the features of the sleep findings of COPD and obstructive sleep apnea (Figs. 11.3-5 to 11.3-7). In the patient with very severe COPD the sleep findings may be related to REM sleep and may then demonstrate hypoventilation and/or apnea (Figs. 11.3-8 to 11.3-10).

Patients with other types of obstructive pulmonary disease (e.g., asthma or cystic fibrosis) may present with findings similar to those described above. There may be audible wheezing during a sleep study (see video images in Chapter 20).

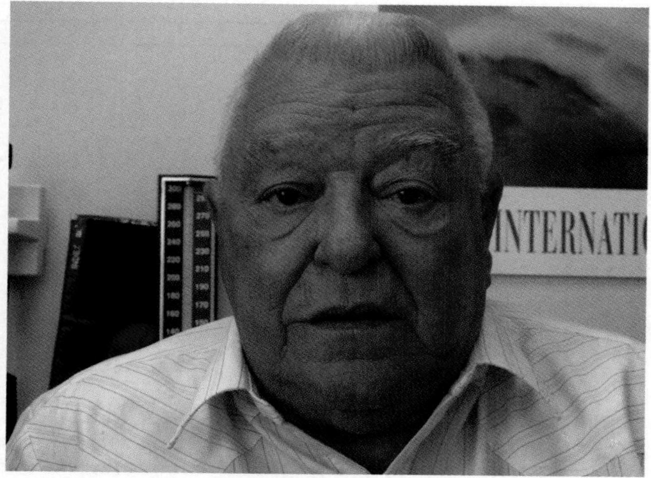

Figure 11.3-5.
This patient has severe COPD and sleep apnea. Note the cyanosis and the bloodshot eyes.

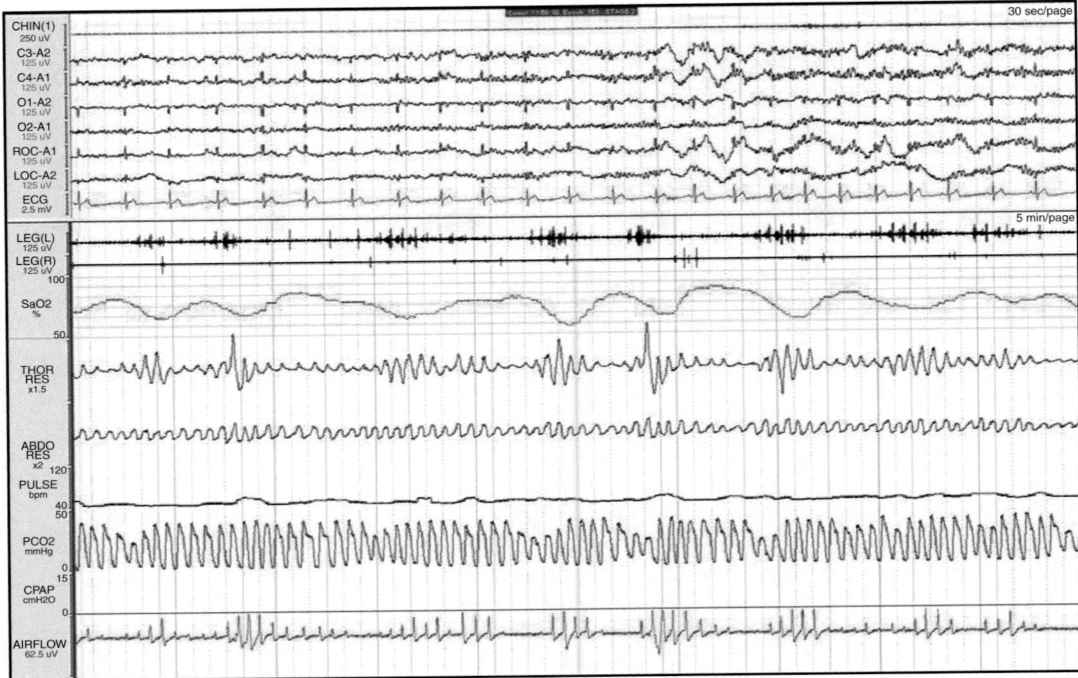

Figure 11.3-6.
The main findings in this patient (see Fig. 11.3-5) are due to repetitive episodes of sleep apnea and hypopnea.

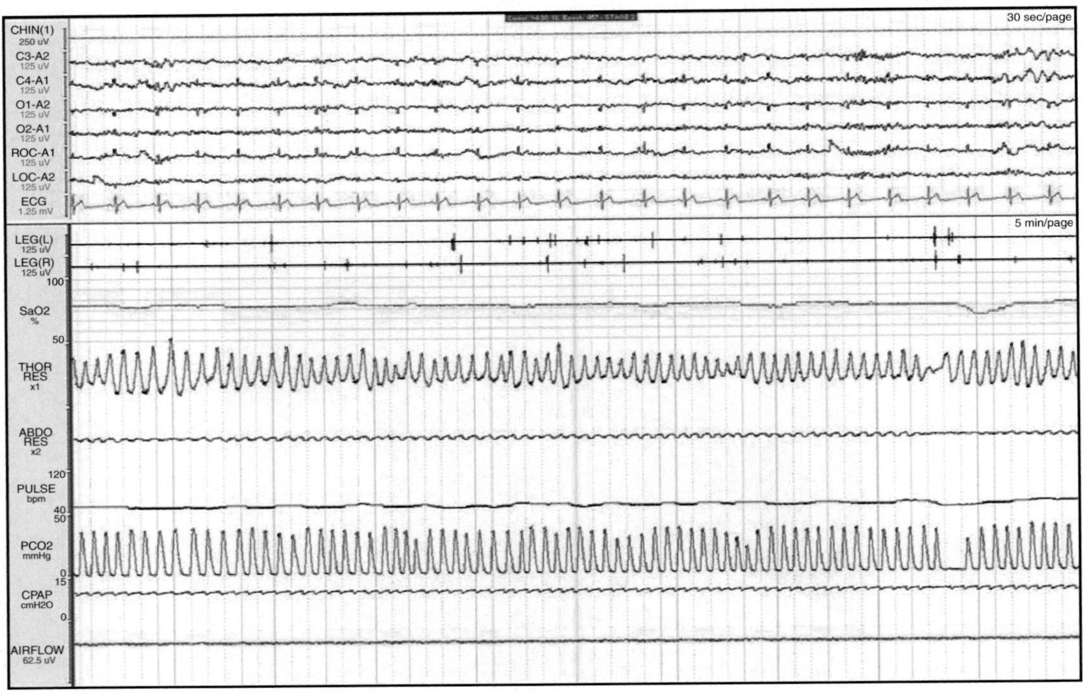

Figure 11.3-7.
Some patients have difficulty tolerating continuous positive airway pressure (CPAP) (or CPAP may make them worse because it may lead to hyperinflation) and thus they may require bilevel positive airway pressure support. CPAP alone was sufficient for this patient (see Fig. 11.3-5).

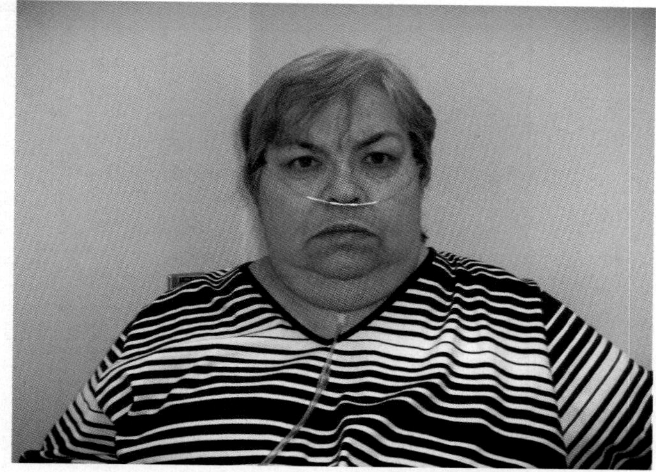

Figure 11.3-8.
This patient had severe COPD and was on 24-hour oxygen therapy.

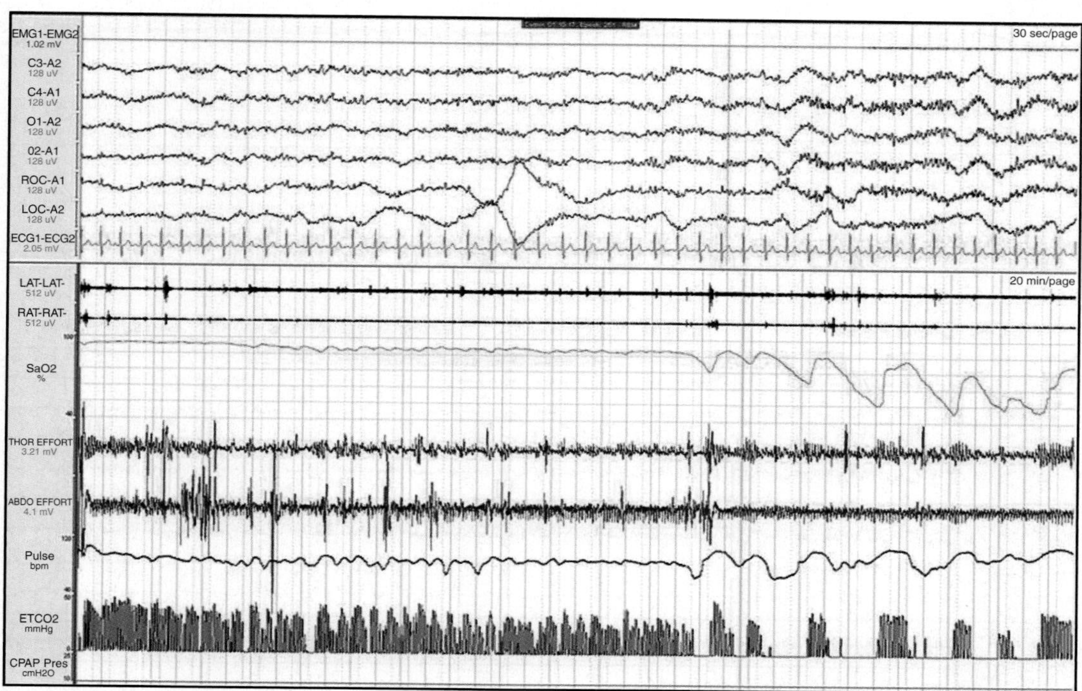

Figure 11.3-9.
The patient (shown in Figure 11.3-8), on entering REM sleep, developed apneic episodes and severe hypoxemia. The top part of the trace shows a 30-second epoch, and the bottom, a 20-minute epoch. The patient was on oxygen. Sleep-disordered breathing is likely related to REM-related respiratory muscle atonia.

Restrictive Lung Diseases

Intrapulmonary lung restriction includes a variety of lung diseases. They include idiopathic pulmonary fibrosis and pulmonary fibrosis related to another medical condition (e.g., rheumatoid lung disease) (Figs. 11.3-11 to 11.3-13). Inhalation of dust may also cause pulmonary fibrosis. Because the pulmonary disease may stimulate lung receptors, such patients may have a rapid, shallow breathing pattern. These patients hyperventilate during most of the course of their disease. In our experience, such patients are referred to sleep clinics when they also develop symptoms such as sleepiness or severe insomnia. In the end-stage of pulmonary fibrosis, sleep may be very difficult to achieve because of the dyspnea superimposed on a sleep breathing disorder.

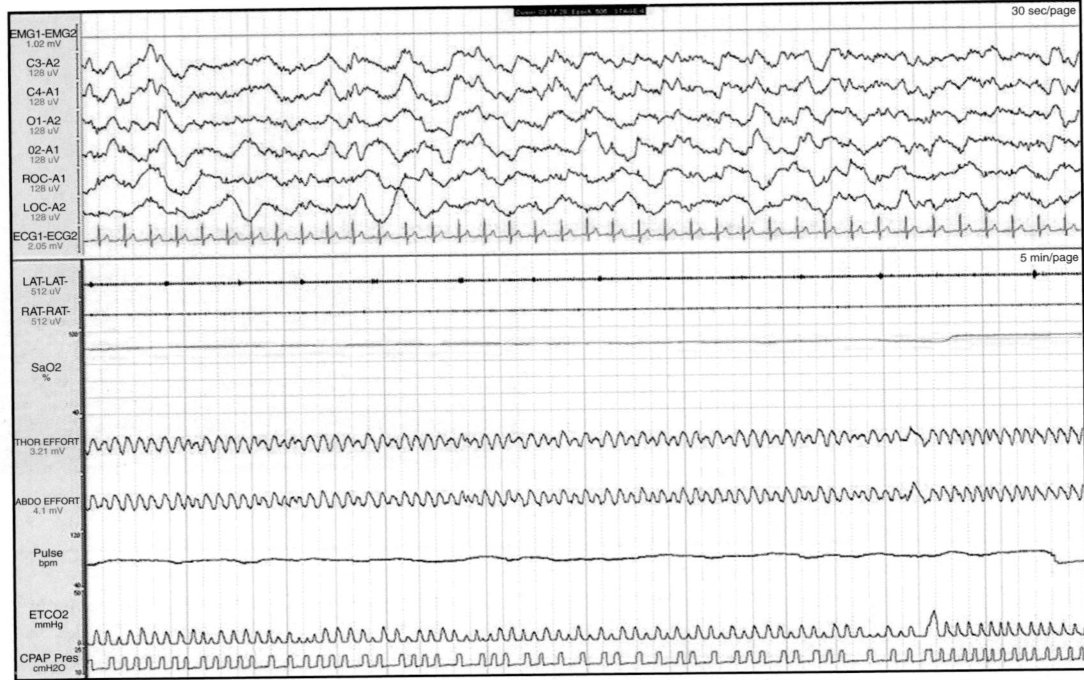

Figure 11.3-10.
The patient (shown in Figure 11.3-8) did best on bilevel positive airway pressure (see lowest channel, which monitors pressure) and oxygen added to the circuit.

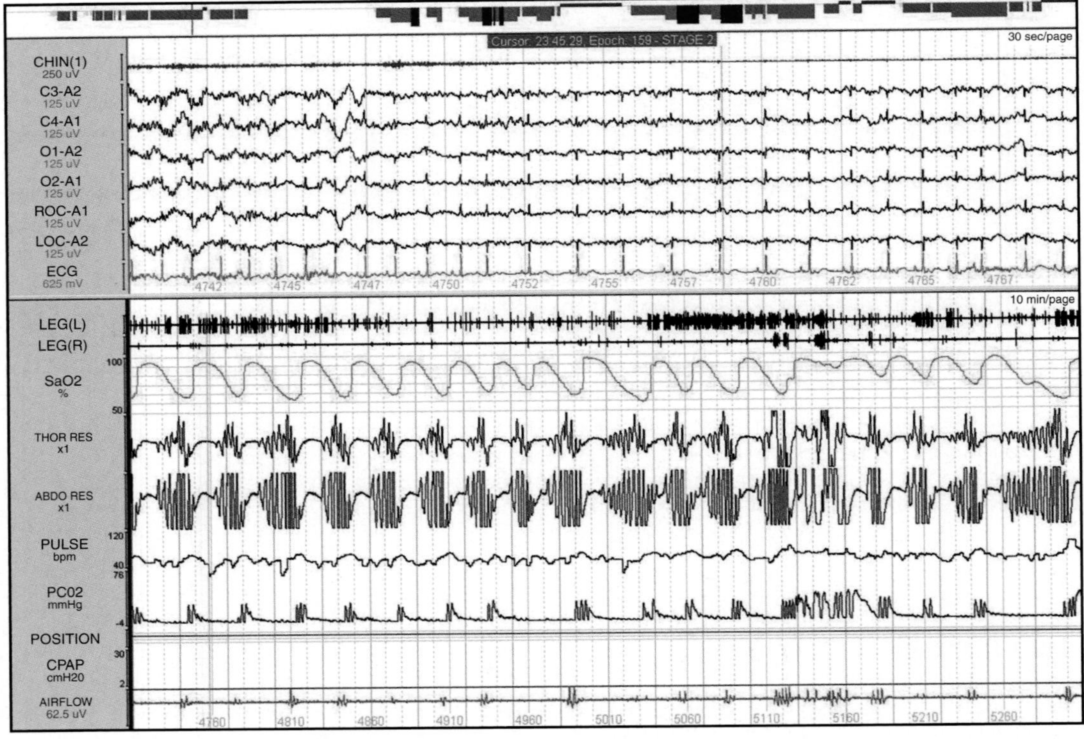

Figure 11.3-11.
This graph represents a 67-year-old male patient who had idiopathic pulmonary fibrosis, a 10-year history of snoring, and an approximately 5-year history of daytime sleepiness. Note the very high apnea index and the very rapid and severe oxygen desaturations and resaturations, likely related to the low lung volumes of his pulmonary disease.

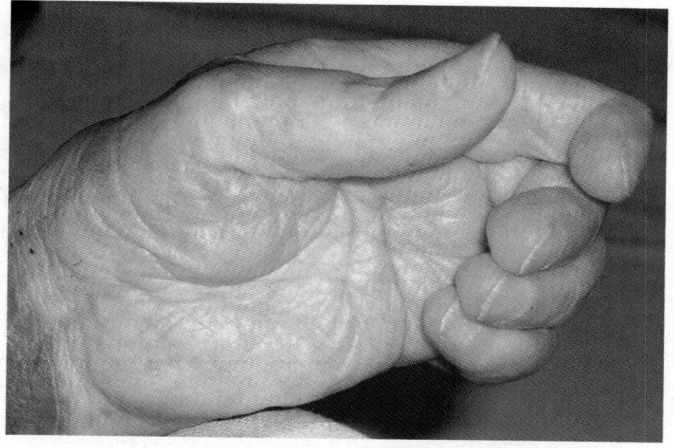

Figure 11.3-12.
This image is of a hand from a patient with rheumatoid arthritis, pulmonary fibrosis, and severe sleepiness (Epworth score 20).

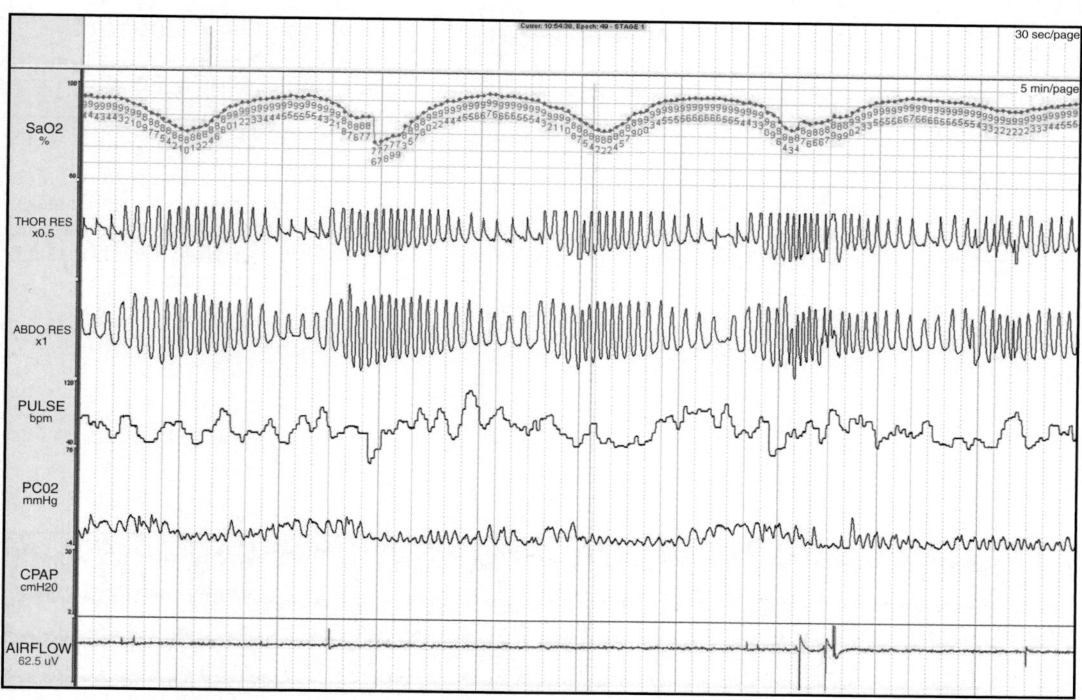

Figure 11.3-13.
This graph represents the female patient in Figure 11.3-12 who had a periodic breathing pattern and, despite very severe sleepiness, was unable to achieve persistent sleep in the sleep disorders center (see video images in Chapter 20). The nasal pressure airflow channel is flat because she breathed with her mouth wide open.

Extrapulmonary Lung Restriction

Extrapulmonary lung restriction includes the diseases that affect the thoracic cage (e.g., kyphoscoliosis) and those that affect the neuromuscular system (e.g., postpolio syndrome, neuromuscular diseases). Such patients may present with hypoventilation and may require bilevel positive airway pressure or intermittent positive pressure ventilation to treat their sleep disorder. Capnography is a useful addition in the monitoring of these patients. The patient's physiology may be further compromised by obesity and medications (Figs. 11.3-14 and 11.3-15). Neuromuscular disorders are reviewed in chapter 10.

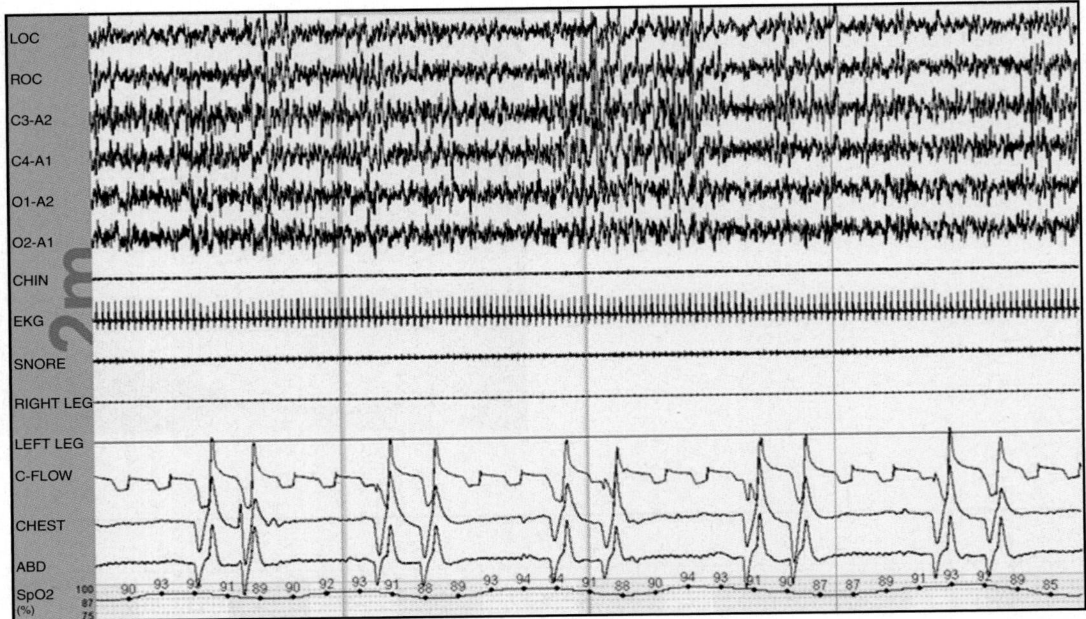

Figure 11.3-14.
Kyphoscoliosis. This graph shows a 2-minute epoch in a patient with kyphoscoliosis. The patient has a body mass index of 40 and is being treated with methadone 40 twice a day. The patient is on noninvasive ventilation (inspiratory pressure 12, expiratory pressure 6), with a backup rate of 12 beats per minute with an oxygen bleed into the circuit. The findings are those of persistent central apneas where the apneas are occurring in the face of a backup rate, suggesting upper airway closure during the central events. (Courtesy Dr. Lisa Wolfe, Northwestern University.)

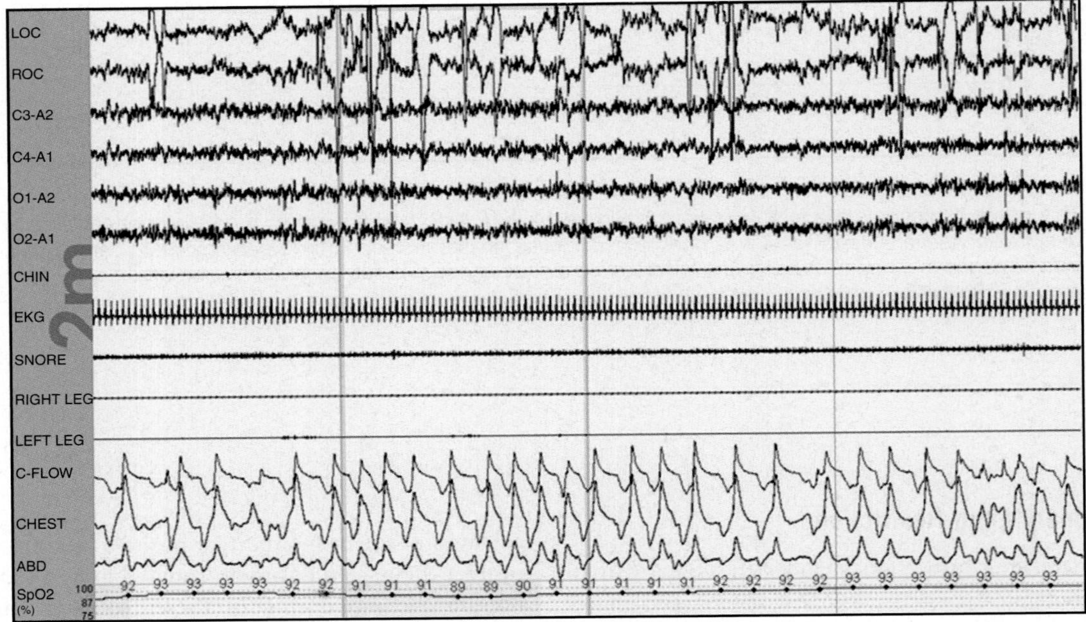

Figure 11.3-15.
Kyphoscoliosis. This graph shows data from the same patient (see Fig. 11.3-14). When the patient entered REM sleep, the central apnea events resolved.

SELECTED READINGS

Bhullar S, Phillips B: Sleep in COPD patients. COPD 2(3):355–361, 2005.

Casey KR, Cantillo KO, Brown LK: Sleep-related hypoventilation/hypoxemic syndromes. Chest 131(6):1936–1948, 2007.

George CF, Kryger MH: Sleep in restrictive lung disease. Sleep 10 (5):409–418, 1987.

Marrone O, Salvaggio A, Insalaco G: Respiratory disorders during sleep in chronic obstructive pulmonary disease. Int J Chron Obstruct Pulmon Dis 1(4):363–372, 2006.

McNicholas WT, Coffey M, Fitzgerald MX: Ventilation and gas exchange during sleep in patients with interstitial lung disease. Thorax 41 (10):777–782, 1986.

Mermigkis C, Chapman J, Golish J, et al: Sleep-related breathing disorders in patients with idiopathic pulmonary fibrosis. Lung 185(3):173–178, 2007.

Ozsancak A, D'Ambrosio C, Hill NS: Nocturnal noninvasive ventilation. Chest 133(5):1275–1286, 2008.

Urbano F, Mohsenin V: Chronic obstructive pulmonary disease and sleep: The interaction. Panminerva Med 48(4):223–230, 2006.

CHAPTER

12 PARASOMNIAS

Mark W. Mahowald, Carlos H. Schenck, and Michel A. Cramer Bornemann

Introduction

The term *parasomnias* refers to undesirable physical, autonomic, or experiential phenomena arising from the sleep period. Parasomnias may be the result of any one of a large number of different conditions which may be divided into two main categories: (1) primary parasomnias, which represent disorders of sleep states per se; and (2) secondary parasomnias, which represent disorders of a number of different organ systems that take advantage of the sleeping state to declare themselves. The most common primary parasomnias represent admixtures of wakefulness and rapid eye movement (REM) sleep (REM sleep behavior disorder, or RBD) or admixtures of wakefulness and non-REM (NREM) sleep (the disorders of arousal). The most common secondary sleep parasomnia is nocturnal seizures. Table 12-1 lists the clinical features of the most common parasomnias.

Disorders of Arousal

Sleep and wakefulness are not mutually exclusive. The primary sleep parasomnias represent dissociated states of being and serve as a reminder that sleep or wakefulness is not necessarily a "whole brain" or "global" phenomenon (see also chapter 3.3). Parts of the brain may be awake and other parts asleep, permitting the simultaneous occurrence of some elements of both sleep and wakefulness, often with dramatic clinical consequences.

Disorders of arousal are common in the general population, occurring on a spectrum ranging from confusional arousals and sleepwalking to sleep terrors. These events are very common in children and occur in up to 4% to 5% of adults (this percentage is likely lower than the true prevalence because of under-reporting of sleepwalking behaviors). Disorders of arousal are due to the admixture of wakefulness and NREM sleep. The brain is awake enough to perform complex behaviors but not awake enough to be aware of the behaviors or to remember them. The behaviors may be extremely complex and prolonged and may result in activities with forensic implications, without conscious awareness or culpability (Table 12-2).

Patients are often difficult to awaken during an event, and if awakening is successful, they are usually confused and disoriented. Unlike awakenings resulting from an REM sleep-related nightmare, patients awakened from a disorder of arousal often report complete amnesia for any mental activity preceding the arousal or, at best, may remember only fragmentary imagery such as a fire, the ceiling falling on them, a frightening face, a monster, or the perception of an ominous presence—not the complex plot of an REM nightmare, which results in full awakening.

Disorders of arousal are not related to underlying psychiatric or psychological problems, and depend on the

Table 12-2. Examples of Disorders of Arousal

Confusional arousals	Patient awakens from sleep confused and disoriented	These disorders of arousal can occur at any age. The patient usually has no recollection of these events the next morning or may have a fleeting recollection.
Sleepwalking	Patient may display behaviors ranging from simple (e.g., wandering) to complex (e.g., cooking)	
Sleep terrors	Patient may appear to awaken and may vocalize loudly, appear aggressive or frightened	

Table 12-1. Clinical Features of the Most Common Parasomnias

CHARACTERISTIC	DISORDER OF AROUSAL	NOCTURNAL SEIZURE	REM SLEEP BEHAVIOR DISORDER
Age of onset	Usually childhood—tending to diminish with increasing age, but may begin in adulthood	Any	Usually > 50 years of age, predominantly males
Frequency	Uncommon more than 1–2 per night, rarely from daytime naps	Often multiple, even very many, episodes nightly. May occur during daytime naps	May occur nightly, rarely from daytime naps
Stereotypy	Low	High	Low
Time of sleep period	Usually within the first third	Any	First episode usually 1–2 hours after sleep onset
Post-event confusion	Typical	Variable	Uncommon

BOX 12-1. CASE 1: COMPLEX SLEEPWALKING

A 21-year-old single male construction worker was referred by his military supervisor for evaluation of complex sleepwalking. He had a history of sleepwalking beginning at age 5 or 6. He had six episodes between the ages of 5 and 8. On one of these occasions, he sleepwalked outside the home in the middle of winter. The spells resolved spontaneously, returning at age 14, and occurring approximately once monthly.

One episode, at age 14, occurred when he was hunting with family members. He fell asleep on a couch while the others remained awake. From sleep, he got up and grabbed a loaded gun from behind the couch and began waving it around. Other family members had to tackle him to take the gun away. He was completely amnestic during the episode.

On numerous occasions he had awakened in a room different from the one he fell asleep in. His girlfriend reported that he talked and acted violently in his sleep—kicking, punching, and thrashing about. Occasionally he fell out of bed. Most recently, while on a National Guard weekend training exercise, he was found sleepwalking with his gun slung over his shoulder. He was then found to crawl into his First Sergeant's bed while sleepwalking.

His past history is otherwise unremarkable. There is no history of seizures, psychiatric disease, or alcohol or recreational drug abuse. Both of his parents have a history of sleepwalking. A detailed neurologic examination was normal.

Because of the potentially violent behaviors (brandishing a gun) and behaviors potentially resulting in forensic issues (crawling into his First Sergeant's bed), formal sleep studies employing a full seizure montage were recommended. It was recommended that he should furnish his bedroom with an alarm device and remove all guns from the house in the interim.

The sleep studies were unremarkable. The final diagnosis was "disorder of arousal."

This patient's behaviors (wielding a gun and ending up in bed with an individual who was practically a stranger) could have resulted in serious legal and forensic issues, which could compromise both personal and public safety and might have had tragic consequences. If such circumstances result in legal ramifications, a sleep forensics evaluation should be considered.

presence of predisposing, priming, and precipitating factors. For example, stress may be a precipitating factor in someone predisposed, but stress in a nonpredisposed individual will not result in a disorder of arousal. Short of capturing an event during a formal sleep study, there are no polysomnographic (PSG) characteristics that reliably indicate that a given individual is prone to have a disorder of arousal. PSG data cannot be used to determine after the fact that a previously occurring event was due to a disorder of arousal.

Inasmuch as disorders of arousal are common and normal, the decision to recommend sleep studies or treatment should be confined to those cases in which the behaviors are potentially injurious or violent or are very disruptive to others in the household. In mild cases, reassurance that these behaviors are normal and unrelated to psychiatric disease is often sufficient. Medications such as clonazepam or imipramine may be effective. Teaching self-hypnosis may also be effective (Boxes 12-1 and 12-2).

Sleep-related eating disorder is a specialized form of disorder of arousal (as is sleep-related sexual activity, sleep sex, or sexsomnia). It is seen most frequently in individuals

BOX 12-2. CASE 2: COMPLEX SLEEPWALKING

A 31-year-old, married, employed, male executive recruiter was referred for injurious sleep-related behaviors. He had experienced sleepwalking and sleep terrors beginning at 3 years of age. These became progressively more frequent and increasingly violent, occurring four to five times weekly. Sleepwalking and sleep terrors typically occur within 2 hours of sleep onset. This patient had gone 1 full month without an episode, and the episodes never occurred more than twice nightly. They did not seem to be related to sleep deprivation, medication, alcohol ingestion, or stress.

He reported precipitous arousals from sleep, often resulting in complex behaviors. He had pushed his wife from the bed, resulting in cuts and scratches, and sustained lacerations when he put his hand through a large aquarium. He had sleepwalked out of the bedroom, but never out of the house. These events are often associated with remembered visual imagery, and if his wife had attempted to awaken or console him during an episode, he might have tried to convince her that what he was visualizing was actually happening. He might have become angry and abusive toward her when she did not acknowledge that she perceived the same danger.

This patient sought medical attention following a sleepwalking episode during which he carried around one of his children, which resulted in great concern over the potential danger he was causing his children. He was placed on clonazepam with some, but incomplete, improvement in his sleepwalking (Fig. 12-1).

with a history of sleepwalking, is more frequently seen in women, and, in the sleep clinic population, is usually not associated with waking eating disorders. It may also be a manifestation of other underlying sleep disorders such as obstructive sleep apnea or restless legs syndrome. Complications include weight gain, eating potentially dangerous substances, and, in patients with diabetes, difficulty in glucose control. Treatment is directed at the underlying cause if the sleep-related eating disorder is associated with obstructive sleep apnea or restless legs syndrome. The idiopathic form often responds to topiramate or a combination of carbidopa/levodopa and opiate medications (Box 12-3; Fig. 12-2).

BOX 12-3. CASE 3: SLEEP-RELATED EATING DISORDER

A 46-year-old male was referred for evaluation of suspected obstructive sleep apnea. In the course of history taking, it became apparent that for the past 10 years he had frequent nocturnal awakenings during which he would eat large amounts of Gummi Bears. He typically ate two bags of Gummi Bears nightly and found that he had to curtail his daytime caloric intake lest he gain weight. He had varying degrees of awareness while eating but was unable to not eat during his nocturnal awakenings.

He underwent a formal sleep study that revealed moderately severe obstructive sleep apnea (apnea-hypopnea index = 29/hr with a nadir saturation of 80%) responding to nasal continuous positive airway pressure (CPAP) of 12 cm H_2O. He was instructed to bring Gummi Bears to the sleep laboratory. During the study there was a prolonged period of eating these candies. Examination of the video monitoring indicated that he was clearly not fully awake, as exemplified by his dozing off and snoring intermittently during the eating episode, for which he was completely amnestic upon awakening in the morning. He was given a therapeutic trial of nasal CPAP to see what effect it might have on his sleep-related eating.

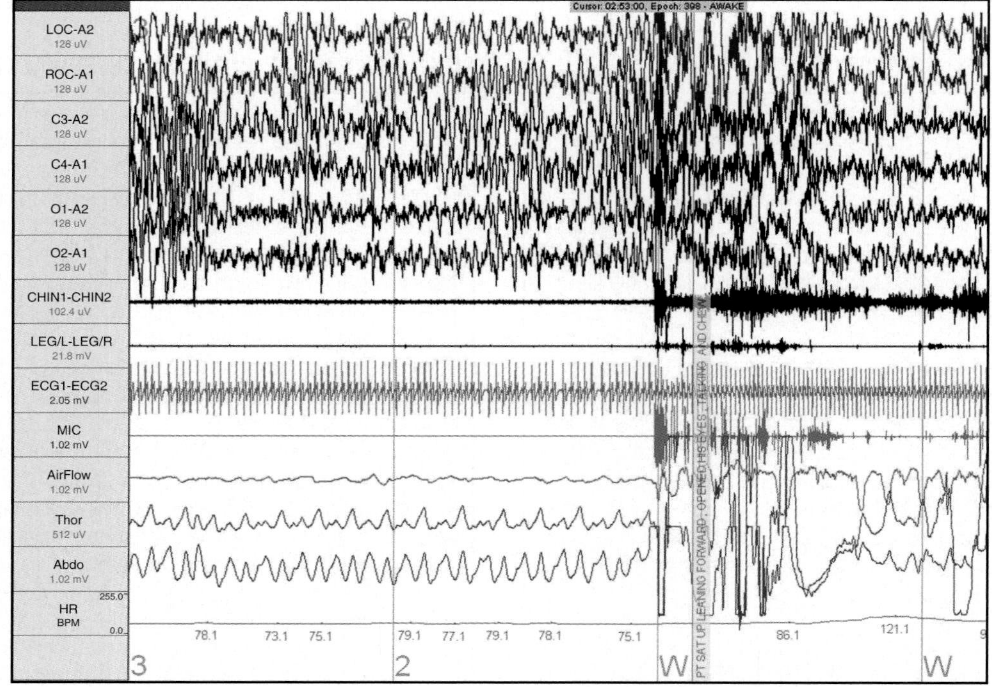

Figure 12-1.
This polysomnograph shows a typical arousal from NREM sleep in a patient with sleep terrors (see Box 12-2). Such arousals are most common from the deepest stages of NREM sleep (slow-wave sleep), but may arise from any stage of NREM sleep, even from relaxed wakefulness. Note the precipitous nature of the arousal with a dramatic increase in heart rate from a baseline of 75 to 121 beat per minute within a few seconds, without a hint of anticipatory change in heart rate or respiratory pattern. This instantaneous autonomic activation, coupled with the fact that disorders of arousal can be triggered de novo by auditory stimulation in susceptible individuals, indicates that these arousals are instantaneous and spontaneous, and not due to the culmination of underlying psychologically or psychiatrically significant sleep-related mentation.

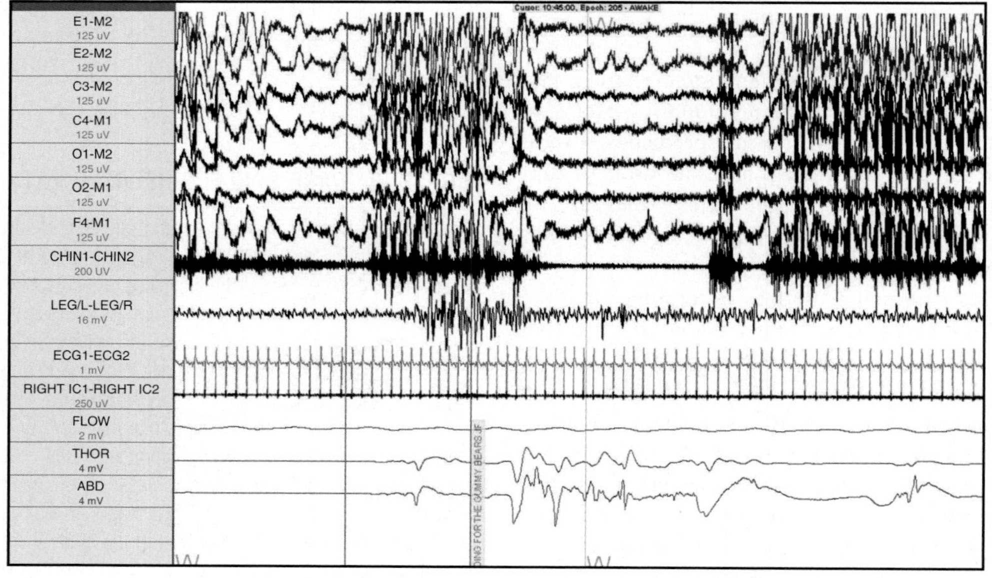

Figure 12-2.
Notice chewing movements during apparent wakefulness as defined by polysomnography. The possibility of dissociation between EEG-defined wakefulness and clinical wakefulness is underscored by the fact that during this period of EEG-defined wakefulness, the patient was clearly dozing and snoring intermittently, and was completely amnestic for this eating episode upon awakening in the morning.

REM Sleep Behavior Disorder

REM sleep behavior disorder, or RBD, is a fascinating experiment in nature, in which the anticipated atonia of REM sleep is absent, resulting in prominent vocalizations and movements and occasionally violent behaviors during REM sleep. Immediately on awakening, unlike patients with disorders of arousal, patients with RBD are completely awake, alert, and oriented, and often report dream mentation, which correlates highly with the observed behaviors (Boxes 12-4 to 12-7). These patients are thought to be "acting out their dreams" (or "dreaming out their acts"—depending on one's concept of dream generation). (See Video images in chapter 19.) RBD is overwhelmingly a male phenomenon (up to 80% to 90% in some series) and is most often seen in men over 50 years of age. RBD may be idiopathic or associated with other diseases (e.g., Parkinson's disease and narcolepsy) and may be a precursor symptom of a neurodegenerative disease. (See Video images in chapter 19.) The movements and behaviors in RBD can range from subtle to violent (see Video images in chapter 20).

BOX 12-4. CASE 4: IDIOPATHIC RBD WITH RUPTURED SPLEEN

A 67-year-old male was referred following a dream-enacting episode occurring during a hospitalization. This resulted in his leaping out of bed, falling on the floor, fracturing ribs, and lacerating his spleen. For the past few years he had been experiencing yelling, vocalizing, and swearing along with punching, kicking, and, on one occasion, putting his hands around his wife's throat during his sleep.

His past history was unremarkable. A detailed neurologic examination revealed no evidence of extrapyramidal disease (Fig. 12-3).

Nocturnal Seizures

Seizures frequently occur predominantly or exclusively during sleep (Boxes 12-8 and 12-9). One explanation for this is that epileptogenesis is state dependent. There are some exceptions, but generally speaking, NREM sleep is the most epileptogenic state, followed by wakefulness, followed by REM sleep. This may reflect the fact that electroencephalogram (EEG) activity of NREM sleep is highly synchronized,

BOX 12-5. CASE 5: RBD WITH PARKINSON'S DISEASE

The patient is an older male with a 5-year history of Parkinson's disease who was referred to the sleep clinic for evaluation of violent and potentially injurious dream-enacting behaviors. Polysomnography revealed prominent, increased tonic and phasic electromyelogram (EMG) activity during REM sleep, with frequent gross body movements and vocalization (Fig. 12-4).

BOX 12-6. CASE 6: DRUG-INDUCED RBD

A middle-aged man was referred to the sleep center for an evaluation of violent dream-enacting behaviors. These began shortly after he was prescribed venlafaxine for depression (Fig. 12-5).

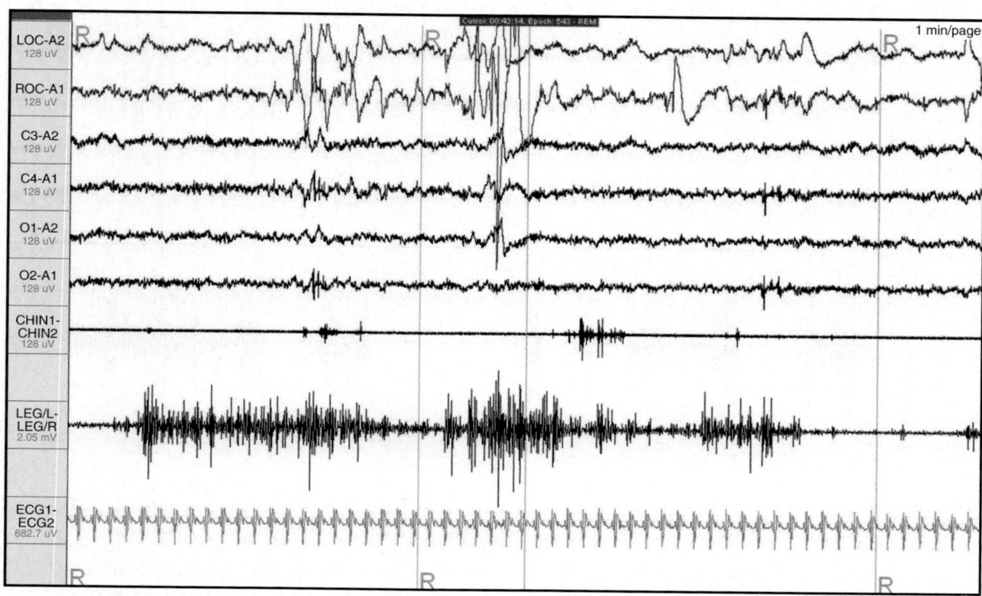

Figure 12-3.
This epoch of REM sleep reveals prominent muscle activity. The pattern is termed *REM sleep without atonia* (RWA). RWA is the polysomnographic marker of RBD; however, RWA may be seen in isolation without a clinical history of RBD.

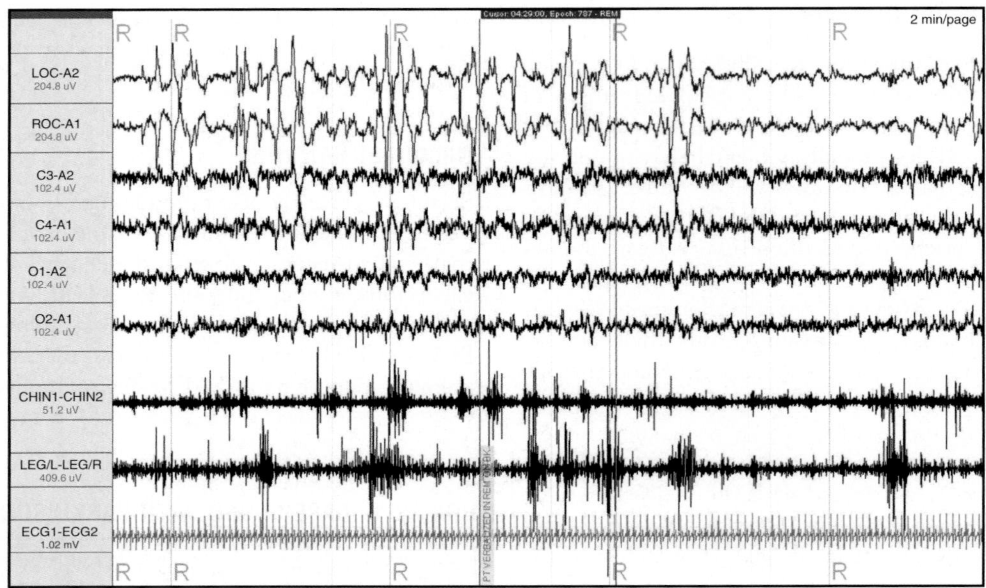

Figure 12-4.
There is a very strong relationship between RBD and neurodegenerative disorders. Approximately 75% of patients initially believed to have idiopathic RBD eventually develop one of the synucleinopathies (Parkinson's disease, dementia with Lewy body disease, or multiple system atrophy). The RBD may precede any other clinical manifestation of the neurodegenerative disorder by over a decade. Therefore, patients with idiopathic RBD must be followed closely for the development of one of these underlying conditions.

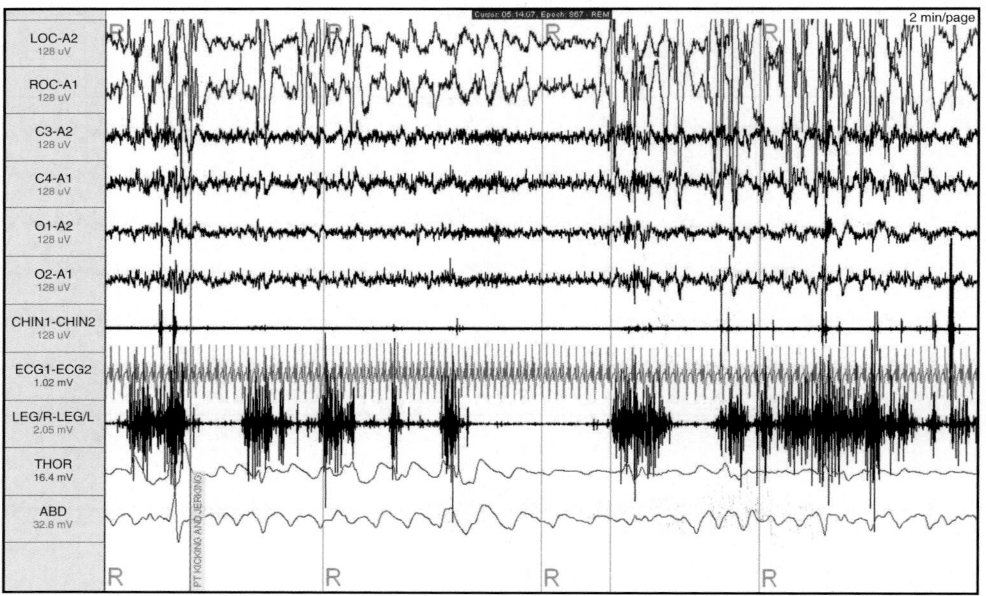

Figure 12-5.
Note the prominent increased EMG activity in the anterior tibialis EMG channels (with relatively little increase in phasic EMG activity in the submental EMG channel). Currently, one of the most common causes of RWA or RBD is iatrogenic, due to frequently prescribed medications such as monoamine oxidase inhibitors (MAOIs), tricyclic antidepressants (TCAs), selective serotonin reuptake inhibitors (SSRIs), and serotonin and norepinephrine reuptake inhibitors (SNRIs).

BOX 12-7. CASE 7: RBD ASSOCIATED WITH NARCOLEPSY

A 28-year-old female with narcolepsy had developed dream-enacting behaviors. She was receiving fluoxetine to treat cataplexy (Fig. 12-6).

as is seizure activity. Most seizures seen in sleep laboratories are associated with very bizarre behaviors, the common features of which are recurrent, stereotyped, and inappropriate.

Treatment of nocturnal seizures is similar to that of other seizures. However, if the seizures are exclusively nocturnal, antiepileptic medication can be given only in the evening, obviating the need for multiple daytime dosing and medication blood-level monitoring.

Bruxism

Although not generally considered a sleep disorder, but rather a dental condition, the excessive motor activity of the muscles that lead to teeth clenching and teeth grinding seems to be activated primarily during sleep. Patients are not generally referred to a sleep clinic unless they have a sleep complaint, the most common being insomnia. After receiving the evaluation from the sleep clinic the referring primary care practitioners are often surprised to learn that the insomnia is caused by bruxism.

BOX 12-8. CASE 8: NOCTURNAL SEIZURES PRESENTING AS SLEEP-RELATED CHOKING

A 3-year, 9-month-old girl was referred to the sleep clinic for evaluation of nighttime gagging and choking spells that had begun at 2 years, 11 months of age, occurring up to five times nightly. There was a history of possible seizures occurring on awakening. She had undergone an adenoidectomy for these spells; the suspicion was that they might have been related to sleep apnea. She had been aggressively treated for gastroesophageal reflux but without benefit. Her father, a nurse anesthetist, was so concerned about these spells, fearing that they might result in respiratory arrest, that he kept an intubation tray at her bedside.

The sleep study was requested in an attempt to identify any "residual" sleep apnea in anticipation of additional upper airway surgery to alleviate these symptoms. The study, including a full electroencephalogram (EEG) seizure montage, revealed a number of choking episodes associated with EEG seizure activity. Between spells, a number of electrical seizures without clinical correlates were present. On the basis of her history, and the presence of prominent electrical seizure activity on the EEG, treatment with carbamazepine was initiated with immediate, complete, and sustained resolution of the nocturnal choking episodes (Fig. 12-7).

The consequence of bruxism is teeth that are ground down and smooth (Figs. 12-8 and 12-9). In the worst cases the teeth are ground down to virtually the gum line. On physical examination of the patient one may see

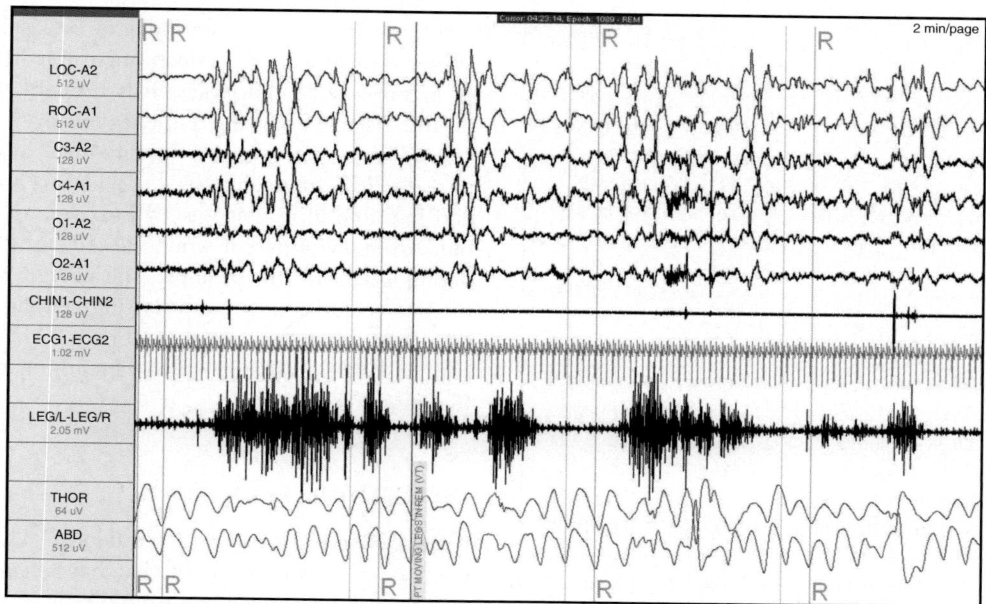

Figure 12-6.
Note the prominent, increased, phasic EMG activity from the anterior tibialis muscles in this patient with narcolepsy (see Box 12-7), with nearly complete sparing of the submental muscle. Up to one third of patients with narcolepsy also have RBD as a manifestation of narcolepsy. Furthermore, many medications prescribed to treat cataplexy (tricyclic antidepressants [TCAs], selective serotonin reuptake inhibitors [SSRIs], and serotonin and norepinephrine reuptake inhibitors [SNRIs]) can cause RBD.

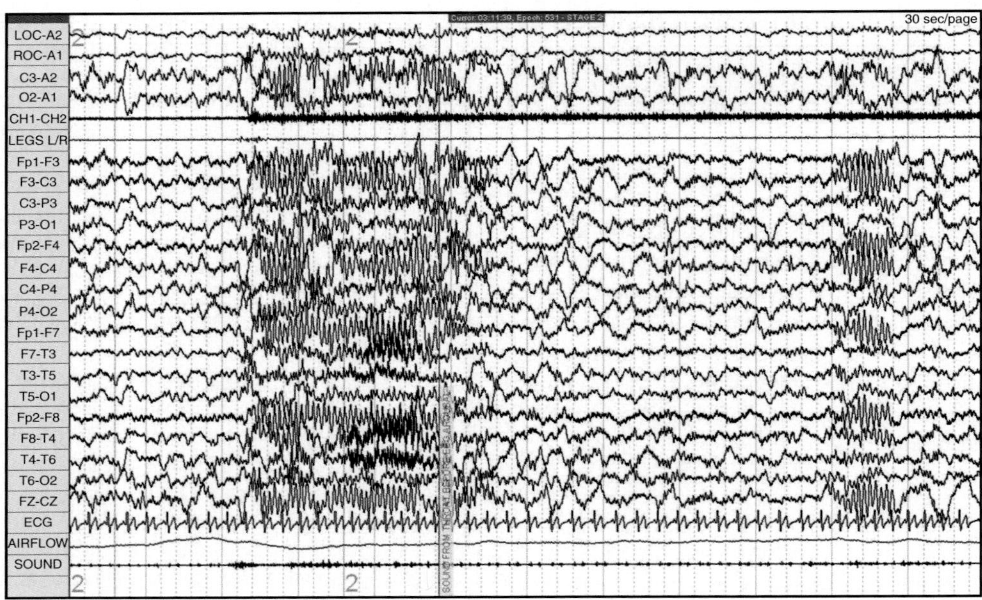

Figure 12-7.
This epoch reveals a run of electrical seizure activity without clinical manifestations. The presence of such activity in this patient (see Box 12-8) suggested the diagnosis of nocturnal seizures.

BOX 12-9. CASE 9: NOCTURNAL SEIZURES MASQUERADING AS SLEEP TERRORS

A 30-year-old employed male with a history of spontaneously resolving sleepwalking episodes occurring in early childhood was referred for evaluation of a recent onset of frequent dramatic behaviors arising from the sleep period. These ranged from simply sitting up abruptly to sitting up with a "blood-curdling" scream with arms and legs flailing. These had resulted in his breaking the footboard of his bed by kicking and sustaining a black eye by falling onto a bedside table. He had awakened to find himself on the floor in the morning. He was unaware of the behaviors; however, he knew that he must have experienced the behaviors because he woke up "foul and tired" and felt "hung over" for much of the morning. These spells typically occur 1 to 2 hours after sleep onset. This patient had gone for up to 2 weeks without a spell, and the maximum number per night had been two.

His past history was unremarkable. Specifically, there was no history of psychiatric disease, seizures, or substance abuse.

No spells occurred during any of the numerous sleep studies (some with full electroencephalogram [EEG] seizure montages) performed at numerous sleep facilities. A magnetic resonance imaging (MRI) study of the brain was normal. He and his fiancée were encouraged to take home videotape recordings, which captured a number of very stereotyped behaviors apparently arising from sleep characterized by sitting up and shouting, for which he was amnestic. Due to the virtually identical clinical behaviors, a clinical diagnosis of nocturnal seizures was made. Antiepileptic medication resulted in a marked reduction in the frequency and severity of the spells.

This is a typical example of nocturnal epilepsy. Formal sleep studies with full EEG seizure montages are often unremarkable, either because an event is not captured or because there may be no surface EEG abnormalities even during a clinical seizure. This case underscores the value of home video monitoring. The identical nature of the spells captured on home video led to the correct diagnosis.

hypertrophy of the masseter muscle. Figure 12-10 shows an example of bruxism that caused multiple awakenings during the night in a woman who believed that she did not sleep.

In the sleep clinic, we have seen patients complaining of severe insomnia whose episodes of bruxism awaken them. When studied with PSG sleep bruxism is frequently missed or incorrectly scored, unless it is brought to the attention of the scorer from the patient's history, or unless it is viewed on a synchronized digital video. In the case shown in three PSG fragments (Figs. 12-11 to 12-13), the patient had multiple long episodes of bruxism, apparent on PSG, but extremely apparent when viewed on the synchronized digital video. In this example, the patient had single, continuous episodes of bruxism lasting as long as 7 to 8 minutes. Note that the episode of bruxism that awakened the patient led to a change in the breathing pattern and yet the patient was awake.

TREATMENT OF BRUXISM

Bruxism is usually treated by a dentist. The goal of treatment is to repair the teeth that have been damaged and to fabricate for the patient a mouth guard to prevent additional damage. A variety of medications have been evaluated anecdotally for patients who continue to have severe sleep complaints, but randomized clinical trials are lacking. Benzodiazepines and muscle relaxants are sometimes tried long term. Often bruxism is a manifestation of stress, and treatment of the stress may be indicated.

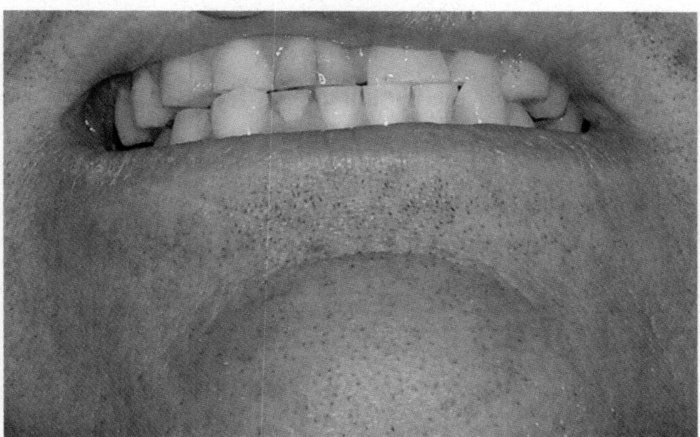

Figure 12-8.
This patient had severe bruxism. In this image the patient was asked to bring the upper and lower teeth together. Note that where the upper and lower teeth ground against each other the bottom of the upper teeth and the top of the lower teeth are flat. The right central incisor has a crack.

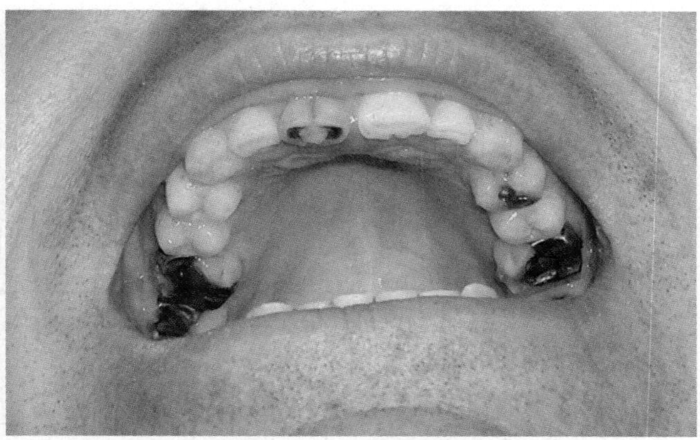

Figure 12-9.
The same patient as seen in Figure 12-8. Notice that the upper anterior teeth are ground down and that the right central incisor has a crack. There is also evidence of a great deal of dental work having been done.

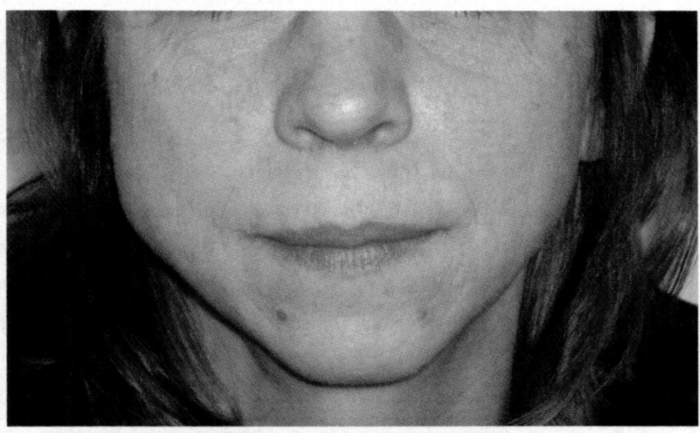

Figure 12-10.
On examination this bruxism patient had a very prominent hypertrophied right masseter muscle.

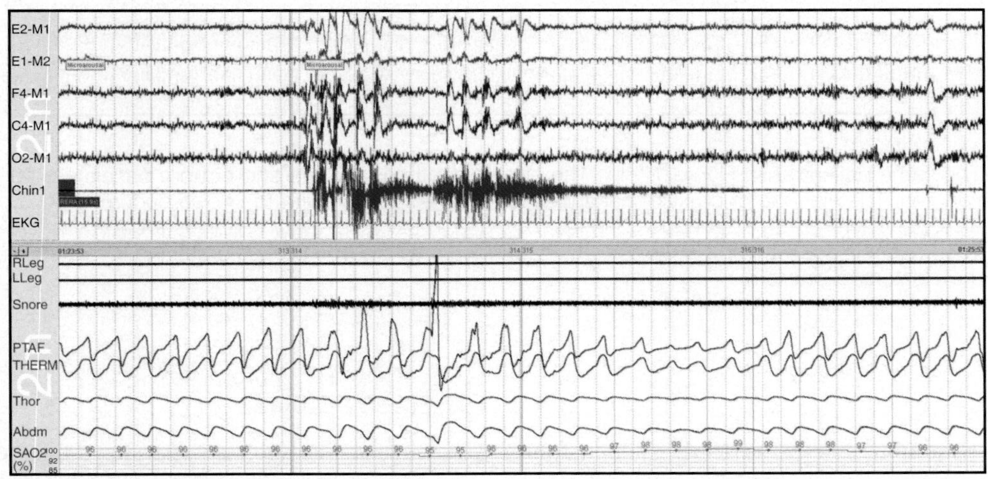

Figure 12-11.
This patient had complained of severe insomnia. The epoch shown here is 2 minutes long. It begins in REM sleep, and there is an abrupt increase in the chin EMG, with transmitted artifact seen in the EEG and EOG. These findings are characteristic in patients with sleep bruxism. By examining the respiratory data *(bottom panel)* separately from the data used for sleep stage scoring *(top panel),* a technician can easily suspect that an episode of hypopnea is present. On synchronized digital video, one can hear the characteristic chattering noise made by the upper and lower teeth striking against each other.

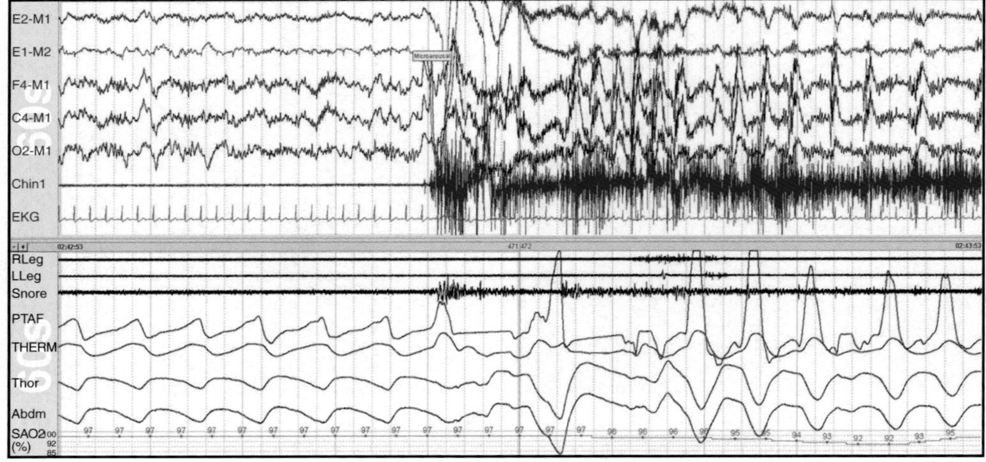

Figure 12-12.
The same patient as in Figure 12-11. The epoch lengths in the top and bottom panels are 60 seconds. Here, the episode of bruxism begins during stage N2 sleep and results in a long awakening. This event could easily have been scored as hypopnea, because one sees changes in the airflow channels and oxygen saturation that meet the criteria for an abnormal respiratory event. Figure 12-13 shows 10 minutes' worth of data beginning with this epoch.

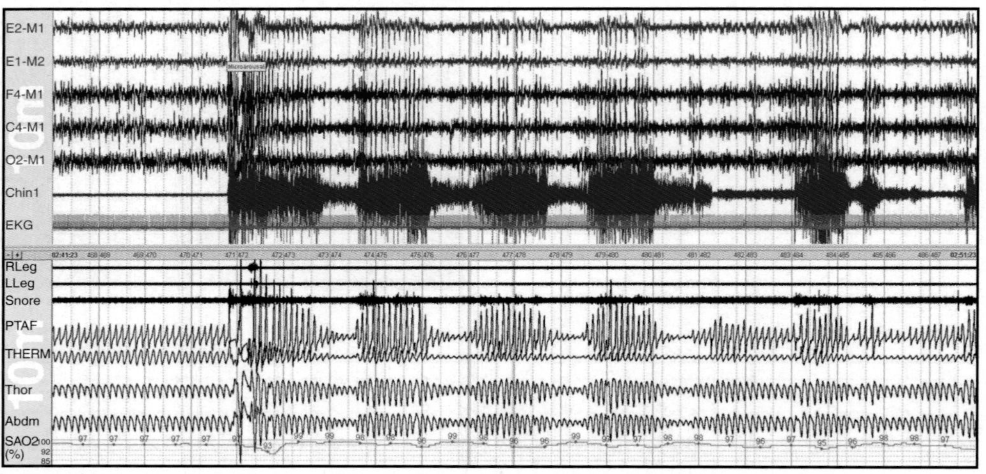

Figure 12-13.
The same patient as in Figure 12-11. The epoch lengths in the top and bottom panels are 10 minutes. The episode of bruxism continues for several minutes with the noise occurring in clusters. There are synchronous changes recorded in the respiratory channels *(bottom panel).* The patient is actually wide-awake, and what appears as Cheyne Stokes breathing is related to the clusters of bruxism.

Summary

The common parasomnias can perfectly mimic one another, making purely clinical diagnosis difficult if not impossible. Parasomnia evaluation should be performed with continuous technologist observation, video recording, and a full EEG seizure montage in a facility with sleep medicine professionals experienced in diagnosis and management.

SELECTED READINGS

Cramer Bornemann MA, Mahowald MW, Schenck CH: Forensic sleep medicine issues: Violent parasomnias. In Smith HR, Comella CL, Hogl B (eds): Sleep Medicine. Cambridge, Cambridge University Press, 2008, pp. 240–255.

Mahowald MW, Schenck CH: NREM sleep parasomnias. Neurol Clin 23:1077–1106, 2005.

Mahowald MW, Schenck CH: Sleep disorders. In Engel J Jr, Pedley TA (eds): Epilepsy: A Comprehensive Textbook. Philadelphia, Lippincott Williams & Wilkins, 2007, pp. 2757–2764.

Nightingale S, Orgill JC, Ebrahim IO, et al: The association between narcolepsy and REM behavior disorder (RBD). Sleep Med 6:253–258, 2005.

Pressman MR: Disorders of arousal from sleep and violent behavior: The role of physical contact and proximity. Sleep 30:1039–1047, 2007.

Pressman MR: Factors that predispose, prime, and precipitate NREM parasomnias in adults: Clinical and forensic implications. Sleep Med Rev 11:5–30, 2007.

Schenck CH, Arnulf I, Mahowald MW: Sleep and sex: What can go wrong? A review of the literature on sleep-related disorders and abnormal sexual behaviors and experiences. Sleep 30(6):683–702, 2007.

Schenck CH, Mahowald MW: REM sleep parasomnias. Neurol Clin 23:1107–1126, 2005.

Schenck CH, Mahowald MW: Review of nocturnal sleep-related eating disorders. Int J Eat Disord 15:343–356, 1994.

Winkelman JW: Treatment of nocturnal eating syndrome and sleep-related eating disorder with topiramate. Sleep Med 4:243–246, 2003.

CHAPTER 13

CARDIOVASCULAR DISORDERS

Shahrokh Javaheri

In this chapter we review cardiovascular diseases encountered in patients presenting with sleep disorders. Both obstructive sleep apnea (OSA) and central sleep apnea (CSA) (see chapter 11.1) may be comorbid with a variety of cardiovascular diseases that continue to be highly prevalent and associated with excess morbidity and mortality and huge economical costs. See chapter 3.7 for a review of the regulation of cardiovascular physiology in sleep.

Impact of Cardiovascular Diseases

It has been estimated that approximately 81 million Americans suffer from one or more cardiovascular diseases. The prevalence of various cardiovascular diseases, including hypertension, coronary heart disease (myocardial infarction and angina pectoris), heart failure, and stroke, is presented in Table 13-1. The associated mortality is presented in Box 13-1.

Since 1900, except in 1918 (the time of an influenza pandemic), cardiovascular diseases have accounted for more deaths than any other cause of death in the United States. Currently cardiovascular disease accounts for 1 out of every 2.8 deaths, with a total of 870,000 deaths annually (36% of all deaths). It is estimated that 2400 adult Americans die of cardiovascular disease each day.

Effect of Sleep Disorders on Cardiovascular Physiology

One of the most significant advances in clinical medicine has been the understanding that obstructive sleep apnea/hypopnea (hitherto referred to as OSA) may be either a cause of or contribute to progression, morbidity, and mortality of various cardiovascular diseases. OSA is characterized by recurrent complete (apnea) or partial (hypopnea) upper airway occlusion. The acute consequences of OSA include recurrent episodes of hypoxemia/reoxygenation, increases and decreases in pCO_2, and large negative swings in intrathoracic pressure. Figure 13-1 shows an example of OSA resulting in desaturation that is followed by reoxygenation with resumption of breathing. There is also an arousal at the termination of the apnea. In this patient we inserted an esophageal balloon to measure intrathoracic pressure. Note the progressively increasing negative swings in intrathoracic pressure that is due to diaphragmatic contraction against the closed upper airway. The negative pressure swings are also reflected outside the cardiac chambers and the intrathoracic aorta, increasing the transmural pressure of the chambers and blood vessels. Increased transmural pressure of the atria may contribute to atrial premature excitation and other arrhythmias such as atrial fibrillation. Increased left ventricular transmural pressure increases its afterload and oxygen consumption. Increased aortic transmural pressure increases the propensity for aortic dilatation and dissection, whereas increased negative interstitial pressure increases the propensity for developing pulmonary edema.

There is increasing evidence that through these acute mechanisms (see Fig. 13-1), OSA leads to activation of redox-sensitive genes, oxidative stress, inflammatory processes, sympathetic overactivity, and hypercoagulability. All of these can contribute to endothelial dysfunction (Fig. 13-2). Endothelial dysfunction is the underlying pathophysiologic mechanism mediating a variety of cardiovascular disorders, including hypertension, atherosclerosis (coronary artery disease as well as cerebrovascular disease), pulmonary hypertension, right and left ventricular systolic and diastolic dysfunction, stroke, and even sudden death (Fig. 13-3).

At times apneas can be very prolonged. This results in severe desaturation, as depicted in Figure 13-4.

Table 13-1. Prevalence of Cardiovascular Diseases in American Adults

	N (MILLIONS)
Total	81
Hypertension	73
Coronary heart disease	17
Angina pectoris	9
Myocardial infarction	8
Heart failure	5.3
Stroke	5.8

Heart disease and stroke statistics—2008 update. Circulation 117:e25–e146, 2008.

BOX 13-1. MORTALITY ASSOCIATED WITH CARDIOVASCULAR DISEASES (CVD)

- 870,000 (36% of all deaths)
- 1 in every 2.8 deaths
- 2400 Americans die of CVD each day
- 1 death every 37 seconds
- In every year since 1900, except 1918, CVD accounted for more deaths than any other cause of death in the U.S.

Heart disease and stroke statistics—2008 update. Circulation 117:e25–e146, 2008.

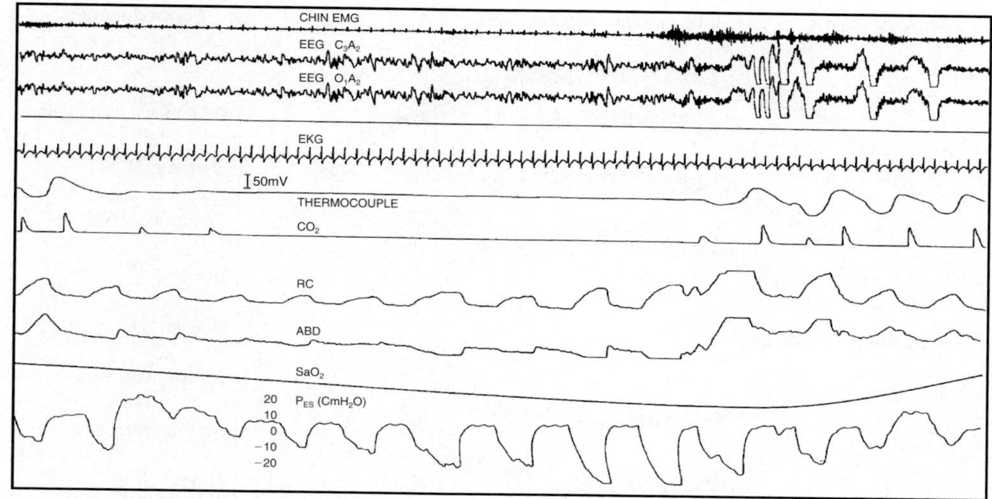

Figure 13-1.
The three immediate nocturnal consequences of obstructive sleep apnea are (1) altered blood gas chemistry characterized by hypoxemia/deoxygenation and hypercapnia/hypocapnia, (2) arousals, and (3) large negative swings in intrathoracic pressure.

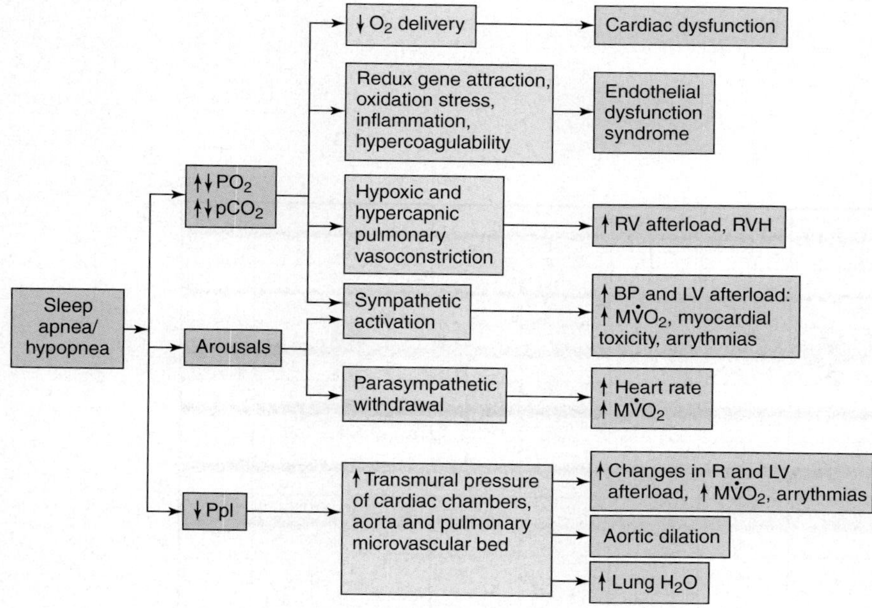

Figure 13-2.
The consequences of recurrent sleep apneas and hypopneas include hypoxemia/reoxygenation in association with hypercapnia and hypocapnia, respectively, during apnea followed by hyperpnea. The other consequences are arousals and negative flows in pleural pressure. These consequences in conjunction could eventually result in significant cardiovascular dysfunction. Hypoxemia may result in diminished oxygen delivery to the myocardium, which could result in arrhythmias and systolic and diastolic dysfunction.

Hypoxemia/reoxygenation could result in activation of redox-sensitive genes, oxidative stress inflammation, and hypercoagulability leading to endothelial dysfunction syndrome. Both alveolar hypoxia and hypercapnia (as a result of sleep apnea/hypopnea) result in hypoxic and hypercapnic pulmonary vasoconstriction that increases right ventricular afterload and its myocardial oxygen consumption. This eventually could result in right ventricular hypertrophy (RVH) and cor pulmonale.

Hypoxemia and hypercapnia, along with arousals, could also lead to sympathetic activation that would increase blood pressure. This would result in increased left ventricular afterload, increased myocardial oxygen consumption, and arrhythmias. In addition, this increase in sympathetic activation and release of myocardial norepinephrine could result in myocardial toxicity and apoptosis. Arousals also result in parasympathetic withdrawal, which increases the heart rate and myocardial oxygen consumption.

Finally, negative swings in pleural pressure (Ppl) increase the transmural pressure of the left ventricle (LV) and right ventricle (RV), both of which increase the wall tension of the ventricles, leading to an increase in myocardial oxygen consumption ($M\dot{V}O_2$). In addition, increasing the transmural pressure also affects the intrathoracic aorta and predisposes to aortic dilatation and potentially dissection. Furthermore, increased pleural pressure of the atria predisposes to development of atrial fibrillation. Finally, a negative interstitial pressure increases transcapillary fluid flow, facilitating the development of pulmonary edema. Overall, therefore, the consequences of sleep apnea and hypopnea in conjunction could result in cardiovascular dysfunction.

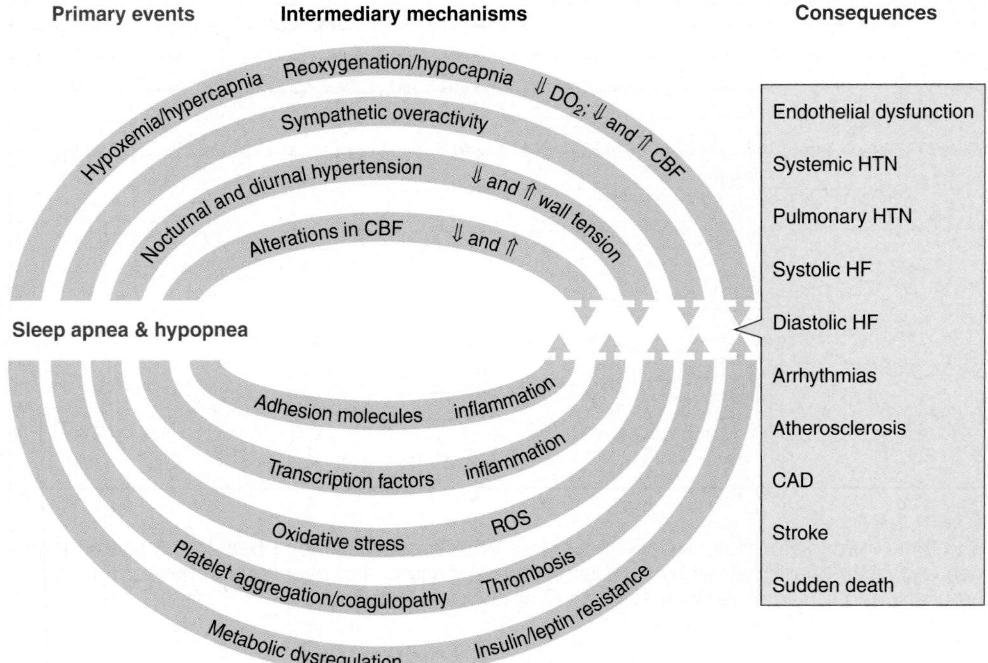

Figure 13-3.
Proposed pathophysiologic pathways in the development of cardiovascular disease in obstructive sleep apnea. CAD, coronary artery disease; CBF, cerebral/coronary blood flow; DO_2, dissolved oxygen; ⇓ decrease; ⇑ increase; HF, heart failure; HTN, hypertension; ROS, reactive oxygen species.

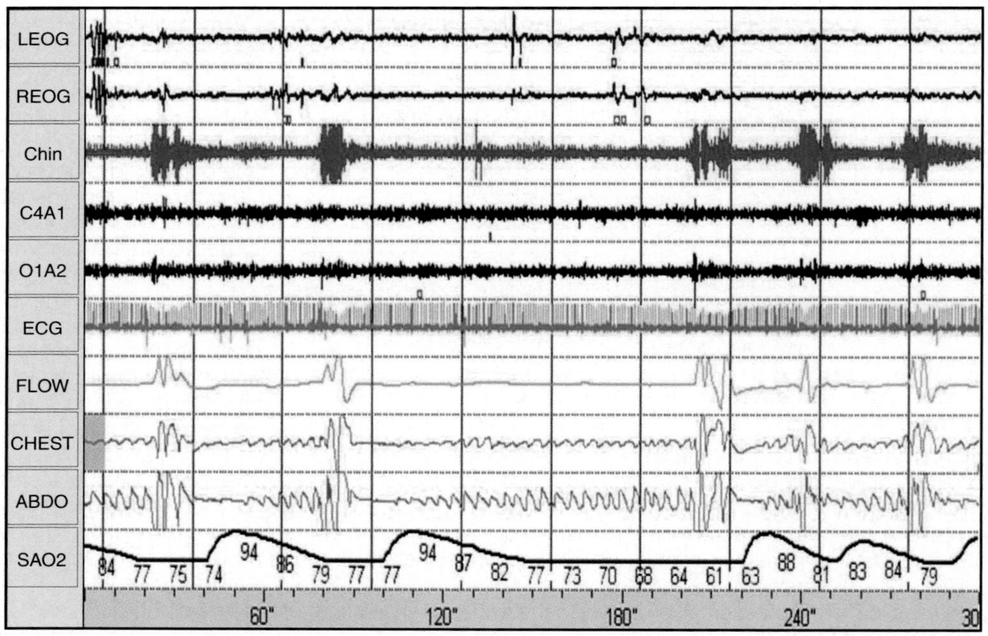

Figure 13-4.
An example of a prolonged obstructive apnea (almost 2 minutes in duration) in REM sleep resulting in significant oxygen desaturation.

OSA as a Cause of Cardiac Arrhythmias

Disorders of cardiac rhythms can occur in patients with OSA. These dysrhythmias may include bradycardia, sinus pause (Fig. 13-5), heart block, ventricular ectopy and tachycardia (Fig. 13-6), and atrial fibrillation. Arrhythmias are apt to occur in patients with severe OSA and in those with cardiac disease. The mechanisms mediating these dysrhythmias relate to a number of consequences of OSA, including altered blood gases (hypoxemia, hyper- and hypocapnia), changes in autonomic tone, and negative swings in intrathoracic pressure (which may distend the atria and ventricles). Particularly in the presence of coronary artery disease, the threshold for developing arrhythmias may be low.

In patients with OSA, nocturnal arrhythmias may contribute to the higher nighttime prevalence of sudden death. In the general population, sudden cardiac death, presumably in part due to ventricular arrhythmias and myocardial infarction, shows a day-night variation with preponderance in the early morning hours of 6:00 A.M. to noon. In contrast, in patients with sleep apnea, the peak in sudden death occurs during sleeping hours between midnight and 6:00 A.M., and the severity of sleep apnea correlates with the risk of nocturnal sudden death. The clinical implications are that the recognition and treatment of OSA may eliminate arrhythmias and improve morbidity and mortality in this population.

OSA as a Cause of Coronary Artery Disease

Through the mechanisms of endothelial dysfunction, which were reviewed earlier (see Figs. 13-2 and 13-3), OSA may either be a cause of or contribute to coronary artery disease or its progression. Evidence is mounting from both population and sleep clinic cohort studies that OSA causes or contributes to the progression of coronary artery disease and eventually to elevated cardiovascular death and all-cause mortality.

OSA has been implicated as a cause of nocturnal ST depression and angina pectoris. These conditions may be particularly more prevalent in patients with established coronary artery disease. We recommend polysomnography for the diagnosis of OSA and continuous positive airway pressure (CPAP) titration, if appropriate, for all patients with nocturnal angina, which should be eliminated with therapy.

In a retrospective sleep laboratory cohort study, Peker and colleagues reported incident coronary artery disease in almost 25% of untreated OSA patients during a 7-year follow-up. The corresponding numbers in treated sleep apnea patients and nonapneic snorers were 4% and 6%, respectively. In a more recent observational sleep laboratory cohort study of 1300 OSA patients and healthy study participants from Spain, Marin and colleagues observed that during a mean follow-up period of approximately 10 years, there was a 3 to 4 times higher incidence of fatal and nonfatal cardiovascular events in the patients with severe OSA (defined as an apnea-hypopnea index of 30

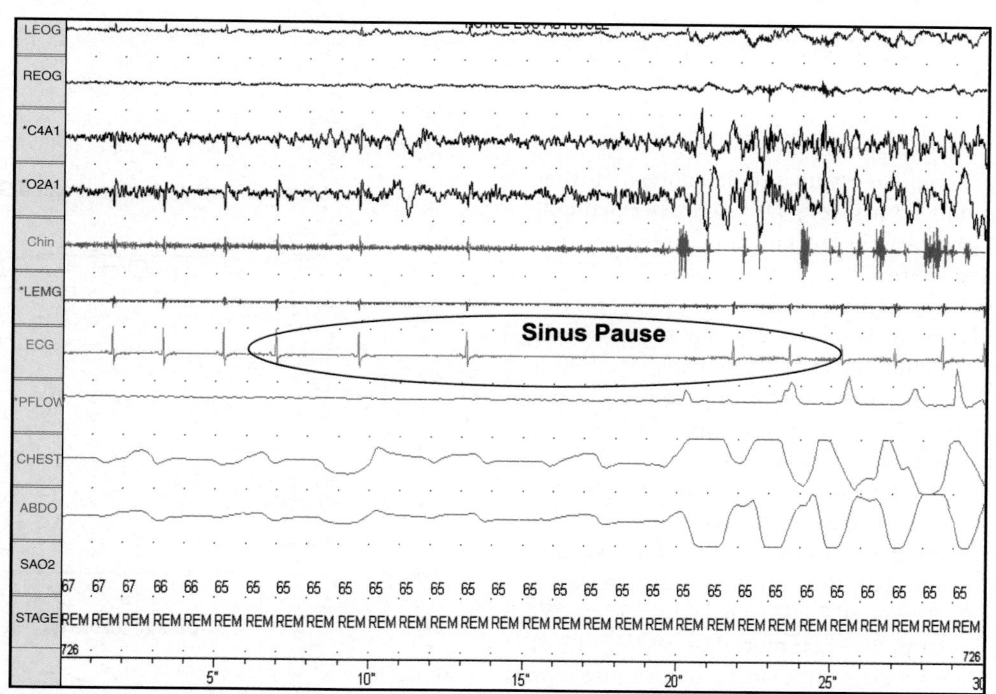

Figure 13-5.
An example of sinus arrest in a patient with obstructive sleep apnea. (With permission from Kapa S, Javaheri S: Constructive sleep apnea and arrhythmias. In Lee Chiong T [ed], Javaheri S [guest ed]: Sleep Medicine Clinics: Sleep and Cardiovascular Disease. Philadelphia, WB Saunders, 2007, pp. 575–581.)

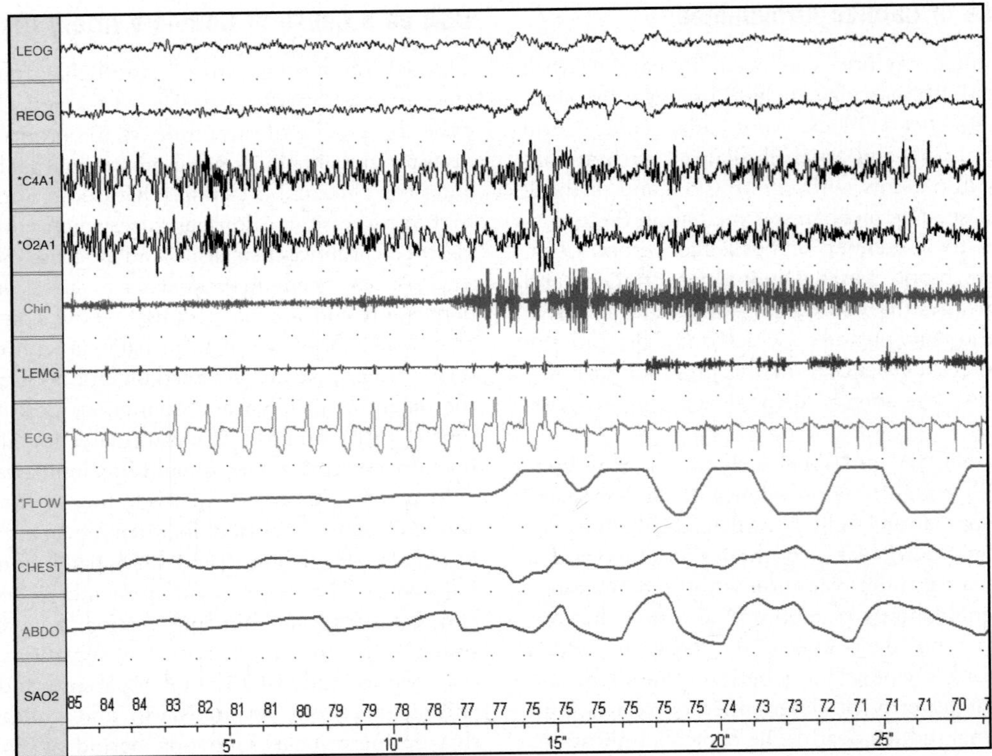

Figure 13-6.
An example of supraventricular tachycardia in a patient with obstructive sleep apnea.

or more per hour) compared with simple snorers. Furthermore, in 372 patients with severe OSA who were compliant with CPAP, cardiovascular event rates were similar to those in nonapneic snorers.

The Wisconsin Sleep Cohort Study is an 18-year mortality follow-up study (mean observation about 14 years) conducted on a cohort sample of 1522 participants aged 30 to 60 years at baseline. The adjusted hazard ratio for all-cause mortality with severe versus no sleep-disordered breathing was 3 (confidence interval [CI] = 1.4, 6.3) (Fig. 13-7). Importantly, after excluding the 126 participants who had used CPAP therapy, the association for all-cause mortality with severe versus no sleep-disordered breathing became stronger, and the adjusted heart hazard ratio increased to 3.8 (CI = 1.6, 9) for all-cause mortality and to 5.2 (CI = 1.4, 19.2) for cardiovascular mortality (see Fig. 13-6).

Thus, severe OSA is a major risk factor for all-cause mortality and cardiovascular disease, and effective treatment of OSA with CPAP improves survival. As reviewed in the next section, the improvement in survival is at least in part due to improvement in hypertension, which has been shown to decrease incident stroke and myocardial infarction.

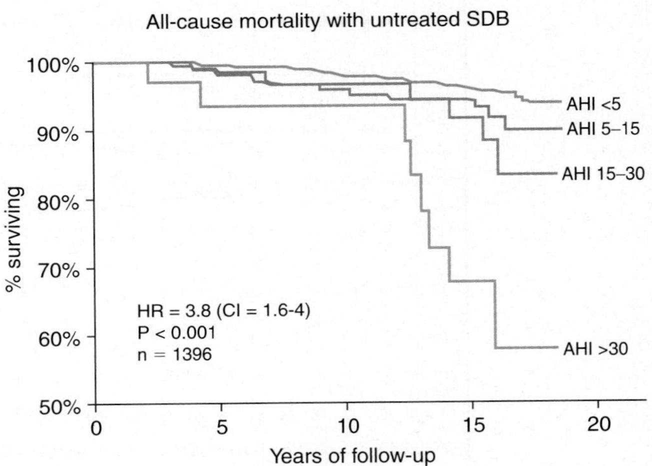

Figure 13-7.
Probability of survival in patients with untreated obstructive sleep apnea. AHI, apnea-hypopnea index; CI, confidence interval; HR, hazard ratio; SDB, sleep-disordered breathing. (Modified from Young T, Finn L, Peppard PE, et al: Sleep-disordered breathing and mortality: Eighteen-year follow-up of the Wisconsin Sleep Cohort. Sleep 31:1071–1078, 2008.)

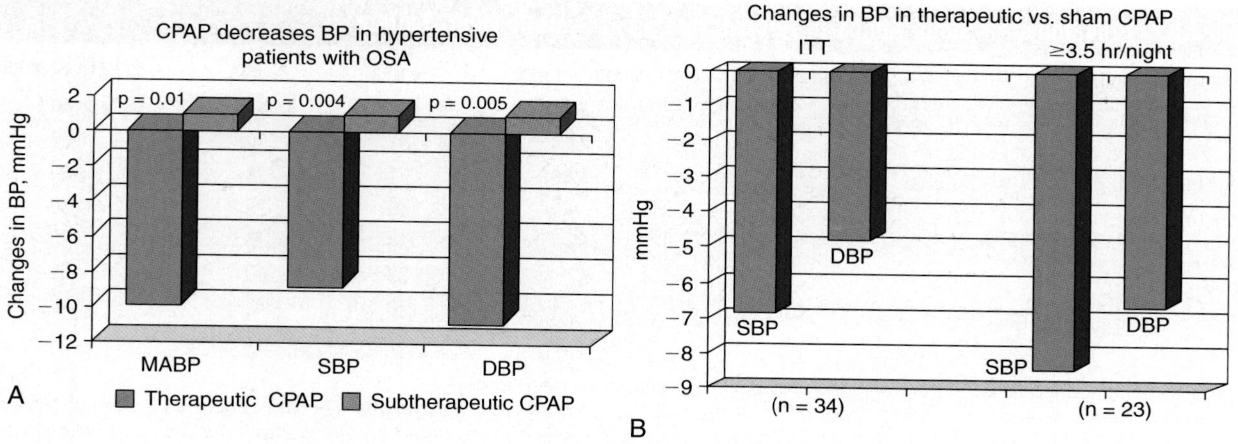

Figure 13-8.
Changes in hypertension induced by obstructive sleep apnea. Note the improvement in hypertension when obstructive sleep apnea (OSA) is effectively treated with continuous positive airway pressure (CPAP) and in those patients who are adherent to therapy. ITT, intention to treat. (A, from Becker HF, Javaheri S: Systemic and pulmonary arterial hypertension in obstructive sleep apnea. In: Lee Chiong T [ed], Javaheri S [guest ed]: Sleep Medicine Clinics: Sleep and Cardiovascular Disease. Philadelphia, WB Saunders, 2007, pp. 549–557; B, Coughlin SR, Mawdsley L, Mugarza JA, et al: Cardiovascular and metabolic effects of CPAP in obese males with OSA. Eur Respir J 29:720–727, 2007.)

OSA as a Cause of Systemic Hypertension

OSA is an independent risk factor for systemic arterial hypertension. Based on biologic plausibility (see Figs. 13-2 and 13-3), animal studies, longitudinal epidemiologic human studies accounting for confounding factors, and therapeutic trials, evidence has evolved indicating that OSA is an important cause of hypertension. In the Seventh Report of the Joint National Committee on Prevention, Detection, Evaluation, and Treatment of High Blood Pressure, OSA is recognized as the first identifiable cause of hypertension.

In a longitudinal study, Peppard and associates reported that the incidence of newly diagnosed arterial hypertension in a 4-year follow-up period increased as the apnea-hypopnea index (AHI) increased (a dose-dependent relationship). There was a twofold increase in the risk for developing hypertension in those with an AHI of 5 to 15 per hour and a threefold increase in risk with an AHI greater than 15 per hour, as compared with study participants without a sleep disorder at baseline.

From a clinical point of view it is important to recognize that approximately half of the 70 million Americans who have systemic hypertension may have OSA. It is further important to note that effective treatment of OSA has been shown to decrease systemic blood pressure. These reports are cited (Fig. 13-8) because of the power of the studies, the presence of a placebo control group (with sham CPAP), and the fact that the patients had hypertension to begin with. Collectively these studies showed the following: there was a small but significant decrease in hypertension in CPAP-treated patients (see Fig. 13-8); hypertension improved the most in patients with the most severe sleep apnea and desaturation index and who used CPAP the most; adherence and adequate therapy of OSA with CPAP are critical for reduction in blood pressure.

In summary, the results of the aforementioned studies indicate that both adequate control of OSA and adherence to CPAP are required elements for OSA-induced hypertension to improve with CPAP therapy. Improvement in hypertension plays a key role in decreasing incident stroke and myocardial infarction, contributing to increased survival.

Systolic Heart Failure

CLINICAL FEATURES

Congestive heart failure with left ventricular systolic dysfunction is a risk factor for sleep apnea. Patients with heart failure may present with insomnia (sleep onset and sleep maintenance). The sleep-onset insomnia may be linked to periodic breathing during relaxed wakefulness, or arousals while nodding off; the sleep-maintenance insomnia may be linked to periodic limb movements or respiratory-related arousals. The latter may be associated with the symptom of paroxysmal dyspnea—awakening with the sensation of intense dyspnea.

EPIDEMIOLOGY

More than 5 million Americans have heart failure. The prevalence of sleep apnea, both central and obstructive, remains high in the era of beta-blockers. Several studies

Table 13-2. Prevalence of Sleep Apnea in Recent Studies of Systolic Heart Failure

COUNTRY (REFERENCE)	N	% AHI ≥ 10/HR	% AHI ≥ 15/HR	% CSA	% OSA	% BETA-BLOCKERS
U.S. (1)	100		49	37	12	10
U.S. (2)	108		61	31	30	82
Canada (3)	287		47	21	26	80
China (4)	126	71		46	25	80
U.K. (5)	55		53	38	15	78
Germany (6)	700		52	33	19	85
Germany (7)	203	71		28	43	90
Germany (8)	102	54		37	17	80

AHI, apnea-hypopnea index; CSA, central sleep apnea; OSA, obstructive sleep apnea.
(1) Javaheri S: Sleep disorders in systolic heart failure: A prospective study of 100 male patients. The final report. Int J Cardiol 106:21–28, 2006; (2) Macdonald M, Fang J, Pitman S, et al: The current prevalence of sleep disordered breathing in congestive heart failure patients treated with beta blockers. J Clin Sleep Med 4:1–5, 2008; (3) Wang H, Parker JE, Newton GE, et al: Influence of obstructive sleep apnea on mortality in patients with heart failure. J Am Coll Cardiol 49:1625–1631, 2007; (4) Zhao Z, Sullivan C, Liu Z, et al: Prevalence and clinical characteristics of sleep apnea in Chinese patients with heart failure. Int J Cardiol 118:122–123, 2007; (5) Vazir A, Hastings PC, Dayer M, et al: A high prevalence of sleep disordered breathing in men with mild symptomatic chronic heart failure due to left ventricular systolic dysfunction. Eur J Heart Failure 9:243–250, 2007; (6) Oldenburg O, Lamp B, Faber L, et al: Sleep-disordered breathing in patients with symptomatic heart failure: A contemporary study of prevalence in and characteristics of 700 patients. Eur J Heart Failure 9:251–257, 2007; (7) Schulz R, Blau A, Borgel J, et al, for the working group "Kreislauf und Schlaf" of the German Sleep Society: Sleep apnoea in heart failure: Results of a German survey. Eur Respir J 29:1201–1205, 2007; (8) Christ M, Sharkova Y, Fenske H, et al: Brain natriuretic peptide for prediction of Cheyne-Stokes respiration in heart failure patients. Int J Cardiol 116:62–69, 2007.

have shown a high prevalence of both obstructive and central sleep apnea in patients with left ventricular systolic dysfunction. Table 13-2 shows the prevalence of central and obstructive sleep apnea in recent studies of patients with systolic heart failure. There has been considerable reported variation in the prevalence of these two forms of sleep apnea. The reported variations are due to a number of issues, such as the differentiation of obstructive from central hypopneas and the enrollment of obese patients, which increases the prevalence of OSA. Combining the results of the most recent series in the literature, as shown in Table 13-2, and using an AHI of 15 hours of sleep as the threshold, 31% of 1250 patients with systolic heart failure have central sleep apnea, or CSA, and 21% have OSA (Fig. 13-9).

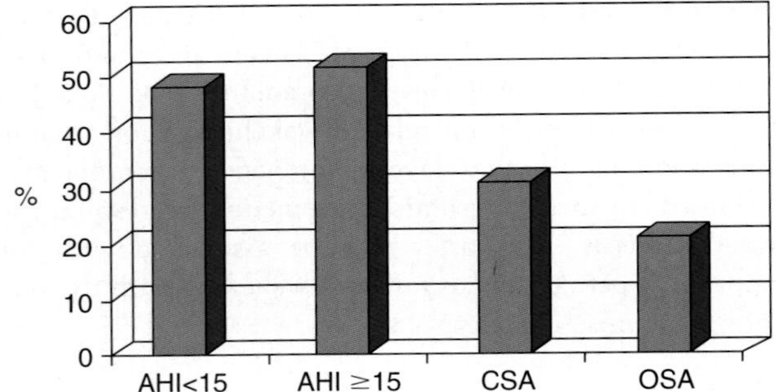

Figure 13-9.
Prevalence of sleep apnea in systolic heart failure (SHF). The data presented combine a series of world sleep studies (referenced in Table 13-2). AHI, apnea-hypopnea index; CSA, central sleep apnea; OSA, obstructive sleep apnea.

The hallmark of OSA in patients with systolic heart failure is similar to that in patients with OSA in the general population, in that such patients are obese and have habitual snoring. In contrast, patients with CSA are normally thinner than patients with OSA and the prevalence of habitual snoring is much less (Fig. 13-10). For these

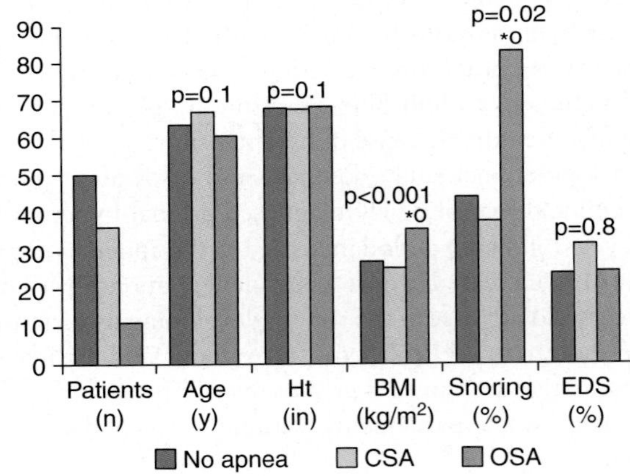

Figure 13-10.
Demographics, historical data, and physical examination findings in heart failure patients without sleep apnea, with central sleep apnea (CSA), and with obstructive sleep apnea (OSA). Patients with obstructive sleep apnea were more obese and had a higher prevalence of habitual snoring than patients with central sleep apnea. There was no difference in prevalence of excessive daytime sleepiness between the patients with heart failure and the patients without sleep apnea. BMI, body mass index; EDS, excessive daytime sleepiness; Ht, height. (Modified from Javaheri S: Sleep disorders in systolic heart failure: A prospective study of 100 male patients. The final report. Int J Cardiol 106:21–28, 2006.)

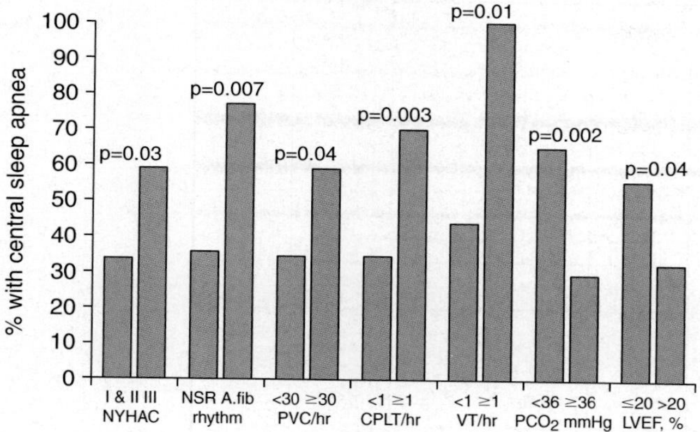

Figure 13-11.
Clinical and laboratory characteristics that are more likely to be associated with central sleep apnea. A.fib, atrial fibrillation; CPLT, couplets; LVEF, left ventricular ejection fraction; NSR, normal sinus rhythm; NYHAC, New York Heart Association Class; PVC, premature ventricular contractions; VT, ventricular tachycardia. (With permission from Javaheri S: Sleep disorders in systolic heart failure: A prospective study of 100 male patients. The final report. Int J Cardiol 106:21–28, 2006.)

reasons, the suspicion for the presence of CSA in cardiology and in primary care clinics is low, and so these patients often go undiagnosed. The risk factors for CSA in patients with systolic heart failure include a high New York Heart Association class, the presence of atrial fibrillation, greater than 30 premature ventricular excitations per hour of sleep, the presence of one or more couplets per hour of sleep, the presence of one or more ventricular tachycardias per hour of sleep, a low steady-state awake pCO_2 of less than 36 mmHg, and a left ventricular ejection fraction of less than 20% (Fig. 13-11). Meanwhile, it is emphasized that in our studies, the prevalence of excessive daytime sleepiness was similar in patients with systolic heart failure with or without CSA and/or OSA (see Fig. 13-10). This further contributes to the under-recognition of sleep apnea in patients with systolic heart failure.

Abnormal Breathing Patterns in Heart Failure

Figures 13-12 and 13-13 show examples of CSA and Hunter–Cheyne Stokes breathing in patients with heart failure. Although usually called Cheyne Stokes breathing, John Hunter was the first physician (37 years before Cheyne) to describe this breathing pattern. The abnormal breathing pattern may occur during wakefulness in such patients. The cycle time of the periodic breathing may be quite long (exceeding a minute) in cases of severe heart failure. Note the decrescendo and crescendo changes in thoracoabdominal excursions, which sandwich the CSA. During CSA (in contrast to OSA; see Fig. 13-2), esophageal pressure remains flat (see Fig. 13-12). Another difference between OSA and CSA is that in the latter arousals occur at the peak of hyperventilation (see Fig. 13-12) and not at the termination of the apnea. In common with OSA, CSA causes hypoxemia (not as

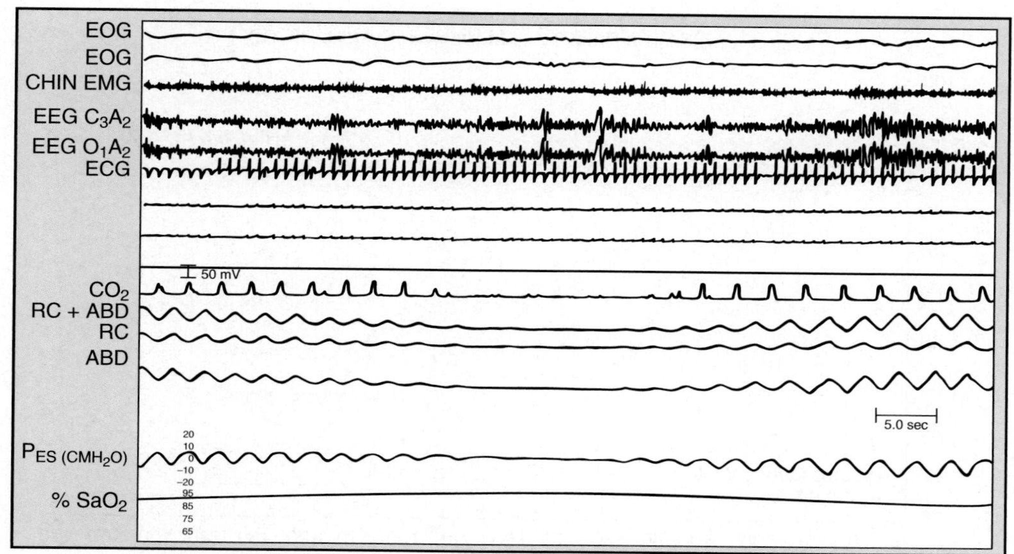

Figure 13-12.
An example of Hunter–Cheyne Stokes breathing in a patient with systolic heart failure. Note the crescendo/decrescendo changes in thoracoabdominal excursion and naso-oral airflow that sandwich central apnea. (With permission from Dowdell WT, Javaheri S, McGinnis W: Cheyne-Stokes respiration presenting as sleep apnea syndrome: Clinical and polysomnographic features. Am Rev Respir Dis 141:871–879, 1990.)

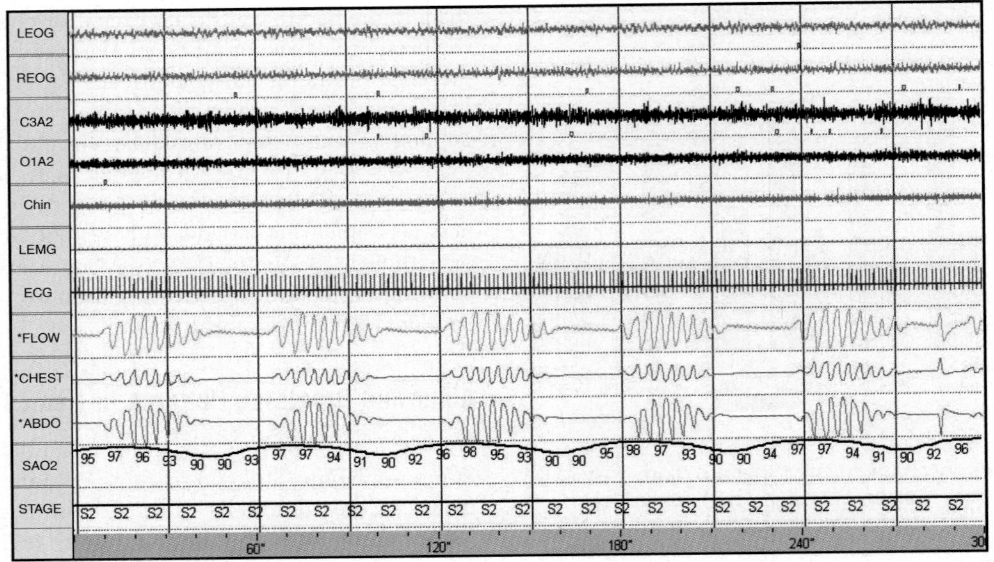

Figure 13-13.
A 10-minute epoch of a patient with systolic heart failure and Hunter–Cheyne Stokes breathing. Note recurrent hypoxia/reoxygenation as a result of central sleep apnea.

severely as does OSA)/reoxygenation (see Fig. 13-13), and negative swings (not as pronounced as in OSA) in intrathoracic pressure during the hyperpneic phase of breathing (see Fig. 13-12). Therefore, similar to OSA, the pathophysiologic consequences of CSA could result in worsening and progression of left ventricular dysfunction in the form of a vicious circle. CSA is a predictor of mortality in patients with systolic heart failure (Fig. 13-14). In this study only three variables independently predicted poor survival: the presence of CSA (see Fig. 13-14), the severity of right ventricular systolic dysfunction, and a low diastolic blood pressure.

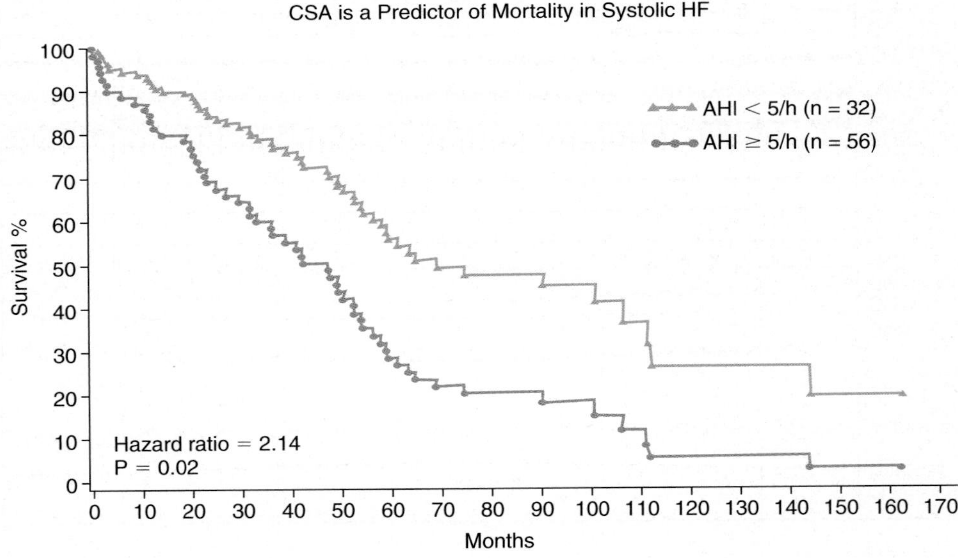

Figure 13-14.
Probability of survival in patients with systolic heart failure according to the presence or absence of central sleep apnea (CSA). AHI, apnea-hypopnea index. (Modified from Javaheri S, Shukla R, Zeigler H, Wexler L: Central sleep apnea, right ventricular dysfunction, and low diastolic blood pressure are predictors of mortality in systolic heart failure. J Am Coll Cardiol 49:2028–2034, 2007.)

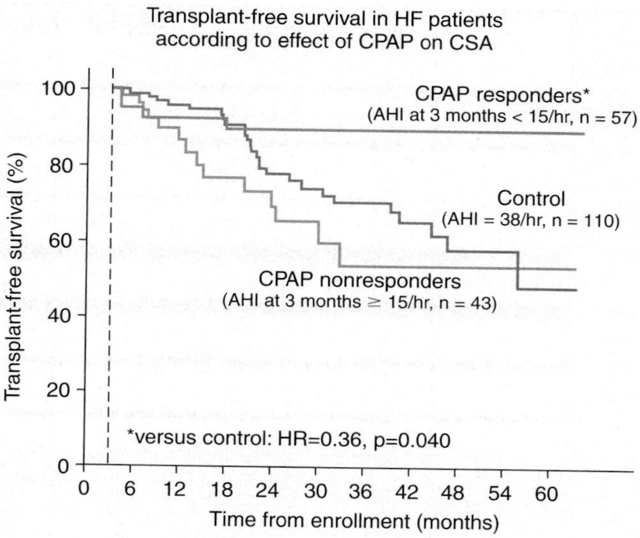

Figure 13-15.
Probability of survival in patients with systolic heart failure (HF) comparing continuous positive airway pressure (CPAP) responders to a control group (patients with systolic heart failure and similar apnea-hypopnea index [AHI]) and to CPAP nonresponders. CPAP responders had a significantly increased probability of survival compared to the control group. CPAP nonresponders tended to have a poor survival when compared to the control group, although this was not significant. CSA, central sleep apnea; HR, hazard ratio. (Modified from Artz M, Floras JS, Logan AG, et al: Suppression of central sleep apnea by continuous positive airway pressure and transplant-free survival in heart failure. Circulation 115:3173–3180, 2007.)

TREATMENT OF THE ABNORMAL BREATHING PATTERN IN HEART FAILURE

Central Apnea

The result of our study showing that CSA is a risk factor for mortality in patients with systolic heart failure is consistent with the result of the post hoc analysis of a continuous positive airway pressure (CPAP) trial examining the effects of treatment. In this study (reported on by M. Artz et al.), CPAP-suppressed CSA patients experienced a greater increase in left ventricular ejection fraction at 3 months and significantly better transplant-free survival (Fig. 13-15). The survival of patients with systolic heart failure who remained CPAP nonresponsive was worse than that of the control group, although the difference was not significant, perhaps because the number of patients was small.

We hypothesize that patients with heart failure who remain unresponsive to CPAP may further suffer from adverse central hemodynamic effects of the CPAP. Specifically, CPAP increases intrathoracic pressure, which could diminish right ventricular venous return and stroke volume resulting in a low diastolic blood pressure. As noted in our study, both right ventricular systolic dysfunction and low diastolic blood pressure were predictors of mortality.

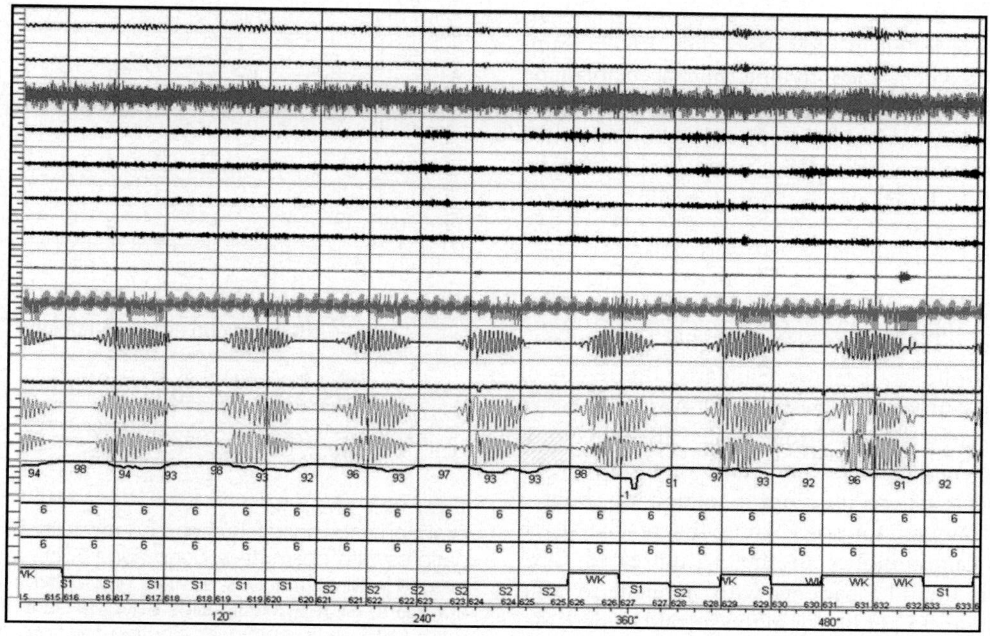

Figure 13-16.
An example of persistent central sleep apnea with Hunter–Cheyne Stokes breathing in a patient with systolic heart failure while on continuous positive airway pressure of 6 cm H_2O.

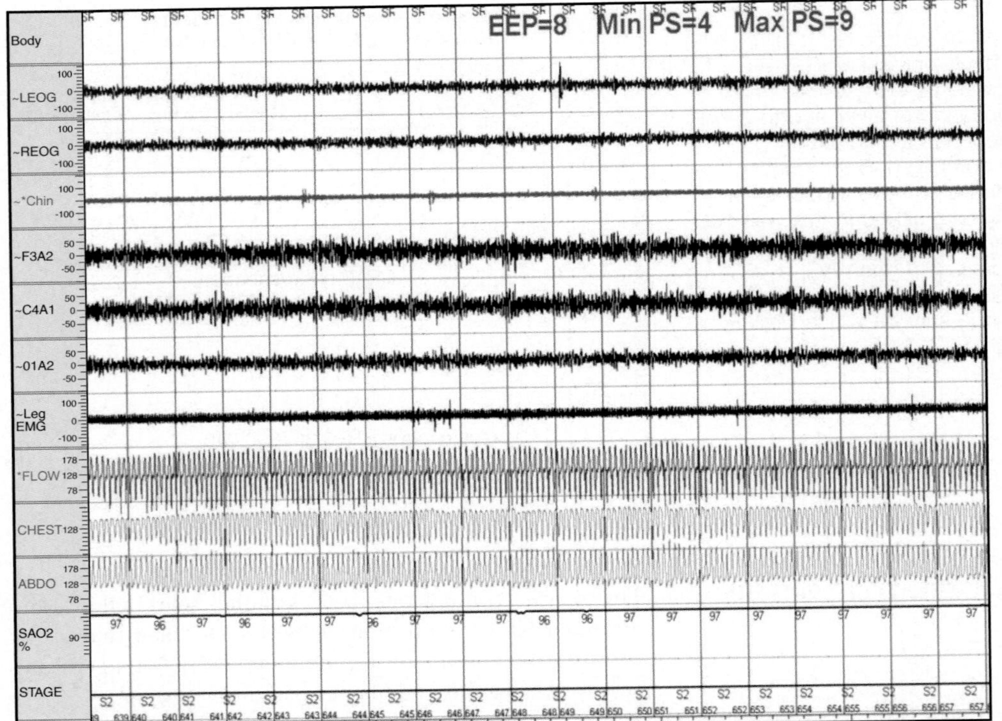

Figure 13-17.
An example of a patient with systolic heart failure on continuous positive airway pressure with persistent central sleep apnea (CSA). The patient's CSA was eliminated by therapy with a pressure support servo-ventilation device. At this time, the end-expiratory pressure (EEP) was 8 cm H_2O, the minimum inspiratory support (PS) was 4, and the maximum inspiratory support was 9 cm H_2O.

Because use of CPAP could affect these hemodynamic parameters adversely, it could increase the mortality of heart failure patients whose CSA remains CPAP nonresponsive. Figure 13-16 shows an example of such a patient with systolic heart failure who continues to have CSA while on CPAP. A new device, pressure support servoventilation, may prove useful in such cases (Fig. 13-17). Supplemental nasal oxygen, theophylline, and acetazolamide have been used to treat CSA in patients with systolic heart failure. Randomized, double-blind, placebo-controlled studies have demonstrated the therapeutic efficacy of these medications. Long-term studies on mortality are not available.

Obstructive Apnea

As noted earlier, OSA, like CSA, is highly prevalent in patients with systolic heart failure. Similarly, the results of two recent studies strongly suggest that OSA is a risk factor for mortality in patients with systolic heart failure. In a prospective study, Wang and associates followed 164 patients with systolic heart failure for a mean period of about 3 years. After accounting for some confounders, the death rate was significantly higher in the 37 untreated OSA patients than in the 113 patients with minimal to mild OSA (AHI less than 15 per hour). In the second study Kasai and associates showed that effective treatment of OSA with CPAP improved survival of heart failure patients. In this observational study, the risk of death and hospitalization

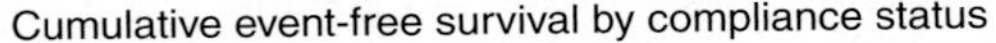

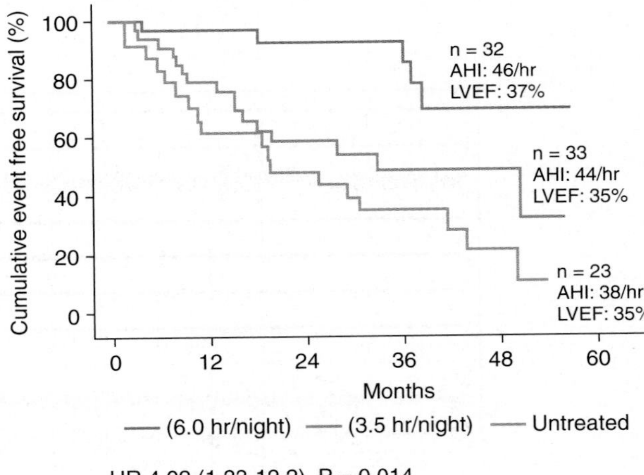

Figure 13-18.
Probability for hospitalization and mortality of heart failure patients with obstructive sleep apnea decrease if they are treated with continuous positive airway pressure (CPAP) and adhere to therapy. AHI, apnea-hypopnea index; HR, hazard ratio; LVEF, left ventricular ejection fraction. (Modified from Kasai T, Narui K, Dohi P, et al: Prognosis of patients with heart failure and obstructive sleep apnea treated with continuous positive airway pressure. Chest 133:690–696, 2008.)

was increased in the untreated compared with the CPAP-treated group (hazard ratio 2.03, CI = 1.07; 23.68, p = 0.03). Furthermore, heart failure patients with OSA who were compliant with CPAP had better survival than those who were noncompliant (Fig. 13-18). Thus, OSA, like CSA, is a risk factor for mortality in patients with systolic heart failure. Also similar to the results seen in CSA, those who are compliant with CPAP and whose sleep apnea is effectively treated by CPAP have better survival.

SELECTED READINGS

Artz M, Floras JS, Logan AG, et al: Suppression of central sleep apnea by continuous positive airway pressure and transplant-free survival in heart failure. Circulation 115:3173–3180, 2007.

Becker HF, Javaheri S: Systemic and pulmonary arterial hypertension in obstructive sleep apnea. In Lee Chiong T (ed): Sleep Medicine Clinics: Sleep and Cardiovascular Disease. Philadelphia, WB Saunders, 549–557, 2007.

Becker HF, Jerrentrup A, Ploch TH, et al: Effect of nasal continuous positive airway pressure treatment on blood pressure in patients with obstructive sleep apnea. Circulation 107:68–73, 2003.

Chobanian AV, Bakris GL, Black HR, et al: Blood Institute Joint National Committee on Prevention, Detection, Evaluation, and Treatment of High Blood Pressure: The JNC 7 report. JAMA 289:2560–2571, 2003.

Coughlin SR, Mawdsley L, Mugarza JA, et al: Cardiovascular and metabolic effects of CPAP in obese males with OSA. Eur Respir J 29: 720–727, 2007.

Gami AS, Howard DE, Olson EJ, et al: Day-night pattern of sudden death in obstructive sleep apnea. New Engl J Med 352:1206–1214, 2005.

Heart disease and stroke statistics—2008 update. Circulation 117: e25–e146, 2008.

Javaheri S. CPAP should not be used for central sleep apnea in congestive heart failure patients. J Clin Sleep Med 2:399–402, 2006.

Javaheri S, Parker TJ, Wexler L, et al: Occult sleep-disordered breathing in stable congestive heart failure. Ann Intern Med 122:487–492, 1995.

Javaheri S, Shukla R, Zeigler H, Wexler L: Central sleep apnea, right ventricular dysfunction, and low diastolic blood pressure are predictors of mortality in systolic heart failure. J Am Coll Cardiol 49:2028–2034, 2007.

Kapa S, Javaheri S, Somers V: Obstructive sleep apnea and arrhythmias. In Javaheri S (ed), Lee Chiong T (guest ed): Sleep Medicine Clinics: Sleep and Cardiovascular Disease. Philadelphia, WB Saunders, 2007, pp. 575–581.

Kasai T, Narui K, Dohi P, et al: Prognosis of patients with heart failure and obstructive sleep apnea treated with continuous positive airway pressure. Chest 133:690–696, 2008.

Marin JM, Carrizo SJ, Vicente E, et al: Long-term cardiovascular outcomes in men with obstructive sleep apnea-hypopnea with or without treatment with continuous positive airway pressure: Observational studies. The Lancet 365:1046–1053, 2005.

Peker Y, Hender J, Norum J, et al: Increased incidence of cardiovascular disease in middle-aged men with obstructive sleep apnea. Am J Respir Crit Care Med 166:159–165, 2002.

Peppard PE, Young T, Palta M, Skatrud J: Prospective study of the association between sleep-disordered breathing and hypertension. N Engl J Med 342(19):1378–1384, 2000.

Pepperell JCT, Ramdassingh-Dow S, Crosthwaite N, et al: Ambulatory blood pressure after therapeutic and subtherapeutic nasal continuous positive airway pressure for obstructive sleep apnea: A randomized parallel trial. The Lancet 359:204–210, 2002.

Wang H, Parker JE, Newton GE, et al: Influence of obstructive sleep apnea on mortality in patients with heart failure. J Am Coll Cardiol 49: 1625–1631, 2007.

Young T, Finn L, Peppard PE, et al: Sleep-disordered breathing and mortality: Eighteen-year follow-up of the Wisconsin Sleep Cohort. Sleep 31:1071–1078, 2008.

Young T, Javaheri S: Systemic and pulmonary hypertension in obstructive sleep apnea. In Kryger MH, Roth T, Dement WC (eds): Principles and Practices of Sleep Medicine, 4th ed. Philadelphia, WB Saunders, 2005, pp. 1192–1202.

CHAPTER 14 OTHER MEDICAL DISORDERS

14.1 Thyroid Disease

Meir Kryger

The main function of the thyroid gland is to produce thyroid hormone, which plays a critical role in metabolism. Sleep can be impacted by three types of thyroid abnormalities: hyperthyroidism, hypothyroidism, and thyroid mass lesions.

Hyperthyroidism

In hyperthyroidism, too much hormone is present, resulting in general symptoms and sleep-related symptoms and findings, which are described in Table 14.1-1, Boxes 14.1-1 and 14.1-2, and Figures 14.1-1 to 14.1-7.

Table 14.1-1. Causes of Hyperthyroidism

CAUSES	FEATURES
Graves' disease	Hyperthyroidism, goiter, ophthalmopathy, pretibial myxedema. May remit
Toxic goiter	Due to hypersecretion of thyroid stimulating hormone. Does not usually remit
Thyroiditis	Hyperthyroidism during acute phase. May "burn out" leading to hypothyroidism
Related to drugs	Lithium and amiodarone are causes

BOX 14.1-2. SLEEP FINDINGS IN HYPERTHYROIDISM

- Nightmares
- Insomnia
- Night sweats
- Tachycardia
- Atrial arrhythmias

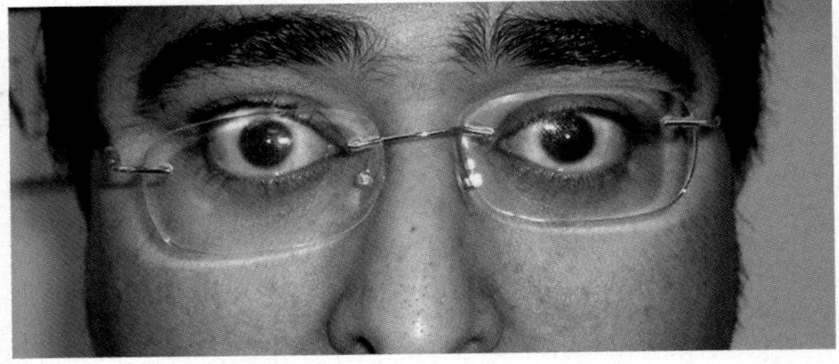

Figure 14.1-1.
The thyroid stare.

BOX 14.1-1. SYMPTOMS OF HYPERTHYROIDISM

RELATED TO EXCESSIVE HORMONE

- Weight loss
- Heat intolerance
- Tremor
- Excessive sweating
- Thyroid "stare"
- Changes in skin and hair
- Palpitations
- Atrial arrhythmias
- Frequent bowel movements
- In elderly may present with "apathetic hyperthyroidism" with symptoms suggesting dementia or depression

RELATED TO GRAVES' DISEASE

- Infiltration of extraocular muscles leads to ophthalmopathy (exophthalmos, lymphocytic infiltration of extraocular muscles); may lead to eye muscle weakness, causing double vision.
- Infiltration of skin over the shins leads to non-pitting pretibial myxedema.

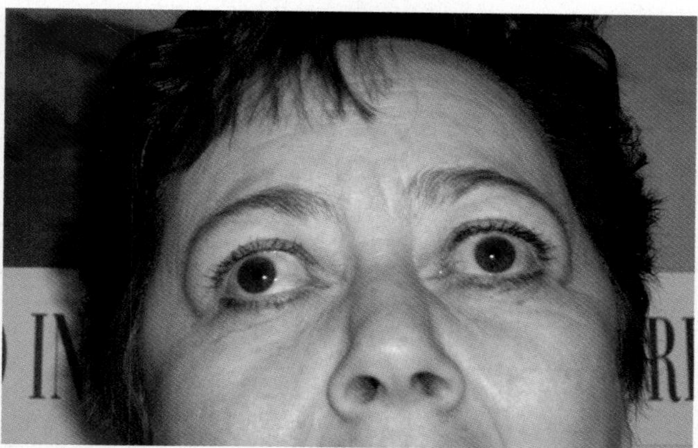

Figure 14.1-2.
Graves' ophthalmopathy; corneal injection and proptosis.

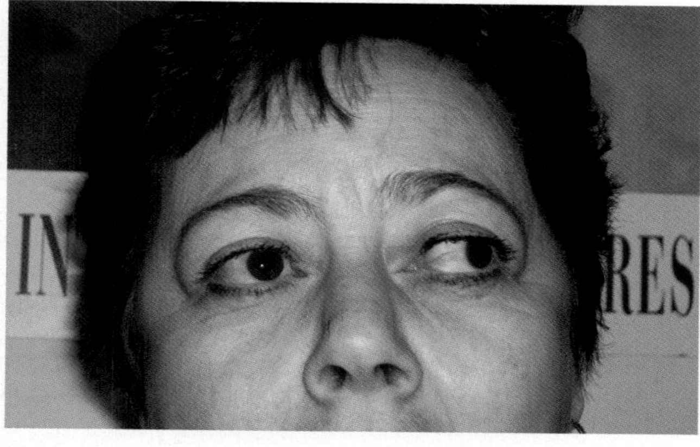

Figure 14.1-3.
Graves' ophthalmopathy; extraocular muscle weakness on left lateral gaze. The patient complained of double vision.

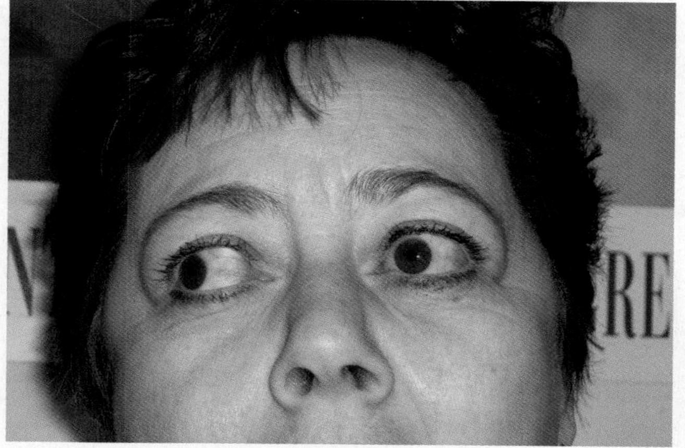

Figure 14.1-4.
Graves' ophthalmopathy; extraocular muscle weakness on right lateral gaze.

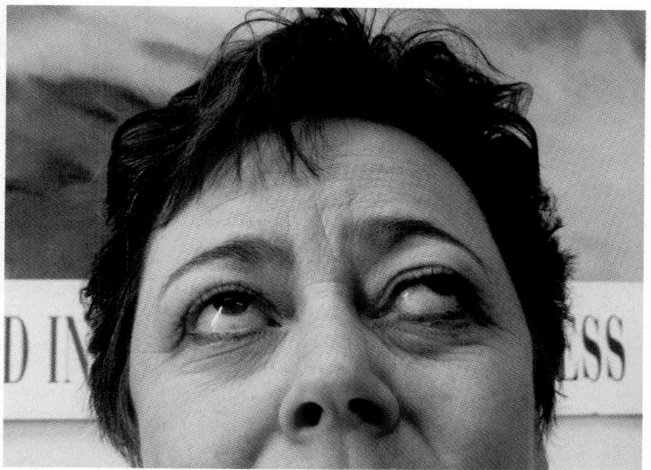

Figure 14.1-5.
Graves' ophthalmopathy; extraocular muscle weakness on upward gaze.

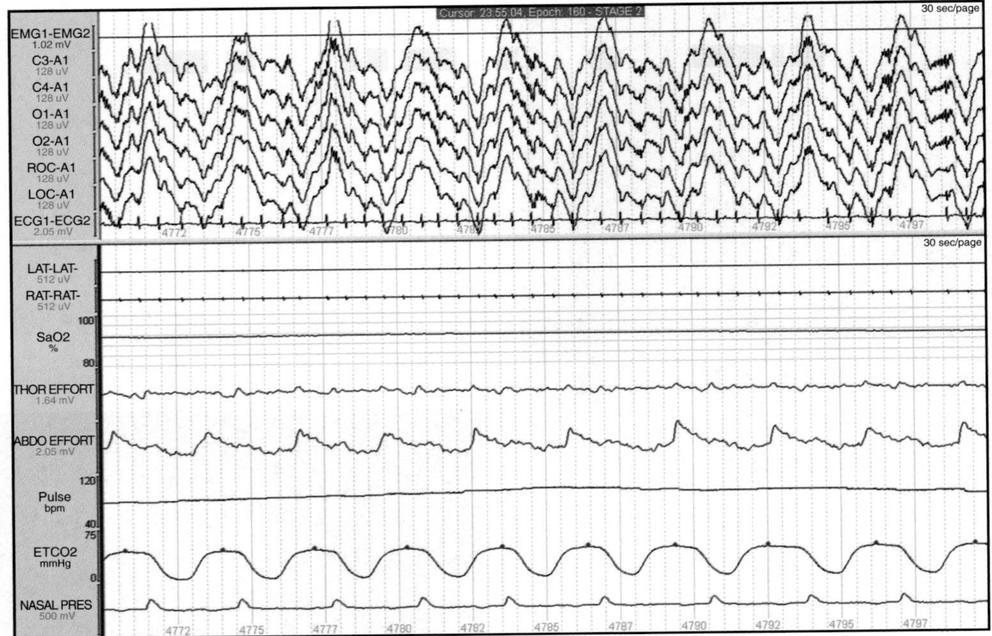

Figure 14.1-6.
Polysomnogram of sweat artifact. Note the high amplitude swings in all the electroencephalogram (EEG) channels in synchrony with breathing. This patient had night sweats. Hyperthyroidism was first suspected from this finding and the newly noted atrial fibrillation. Top and bottom windows are 30-second epochs.

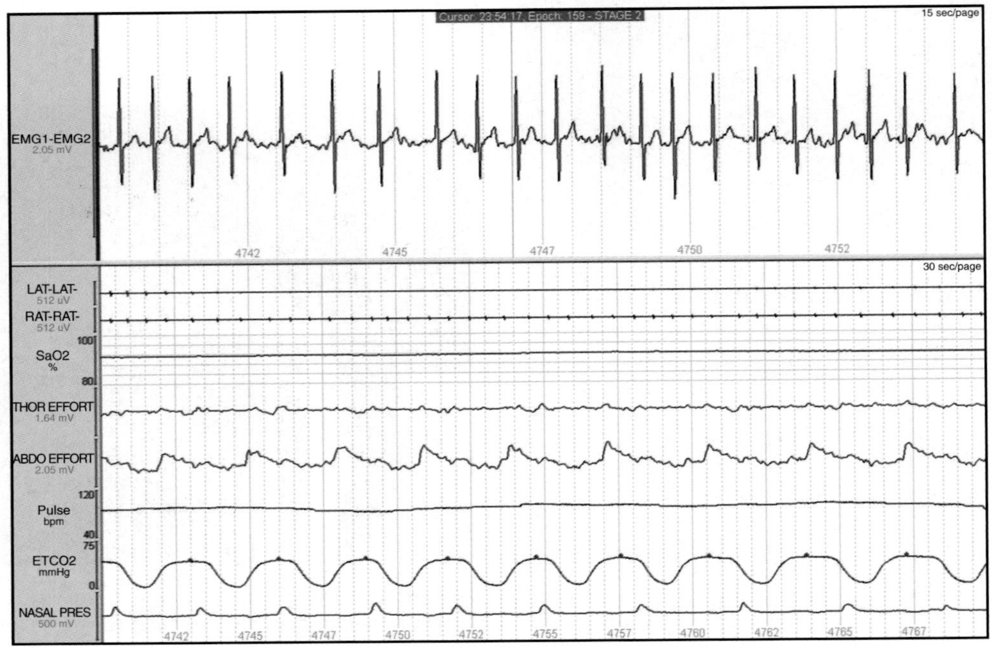

Figure 14.1-7.
Same patient as Figure 14.1-6. This figure highlights the finding of atrial fibrillation. The electrocardiogram (EKG) panel shows a 15-second epoch.

Hypothyroidism

The features of hypothyroidism are described in Table 14.1-2, Boxes 14.1-3 and 14.1-4, and Figures 14.1-8 to 14.1-14.

Table 14.1-2. Causes of Hypothyroidism

CAUSES	FEATURES
Primary	May occur after "burnt out" thyroiditis
Secondary to radio- or medical therapy of thyroid disease	
Iodine deficiency	
Drug induced	Lithium, amiodarone

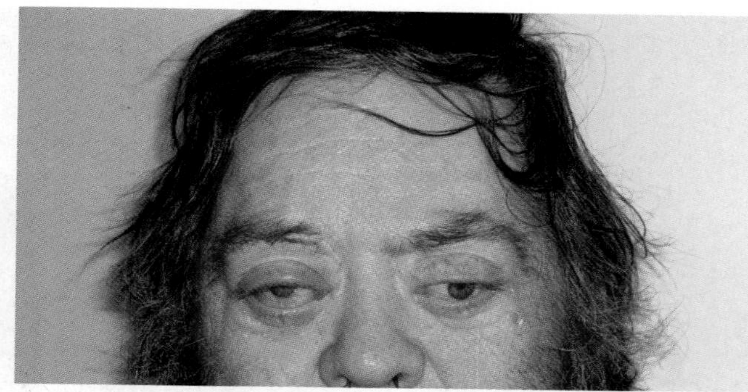

Figure 14.1-8.
"Burnt-out" Graves' disease. This patient who had been treated for Graves' disease developed severe hypothyroidism with obesity and sleepiness and was found to have severe obstructive sleep apnea. Note the conjunctival injection and the droopy lids.

BOX 14.1-3. SYMPTOMS OF HYPOTHYROIDISM

- Weight gain
- Cold intolerance
- Changes in skin and hair (dry, coarse, hair loss)
- Macroglossia
- Hoarse voice
- Puffiness around eyes
- Constipation
- Changes in personality

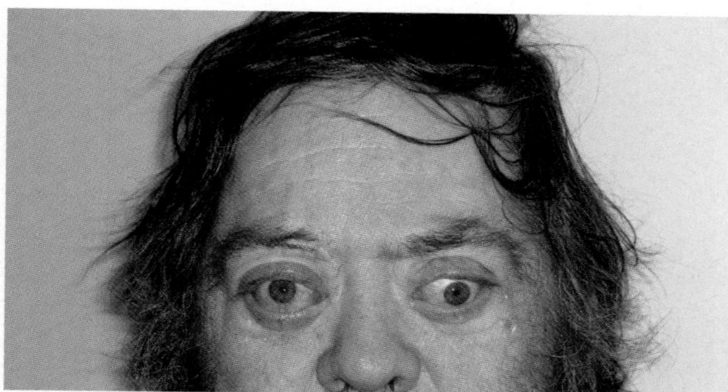

Figure 14.1-9.
When the patient is focusing and alert the eye signs of proptosis and the asymmetry of eye movements become apparent.

BOX 14.1-4. SLEEP FINDINGS IN HYPOTHYROIDISM

- Obstructive sleep apnea
- May develop respiratory failure
- Excessive sleepiness
- Bradycardia

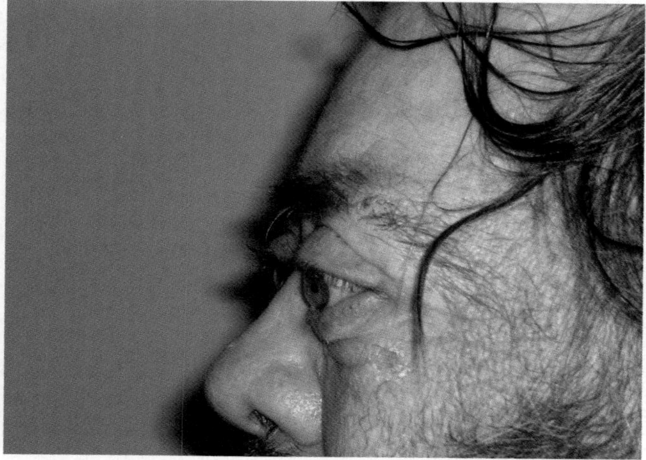

Figure 14.1-10.
The bulging eyes (exophthalmos) of Graves' disease.

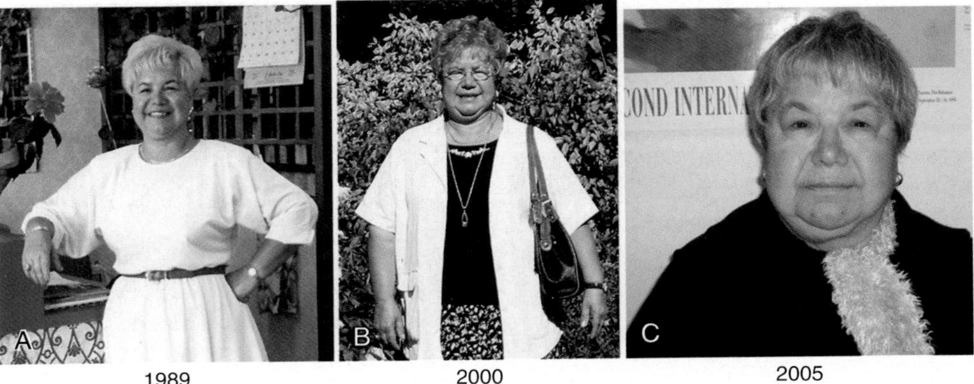

Figure 14.1-11.
A to **C,** This figure shows the development of hypothyroidism over time. The patient developed coarse facial features, puffy eyes, and cold intolerance. Note that the patient is wearing a scarf indoors.

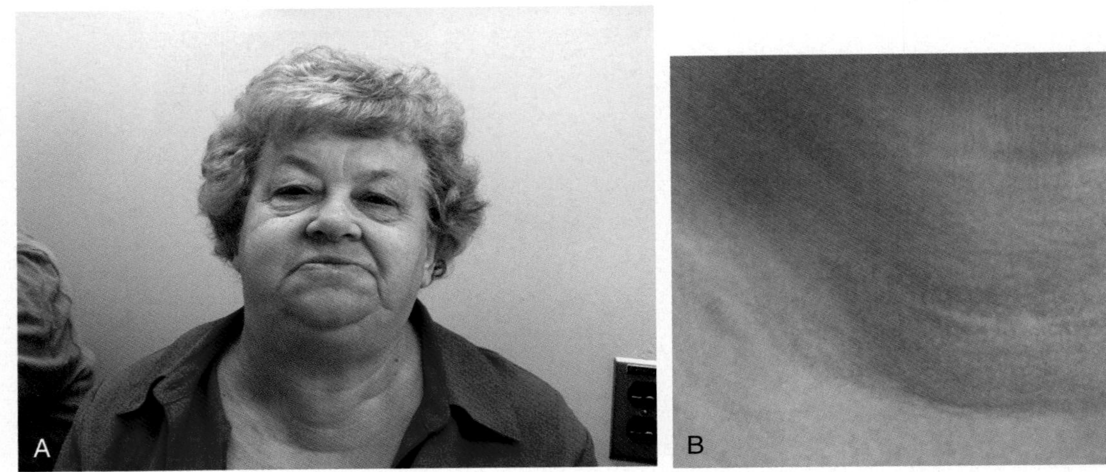

Figure 14.1-12.
Features of hypothyroidism. **A,** Puffy eyes. **B,** Fullness in neck and scar from thyroid surgery.

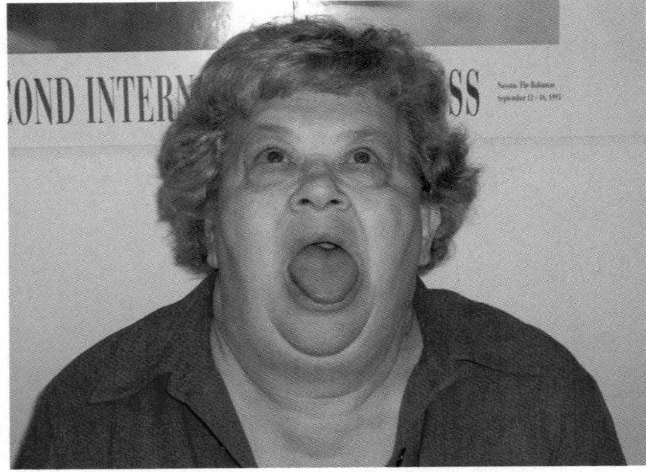

Figure 14.1-13.
Features of hypothyroidism. Macroglossia fills up the mouth, impinging on the oropharyngeal airway.

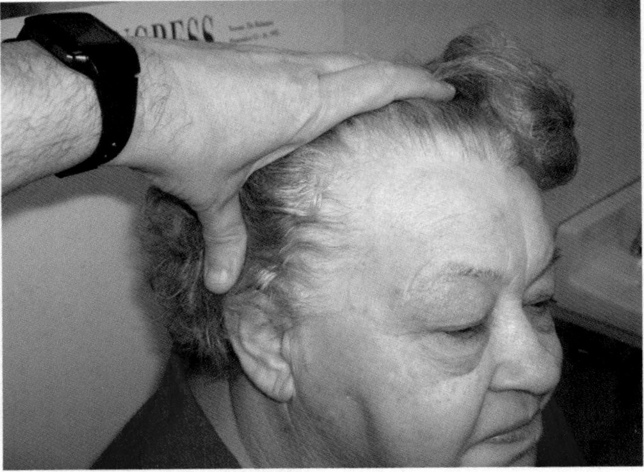

Figure 14.1-14.
Features of hypothyroidism. Brittle, sparse hair and receding hairline. Loss of hair on eyebrows.

Thyroid Mass Lesions

See Boxes 14.1-5 and 14.1-6 and Figures 14.1-15 and 14.1-16.

BOX 14.1-5. TYPES OF THYROID MASS LESIONS

- Idiopathic goiter
- Secondary to radiotherapy or medical therapy of thyroid disease
- Iodine deficiency
- Tumors

BOX 14.1-6. SLEEP FINDINGS WITH THYROID MASS LESIONS

- Snoring
- Apnea
- Stridor

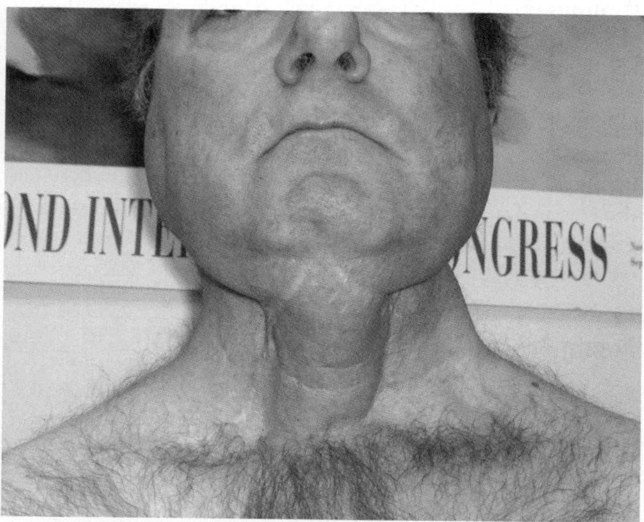

Figure 14.1-15.
This patient had severe sleep apnea with stridor. He had previously had a radical neck dissection for thyroid cancer that had invaded the trachea. The sternocleidomastoid muscles had been removed.

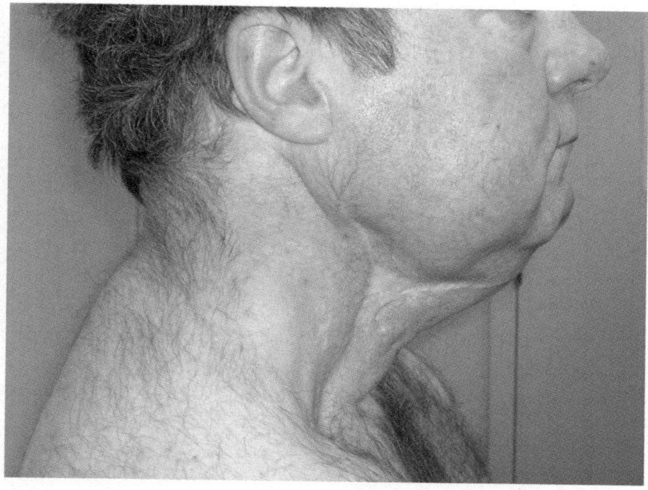

Figure 14.1-16.
Lateral view of same patient as in Figure 14.1-15.

SELECTED READINGS

Erden S, Cagatay T, Buyukozturk S, et al: Hashimoto thyroiditis and obstructive sleep apnea syndrome: Is there any relation between them? Eur J Med Res 9(12):570–572, 2004.

Misiolek M, Marek B, Namyslowski G, et al: Sleep apnea syndrome and snoring in patients with hypothyroidism with relation to overweight. J Physiol Pharmacol 58(Suppl1):77–85, 2007.

Resta O, Carratù P, Carpagnano GE, et al: Influence of subclinical hypothyroidism and T4 treatment on the prevalence and severity of obstructive sleep apnoea syndrome (OSAS). J Endocrinol Invest 28(10):893–898, 2005.

Resta O, Pannacciulli N, Di Gioia G, et al: High prevalence of previously unknown subclinical hypothyroidism in obese patients referred to a sleep clinic for sleep disordered breathing. Nutr Metab Cardiovasc Dis 14(5):248–253, 2004.

Meir Kryger

14.2 Growth Hormone Hypersecretion

Pathophysiology

Hypersecretion of growth hormone can result in metabolic abnormalities and anatomic changes of skeletal and soft tissue structures. These may result in obstructive sleep apnea (OSA). The most common cause of excess secretion of growth hormone is a pituitary tumor (Fig. 14.2-1), and the clinical presentation (Box 14.2-1) is related to the age of the patient, the local effects of the enlarging tumor on the structures in and around the pituitary gland, and the resulting metabolic and anatomical changes. When these result in orofacial changes (Figs. 14.2-2 to 14.2-5) the patient may develop OSA.

About 60% to 80% of acromegaly patients have sleep apnea. In about two thirds of the cases with sleep-disordered breathing the apnea is obstructive, while in a third it is central. Some

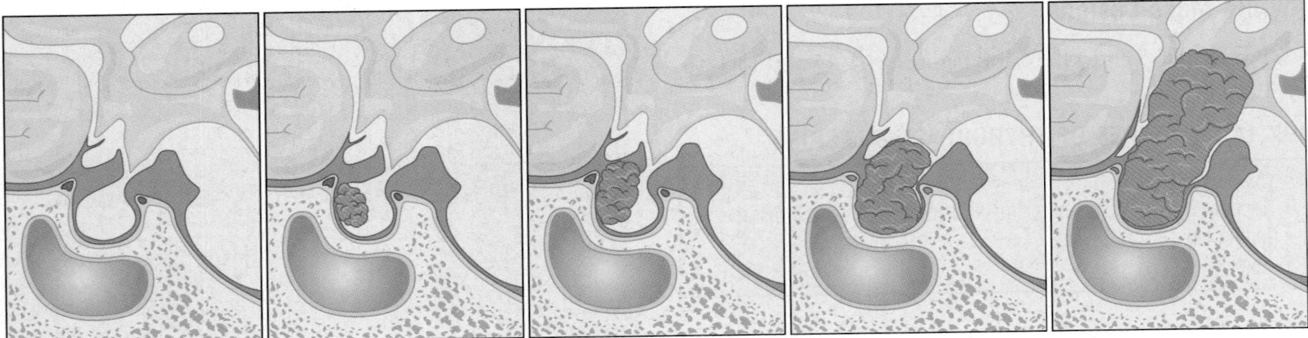

Figure 14.2-1.
An enlarging pituitary adenoma compresses structures in and around the pituitary gland.

patients may have a waxing and waning breathing pattern. The finding that many cases do not have obstructive apnea suggests that abnormal control of breathing may be present.

When growth hormone excess occurs while a child is still growing, there is a marked increase in height, and the condition is termed *gigantism*. When the growth hormone hypersecretion occurs after growth has ceased, the condition is called *acromegaly* (see Fig. 14.2-1).

Clinical Findings

Patients with growth hormone excess have characteristic physical and laboratory findings, some of which remain after successful surgical treatment. Some of the changes evolve slowly with time (Figs. 14.2-6 and 14.2-7).

Diagnosis

Patients with acromegaly or gigantism generally require multispecialty management especially if they are initially untreated. Collaboration between specialists in endocrinology and neurosurgery is usually necessary. Sleep specialists are often involved when sleep symptoms develop. Usually they are the classical ones of OSA and will usually require polysomnography (see chapter 11.2). Confirmation of sleep apnea is generally identical to what is done for the typical OSA patient.

Treatment

Besides the treatment of the pituitary adenoma, treatment of the chemical abnormalities has been reported. With bromocriptine the percentage of sleep time in apnea or hypopnea

BOX 14.2-1. CLINICAL FEATURES OF ACROMEGALY

- Sleep apnea syndrome
- Due to compression caused by pituitary adenoma
  - Visual field defects
  - Hypopituitarism, hyperprolactinemia, hypogonadism, galactorrhea
- Direct growth hormone consequences
  - Impaired glucose tolerance and diabetes mellitus
- Soft tissue abnormalities (see Figs. 14.2-3 and 14.2-5)
  - Myopathy
  - Soft tissue enlargement of nose, tongue, larynx, visceral organs
  - Thick skin
- Bony changes (see Figs. 14.2-4,14.2-6, and 14.2-7)
  - Enlargement of hands and feet
  - Osteoarthritis
  - Prognathia and increased interdental spacing
  - Frontal bossing
- Others
  - Hypertension
  - Enlarged heart
  - Heart failure

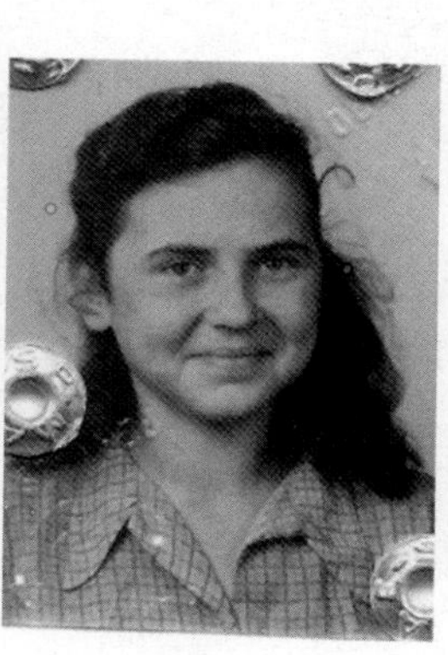

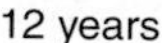

12 years

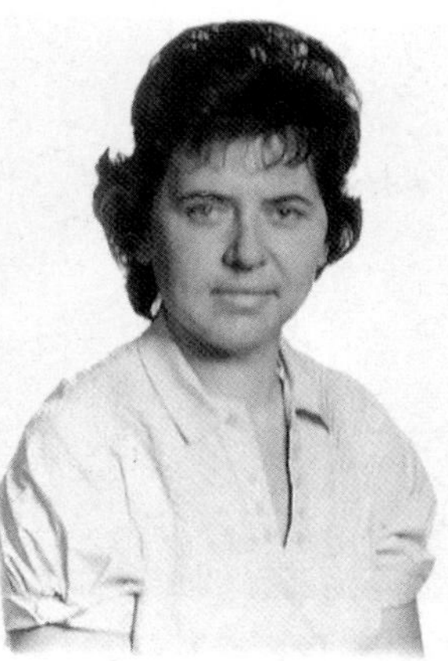

25 years

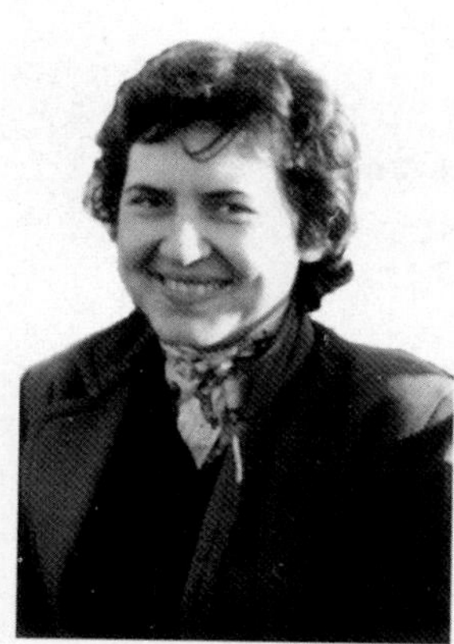

30 years

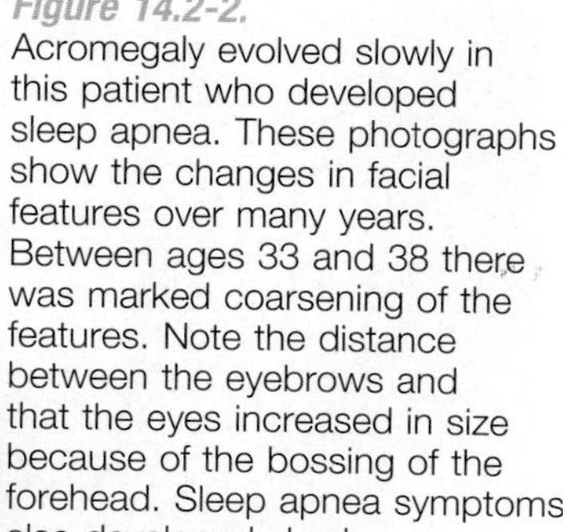

Figure 14.2-2.
Acromegaly evolved slowly in this patient who developed sleep apnea. These photographs show the changes in facial features over many years. Between ages 33 and 38 there was marked coarsening of the features. Note the distance between the eyebrows and that the eyes increased in size because of the bossing of the forehead. Sleep apnea symptoms also developed slowly.

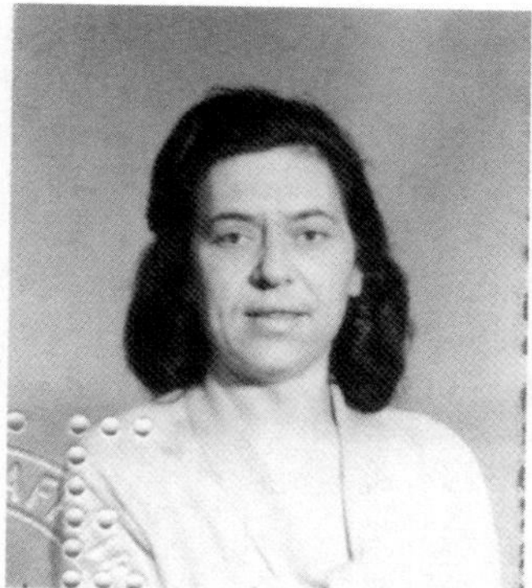

33 years

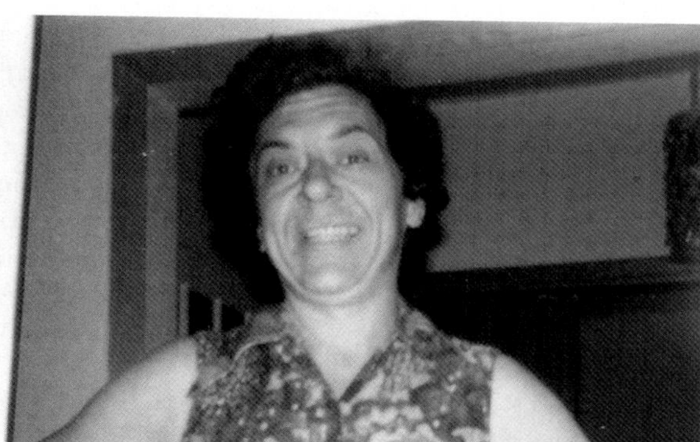

38 years

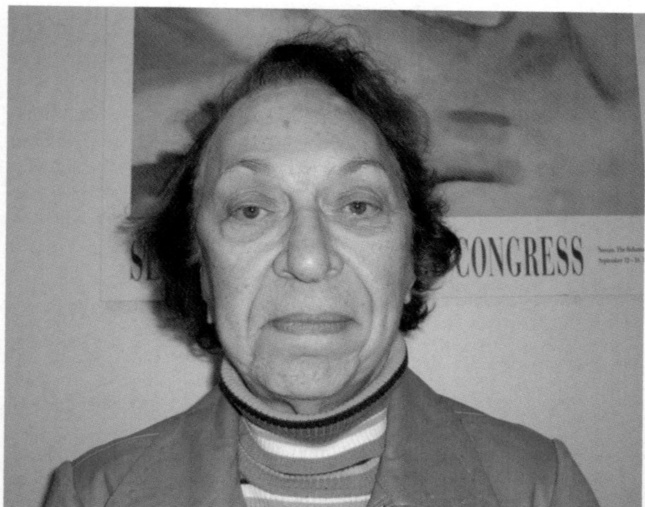

Figure 14.2-3.
The same patient as in Figure 14.2-2. She is now in her sixties. There is a large jaw, large nose, frontal bossing, coarse facial features, thick skin, and deep facial creases. The sleep apnea is believed to be due to the anatomic changes including the enlarged tongue and the abnormal jaw structure. This patient has severe obstructive sleep apnea and has been on nasal continuous positive airway pressure for several years.

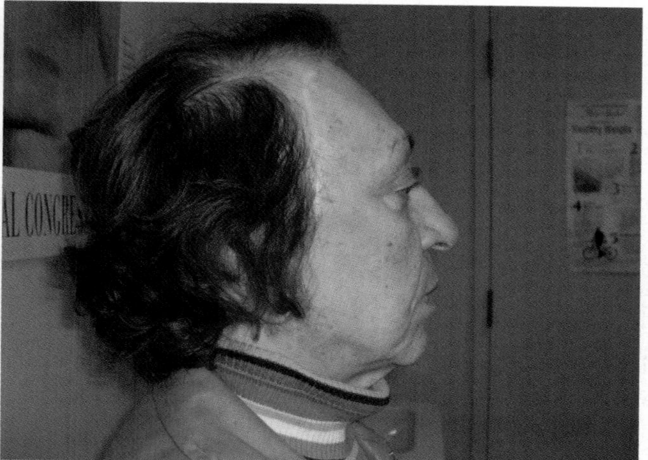

Figure 14.2-4.
Note the frontal bossing and the healed scar from the surgery she had to treat the pituitary tumor. In some patients the lower jaw juts forward (prognathism).

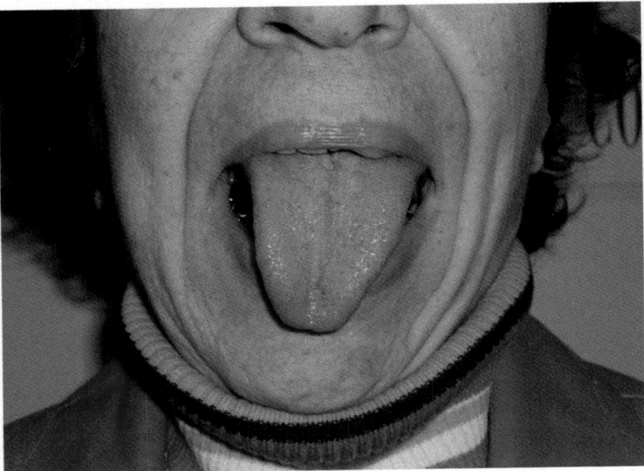

Figure 14.2-5.
The patient has a large tongue.

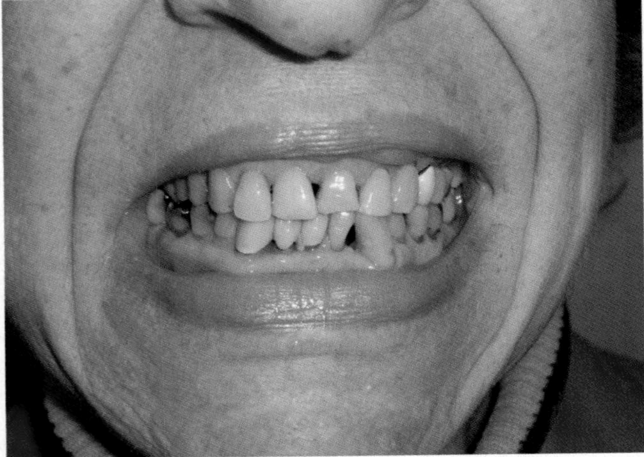

Figure 14.2-6.
Examination of the lower jaw and dental structures reveals the changes of acromegaly, which include increased space between teeth caused by enlargement of the jaw.

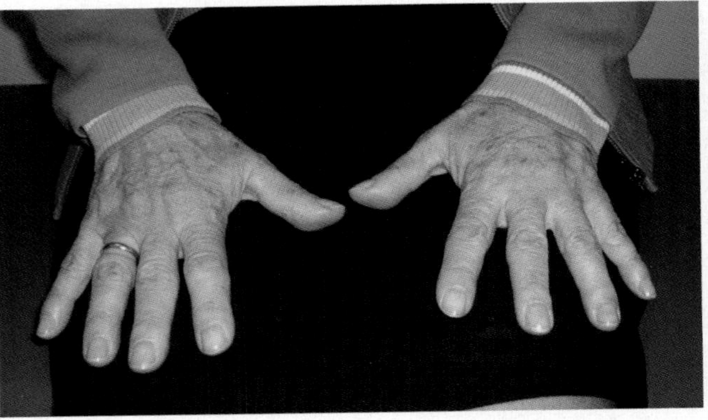

Figure 14.2-7.
One of the first symptoms the patient noted was enlargement of her hands.

dropped by 75%. Octreotide, a somatostatin analog, reduced the apnea-hypopnea index from 39 to 19. Normalization of growth levels following transsphenoidal adenomectomy may cure sleep apnea and improve insulin resistance and hypertension. However, the acromegalic skeletal abnormalities may be irreversible. Also, apneic episodes may continue after normalization of hormonal levels, and thus patients may require continuous positive airway pressure therapy.

SELECTED READINGS

Sze L, Schmid C, Bloch KE, et al: Effect of transsphenoidal surgery on sleep apnoea in acromegaly. Eur J Endocrinol 156(3):321–329, 2007.

Tolis G, Angelopoulos NG, Katounda E, et al: Medical treatment of acromegaly: Comorbidities and their reversibility by somatostatin analogs. Neuroendocrinology 83(3–4):249–257, 2006.

van Haute FR, Taboada GF, Corrêa LL, et al: Prevalence of sleep apnea and metabolic abnormalities in patients with acromegaly and analysis of cephalometric parameters by magnetic resonance imaging. Eur J Endocrinol 158(4):459–465, 2008.

Veasey SC, Guilleminault C, Strohl KP, et al: Medical therapy for obstructive sleep apnea: A review by the Medical Therapy for Obstructive Sleep Apnea Task Force of the Standards of Practice Committee of the American Academy of Sleep Medicine. Sleep 29(8):1036–1044, 2006.

Watson NF, Vitiello MV: Management of obstructive sleep apnea in acromegaly. Sleep Medicine 8(5):539–540, 2007.

14.3 Gastrointestinal Disorders

William C. Orr

Nocturnal Gastrointestinal Symptoms

The manifestation of gastrointestinal symptoms during sleep is quite familiar to the practicing gastroenterologist. Perhaps the most obvious and common example is the occurrence of epigastric pain characteristically awakening the patient from sleep in the early morning hours. Patients may also have awakenings from sleep with symptoms that ostensibly are not related to gastrointestinal disorders. For example, sleep disturbance is a common symptom among patients with irritable bowel syndrome (IBS) and dyspepsia.

BOX 14.3-1. EXAMPLES OF NOCTURNAL GASTROINTESTINAL SYMPTOMS

- Epigastric pain
- Gastroesophageal reflux
- Peptic ulcer disease
- Nocturnal diarrhea
- Diabetic neuropathy
- Inflammatory bowel diseases
- Nocturnal exacerbation of respiratory diseases
- Gastroesophageal reflux worsening asthma
- Abnormal nocturnal behaviors or seizures
- Insulinoma causing hypoglycemia
- Insomnia
- Pancreatic cancer causing pain

Asthmatics may awaken from sleep by the exacerbation of bronchial asthma, which can be secondary to sleep-related gastroesophageal reflux (GER) disease (GERD). Numerous studies are accumulating to suggest that respiratory complications secondary to GERD are common, and that these symptoms are noted primarily as secondary to sleep-related GER (Box 14.3-1).

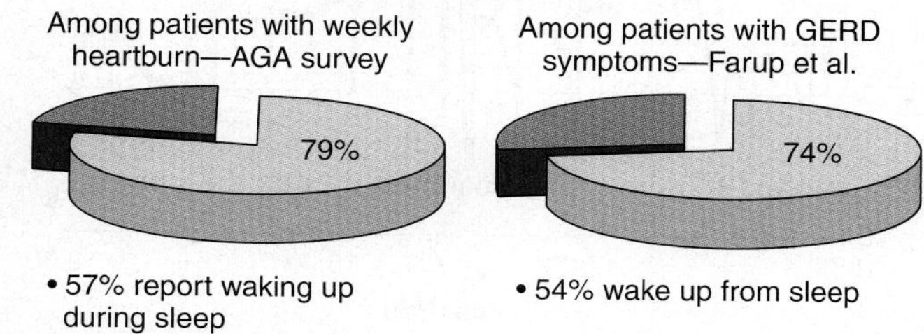

Figure 14.3-1.
Data from two studies. Each study surveyed 1000 patients with gastroesophageal reflux disease (GERD). Both studies demonstrated that nighttime heartburn is common in patients with GERD, and that in patients with nighttime heartburn, complaints of sleep disturbance are common. (Data from the American Gastroenterological Association [AGA], Gallup Survey, May 2000; Farup C, Leinman L, Sloan S, et al: The impact of nocturnal symptoms associated with gastroesophageal reflux disease on health-related quality of life. Arch Intern Med 161:45–52, 2001.)

THE UPPER GASTROINTESTINAL TRACT

Patients with duodenal ulcer disease maintain a circadian pattern of gastric acid secretion, and studies have shown that the levels of secretion are enhanced in the early part of the sleeping interval. Howden and colleagues reviewed the published data on nocturnal dosing of H_2 receptor antagonists in more than 12,000 patients with duodenal ulcer disease. They concluded that nocturnal dosing showed a clear advantage over multiple daily doses. These data strongly support the notion that nocturnal acid suppression alone is sufficient to heal a duodenal ulcer.

GERD, along with its familiar symptom of heartburn, is common. Most normal people experience occasional bouts of heartburn. About 7% of the general population experience heartburn nearly every day. Furthermore, the majority of patients with frequent heartburn complain of nighttime GER symptoms, and a substantial proportion (over 50%) of these patients report that their symptoms disrupt their sleep and affect their daytime functioning (Fig. 14.3-1). In Figure 14.3-2 it can be seen that the prevalence of sleep disturbance clearly increases with increasing frequency of nighttime heartburn. There are also data to suggest that complications appear to be the result of recurrent episodes of sleep-related GER.

Attention has been focused on the importance of different patterns of GER associated with waking and sleeping. These patterns were documented in studies involving 24-hour monitoring of the distal esophageal pH. GER is identified when the pH falls below 4 for a period of more than 30 seconds, and the reflux episode is arbitrarily terminated when the pH reaches 4 or 5. There are two different patterns of reflux. Reflux in the upright position occurs most often postprandially and usually consists of two or three reflux episodes that are rapidly cleared (Fig. 14.3-3). Reflux

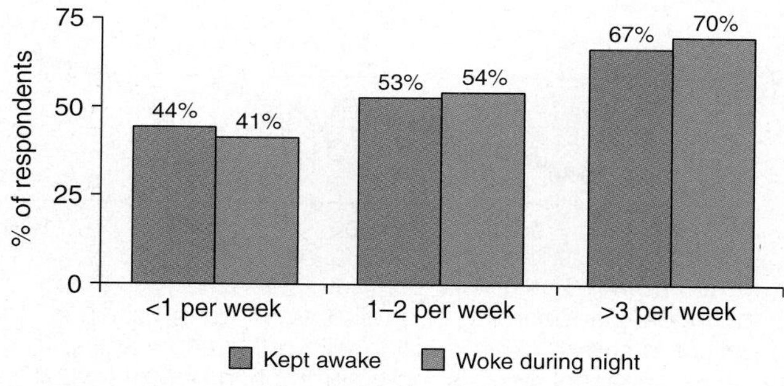

Figure 14.3-2.
Relation between the frequency of nighttime sleep disturbance and the percentage of individuals reporting sleep disturbance. This figure demonstrates that the percentage of patients complaining of sleep disturbance is greater in groups who indicate more frequent nighttime heartburn. (Data from Shaker R, Castell DO, Schoenfeld PS, Spechler SJ. Nighttime heartburn is an under-appreciated clinical problem that impacts sleep and daytime function: The results of a Gallup survey conducted on behalf of the American Gastroenterological Association. Amer J Gastroenterol, July 1487–1493, 2003.)

in the supine position is usually associated with sleep and with more prolonged clearance time (Fig. 14.3-4).

There are significant increases in acid mucosal contact time in patients with esophagitis, especially in the recumbent position as opposed to the upright position. Typically, data from the upright position reflect waking and data from the recumbent position reflect the sleeping interval. It is likely that the prolonged acid clearance times associated with sleep result in greater damage to the esophageal mucosa. Similar results have been reported in patients with severe complications of GERD, including erosive esophagitis, stricture, and Barrett's esophagus.

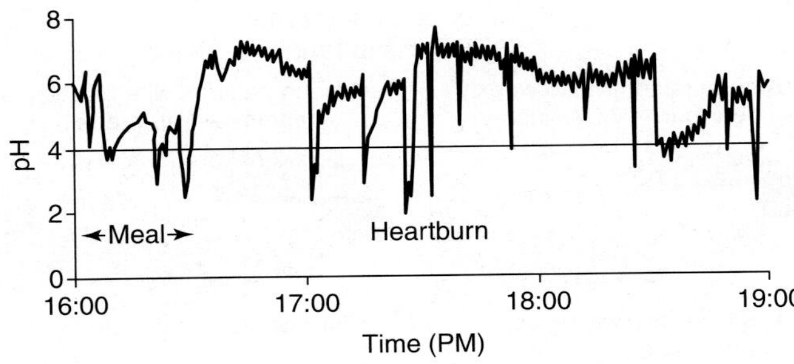

Figure 14.3-3.
Esophageal pH recording showing gastroesophageal reflux subsequent to a meal in a normal individual (pH less than 4 designates a reflux event). Gastroesophageal reflux in normal individuals during the daytime is largely related to short episodes occurring postprandially.

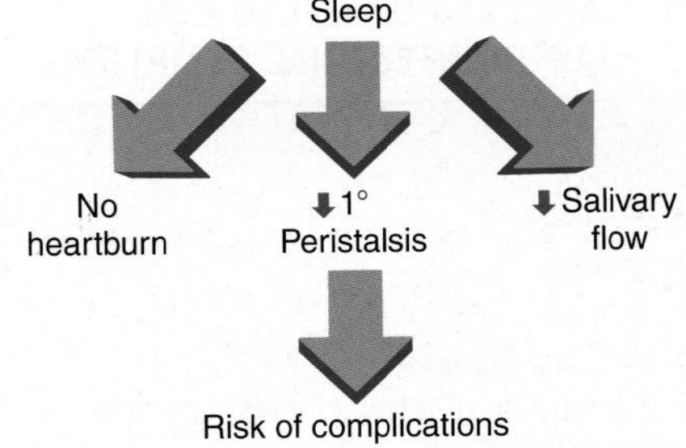

Figure 14.3-6.
Acid mucosal response. Illustration of the alterations in the response to acid mucosal contact during sleep. This figure shows that sleep is associated with the alterations in responses that are essential in the acid clearance process. These essential alterations include a marked reduction in swallowing rate and salivation.

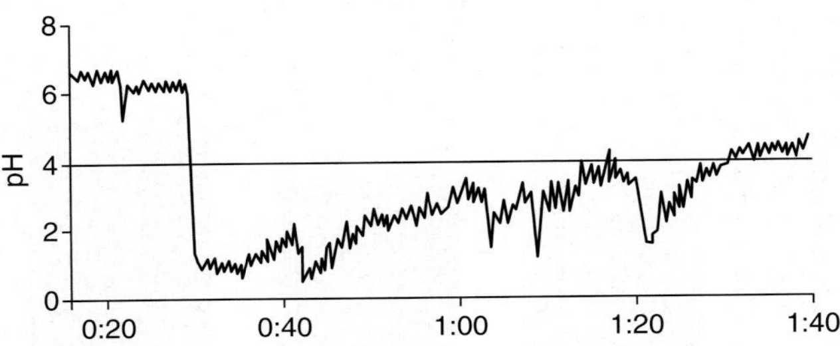

Figure 14.3-4.
Esophageal pH recording of a reflux event during sleep in a patient in supine sleep position with reflux esophagitis. Gastroesophageal reflux is more common in patients with esophagitis and is distinguished by lengthy episodes that occur during the sleeping interval.

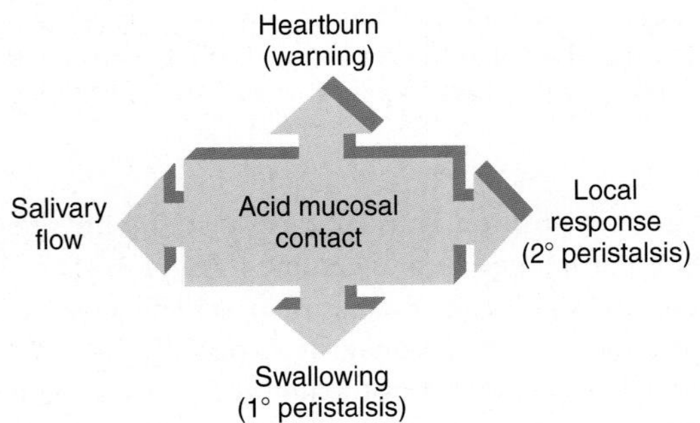

Figure 14.3-5.
Normal defense mechanisms against acid load. Illustration of the events associated with acid mucosal contact in a normal individual. The orchestrated response to acid mucosal contact is complicated and involves waking conscious responses such as swallowing and the experience of heartburn.

Figure 14.3-5 shows the orchestrated response to acid mucosal contact in a normal individual. Swallowing and salivation are reflexive responses that provide the salivary buffer to the distal esophagus and bring the esophagus from an acidic to a more normal alkaline pH. In addition, secondary peristalsis (a normal peristaltic wave not initiated by a swallow) is activated by the noxious acidic contents of the stomach, and heartburn may occur, providing a warning signal that acid is present in the esophagus and stimulating swallowing. Figure 14.3-6 describes how these responses are altered by sleep. Swallowing decreases approximately tenfold and salivation is nearly nonexistent. There is no "warning signal" during sleep because the sensation of heartburn is a waking, conscious phenomenon. These changes in combination result in a prolongation of acid clearance, which appears to be the result of the sleeping state.

THERAPEUTIC CONSIDERATIONS

Sleep-related reflux produces a pattern of prolonged acid clearance during waking and sleep. Documentation of this pattern comes from studies showing that the back-diffusion of hydrogen ions in the esophagus is directly related to the duration of acid mucosal contact time (Fig. 14.3-7). Further evidence of nocturnal GER comes from a clinical study of individuals with symptoms of nocturnal heartburn as well as dysphagia and chest pain. The study showed that these individuals were much more likely to have demonstrable esophageal disease.

To summarize, studies on acid clearance during sleep lend increasing support to the idea that sleep is a time of considerable risk for the development of reflux esophagitis and that sleep itself imposes changes in acid mucosal responses that prolong acid contact time. Sleep-related acid contact time appears to play a major role in the development of reflux esophagitis, and reflux during sleep itself can serve as a stimulus associated with sleep disturbances.

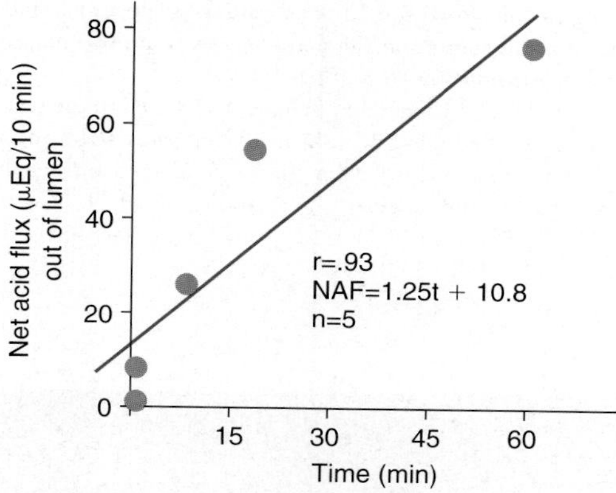

Figure 14.3-7.
Flux and duration of acid exposure. Hydrogen ion back-diffusion into the esophageal mucosa as a function of the time of acid contact. This figure illustrates animal data showing that increasing acid mucosal contact results in greater back-diffusion of hydrogen ions, which causes damage to the esophageal mucosa. NAF, net acid flux; r, Pearson product-moment correlation. (Data from Johnson LF, Harmon JW: Experimental esophagitis in a rabbit model: Clinical relevance. J Clin Gastroenterol 8(Suppl 1):S26–S44, 1986.)

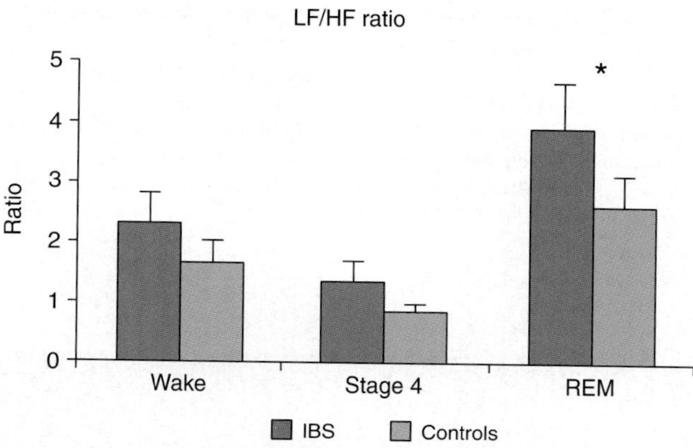

Figure 14.3-8.
Sympathetic dominance (measured by low frequency/high frequency ratio) during stages of sleep in patients with irritable bowel syndrome (IBS) and controls. This figure shows the results of a study documenting that patients diagnosed with IBS, when compared to a group of normal individuals, show enhanced sympathetic activity during REM sleep *(asterisk)*.

Pulmonary Complications

Individuals who reported GER symptoms one to two times per week were significantly more likely to report symptoms of sleep-disordered breathing, and those with a combination of asthma and GER had a higher prevalence of nocturnal cough and sleep-related symptoms. Thus, the occurrence of nocturnal GER is strongly associated with both asthma and respiratory symptoms, as well as symptoms of obstructive sleep apnea syndrome. Symptoms of nocturnal GER are also associated with daytime sleepiness and daytime tiredness and fatigue. Nocturnal wheezing in persons with asthma and chronic nocturnal cough are pulmonary symptoms that have been linked to the occurrence of GERD. GERD may be clinically "silent," that is, not associated with a clinical symptom of heartburn, and the treatment of GER may reduce nocturnal asthma symptoms.

Intestinal Motility and Irritable Bowel Syndrome

Attempts to measure bowel motility patterns in patients with IBS have not revealed any discernible pattern that distinguishes this group. However, it has been shown that both arousal from sleep and awakening from sleep are associated with high-amplitude propagating pressure waves in the colon, commonly associated with an urge to defecate.

Patients with functional dyspepsia (characterized by epigastric postprandial bloating, nausea, or early satiety) often complain of general sleep disturbances suggestive of nonrestorative sleep (i.e., numerous awakenings after sleep onset, morning awakenings without feeling rested), and it has been shown that there is a marked increase in sleep complaints in patients with functional bowel disorders, such as IBS and functional dyspepsia, compared to normal controls. In addition, the dyspeptic patients had more complaints of sleep disturbance, perhaps due to more intense abdominal pain. Some studies suggest abnormalities in rapid eye movement (REM) sleep, and some have shown autonomic imbalances in IBS patients during REM sleep (Fig. 14.3-8) wherein increased sympathetic dominance was evident. Exacerbation of IBS symptoms and poor sleep show a strong correlation. Thus, not only are there sleep disturbances in this patient population, but also the sleep disturbances may be contributing to altered gastrointestinal functioning. These studies confirm the notion that there are central nervous system alterations in patients with functional bowel disorders and that these alterations are perhaps uniquely identified during sleep.

Conclusions

It appears that there is an important relation between sleep and the development of various acid peptic diseases, such as duodenal ulcer disease and GERD. The pathogenesis and treatment of these disorders relate in large measure to the control of acid secretion during sleep. Functional bowel disorders, including nonulcer dyspepsia and IBS, appear to be associated with an increased incidence of sleep complaints, and autonomic dysfunction specifically noted during REM sleep appears to characterize a subset of patients diagnosed with IBS.

SELECTED READINGS

DeMeester TR, Johnson LF, Guy JJ, et al: Patterns of gastroesophageal reflux in health and disease. Ann Surg 184:459–470, 1976.

Fass R, Fullerton S, Tung S, et al: Sleep disturbances in clinic patients with functional bowel disorders. Am J Gastro 95:1195–2000, 2000.

Gisalson T, Janson C, Vermeire P, et al: Respiratory symptoms and nocturnal gastroesophageal reflux. Chest 121:158–163, 2002.

Goldsmith G, Levin JS: Effect of sleep quality on symptoms of irritable bowel syndrome. Dig Dis Sci 38:1809–1814, 1993.

Howden CW, Jones DB, Hunt RH: Nocturnal doses of H_2 receptor antagonists for duodenal ulcer. The Lancet 1:647–648, 1985.

Orr WC: Sleep-related gastroesophageal reflux: Clinical and physiologic consequences. Curr GERD Rep 1:59–64, 2007.

Orr WC, Allen ML, Robinson M: The pattern of nocturnal and diurnal esophageal acid exposure in the pathogenesis of erosive mucosal damage. Am J Gastro 89:509–512, 1994.

Shaker R, Castell DO, Schoenfeld PS, Spechler SJ: Nighttime heartburn is an under-appreciated clinical problem that impacts sleep and daytime function: The results of a Gallup survey conducted on behalf of the American Gastroenterological Association. Amer J Gastroenterol 1487–1493, 2003.

14.4 Diabetes Mellitus

Charles George

Diabetes mellitus is a disease of abnormal glucose metabolism caused by impaired insulin secretion and/or insulin resistance. Characteristics of diabetes types are given in Table 14.4-1.

Key Symptoms Related to High Blood Sugar

The osmotic acute diuresis that is caused by glycosuria leads to polyuria and polydipsia, which may lead to hypotension and dehydration. This may be followed by nausea and vomiting (especially if ketoacidosis occurs). Over the longer term, there may be weight loss.

Sleep in Diabetics

Sleep deprivation may lead to insulin resistance and diabetes mellitus (Fig. 14.4-1; see also chapter 3.10).

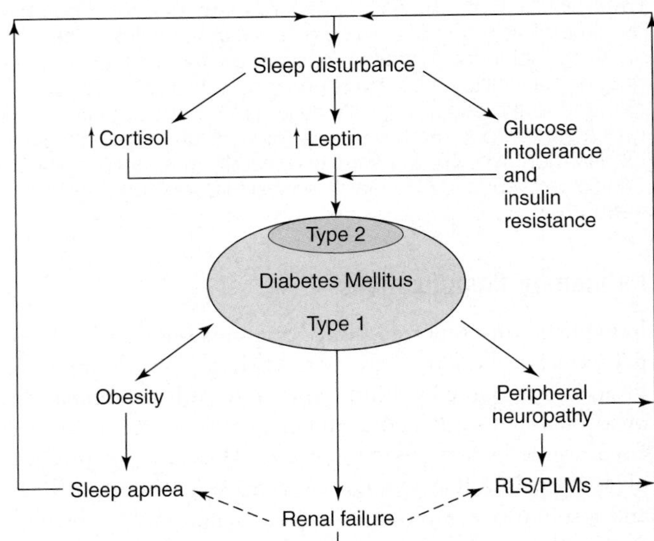

Figure 14.4-1.
Interactions between sleep disturbances and diabetes. Solid arrows indicate known interactions. Dashed arrows indicate where pathogenetic mechanisms is not yet clear. PLMs, periodic limb movements; RLS, restless legs syndrome.

Table 14.4-1. Clinical Features of Diabetes

FEATURE	TYPE 1	TYPE 2
Age at onset	Mostly in ages under 30 yr	Mostly in ages over 30 yr
Obesity	No	Very common
Level of endogenous insulin	Low to absent	May be low, normal, or high
Islet cell antibodies or abnormalities	Yes	No
Prone to develop ketoacidosis	Yes	No
Risk of developing complications involving eyes, kidneys, nervous system, and cardiovascular system	Yes	Yes
Response to oral antihyperglycemic drugs	No	Yes, initially in many patients

SLEEP APNEA

Obesity is a risk factor for diabetes and sleep apnea. Many patients therefore have both conditions. Sleep apnea may lead to insulin resistance.

INSOMNIA

About 50% of diabetes patients have problems with sleep.

NOCTURNAL AWAKENINGS

Sleep can be impacted as a result of the osmotic diuresis (nocturia, polyuria, polydipsia). Sleep can be affected if a patient has chronic complications of diabetes (Table 14.4-2; see Fig. 14.4-1).

Table 14.4-2. Potential Sleep Outcomes as a Result of Diabetes Complications

COMPLICATION OF DIABETES	SLEEP DISTURBANCE
Chronic renal failure	May develop Cheyne Stokes respiration
Peripheral neuropathy	Sleep may be impacted by pain, numbness, and restless legs syndrome. Some patients may have nocturnal diarrhea
Autonomic neuropathy	May demonstrate "fixed cardiac rate" during sleep and painless nocturnal cardiac ischemia

SELECTED READINGS

Knutson KL, Spiegel K, Penev P, Van Cauter E: The metabolic consequences of sleep deprivation. Sleep Med Rev 11:163–178, 2007.

Lopes LA, Lins CMM, Adeodato VG, et al: Restless legs syndrome and quality of sleep in type 2 diabetes. Diabetes Care 28:2633–2636, 2005.

Parish JM, Adam T, Facchiano L: Relationship of metabolic syndrome and obstructive sleep apnea. J Clin Sleep Med 3(5):467–472, 2007.

Skomro RP, Ludwig S, Salamon E, Kryger MH: Sleep complaints and restless legs syndrome in adult type 2 diabetics. Sleep Med 2:417–422, 2001.

Tasali E, Mokhlesi B, Van Cauter E: Obstructive sleep apnea and type 2 diabetes: Interacting epidemics. Chest 133:496–506, 2008.

Charles George

14.5 *Sleep Disorders in Chronic Renal Disease*

Sleep disorders are common in patients with chronic kidney disease (CKD) (Table 14.5-1). Initially sleep disturbances were reported only in advanced cases with severe uremia, on dialysis, or both; however, subsequent reports suggest that similar problems develop soon after a diagnosis of early chronic renal failure has been established.

There is no one single cause for sleep disturbance in CKD patients. Evidence exists for multiple factors, some of which are summarized in Figure 14.5-1. Careful attention to history and modification of contributing factors is important in both diagnosis and treatment of sleep disorders in this population.

Obstructive sleep apnea is common in patients in longstanding hemodialysis. While comorbidity (e.g., obesity) may be the major pathogenetic factor, obstructive sleep apnea occurs in the patient with uremia independent of obesity and sometimes resolves with correction of the uremia by transplant.

Symptoms of restless legs syndrome are common in CKD patients, and periodic limb movements (PLM) during sleep are sometimes a major factor in sleep disturbance. PLM indices are often very high in these patients (Fig. 14.5-2). When these high PLM indices create instability of sleep, ventilation may become unstable, resulting in cyclical apneas (Fig. 14.5-3). Treatment with dopamine agonists or gabapentin is usually helpful.

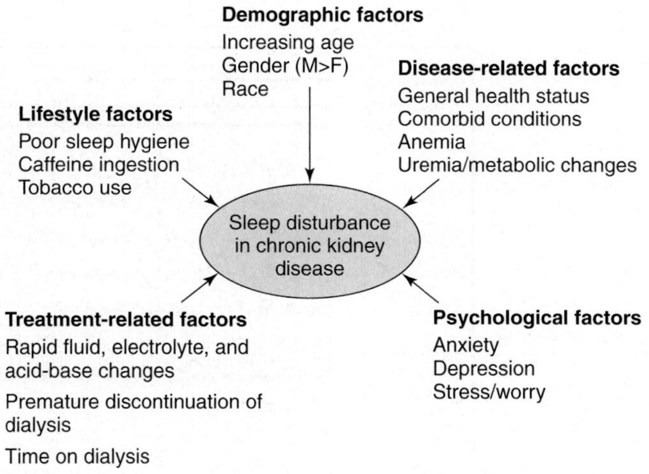

Figure 14.5-1.
Factors that may influence the development of sleep disturbances in chronic kidney disease.

Table 14.5-1. Common Sleep Complaints in Patients with Chronic Kidney Disease and Percentage (Range) of Patients with Each Complaint

SLEEP COMPLAINTS	PATIENTS REPORTING POSITIVE (%)
Prolonged sleep latency (greater than 30 min)	40–45
Frequent awakenings	50–65
Early awakenings	55–60
Nonrefreshing sleep	50
Snoring	10–15
Obstructive sleep apnea	6–10
Nightmares	25–30
Somnambulism	7–8

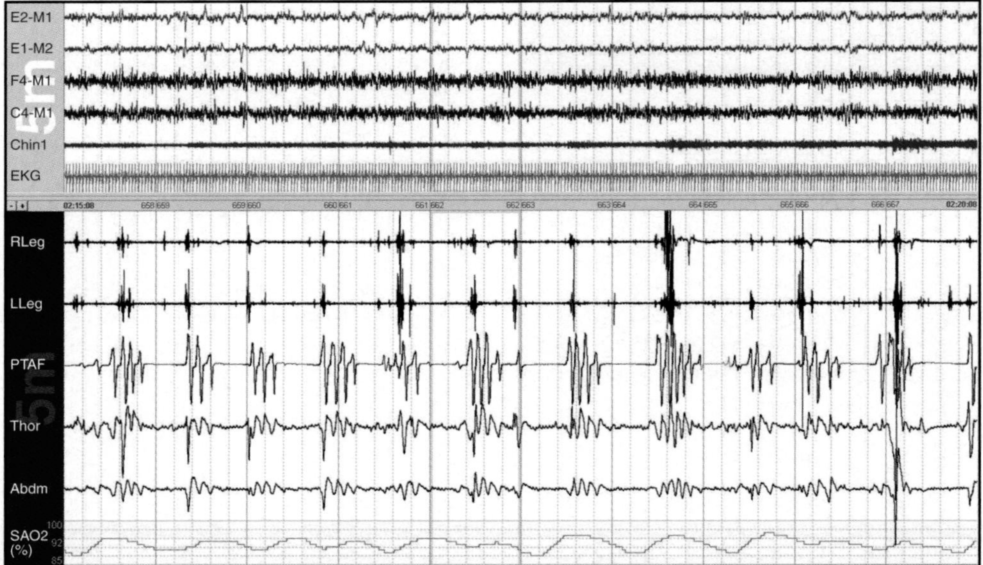

Figure 14.5-2.
Periodic limb movements in a patient on chronic hemodialysis. Some periodic movements appear to promote ventilatory instability and produce repetitive apneas.

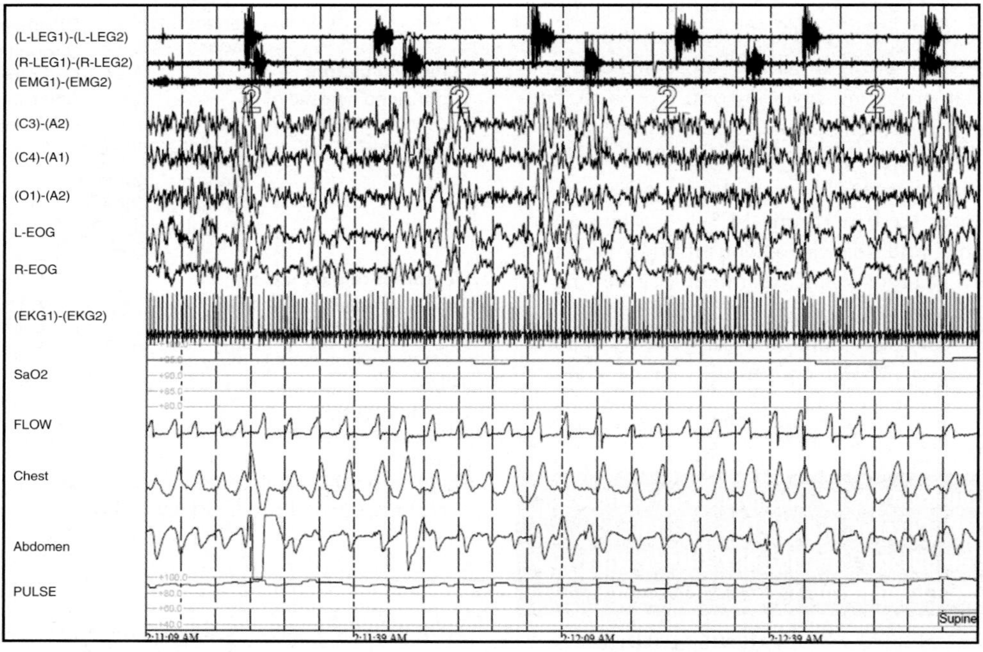

Figure 14.5-3.
Frequent periodic limb movements with fairly regular respiration and increased cyclic alternating pattern (CAP).

SELECTED READINGS

Gigli GL, Adorati M, Dolso P, et al: Restless legs syndrome in end-stage renal disease. Sleep Med 5:309–315, 2004.

Hanly PJ, Pierratos A: Improvement of sleep apnea in patients with chronic renal failure who undergo nocturnal hemodialysis. N Engl J Med 344:102–107, 2001.

Iliescu EA, Yeates KE, Holland DC: Quality of sleep in patients with chronic kidney disease. Nephrol Dial Transplant 19:95–99, 2004.

Parker KP, Bliwise DL, Bailey JL, Rye DB: Polysomnographic measures of nocturnal sleep in patients on chronic, intermittent daytime haemodialysis vs. those with chronic kidney disease. Nephrol Dial Transplant 20:1422–1428, 2005.

Tada T, Kusano KF, Ogawa A, et al: The predictors of central and obstructive sleep apnoea in haemodialysis patients. Nephrol Dial Transplant 22(4):1190–1197, 2007.

WOMEN'S HEALTH

CHAPTER 15

Kathryn Lee

The Menstrual Cycle 15.1

Menstrual Cycle Sleep Changes

The menstrual cycle starts with menses, or 2 to 5 days of menstrual bleeding, followed by a follicular or preovulation, phase, a brief ovulation phase that lasts between 13 and 15 days after the start of menses, and a postovulation phase that lasts about 14 days and ends with the onset of menses. The postovulation phase is also known as the luteal phase because there is substantial secretion of gonadal hormones (progesterone and estrogen) from the corpus luteum of the ovary if ovulation occurs. If ovulation does not occur, the cycle is likely irregular with either a substantially shorter (less than 25 days) or longer (more than 35 days) length.

Healthy menstruating women report more problems with their sleep during the premenstrual week and during the first few days of menses compared with other days. Their sleep problems are likely due to menstrual cramps and pain of dysmenorrhea, although there is little research on possible mechanisms. Sleep problems may also be from rapid withdrawal of the sedating effects of progesterone prior to menses onset. Objective sleep measures in controlled laboratory settings, however, show little change in rapid eye movement (REM) and non-REM (NREM) sleep stages from one phase of the cycle to another; of course, only small numbers of women participate in these longitudinal studies. When ovulation has occurred and the increased progesterone raises core body temperature during the luteal phase, a woman's REM latency is often shorter compared with her own follicular phase (Fig. 15.1-1).

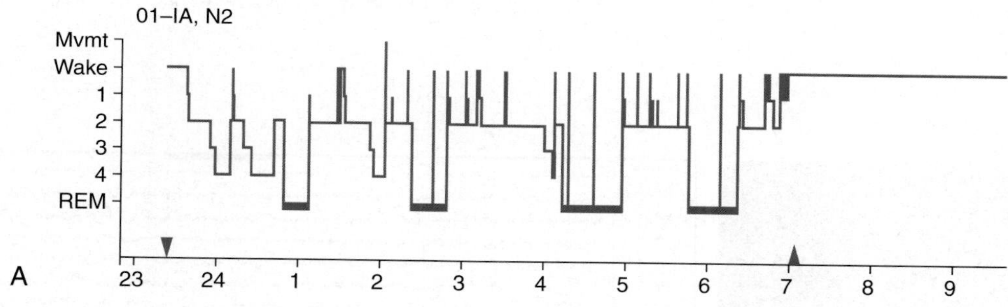

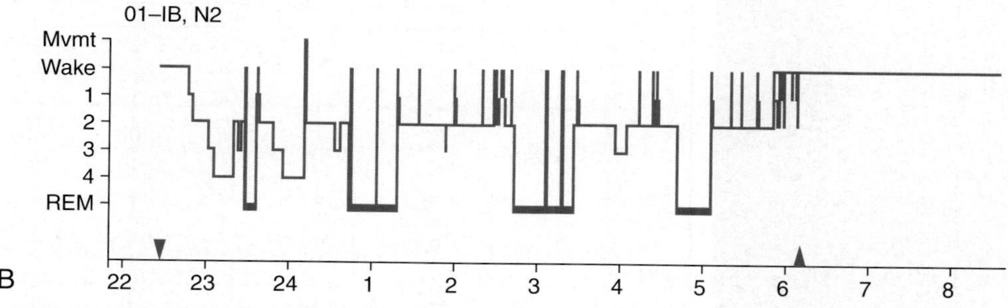

Figure 15.1-1.
Hypnograms from ambulatory polysomnography in the home setting. The patient is a 29-year-old woman with a history of premenstrual syndrome. **A**, Follicular phase (day 8 of the menstrual cycle), night 2 of polysomnography recording: total sleep time = 425 minutes; REM latency from stage 2 sleep = 87 minutes; REM = 27%; stage 2 = 52%; stage 3-4 sleep = 12.5%; sleep efficiency = 96%. **B**, Luteal phase (day 20 of the menstrual cycle), night 2 of polysomnography recording: total sleep time = 420 minutes; REM latency from stage 2 sleep = 62 minutes; REM = 24%; stage 2 = 53%; stage 3-4 sleep = 12.9%; sleep efficiency = 95%. Mvmt, movement.

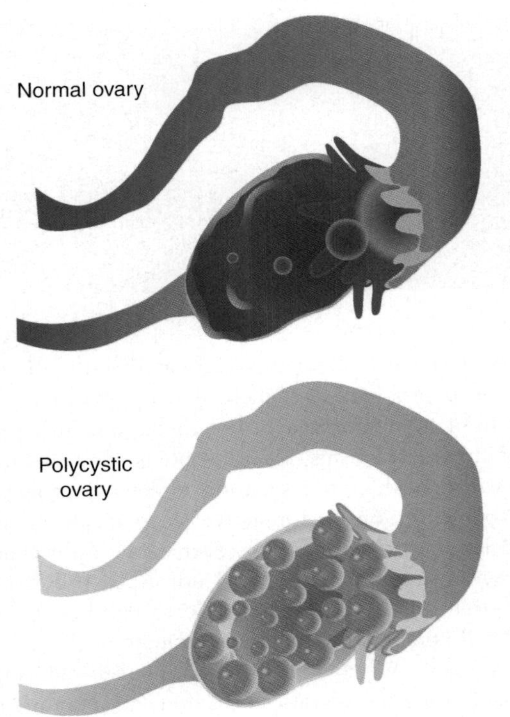

Figure 15.1-2.
A normal ovary and fallopian tube compared to a polycystic ovary.

Premenstrual Mood and Sleep

There is some evidence that women with premenstrual syndrome (PMS) may have substantially less slow-wave deep sleep (10% or less) than do other women of the same age who have about 20%. Figure 15.1-1 depicts hypnograms for a woman with PMS. At each phase she had only 13% slow-wave deep sleep. Note in the figure the earlier REM latency during the luteal phase (62 minutes) compared with the follicular phase (87 minutes). Oral contraceptives maintain low levels of hormones during the menstrual cycle, and, in addition to preventing ovulation, this therapy may be useful for severe sleep complaints in young women.

Polycystic Ovary Syndrome

Polycystic ovary syndrome, or PCOS, occurs in about 5% of young women and is usually diagnosed when infertility becomes a concern. In addition to the presence of bilateral polycystic ovaries (Fig. 15.1-2), the women often experience irregular and anovulatory menstrual cycles, as well as androgen excess with hirsutism and acne (Fig. 15.1-3). About half of this patient population is also obese and at risk for insulin resistance. They have lower sleep efficiency, with less REM and NREM sleep, and they are much more likely to experience sleep-disordered breathing and daytime sleepiness compared with ovulating women of similar age and body weight. It is likely that between 20% and 40% of obese women with PCOS have sleep apnea.

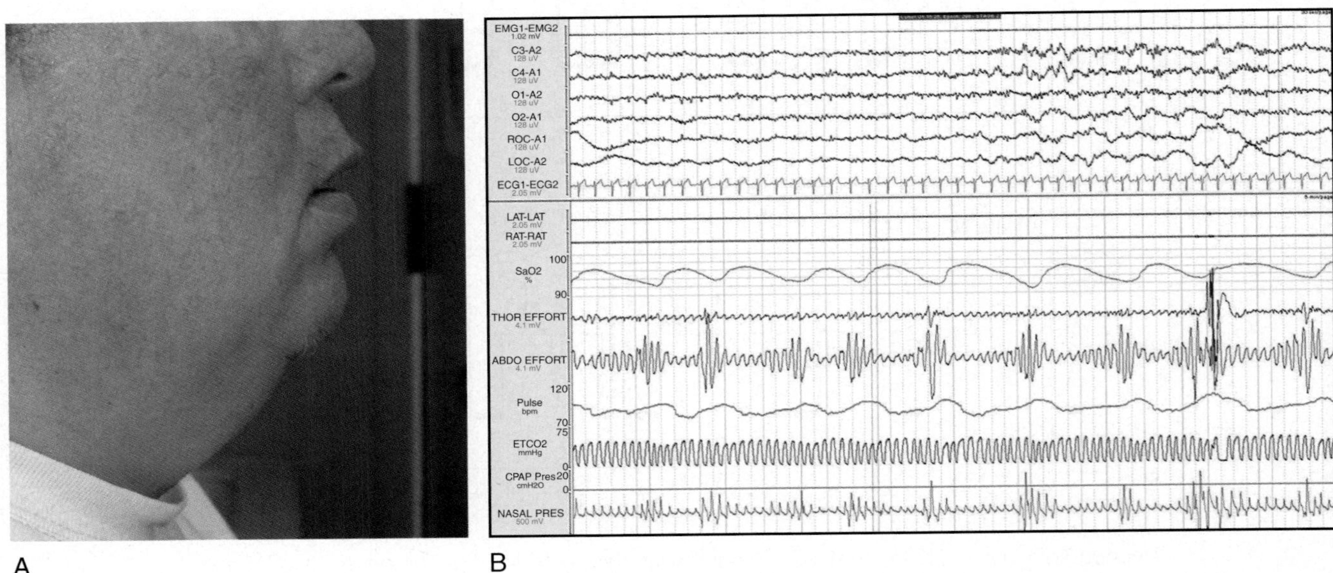

Figure 15.1-3.
A, A woman with polycystic ovary syndrome (PCOS). Note the facial features (hirsutism and acne) characteristic of androgen excess. **B**, Polysomnogram segment showing severe sleep apnea in a 48-year-old woman who had symptoms of PCOS for over a decade and who was first diagnosed with PCOS when assessed for sleep apnea. The patient is obese and has angina pectoris, arterial hypertension, and diabetes mellitus.

SELECTED READINGS

Baker FC, Driver HS: Self-reported sleep across the menstrual cycle in young, healthy women. J Psychosom Res 56:239–243, 2004.

Guzick D: Polycystic ovary syndrome. Obstet Gynecol 103:181–193, 2004.

Lee KA, Shaver JF, Giblin ED, Woods NF: Sleep patterns related to menstrual cycle phase and premenstrual affective symptoms. Sleep 13:403–409, 1990.

Vgontzas AN, Legro RS, Bixler EO, et al: Polycystic ovary syndrome is associated with obstructive sleep apnea and daytime sleepiness: Role of insulin resistance. J Clin Endocrinol Metab 86:517–520, 2001.

Kin M. Yuen

Pregnancy and Postpartum 15.2

Blood volume, hormone effects, and physical changes during pregnancy impact a woman's sleep. During the first trimester, with a rapidly expanding blood volume and progesterone-induced hyperventilation, there is a sense of shortness of breath. The added estrogen increases pliability and hyperemia, causing nasal passages to become more collapsible. Both changes contribute to the heightened sensation of dyspnea. The added progesterone is also likely to

Table 15.2-1. Features of Sleep Disturbances in Pregnancy and Postpartum

TRIMESTER	COMPLAINTS	PSG FINDINGS	HORMONAL CORRELATES	SLEEP DISORDERS*
First (mo 1–3)	Excessive daytime sleepiness Insomnia Urinary frequency	↑naps ↑TST ↑wake time, ↓SWS	↑progesterone: hyperventilation, sedation, smooth muscle relaxation ↑prolactin ↑REM ↑estrogen Melatonin not affected**	Snoring/OSA Less bruxism than baseline More sleep starts
Second (mo 4–6)	↑awakenings	↓SWS ↓REM	↑progesterone ↑estrogen	Snoring/OSA More sleep paralysis Less somnambulism Less somniloquy
Third (mo 7–9)	3–5 Awakenings/night ↓daytime alertness Leg cramps Dyspnea Backache Heartburn Abdominal discomfort Fetal movement Frequent nocturia	↓TST ↓SWS ↓REM ↑wake after sleep onset ↑stage 1 sleep	↑estrogen ↓progesterone at parturition Oxytocin at parturition Lower cortisol	Snoring/OSA Preeclampsia Restless legs Leg cramps Recurrence of somnambulism More sleep paralysis
Preeclampsia	Poor sleep Nausea Edema Headaches Dizziness Changes in vision Sleepiness	↑sleep fragmentation ↑time out of bed ↑body movements	↑cytokines ↑C-reactive protein ↑TNF	Snoring/OSA
Postpartum†	Poor sleep	↓TST‡ ↓REM ↓REM latency ↓stage 2 sleep ↑SWS ↑awake time ↓sleep efficiency	↓estrogen ↓progesterone	Blues: 50%–80% Depression: 10%–20% Psychosis (rare): 0.1%

*Narcoleptic symptoms can continue during pregnancy.
**Beta HCG, rennin, nitric oxide, interleukin-1, tumor necrosis factor, and interferon may also facilitate sleepiness.
†Multiparous mothers with fewer symptoms compared to nulliparous mothers.
‡Mothers caring for premature infants with more WASO and even less TST.
OSA, obstructive sleep apnea; PSG, polysomnography; REM, rapid eye movement; SWS, slow-wave sleep; TNF, tumor necrosis factor; TST, total sleep time, WASO, wake after sleep onset.

increase daytime sleepiness and napping, thereby increasing overall total sleep time. Persistent nighttime or early morning nausea and vomiting of pregnancy can also worsen sleep. The second trimester brings some normalization to total sleep time. Table 15.2-1 summarizes common complaints, polysomnographic findings, and sleep disorders found during the three trimesters of pregnancy.

Frequent snoring affects fewer than 5% of nonpregnant women, but 15% to 20% of pregnant women. A higher incidence of snoring has been reported in the second trimester.

Although most parasomnias purportedly decrease during pregnancy, the prevalence of sleep paralysis has been reported to increase in the second and third trimester to about 13% from a prepregnancy rate of 6%. Sleep fragmentation has been suggested as the cause; sleep paralysis resolves upon delivery.

During the third trimester women have further decrements in total sleep time. More awakenings are reported, and sleep efficiency is lower. Other physical discomforts arise because of the expanding abdominal girth and anatomical changes. They include frequent urination, heartburn, and dyspnea, which further decrease sleep efficiency. Since functional residual capacity is now greatly reduced due to elevation of the diaphragm, dyspnea again returns.

Sleep-disordered Breathing

A higher risk of preeclampsia has been reported among frequent snorers (Table 15.2-2). Aside from systemic hypertension, pedal edema, and proteinuria, babies born to preeclamptic women who snore may be more likely to have intrauterine growth retardation and lower Apgar scores. Studies further document an increase in cytokine markers, tumor necrosis factor, and interleukin-6 among preeclamptic snorers.

Sleep apnea impacts pregnancy in several situations. For example, a woman who has sleep apnea becomes pregnant; apnea starts during pregnancy, especially in cases where there has been marked weight gain; and sleepiness from untreated apnea affects the new mother's ability to care for the newborn.

Nasal positive airway pressure application during pregnancy has been reported to be effective in treating obstructive sleep apnea with no adverse effects on the fetus.

Table 15.2-2. Pregnancy and Sleep-disordered Breathing

	PRIOR TO PREGNANCY	PREGNANCY	PREECLAMPSIA
Snore (self-report)	5%	15%–30%	
Snore (partner report)	25%–35%	55%	85%

Restless Legs Syndrome

Restless legs syndrome (RLS), originally reported in individuals with iron or folate deficiency, affects 15% to 25% of women in the third trimester. This is independent of the often-reported severe leg cramps that awaken women from sleep. Because of the rapid blood volume expansion by 2 to 3 liters during pregnancy, and despite oral iron and folate prenatal supplementation, some women continue to have iron deficiency anemia. Because RLS in pregnancy is short term, conservative measures, such as evening massage, are advised. In severe cases, further iron supplementation is usually recommended prior to the use of dopaminergic agents.

Labor and Delivery

Few polysomnographic sleep studies have been done on women in labor, for obvious reasons (Fig. 15.2-1). When women expecting their first child were monitored with wrist actigraphy for 5 nights before onset of labor, results were surprising. Sleep deteriorates progressively from an average of 7.5+1.0 hours and 15% wake time to 4.5+2.0 hours with about 30% wake time the night before the onset of labor and hospital admission. This also occurs to a lesser extent in women scheduled for induction of labor. Anxiety about labor may be a key factor. Having most of one's active labor during the night may be related to depressed mood during the first few weeks after delivery.

When women expecting their first child had their sleep monitored by wrist actigraphy at about 3 weeks before onset of labor, 15% slept less than 6 hours. Compared with those who slept 7 hours or more, these short sleepers were in labor almost 12 hours longer on average, and were 4.5 times more likely to have a cesarean delivery (Tables 15.2-3 and 15.2-4).

Postpartum Sleep

The postpartum period allows for some recovery of slow-wave deep sleep and rapid eye movement (REM) sleep. Although all new mothers exhibit lower sleep efficiency while caring for a newborn, multiparous women are more likely to enter into stable sleep during the infant's first few weeks of life than are first-time mothers. A few studies have shown that breastfeeding mothers sleep better than formula-feeding mothers, with polysomnography indicating more slow-wave deep sleep, and actigraphy indicating about 45 minutes more sleep during the night. Further research is needed, but prolactin hormone level in lactating mothers is thought to be responsible for these findings. New mothers caring for premature infants, or infants with special needs, have persistently less total sleep time, with more frequent awakenings and longer wake episodes at night.

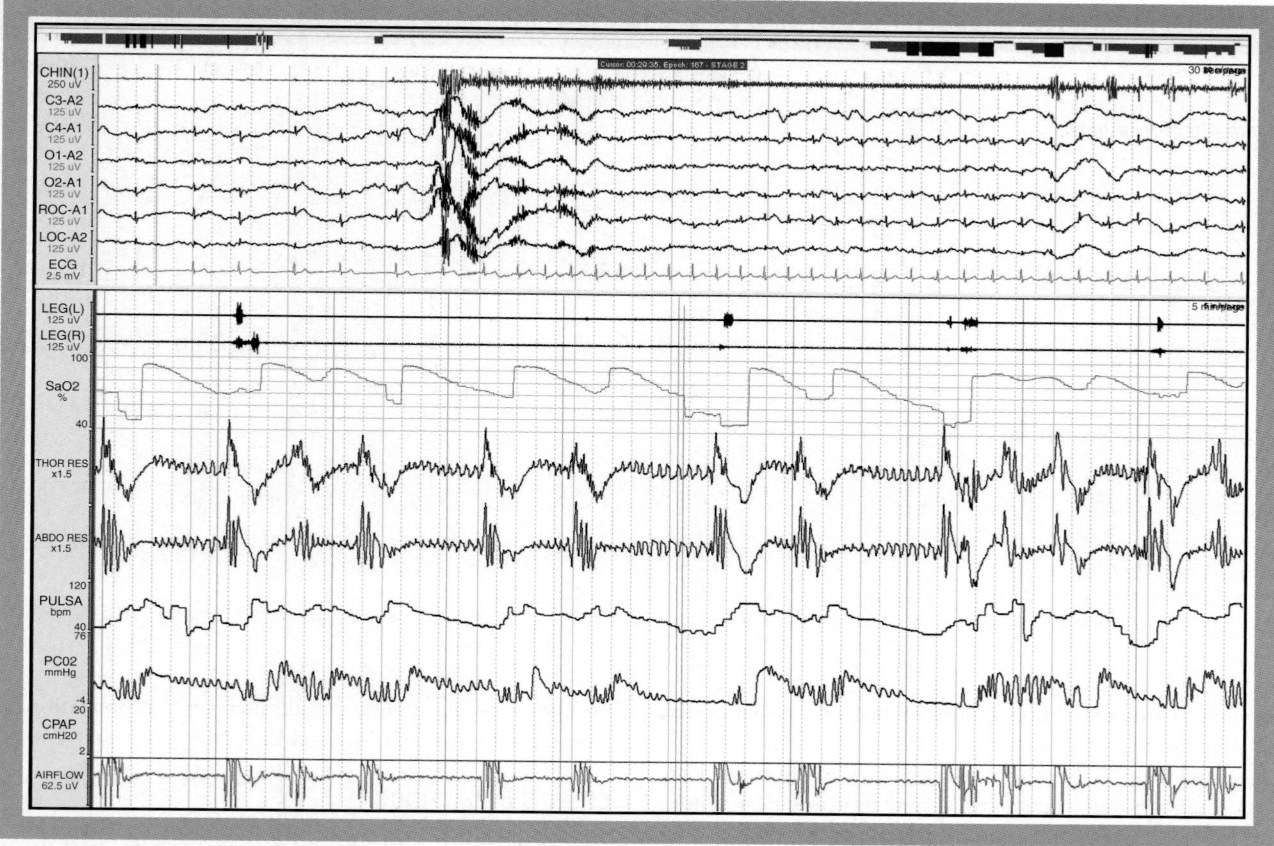

Figure 15.2-1.
Postcesarean polysomnography in patient with apnea. This PSG fragment was taken from a 38-year-old woman immediately after cesarean section. She had a difficult pregnancy with arterial hypertension, peripheral edema, and gastroesophageal reflux. There was also a history of snoring, observed apnea, and daytime sleepiness. Immediately after the cesarean section she was noted to have life-threatening hypoxemia. She had an apnea-hypopnea index of 167 and her SaO_2 approached 40%.

Table 15.2-3. Differences in Labor Duration by Total Sleep Time and Wake after Sleep Onset (n = 131)

	n	LABOR DURATION* (M ± SD)
Wake after sleep onset		
15%+	41	26.0 ± 11.7**
10%–14.9%	32	16.3 ± 12.9
<10%	58	18.3 ± 14.6
Total sleep time		
<6 hours	19	29.0 ± 12.5**
6–6.9 hours	38	20.5 ± 11.3
7+ hours	74	17.7 ± 15.6

**In hours, adjusted for infant birth weight.*
***Significantly longer labor than other two groups.*
M, mean; SD, standard deviation.
Data from Lee KA, Gay CL: Sleep in late pregnancy predicts length of labor and type of delivery. Am J Obstet Gynecol, 191:2041–2046, 2004.

Postpartum Sleep and Mental Health

Postpartum "baby blues"—commonly reported in new mothers (50% to 80%)—is thought to be due to the rapid drop in placental hormones. Most women recover from postpartum depression in 2 to 3 weeks. However, in 10% to 20% of new mothers, postpartum depression remains a problem. A history of depression before pregnancy is the biggest risk factor. Studies have found that continuing serotonin reuptake inhibitor antidepressants in depressed mothers does not significantly affect fetal outcome, except for some "jitteriness" in the newborn infant immediately after birth. In 0.1% of new mothers, postpartum psychosis is diagnosed, and these women are likely to have a history of bipolar disorder.

Narcolepsy and Pregnancy

The management of narcolepsy in pregnant women remains a challenge. The general consensus is that supportive changes in work schedules should, if necessary, be provided, so that daytime naps can be included. For others who might be affected by frequent cataplexy or sleep attacks, the judicious use of medication for alertness and

Table 15.2-4. Differences in Cesarean Rates by Wake after Sleep Onset ($n = 131$)

	N	CESAREAN RATE	ODDS RATIO*	95% CI	P-VALUE
Wake after sleep onset					
15%+	41	39.0%	5.19	1.77–15.18	.003
10%–14.9%	32	18.8%	1.90	0.55–6.63	.312
<10%	58	10.3%	ref		
Total sleep time					
<6 hours	19	36.8%	4.54	1.36–15.21	.014
6–6.9 hours	38	34.2%	3.67	1.33–10.18	.012
7+ hours	74	10.8%	ref		
GSDS sleep quality subscale					
Poor sleep 5+ days/wk	48	31.3%	5.33	1.40–20.36	.014
Poor sleep 3–4 days/wk	39	25.6%	4.21	1.05–16.93	.043
Poor sleep 0–2 days/wk	44	6.8%	ref		

*Adjusted for infant birth weight.

CI, confidence interval; GSDS, general sleep disturbance scale; ref, reference group.

Data from Lee KA, Gay CL: Sleep in late pregnancy predicts length of labor and type of delivery. Am J Obstel Gynecol, 191:2041–2046, 2004.

cataplexy needs to be considered in order to enhance the safety of mother and fetus.

In conclusion, pregnancy encompasses many rapid hormonal, hematologic, mechanical, and physiologic changes (see Table 15.2-1). Parasomnias generally decrease during pregnancy. Snoring should be evaluated for obstructive sleep apnea. Restless legs syndrome is common in the third trimester and resolves after delivery without further intervention. Pharmacologic interventions are rarely considered due to the potential adverse effects on the fetus or breast-feeding newborn. Nonpharmacologic interventions, such as nasal continuous positive airway pressure, has the potential to minimize fetal/newborn complications in women with sleep-disordered breathing.

SELECTED READINGS

Blyton DM, Sullivan CE, Edwards N: Lactation is associated with an increase in slow-wave sleep in women. J Sleep Res 11:297–303, 2002.

Iczi B, Vennelle M, Liston WA, et al: Sleep-disordered breathing and upper airway size in pregnancy and post-partum. Eur Respir J 27:321–327, 2006.

Lee KA, Caughey AB: Evaluating insomnia during pregnancy and postpartum. In Attarian HP (ed): Sleep Disorders in Women: A Guide to Practical Management. Totowa, NJ, Humana Press, 2006, pp. 185–198.

15.3 Midlife Transition and Menopause

Kathryn Lee

For women, midlife is defined as the period between 40 and 60 years of age. With technological advances, however, some women in their 40s are having their first child, while others are becoming grandmothers. Socioeconomic situations may require some women to welcome their adult children back home to live; others may be launching children out of the home with great trepidation and stress. For the average American or European woman, menopause occurs at about 51 years of age, when there has been no menses for 12 months. The age range is quite broad, and the transition can begin with irregular cycles and hormonal fluctuations for 8 to 10 years before the actual cessation of menses. Sleep studies of older adults conducted in laboratory settings conclude that women retain more slow-wave deep sleep compared with men of the same age; however, epidemiologic studies of self-reported sleep problems conclude that women experience more sleep problems than men.

Thermoregulation and Vasomotor Symptoms

When the ovaries cease to function and there is no longer ovarian estrogen production, hypothalamic secretion of follicle-stimulating hormone and luteinizing hormone continues and serum levels rise. Estrogen plays a role in maintaining a broad thermoneutral zone. The absence of estrogen is thought to be responsible for the disruptions in thermoregulation, narrowing the zone between sweating to cool off and shivering to stay warm. Attenuation of the thermoneutral zone also occurs with stress (Fig. 15.3-1).

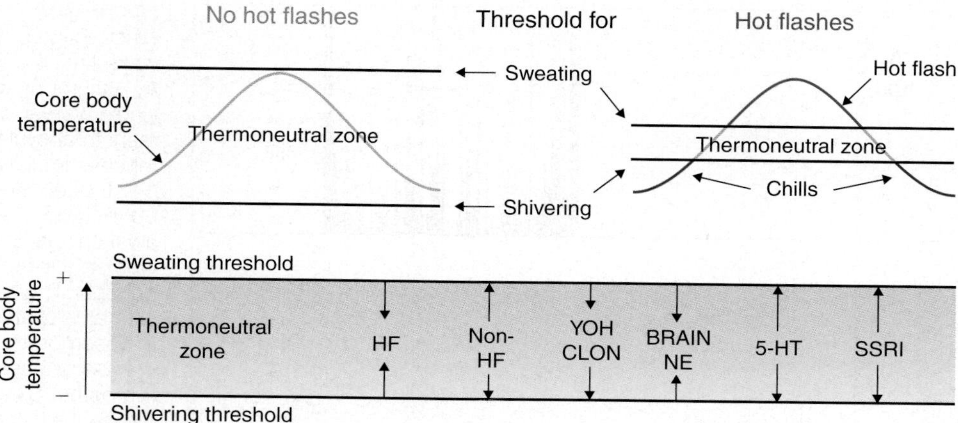

Figure 15.3-1.
The thermoneutral zone changes in women with hot flash (HF) symptoms. Small core body temperature elevations acting within a reduced thermoneutral zone trigger HFs in symptomatic postmenopausal women. The thermoneutral zone is narrowed in symptomatic women (with HF) compared with asymptomatic women (non-HF). In animals, elevated brain norepinephrine (NE) reduces this zone. Yohimbine (YOH) elevates brain NE and should reduce the zone. Conversely, clonidine should widen it. 5-HT, serotonin; SSRI, serotonin selective reuptake inhibitor. (Adapted from Freedman RR: Hot flashes: Behavioral treatments, mechanisms, and relation to sleep. Am J Med 118[Suppl 12B]:124–130, 2005.)

Vasomotor symptoms of menopause include hot flashes and night sweats and are thought to occur when the hypothalamic thermoregulatory system is poorly regulated. Although in some cultures, these vasomotor symptoms are experienced by less than 10% of the population (in Asia), it is estimated that up to 80% of American and European women have these symptoms and are most distressed when the symptoms interfere with sleep.

Hot flashes occur day and night, but are more frequent in the evening (Fig. 15.3-2). In laboratory settings, polysomnography data indicate that cortical arousals from sleep occur just prior to the onset of a hot flash. Some women have a measurable hot flash while sleep is being monitored in the laboratory but have no cognitive awareness of the experience. Other women have such extensive diaphoresis that bed linens must be changed before sleep can resume.

Figure 15.3-3 includes wrist actigraphy sleep and wake time for a woman while premenopausal with 90% sleep efficiency. When she became perimenopausal over a year

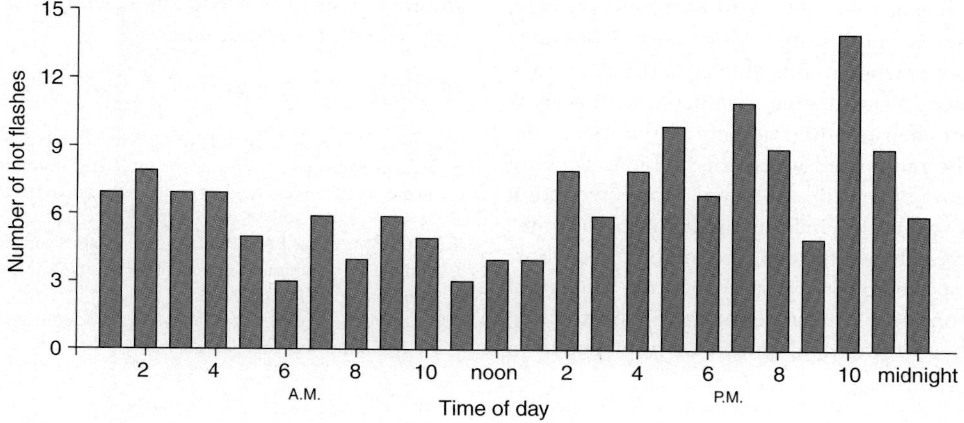

Figure 15.3-2.
Pattern of hot flash frequency across 24 hours. (Adapted from Woodward S, Freedman RR: The thermoregulatory effects of menopausal hot flashes on sleep. Sleep 17:499, 1994.)

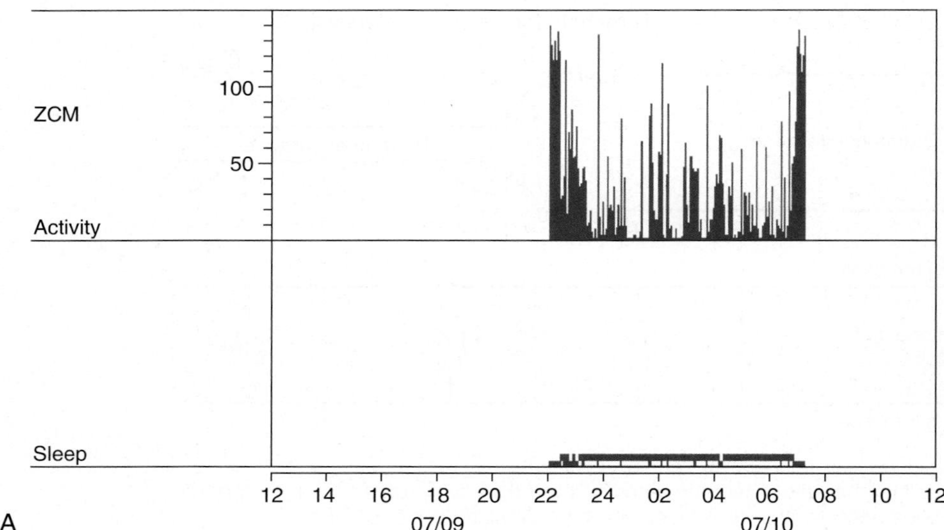

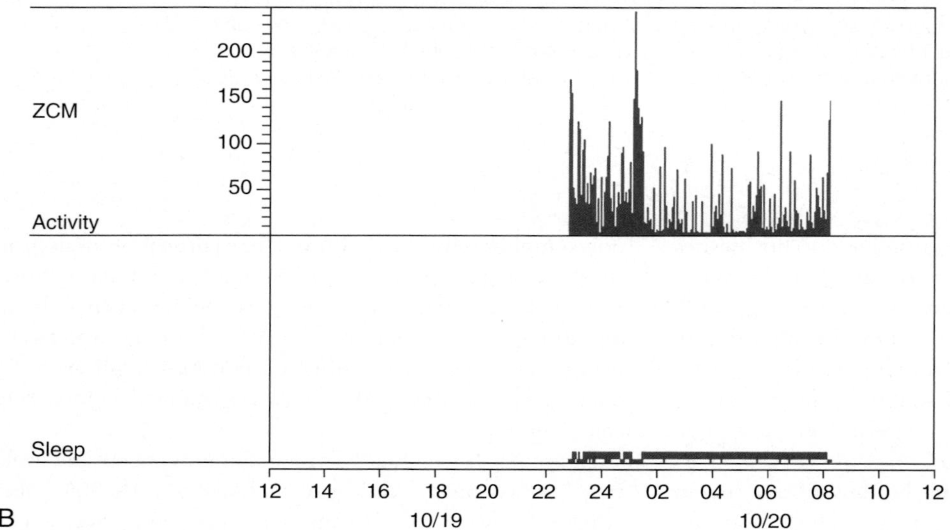

Figure 15.3-3. Wrist actigraphy sleep and wake time for a midlife woman. **A,** Actigraphy for a premenopausal single woman with regular menstrual cycles and low follicle-stimulating hormone (FSH) level. Sleep efficiency is 90.4% and she reported no awakenings. **B,** The same woman's sleep 15 months later, on night 1, when perimenopausal with an elevated FSH and reports of vasomotor symptoms and irregular menstrual cycles for 3 months. Sleep efficiency was 82.2% and she reported no awakenings.

later, her sleep efficiency was 82% and 88%, respectively, on the two nights of monitoring. Most sleep laboratory studies of menopausal women indicate very little difference in wake time or sleep stage changes compared with asymptomatic women or menstruating women of the same age. Hot flashes can be minimized when the ambient sleeping environmental temperature is cool, and stress reduction therapeutics may be useful in minimizing hot flash frequency or severity during the day and night. Since hormone replacement therapy is controversial and studies of estrogen's effect on sleep are not conclusive, short-acting hypnotics have been tested and shown to be effective in improving sleep in menopausal women who are experiencing vasomotor symptoms.

SELECTED READINGS

Dorsey CM, Lee KA, Scharf MB: Effect of zolpidem on sleep in women with perimenopausal and postmenopuasal insomnia: A 4-week, randomized, multicenter, double-blind, placebo-controlled study. Clin Ther 26:1578–1586, 2004.

Kravitz HM, Ganz PA, Bromberger J, et al: Sleep difficulty in women at midlife: A community survey of sleep and the menopausal transition. Menopause 10:19–28, 2003.

Ohayon MM: Severe hot flashes are associated with chronic insomnia. Arch Intern Med 166:308–317, 2006.

Carol A. Landis

15.4 Chronic Fatigue and Fibromyalgia Syndromes

Chronic fatigue syndrome (CFS) and fibromyalgia (FM) are complex, chronic illnesses of unknown etiology and pathogenesis with a much higher prevalence in women than in men. Both are characterized by symptoms that include pain, fatigue, and sleep disturbance. Individuals who develop these disorders may have a genetic component that renders them susceptible to activation of central nervous system mediators by a "trigger" such as an acute infection or traumatic event. Characteristics of CFS and FM are listed in Box 15.4-1. Individuals with CFS and FM are likely to suffer from comorbid conditions such as irritable bowel syndrome, multiple chemical sensitivity, temporomandibular joint disorder, myofascial pain syndrome, tension headaches, and chronic sinusitis.

CFS is characterized by severe disabling fatigue not attributed to another medical or psychiatric cause. It must coexist with a combination of symptoms including impaired cognition, sleep disturbance, and musculoskeletal pain, and does not exclude conditions such as fibromyalgia, anxiety, somatoform disorders, subsyndromal depression, and chemical sensitivity disorder.

FM is based on symptoms and tenderness at nine paired sites on the body (Fig. 15.4-1). Its prevalence in the adult population is estimated to be 2% to 4% in the United States and is nine times higher in women than in men, affecting nearly 7% of women over 60 years of age. Greater sensitivity to pain may place women at higher risk for developing FM.

BOX 15.4-1. DIAGNOSTIC CRITERIA FOR FIBROMYALGIA AND CHRONIC FATIGUE SYNDROME

FIBROMYALGIA

- Widespread pain (bilateral above and below waist) for at least 3 months' duration in combination with tenderness at 11 or more of 18 specific bilateral tender point sites. Tenderness is defined as mild or greater pain at occiput, low cervical, trapezius, supraspinatus, second rib, lateral epicondyle, gluteal, greater trochanter, and knee. Digital palpation is performed with approximately 4 kg force.
- The presence of a second clinical disorder does not exclude the diagnosis of fibromyalgia.

CHRONIC FATIGUE SYNDROME

Chronic severe fatigue persists or relapses for 6 months or longer. Fatigue is new or of defined onset, not substantially alleviated by rest, and results in substantial reduction in previous levels of social and personal activities.

Classify as chronic fatigue syndrome if four or more of the following symptoms present for at least 6 months and developed after the onset of fatigue:

- Impaired memory or concentration
- Sore throat
- Tender cervical or axillary lymph nodes
- Muscle pain, multi-joint pain
- New headaches
- Unrefreshing sleep
- Postexertion exercise

Classify as idiopathic chronic fatigue if the above criteria for chronic fatigue syndrome are not met.

Sleep Disturbance in CFS and FM

Insomnia, sleep-disordered breathing, restless legs syndrome, and periodic leg movement disorder are common in CFS and FM. Self-report of sleep disturbance is one of eight possible

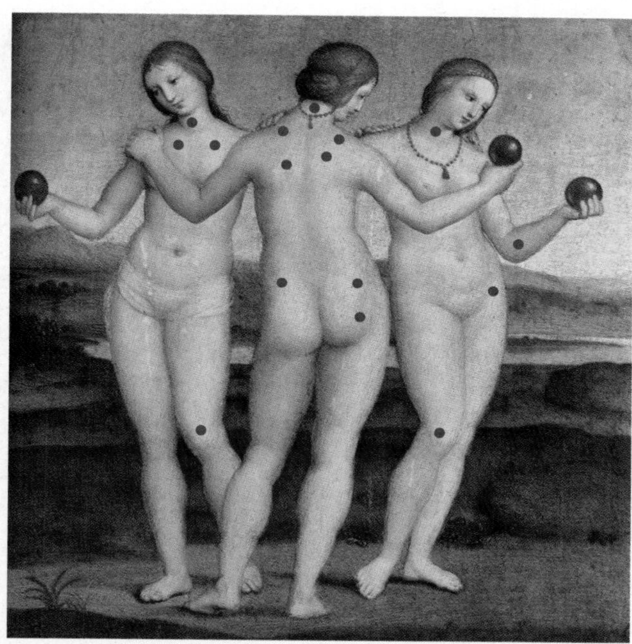

Figure 15.4-1.
Tender point locations for fibromyalgia from *Three Graces* by Raphael (Musèo Conde). Low cervical, front neck area: At the anterior aspect of the interspaces between the transverse processes of C5 and C7 *(1, 2);* Front chest area: Just lateral to the second costochondral junctions *(3, 4);* Elbow area: 2 cm distal to the lateral epicondyle *(5, 6);* Knee area: At the medial fat pad proximal to the joint line *(7, 8);* Occiput, back of the neck: At the insertions of one or more of the following muscles: trapezius, sternocleidomastoid, splenius capits, semispinalis capítis *(9, 10);* Trapezius muscle, back of shoulder: At the midpoint of the upper border *(11, 12);* Supraspinatus muscle, shoulder blade area: Above the scapular spine near the medial border *(13, 14);* Gluteal, rear end: At the upper outer quadrant of the buttocks at the anterior edge of the gluteus maximus *(15, 16);* Greater trochanter, rear hip: Posterior to the greater trochanteric prominence *(17, 18).*

symptoms characteristic of CFS, and occurs in 78% of those with FM. Poor sleep adversely affects pain and mediates the relation between pain and fatigue. Fatigue in FM has been directly related to actigraphy-derived poor sleep efficiency. Evidence for altered circadian rhythms in CFS is mixed, but a constant routine study showed no difference in melatonin or cortisol between women with and without FM.

The most consistent polysomnographic findings for FM show lower sleep efficiency, with slightly longer sleep-onset latency and more wakefulness in the first half of the night. In CFS, there is also a longer sleep-onset latency and rapid eye movement (REM) sleep latency, and less REM sleep, whereas evidence for fragmented sleep is mixed.

Women with CFS or FM often complain of nonrestorative sleep, and this complaint has been linked to alpha activity in non-REM sleep in FM (Fig. 15.4-2). The alpha-delta hypothesis of nonrestorative sleep assumes that increased alpha activity represents pain during sleep. However, this pattern was first described in psychiatric disorders and is also seen in primary insomnia. Alpha activity has not been correlated with symptom severity.

Rather than alpha-delta activity, FM patients consistently demonstrate fewer sleep spindles per minute of stage 2 sleep (Fig. 15.4-3). Pain tender point pressure threshold predicts the number of spindles after controlling for age and depression, two variables also associated with fewer sleep spindles.

Summary

Women's health is associated with various aspects of reproductive stages in life. This chapter briefly highlights how sleep can be altered by menstrual cycle and hormonal fluctuations that also affect mental health. Pregnancy and postpartum are brief events in women's lives but bring about dramatic changes in sleep during childbearing years.

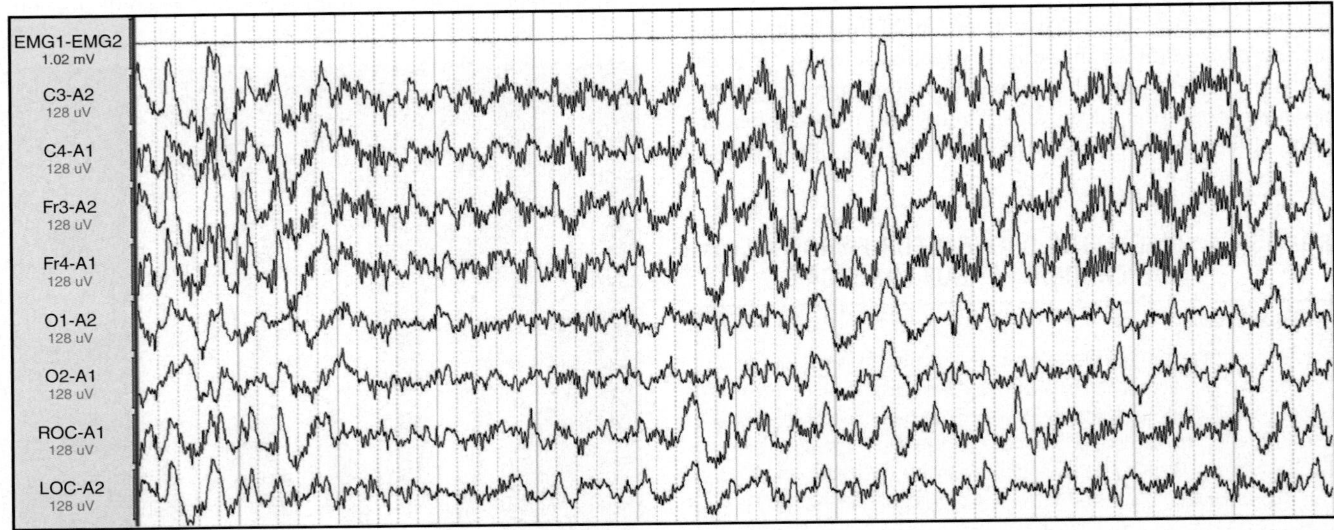

Figure 15.4-2.
An example of alpha-delta sleep. (Courtesy of M. H. Kryger.)

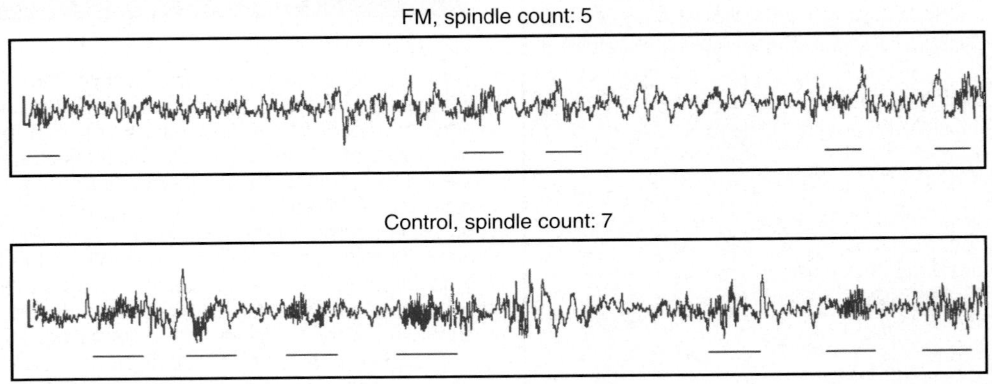

Figure 15.4-3.
Sleep spindle activity in a woman with fibromyalgia (spindle count = 5) compared with a healthy age-matched control (spindle count = 7). (From Landis CA, Lentz MJ, et al: Decreased sleep spindles and spindle activity in midlife women with fibromyalgia. Sleep 27[3]:741–750, 2004.)

Menopausal transition is also a time during which women experience changes in their sleep, but there are discrepancies between objective and self-report indicators. Midlife women are also more likely than men to experience chronic illnesses that impact sleep. FM and CFS are presented here as two examples of relevance to women's health and sleep. Other chronic illnesses that also impact women are reviewed in chapters 13 and 14.

SELECTED READINGS

Clauw DJ, Crofford LJ: Chronic widespread pain and fibromyalgia: What we know, and what we need to know. Best Prac Res Clin Rheum 17: 685–701, 2003.

Klerman EB, Goldenberg DL, Brown EN, et al: Circadian rhythms of women with fibromyalgia. J Clin Endocrinol Metab 86:1034–1039, 2001.

Landis CA, Lentz MJ, Rothermel J, et al: Decreased sleep spindles and spindle activity in midlife women with fibromyalgia. Sleep 27(3):741–750, 2004.

Landis CA, Lentz MJ, Tsuji J, et al: Pain, psychological variables, sleep quality and natural killer cell activity in midlife women with and without fibromyalgia. Brain Behav Immun 18:304–313, 2004.

Wolfe F, Smythe H, Yunus M, et al: The American College of Rheumatology 1990 criteria for the classification of fibromyalgia. Report of the multicenter criteria committee. Arthritis Rheum 33:160–172, 1990.

CHAPTER 16

SLEEP AND PSYCHIATRIC DISEASE

Philip Saleh, Negar Ahmadi, and Colin Shapiro

Sleep disturbances of various forms are common symptoms of many psychiatric disorders. For instance, the prevalence of insomnia among psychiatric patients is 18.6% compared to 10% in the primary care population (Fig. 16-1). Conversely, psychiatric illnesses are common among patients with sleep disorders, suggesting a bidirectional relation (Fig. 16-2).

Investigations of chronic insomnia among sleep clinic patients show that in about 45% of patients, their chronic insomnia is due to a mental disorder. Furthermore, sleep disorders, particularly insomnia, are considered risk factors for several psychiatric disorders (Fig. 16-3). In over 50% of patients with recurrent mood disorders, insomnia precedes the mood disorder, and among patients suffering from insomnia, the prevalence of depression, anxiety, and drug abuse is significantly higher than in those with no insomnia.

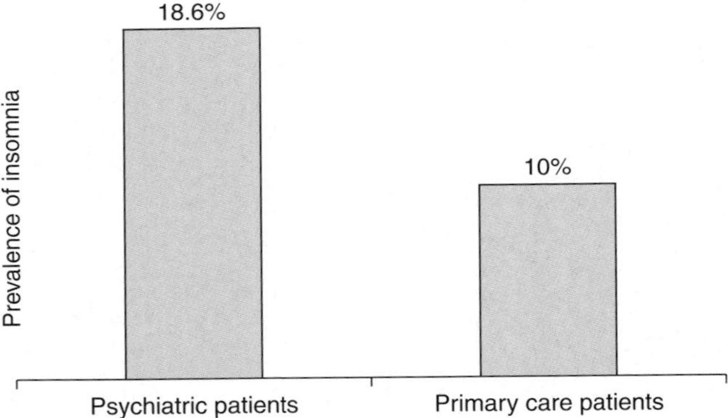

Figure 16-1.
Prevalence of insomnia in psychiatric patients compared with primary care patients. (Adapted from Ohayon MM, Roth T: Place of chronic insomnia in the course of depressive and anxiety disorders. J Psychiatr Res 37:9–15, 2003.)

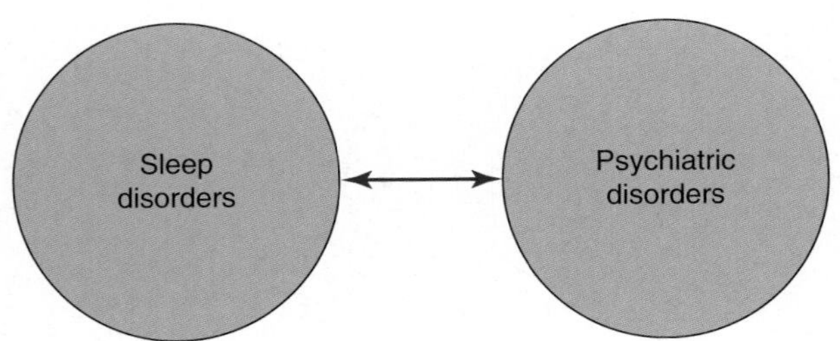

Figure 16-2.
There is a bidirectional relation between sleep disorders and mental illness.

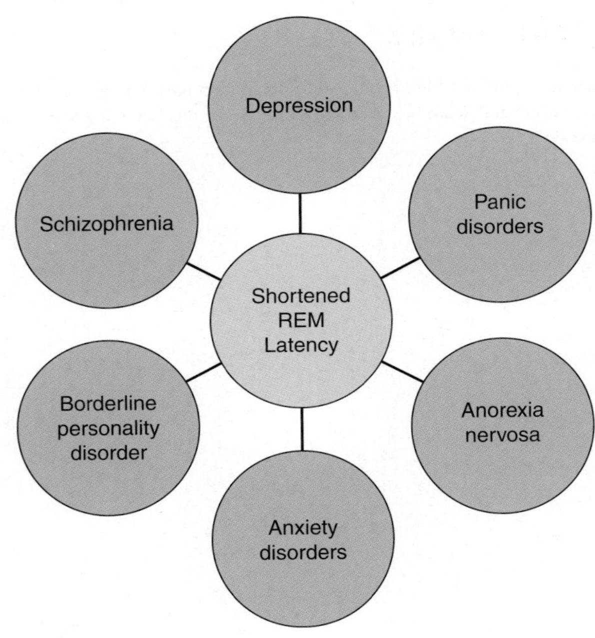

Figure 16-3.
Shortened REM sleep is found in patients suffering from these disorders.

On the other hand, patients with depression also report higher levels of daytime sleepiness. Problems related to the circadian timing of sleep, such as delayed sleep phase syndrome (DSPS), are also found to be more prevalent among patients with mood disorders, and our own unpublished studies support the notion that free-running rhythms commonly coexist with psychiatric problems. Although not commonly seen in children with phase delay, in adults, psychiatric problems are frequently comorbid with DSPS.

The close association between sleep and psychiatric problems can further be observed in polysomnographic (PSG) studies and treatment outcomes. Many psychiatric disorders are associated with certain changes in sleep architecture observed using PSG (Table 16-1). For instance, shortened rapid eye movement (REM) latency is found in patients suffering from a variety of psychiatric disorders, but especially in depression, these sleep changes are more defined (see Table. 16-2).

The close relation between sleep and psychiatry is further found in treatment. Thase and colleagues in 1997

Table 16-1. Polysomnographic Features of Mood Disorders, Anxiety Disorders, Alcohol Abuse, and Schizophrenia

	TOTAL SLEEP TIME	SLEEP LATENCY	SLOW-WAVE SLEEP (%)	REM LATENCY	REM (%)
Mood disorders	↓	↑	↓	↓	↑
Anxiety disorders	↓	↑	↔	↔	↔
Alcohol abuse	↓	↑	↓	↑	↓
Schizophrenia	↓	↑	↓	↓	↔

↓, decreased; ↑ increased; ↔, no change.
Data from Benca RM, Obermeyer WH, Thisted RA, Gillin JC: Sleep and psychiatric disorders: A meta-analysis. Arch Gen Psychiatr 49:651–668, 1992.

Table 16-2. Sleep Changes Associated with Major Depressive Disorder

SLEEP DISTURBANCE CATEGORY	POLYSOMNOGRAPHIC DISTURBANCE
NREM sleep	Decreased slow-wave sleep Decreased delta sleep in NREM-1 vs. NREM-2
REM sleep	Reduced REM latency Increased REM during first half of the night Increased REM density Increased overall REM
Sleep continuity	Increased sleep-onset latency Increased wake time Early morning awakenings Sleep fragmentation Decreased sleep efficiency

The sensitivity and specificity of these changes are approximately 80% (similar to the electrocardiographic changes in the diagnosis of myocardial infarction).

reported that a disturbed sleep pattern is a better predictor of poor response to psychotherapy than is the severity of the depression. Furthermore, treatment of sleep disorders has been shown to alleviate psychiatric illness in many cases. With this in mind, understanding sleep in patients with psychiatric problems and how it relates to their particular psychopathology could be essential in selecting the appropriate course of treatment. Treating the sleep disorder first or concurrently may be a necessary prerequisite to successful treatment of the psychiatric condition (Fig. 16-4). For this reason, a simple screening for specific sleep disorders is essential (Table 16-2).

Sleep and Depression

Patients who are clinically depressed almost uniformly complain of disturbed sleep. Of those individuals, approximately four-fifths have insufficient sleep, with the other fifth complaining of excessive sleep (Fig. 16-5). When the depression is treated using either cognitive therapy or pharmacotherapy, improvements in sleep quality and sleep efficiency, with reductions in latency to sleep onset and time awake after sleep onset, have been observed. From the opposite perspective, as sleep disorders are risk factors for development of depression, treatment of sleep disorders can often prevent depression from occurring in the first place. One of the clearest demonstrations of this was a study of patients treated for their depression with cognitive behavioral therapy that showed an increase in relapse rates for those who developed insomnia while in remission. This

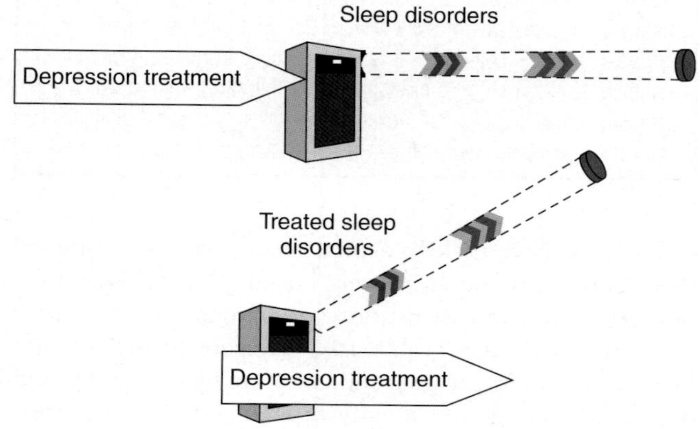

Figure 16-4.
Sleep disorders act as a barrier to the treatment of depression. Once the sleep disorder is treated, previous ineffective depression treatment may become active.

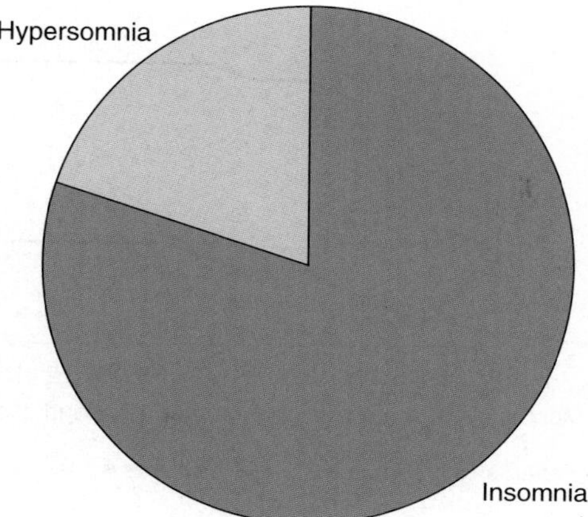

Figure 16-5.
Sleep complaints among depressed patients. Approximately four fifths of depressed patients complain of insomnia and one fifth complain of hypersomnia. (Adapted from Kennedy S, Parikh SV, Shapiro CM: Defeating Depression. Thornhill, ONT: Joli Joco Publications, 1998.)

study added weight to the notion of comorbidity; insomnia was not merely a prodrome to relapse. The treatment implication is that a formerly depressed patient who has insomnia should be vigorously treated with hypnotics. Ironically, many antidepressants lead to sleep disruption and may be deleterious at this juncture. In this context, it should be noted that sleep apnea appears to act as a block to the effective action of both antidepressants and antihypertensive agents (see Fig. 16-4).

Specific patterns of change in the architecture of sleep, as measured by overnight PSG, have been commonly although not consistently observed among patients with major depressive disorder (MDD). Continuing sleep disruption when patients appear euthymic increases the rate of relapse twofold (Fig. 16-6), and of the vegetative features of depression (sleep, appetite, libido, diurnal variation, and concentration), sleep stands out as a key variant. The resolution of sleep problems is therefore critical in terms of recovery and continued well-being. Broadly defined, the sleep architecture changes can be classified as disturbances of non-REM (NREM) sleep, disturbances of REM sleep, and decreased sleep continuity, with each category consisting of several PSG variables observed in multiple studies to differ between MDD patients and nondepressed controls (see Table 16-2).

For the most part, however, individual disturbances of sleep, such as decreased REM latency (once thought to be a candidate-specific marker for depression), decreased slow-wave sleep, or decreased sleep efficiency, cannot on their own specifically predict who is and who is not depressed. A meta-analysis in 1992 indicated that no single sleep parameter known at that time to be associated with MDD can reliably identify those who are and are not depressed. Our experience is that if there are multiple features and specific "representatives" from each of the three major categories of sleep change, further inquiry often leads to evidence of depression even when initially denied or not expected. A treatment trial of an antidepressant is merited in this situation (see Vignette 16-1 and Fig. 16-8).

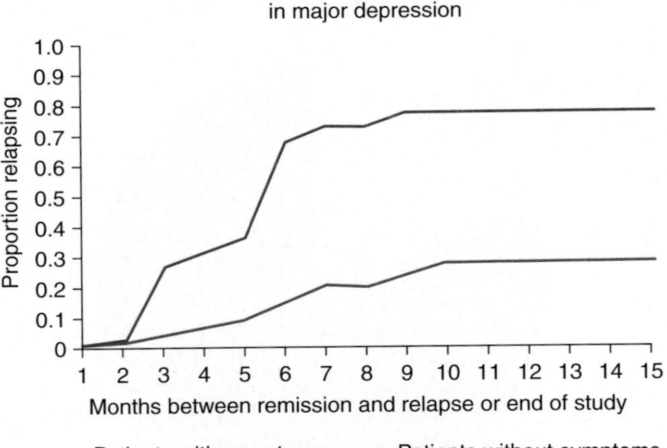

Figure 16-6.
Rates of relapse of depression increase dramatically when any of the vegetative symptoms of depression (including poor sleep) remain following treatment. (Adapted from Kennedy S, Parikh SV, Shapiro CM: Defeating Depression. Thornhill, ONT: Joli Joco Publications, 1998.)

VIGNETTE 16-1. MASKED DEPRESSION AND TREATMENT-RESISTANT INSOMNIA

A 38-year-old woman who had adopted a child when she was 19 years of age presents to the sleep clinic having been seen and treated previously. Her major complaint is that of insomnia. A detailed assessment shows clear current features of initial and maintenance insomnia. She describes a history of having been tried in the past on a benzodiazepine hypnotic by her family physician and having received brief counseling at a previous sleep clinic as well as sequentially a treatment with zopiclone. None of these interventions had any benefit.

Her history is noncontributory from a medical, psychiatric, or substance abuse perspective. A suggestion is made that she enter a brief (eight-session) cognitive behavioral therapy group program for insomnia that occurs with a psychiatrist and occupational therapist and seven other patients. She participates enthusiastically but has no benefit. A repeat attempt at a trial of a hypnotic is made, and subsequently a trial of tryptophan is also attempted, all to no avail. At this point a sleep assessment is carried out, which shows characteristic features of depression. When the patient is seen at follow-up and the possibility of depression, which did not show up in standardized questionnaires, is raised, she claims to have always "hid my feelings." A trial of treatment with mirtazapine is instituted, and within 3 weeks she has no residual insomnia. The trial is continued for a period of 6 months with no further change. At no point did she have other vegetative features of depression. She is discharged from treatment.

Six years later she re-presents with a number of personal stressors and significant insomnia. There are no other features of depression. She has already been to her family physician and had a trial of a hypnotic. On this occasion a sleep study is again suggested, although the patient says that on this occasion the experience is very different and she does not believe that she is at all depressed. The sleep study is carried through, and again there are clear sleep markers of depression including short REM latency, fragmentation of sleep, no initial insomnia, and reversal of slow-wave sleep. She is given a trial of venlafaxine, which again is dramatically effective in resolving her sleep complaints. This case is a clear indication that sleep markers of depression may be helpful, for example, in cases of masked depression that might be viewed as treatment-resistant insomnia.

There is, nevertheless, a physiologic basis for thinking that sleep and mood are closely linked. The REM suppressant action of the vast majority of antidepressant medications (summarized in Table 16-3) is cause to believe that increasing noradrenergic and serotonergic activity and decreasing cholinergic activity brought on by antidepressants is a possible common pathway through which normalization of sleep reflects improvement in depressive symptoms (Fig. 16-7). In 1975 it was suggested that REM

Table 16-3. Degree of REM Suppression of Selected Antidepressant Medications

CLASS OF ANTIDEPRESSANT	NAME OF DRUG	REM EFFECT	REML EFFECT
TCAs	Amitriptyline	↓↓↓	↑
	Doxepin	↓↓	?
	Imipramine	↓↓	?
	Desipramine	↓↓	↑
	Clomipramine	↓↓↓↓	/
	Trimipramine	↔	↑
	Amineptine	↑	↓
	Nortriptyline	↓	↔
MAOIs	Phenelzine	↓↓↓↓	/
	Tranylcypromine	↓↓↓↓	↑
	Moclobemide	?	↑
	Brofaromine	↓?	↑
	Paragyline	↓↓↓↓	/
SSRIs	Fluoxetine	↓	↑
	Paroxetine	↓↓	?
	Sertraline	↔	↔
	Fluvoxamine	↓↓	↑
	Zimelidine	↓?	↑
	Vilazodone	↓↓↓↓	/
	Citalopram	↓	↑
SNRIs	Duloxetine	↓↓	↑
	Nefazodone	↑	↔
	Venlafaxine	↓?	↑
NRIs	Atomoxetine	↓	↔
	Reboxetine	↓	↑
	Viloxazine	↓↓	↑
	Bupropion	↔	↔
Other	Trazodone	↓	?
	Mirtazapine	↓?	↑
	Mianserin	↔	↑
	Melatonin	↑	↔

REM effect = amount of REM sleep over the course of a night; REML effect = change in REM latency.
MAOIs, monamine oxidase inhibitors; NRIs, noradrenaline reuptake inhibitors; SNRIs, serotonin and norepinephrine reuptake inhibitors; SSRIs, selective serotonin reuptake inhibitors; TCAs, tricyclic antidepressants.
↓to ↓↓↓↓: Mild suppression to complete or near complete suppression; decrease in REM latency.
↑: Increase in REM/REM latency.
↔: No change.
↓?: Suppression of REM sleep, degree unknown.
?: Trend unknown.
/: Not applicable due to complete or near complete suppression of REM sleep.
Suggested readings: Mayers AG, Baldwin DS: Antidepressants and their effect on sleep. Hum Psychopharmacol 20:533–559, 2005; Sandor P, Shapiro CM: Sleep patterns in depression and anxiety: Theory and pharmacological effects. J Psychosom Res 38(Suppl 1):125–139, 1994.

suppression could be important in the treatment of depression. The theory was subsequently modified to indicate that REM suppression may only be one mechanism of treatment (Table 16-4). In healthy patients, the administration of serotonin agonists has been shown to cause increases in slow-wave sleep, and, conversely, in neuroimaging and postmortem studies, it has been shown that decreased serotonergic activity in the brain is associated with depression and suicide. This is again consistent with commonly observed sleep markers.

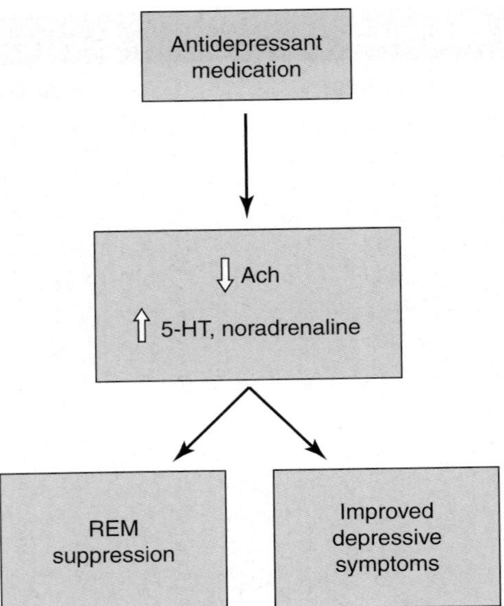

Figure 16-7.
Hypothesized activity of a typical antidepressant medication. Ach, acetylcholine; 5-HT, serotonin.

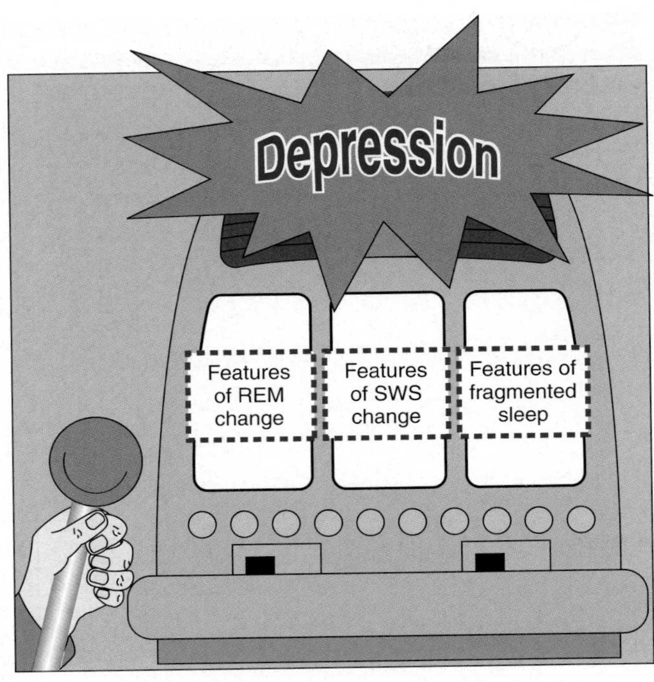

Figure 16-8.
When one or more features of these categories (see Table 16-2) is present then the likelihood of depression is high.

Interestingly, when sleep in depression is approached from a multitude of perspectives, the link between sleep architecture and MDD becomes more specific and reliable. Several studies that examined the ability of multiple sleep parameters to distinguish MDD patients from healthy controls in the 1980s have been much more successful than studies that looked at one parameter alone (Fig. 16-8). A broader set of sleep markers may more specifically characterize depression. Sleep in depression may instead be thought of as an orchestra, in which a performance could be salvaged with a mediocre string section, but the cumulative effect of poor performance by the woodwinds and the brass will be a severe handicap. In the same vein, decreased latency to the first REM period, for example, may not in itself be linked to depression, but if seen in conjunction with both abnormalities in slow-wave sleep and decreased sleep continuity, the likelihood that a patient is or will become depressed may be increased.

Table 16-4. REM Sleep Effects of Various Pharmacologic and Nonpharmacologic Treatments

Treatment of depression can be thought of in many ways, for example, pharmacologic and psychological (or combined). One way is to consider which treatments do and do not suppress REM sleep. In general, if one treatment does not work, a treatment from a different category should be tried.

TREATMENT TYPE	SUPPRESSES REM SLEEP	DOES NOT SUPPRESS REM SLEEP
Pharmacologic	Most antidepressants (see Table 16-3)	Nefazodone Amineptine
Nonpharmacologic	Sleep deprivation (esp. REM sleep deprivation) Electroconvulsive therapy Psychosurgery	Cognitive therapy Bright light treatment

More recently, the use of quantitative electroencephalogram (EEG) analysis to delve deeper into the microarchitecture of sleep has yielded a potential new layer of insight into the neurophysiology of MDD. Primarily using the techniques of power spectral analysis and period amplitude analysis, the energy and variation in polarity of an EEG signal can be quantified. Recent studies have demonstrated that sleep microarchitecture may be the most specific measure of the susceptibility to developing depressive symptoms, particularly in adolescents. Overall, quantitative EEG trends have differed across genders. In women, we tend to see decreases in temporal coherence, that is, the degree of synchrony or coupling between all-night brain EEG rhythms. In men, the microarchitecture of slow-wave sleep may be more characteristic of their depressive state, with lower delta counts and slower time course of accumulation and dissipation of slow-wave activity (Fig. 16-9). The use of quantitative EEG analysis has thus far provided some basis for suggesting that on average, depression represents distinct pathophysiologies among men and women.

There still remains much to be discovered about the specificity of sleep markers for depression. What is clear after decades of study is that sleep holds at least some of the answers to both why and how we become depressed.

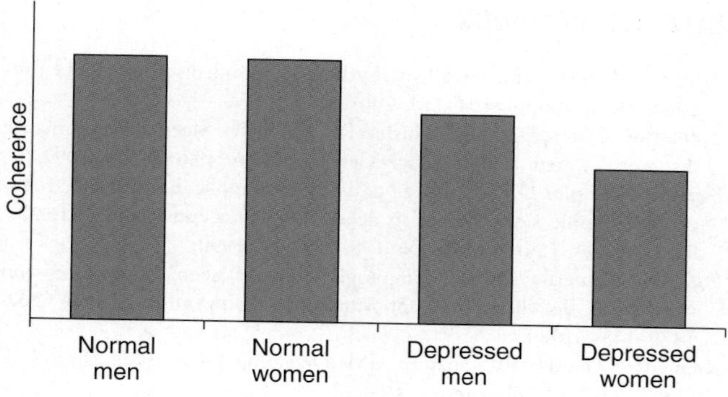

Figure 16-9.
Depressed individuals have lower coherence compared with normal controls. Among depressed individuals, depressed women have lower coherence than depressed men. (Adapted from Armitage R: Sleep and circadian rhythms in mood disorders. Acta Psychiatr Scand (Suppl):104–115, 2007.)

Sleep and Post-Traumatic Stress Disorder

Post-traumatic stress disorder (PTSD) is another psychiatric disorder that is often associated with poor sleep and nightmares. Some of the PSG features associated with PTSD include decreased total sleep time, reduced sleep efficiency, increased sleep latency, decreased REM and non-REM dream recall, increased motor activity in REM and non-REM, and increased fast-frequency EEG activity during sleep. However, the evidence in regard to the amount of REM sleep and REM latency among PTSD patients seems to be contradictory. Several studies have shown improvements in PTSD symptoms after sleep treatments and nightmare reductions. Some have further suggested that the delay in the onset of REM sleep is indicative of an adaptive adjustment to PTSD. Sleep architecture can be a useful clue in this diagnosis (see Vignette 16-2).

VIGNETTE 16-2. PTSD DIAGNOSIS FACILITATED BY SLEEP EVALUATION

An 11-year-old girl who is seen by a clinical neuropsychologist and at an inpatient psychiatric service is found to have attention deficit disorder and significant sleep complaints. The patient has been admitted for a period of a month and no clear psychiatric diagnosis has been made. There is a marked degree of acting out by the child, including a couple of known episodes of fire setting. The sleep evaluation shows markedly delayed onset of REM sleep and very fragmented sleep. In the follow-up interview when the child is seen with her nurse, the suggestion is made to the child that it would appear from the sleep evaluation that there might have been some significant traumatic experience in her past life. At this point her facial expression changes dramatically with significant pallor, and after a lengthy pause she comments, "How did you know?" The sleep specialist/psychiatrist asks her what the "worst thing that had happened in your life" was and at this point for the first time the child opens up and describes sexual abuse by her father and violent physical abuse by her mother.

The ensuing few weeks in the inpatient psychiatric unit are dramatically different with a formulation of post-traumatic stress disorder and a psychotherapeutic approach being taken to deal with the past traumas. The child eventually returns to a foster home with improved sleep, fewer features of attention deficit, and an apparent, dramatic subjective improvement. This case gives an indication that the sleep study can facilitate an understanding of traumas when for whatever reason the patient may be resistant to discussing negative past experiences.

Sleep and Anxiety

Many patients suffering from anxiety disorders complain of difficulty initiating and maintaining sleep. PSG studies of these patients show longer sleep latency, increased time awake, reduced sleep efficiency, reduced slow-wave sleep, and an increased arousal index compared to normal individuals. Alcohol dependence is also associated with several sleep disturbances, including insomnia, obstructive sleep apnea, and circadian rhythm disturbances. Some of the PSG features of alcohol dependence include decreased sleep efficiency, decreased total sleep time, increased stage changes, decreased slow-wave sleep, and decreased REM latency. Alcoholism is further associated with suppression of growth hormone, which is predominantly secreted during sleep and specifically related to slow-wave sleep. The suppression of slow-wave sleep may lead to unrefreshing sleep, a common complaint among drinkers. There is an extensive literature concerning the link between slow-wave sleep and restorative experience, and the lack of refreshing sleep may lead drinkers to increase consumption. Therefore, one suspects that the PSG features observed in alcohol dependence might be due to the suppression of growth hormones during sleep.

Sleep and Schizophrenia

Schizophrenia is similarly associated with sleep disturbances, including insomnia, disturbed circadian rhythm, and daytime sleepiness. The observed PSG features of schizophrenia include increased sleep latency, decreased sleep efficiency, decreased slow-wave sleep, and decreased REM latency. PSG features associated with schizophrenia, like other psychiatric conditions, may be confounded by medication effects, and drug-free study participants are difficult to find. Furthermore, treatments of both alcohol dependence and schizophrenia are associated with improved sleep.

Consequences of Untreated Sleep Disorders

If left untreated, sleep disorders can cause onset or recurrence of psychiatric disorders. Table 16-5 summarizes the consequences of untreated sleep disorders.

Table 16-5. Psychiatric Consequences of Untreated Sleep Disorders

SLEEP DISORDER	PSYCHIATRIC CONSEQUENCES
Insomnia	Depression Anxiety disorders Substance use disorder
Obstructive sleep apnea	Depression Impaired cognition Fatigue Daytime sleepiness
Narcolepsy	Depression Hallucinations Fatigue Daytime sleepiness
Restless legs syndrome	Depression Akathisia Anxiety disorders Attention deficit hyperactivity disorder
Circadian rhythm sleep disorder	Depression Anxiety disorders Personality disorder

Conclusions

There remains much to be found out regarding the specificity of sleep disturbances for depression and other psychiatric conditions. What is clear after decades of study is that sleep has an important role in both the development of psychiatric problems and the selection of effective ways to treat them.

SELECTED READINGS

Armitage R: Sleep and circadian rhythms in mood disorders. Acta Psychiatr Scand (Suppl):104–115, 2007.

Benca RM, Obermeyer WH, Thisted RA, Gillin JC: Sleep and psychiatric disorders: A meta-analysis. Arch Gen Psychiatry 49:651–668, 1992.

Buysse DJ, Kupfer DJ: Diagnostic and research applications of electroencephalographic sleep studies in depression: Conceptual and methodological issues. J Nerv Ment Dis 178:405–414, 1990.

Ford DE, Kamerow DB: Epidemiologic study of sleep disturbances and psychiatric disorders: An opportunity for prevention? JAMA 262: 1479–1484, 1989.

Kennedy S, Parikh SV, Shapiro CM: Defeating Depression. Thornhill, ONT, Joli Joco Publications, 1998.

Mayers AG, Baldwin DS: Antidepressants and their effect on sleep. Hum Psychopharmacol 20:533–559, 2005.

Ohayon MM, Roth T: Place of chronic insomnia in the course of depressive and anxiety disorders. J Psychiatr Res 37:9–15, 2003.

Ross RJ, Ball WA, Dinges DF, et al: Rapid eye movement sleep disturbance in posttraumatic stress disorder. Biol Psychiatr 35:195–202, 1994.

Sandor P, Shapiro CM: Sleep patterns in depression and anxiety: Theory and pharmacological effects. J Psychosom Res 38(Suppl 1):125–139, 1994.

Shapiro CM: Growth hormone—sleep interaction: A review. Res Commun Psychol Psychiatr Behav 6:115–131, 1981.

Shapiro CM, Ohayon MM, Huterer N, Grunstein R: Fighting Fatigue and Sleepiness. Thornhill, ONT, Joli Joco Publications, 2005.

Shapiro GK, Shen J, Shapiro CM: Sleep changes in the depressed older adult: Implications for management. Geriatric and Aging (Suppl 7):25–31, 2004.

Shen J, Kennedy SH, Levitan RD, et al: The effects of nefazodone on women with seasonal affective disorder: Clinical and polysomnographic analyses. J Psychiatr Neurosci 30:11–16, 2005.

Thase ME, Buysse DJ, Frank E, et al: Which depressed patients will respond to interpersonal psychotherapy? The role of abnormal EEG sleep profiles. Am J Psychiatr 154:502–509, 1997.

Yang C, Winkelman JW: Clinical significance of sleep EEG abnormalities in chronic schizophrenia. Schizophr Res 82:251–260, 2006.

DIAGNOSTIC ASSESSMENT METHODS

CHAPTER 17

Max Hirshkowitz and Amir Sharafkhaneh

Introduction

As you read this, thousands of people are having their sleep recorded. These digital electrophysiologic data will be collected in hospitals, specialized sleep disorders centers, and patients' homes. The vast majority of these "sleep studies" will focus on determining the presence, type, and severity of sleep-disordered breathing. Recordings will also be made to diagnose narcolepsy, seizures, parasomnias, and other sleep disorders. Other studies will be conducted for research. However, unlike most major medical diagnostic procedures, the parameters recorded, how tests are conducted, techniques applied for record review, and procedures used for data reduction will vary substantially from one test facility to another. In an attempt to standardize recordings used in sleep medicine, the American Academy of Sleep Medicine (AASM) developed and published a standardized clinical polysomnography (PSG) manual, and that is what is largely described in this chapter.

The diversity in methods and techniques arises from "sleep medicine's" foundation as a research endeavor. Discovering recordable bioelectric correlates for suspected sleep problems paved the way for adopting PSG (a psychophysiologic research method) as the "big clinical procedure" in sleep medicine. As is common in science, methods were diverse. Furthermore, methods were continually modified to increase sensitivity depending on the focused questions under study. Nevertheless, as clinical utility for PSG grew, de facto standards gained acceptance and expert panels developed guidelines. The AASM manual was based largely on existing techniques, and its content represents the efforts of a great many individuals. Previous guidelines included the standardized manual for terminology, techniques, and scoring (see next section); the guidelines developed by the American Sleep Disorders Association (ASDA) task forces on arousal scoring and periodic leg movements scoring; and the "Chicago Group's" work on sleep-related breathing. The AASM manual, developed through the use of evidence-based research techniques, provides a single source for information on how to record, score, and reduce sleep data.

Sleep Staging

Loomis and colleagues recorded the first known, continuous, all-night, electrophysiologic sleep study, and distilling their mass of collected data down to a manageable form became immediately imperative. Thus, sleep staging was developed. During the following three decades an assortment of sleep stage classification schemes emerged, culminating in the standardized technique described in *A Manual of Standardized Terminology, Techniques and Scoring System for Sleep Stages in Human Subjects*. Drs. Allan Rechtschaffen and Anthony Kales chaired this project and consequently the manual is nicknamed the *R&K manual*. The *R&K manual* focused on normal sleep and mainly addressed sleep staging. As pointed out in the AASM scoring manual preface, "the rapidly emerging field of sleep medicine requires a more comprehensive system of standardized metrics that considers events occurring outside of normal brain activity."

RECORDING

Three types of measures are recorded and are used to stage sleep: (1) brain activity, (2) eye movements, and (3) skeletal muscle tone.

Electroencepahalogram for Brain Activity

For classifying sleep stages, the AASM manual recommends recording frontal, central, and occipital electroencephalograms (EEGs)—specifically, monopolar derivations from F_4, C_4, and O_2, linked to the contralateral mastoid (M). Backup electrodes are placed at homologous sites at left scalp loci. An alternative recording montage allows for substitution of midline bipolar recordings from frontal and occipital derivations (Table 17-1, Figs. 17-1 to 17-3).

Eye Movements

To detect eye movements, electrodes are placed near the eyes' right and left outer canthi (E_2 and E_1, respectively). The manual recommends a monopolar electro-oculographic (EOG) montage, with E_2 placed 1 cm above and E_1 placed 1 cm below the outer canthus. When a lateral eye movement occurs, the positive corneal potential moves toward one electrode and away from the other. Therefore, this electrode arrangement produces robust right versus left EOG out-of-phase activity when horizontal eye movements occur. Consequently, eye movements are easily differentiated by frontal EEG activity proximal to the EOG electrodes (which appears as an in-phase signal). Staggering the electrode placements slightly above and slightly below each eye's horizontal plane allows for some limited appreciation of vertical eye movements on the PSG. An alternative recording montage allowing better visualization of vertical eye movements

Table 17-1. Recording Montage for Sleep Staging and Respiratory Monitoring

			SAMPLING RATE (Hz)		FILTER SETTING (Hz)	
RECORDED ACTIVITY	STANDARD SITE	ALTERNATE SITE	PREFERRED	MINIMAL	LOW *f*	HIGH *f*
Central EEG	C_4-M_1		500	200	0.3	35
Occipital EEG	O_4-M_1	C_z-Oz	500	200	0.3	35
Frontal EEG	F_4-M_1	F_z-Cz	500	200	0.3	35
Left EOG	E_1*-M_2	E_1*-F_p	500	200	0.3	35
Right EOG	E_2**-M_2	E_2*-F_p	500	200	0.3	35
Muscle tone	Submental EMG		500	200	10	100
EKG	Lead II		500	200	0.3	70
Airflow thermistor	Nares and mouth		100	25	0.1	15
Oximetry	Earlobe or finger		25	10	0.1	15
Nasal pressure	Nose		100	25	0.1	15
Esophageal pressure	[Inserted]		100	25	0.1	15
Body position	Various		1	1		
Snoring sounds	Microphone		500	200	10	100
Respiratory effort	Rib cage and abdominal movement		100	25	0.1	15
		Intercostal EMG	500	200	10	100

*Place electrode 1 cm below the eye's outer canthus.
**Place electrode 1 cm above the eye's outer canthus.
C_z, central zero (midline); E_1, left eye; E_2, right eye; EEG, electroencephalogram; EKG, electrocardiogram; EOG, electro-oculography; f, frequency; Fp, frontal pole; Hz, Hertz; M, mastoid; O_z, occipital zero (midline).

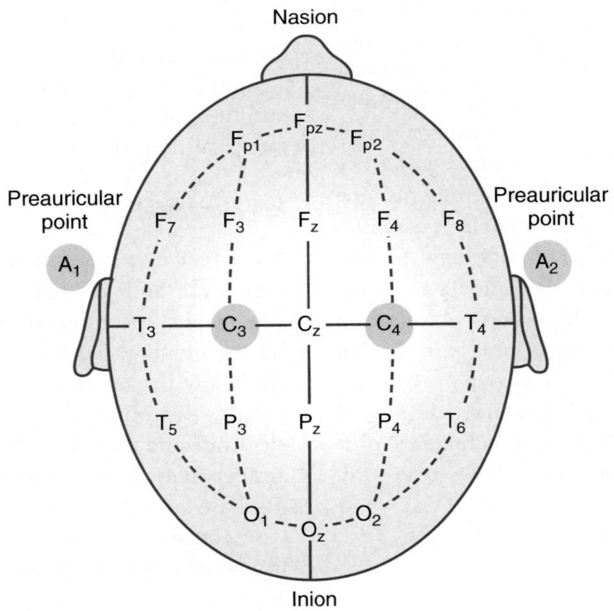

Figure 17-1.
Classic Rechtschaffen and Kales derivations for recording the EEG. Electrode locations as recommended in 1969. Electrode pairs are indicated by the same colors.

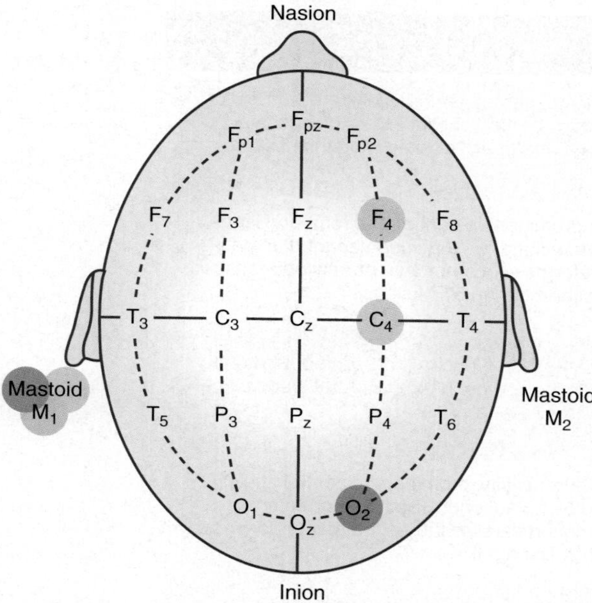

Figure 17-2.
Updated AASM recommended derivations for recording the EEG. Electrode locations as recommended in 2007 by the American Academy of Sleep Medicine.

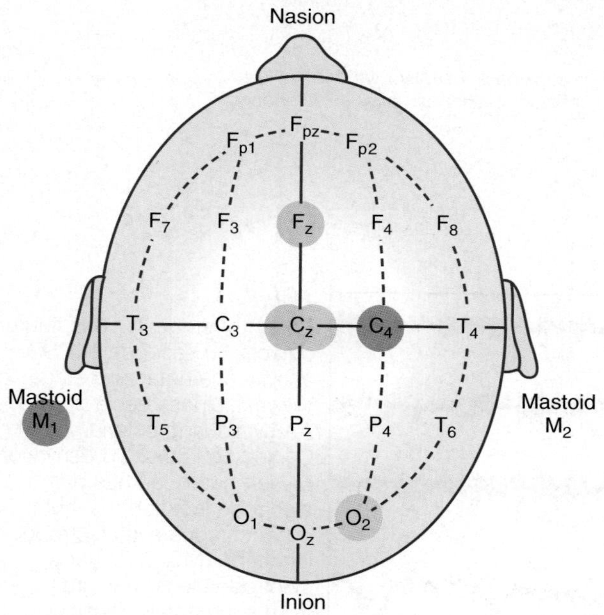

Figure 17-3.
Updated AASM alternative derivations for recording the EEG. Alternative electrode locations as recommended in 2007. Backup electrode substitutions: O_1 for O_z, F_{pz} for F_z, and C_3 for C_z.

(albeit sacrificing the in-phase/out-of-phase differentiation by frontal EEG activity) has both EOG placements 1 cm below the outer canthi and referenced to the middle of the forehead (see Table 17-1).

Electromyogram for Skeletal Muscle Tone

Finally, to record a submentalis electromyogram (EMG), one electrode is placed 1 cm above the mandible's inferior edge (on the midline) and the other two are placed 2 cm below and 2 cm to the right and left of midline, respectively. Recordings should reference one of the two electrodes below the mandible to the one above (with the remaining electrode for backup).

STAGING

Classification

The AASM manual sets epoch length at 30 seconds. Overall, three categories representing distinct, overall organizational states of the central nervous system (CNS) are conceptualized: wakefulness, rapid eye movement sleep (REM sleep), and non-REM sleep (NREM sleep). On the basis of EEG, EOG, and EMG activity, each recorded epoch is classified as either stage N1 (NREM 1), N2 (NREM 2), N3 (NREM 3), R (REM), or W (wakefulness).

Waves

Six EEG waveforms are commonly used to differentiate state and classify sleep stages: (1) α (alpha) activity, (2) θ (theta) activity, (3) vertex sharp waves, (4) sleep spindles, (5) K complexes, and (6) slow-wave activity (Table 17-2).

Stages

Stage W. In patients with well-defined alpha activity, wakefulness and sleep are easily differentiated. Stage W is scored when alpha activity occupies 15 or more seconds of an epoch (Fig. 17-4). By contrast, in the absence of clear alpha activity, staging can be difficult.

Stage N1. Vertex sharp waves that often herald sleep onset provide a valuable landmark for recognizing stage N1 sleep. Wakefulness usually transitions to either stage N1 or N2. Stage N1 is marked by a general slowing of the background activity with the appearance of theta and vertex short waves. N1 may also be marked by the cessation of blinking and saccadic eye movements and by the appearance of slow eye movements (Fig. 17-5). While not required, N1 can be discerned by its low-voltage, mixed-frequency background EEG containing theta activity in the absence of slow waves, sleep spindles, K complexes, prominent alpha activity, or REMs. Inter- and intra-scorer reliability is lowest for stage N1 because it is defined largely by rules of exclusion rather than by clearly recognizable electrophysiologic events.

Table 17-2. Sleep EEG Waveforms

Sample	Label	Definition
	Alpha activity	8–13 Hz rhythm, usually most prominent in occipital leads. Thought to be generated by cortex, possibly via dipole located in layers 4 and 5. Used as a marker for relaxed wakefulness and CNS arousals.
	Theta activity	4–8 Hz waves, typically prominent in central and temporal leads. Sawtooth activity (shown in figure) is a unique variant of theta activity (containing waveforms with a notched or *sawtooth-shaped* appearance) frequently seen during REM sleep.
	Vertex sharp waves	Sharply contoured, negative-going bursts that stand out from the background activity and appear most often in central leads placed near the midline.
	Sleep spindle	A phasic burst of 11–16 Hz activity, prominent in central scalp leads; typically last for 0.5–1.5 seconds. Spindles are a scalp representation of thalamocortical discharges; the name derives from their shape (which is spindle-like).
	K complex	Recently redefined in the AASM manual as *an EEG event consisting of a well-delineated negative sharp wave immediately followed by a positive component standing out from the background EEG with total duration ≥ 0.5 seconds, usually maximal in amplitude over the frontal regions.*
	Slow waves	High-amplitude (≥ 75 μvolts) and low-frequency (≤ 2 Hz) variants of delta (1–4 Hz) activity. Slow waves are the defining characteristics of stage N3 sleep.
	REM	Rapid eye movements are conjugate saccades occurring during REM sleep correlated with the dreamer's attempt to look at the dream sensorium. They are sharply peaked with an initial deflection usually < ½ second in duration.
	SEM	Slow eye movements are conjugate, usually rhythmic, rolling eye movements with an initial deflection usually ≥ ½ second in duration.

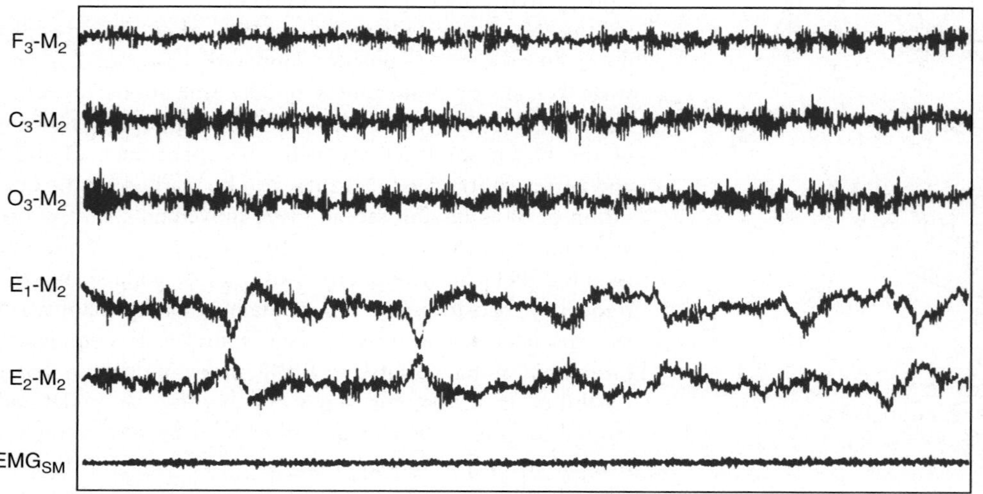

Figure 17-4. Epoch of stage W. This figure depicts 30 seconds of PSG activity characterizing stage W wakefulness according to AASM scoring criteria. C_3, left central scalp derivation; E_1, left outer canthus eye electrode location; E_2, right outer canthus eye electrode location; EMG_{SM}, surface electrode electromyogram from submentalis muscle; F_3, left frontal scalp derivation; M_2, right mastoid electrode location; O_3, left occipital scalp derivation.

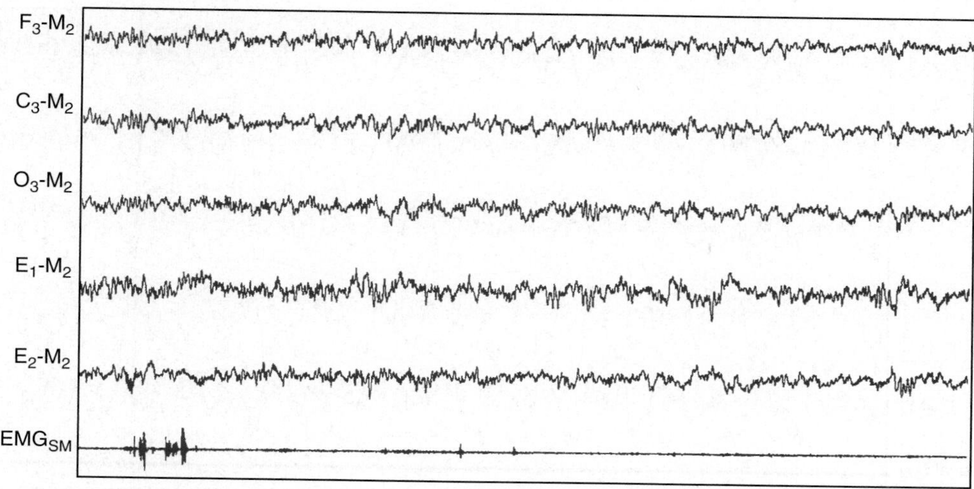

Figure 17-5.
Epoch of stage N1. This figure depicts 30 seconds of PSG activity characterizing stage N1 sleep according to AASM scoring criteria. C_3, left central scalp derivation; E_1, left outer canthus eye electrode location; E_2, right outer canthus eye electrode location; EMG_{SM}, surface electrode electromyogram from submentalis muscle; F_3, left frontal scalp derivation; M_2, right mastoid electrode location; O_3, left occipital scalp derivation.

Stage N2. By contrast, stage N2 is easily recognized by sleep spindles or K complexes (Fig. 17-6) occurring on a low-voltage, mixed-frequency background EEG in the absence of significant slow-wave activity (i.e., less than 6 seconds of 75 or more μvolts).

Stage N3. When 6 or more seconds of slow-wave activity are present in an epoch, it is scored as stage N3 (Fig. 17-7). The designation N3 conforms to what used to be called slow-wave sleep because of the highly synchronized low-frequency activity. If the alternate bipolar montage is used (F_z-C_z), amplitudes would be lower, and the current AASM manual does not provide a guideline for amplitude adjustment. Therefore, stage N3 should be scored with the monopolar central lead included as part of the alternate montage.

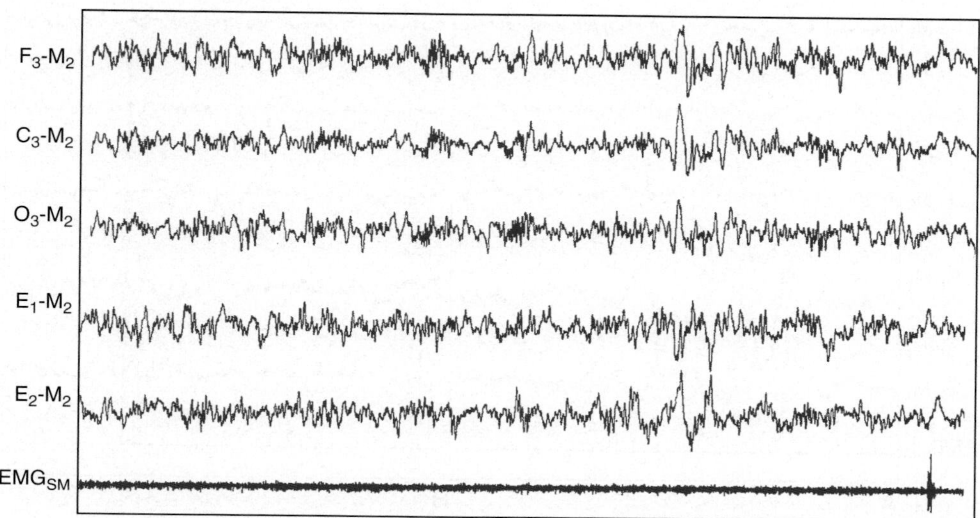

Figure 17-6.
Epoch of stage N2. This figure depicts 30 seconds of PSG activity characterizing stage N2 sleep according to AASM scoring criteria. C_3, left central scalp derivation; E_1, left outer canthus eye electrode location; E_2, right outer canthus eye electrode location; EMG_{SM}, surface electrode electromyogram from submentalis muscle; F_3, left frontal scalp derivation; M_2, right mastoid electrode location; O_3, left occipital scalp derivation.

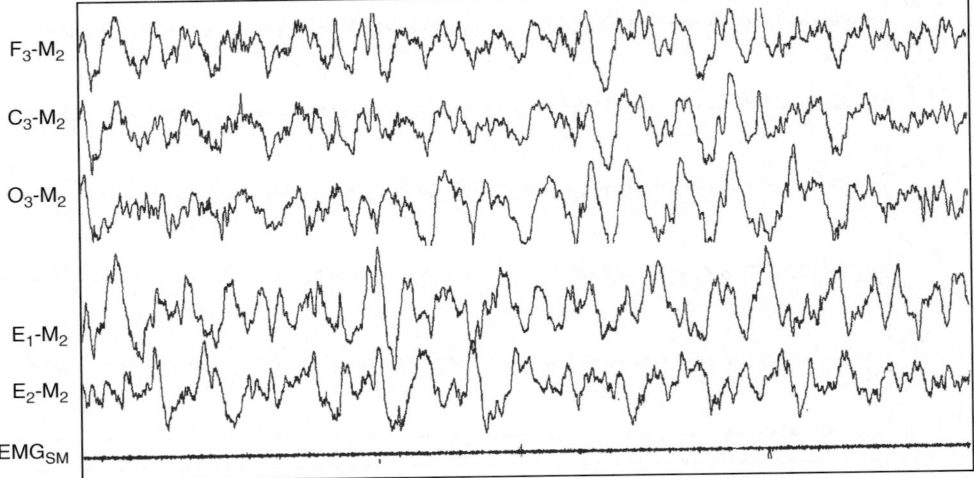

Figure 17-7.
Epoch of stage N3. This figure depicts 30 seconds of PSG activity characterizing stage N3 sleep according to AASM scoring criteria. C_3, left central scalp derivation; E_1, left outer canthus eye electrode location; E_2, right outer canthus eye electrode location; EMG_{SM}, surface electrode electromyogram from submentalis muscle; F_3, left frontal scalp derivation; M_2, right mastoid electrode location; O_3, left occipital scalp derivation.

Stage R. Essentially, criteria for scoring REM sleep (or stage R, as it has been renamed—although most people will likely continue to call it REM sleep) have remained the same. Stage R is characterized by low-voltage, mixed-frequency EEG, very low chin EMG levels, and REMs (Fig. 17-8). Sawtooth activity is a unique variant of theta activity (containing waveforms with a notched or sawtooth-shaped appearance) frequently seen in stage R (Table 17-3).

Smoothing Rules

When an epoch contains characteristic features for more than one sleep stage, it is scored according to the characteristics that make up its majority. One source of scoring difficulty arises when epochs without REMs are contiguous with REM sleep. The AASM manual does not address the concept of differentiation between phasic and tonic REM sleep (see Fig. 17-8). Nevertheless, this concept is widely

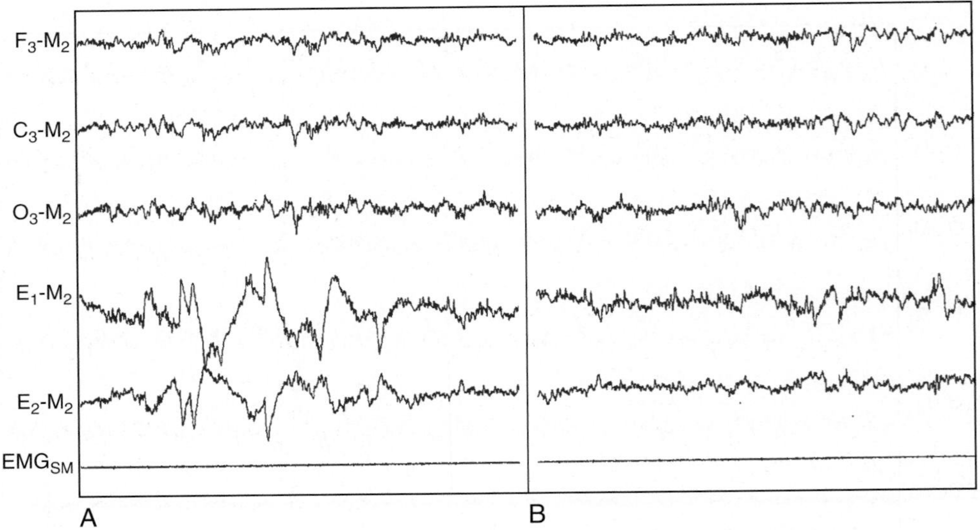

Figure 17-8.
Phasic and tonic REM sleep. This figure depicts PSG activity characterizing stage R sleep according to AASM scoring criteria. **A** illustrates stage R with phasic bursts of rapid eye movements (phasic REM); **B** shows a quiescent period of stage R sleep (tonic REM). C_3, left central scalp derivation; E_1, left outer canthus eye electrode location; E_2, right outer canthus eye electrode location; EMG_{SM}, surface electrode electromyogram from submentalis muscle; F_3, left frontal scalp derivation; M_2, right mastoid electrode location; O_3, left occipital scalp derivation.

Table 17-3. Electrophysiologic Characteristics of Each Sleep Stage

	SLEEP STAGE				
ELECTROPHYSIOLOGIC ACTIVITY	***W****	***N1***	***N2***	***N3***	***R***
Low-voltage, mixed-frequency EEG		√	√		√
Vertex sharp waves		√	√		
Sleep spindles			√	√	
K complexes			√	√	
EEG β bandwidth activity	√	√			√
EEG α bandwidth activity	≥ 15 s	< 15 s	< 15 s	< 15 s	< 15 s
EEG θ bandwidth activity		√	√	√	√**
EEG Δ bandwidth activity		√	√	√	
Slow-wave activity†		< 6 s	< 6 s	≥ 6 s	< 6 s
Eye movements activity	Slow and rapid	Slow			Rapid
EMG activity level	Variable	Low	Low	Low	Atonic

*With eyes closed

**Special form of theta called sawtooth owing to its appearance

†For purposes of sleep staging, monopolar slow-wave activity from frontal or central derivations must be 75 μvolts or more.

EEG, electroencephalographic; EMG, electromyographic; s, seconds.

used in research and can serve as a pedagogic aid in this matter. Phasic REM sleep encompasses epochs scored as stage R clearly accompanied by eye movements (and sometimes other phasic events). By contrast, tonic REM sleep has the same background EEG activity with completely diminished chin EMG but lacks eye movements. If such an epoch occurred in isolation, it would likely be scored as N1; however, when surrounded by epochs of phasic REM sleep, it is considered stage R. In fact, eye-movement-less N1-like epochs contiguous with REM sleep continue to be scored as stage R until a spindle, a K complex, arousal, increase in chin EMG, a body movement followed by slow eye movements, or another sleep stage appears (in the first half of the epoch). The AASM manual provides examples to guide scoring decisions at stage transitions.

Arousal Scoring

EEG SPEEDING AND CNS AROUSALS

Sleep staging forms what may be called the building blocks of sleep macroarchitecture. Staging can be useful in getting a general impression of sleep's overall continuity and integrity, detecting gross disturbances, and correlating pathophysiology with the CNS's organizational state (i.e., REM, NREM, or wakefulness). Staging parameters, however, fail to capture transient sleep disturbances (those less than 15 seconds in duration). Therefore, techniques were developed to score brief CNS arousals. In general, arousal scoring applies the concept of "EEG speeding." That is, an abrupt *shift* during sleep to faster EEG activities (including theta, alpha, and beta but not sleep spindles) for 3 seconds or longer, constitutes a sleep alteration. Usually, the shift manifests as alpha activity and is best visualized in occipital leads. For the shift to qualify as an arousal, the person must have been asleep for at least 10 seconds. Finally, during REM sleep, the EEG shift must be accompanied by at least 1 second of increased chin EMG tone (Fig. 17-9) because alpha bursts routinely appear during REM sleep and do not necessarily represent a pathophysiology. The 3-second duration was not arbitrary; it was the minimum arousal duration reliably scored by hand among the task force members. Undoubtedly digital systems could reliably score shorter arousals, but the clinical significance of such events is not known.

CYCLIC ALTERNATING PATTERN

The cyclic alternating pattern (CAP) refers to an EEG pattern seen during sleep (Fig. 17-10). It is composed of EEG activity bursts (usually high-amplitude slow, sharp, or polymorphic wave burst) alternating with periods of quiescence. The "Parma Group's" untiring work with CAP, led by Terzano and Parrino, resulted in an international workshop during which recording and scoring techniques were codified. Essentially, the burst, or "A phase," was subcategorized into three types. Type A1

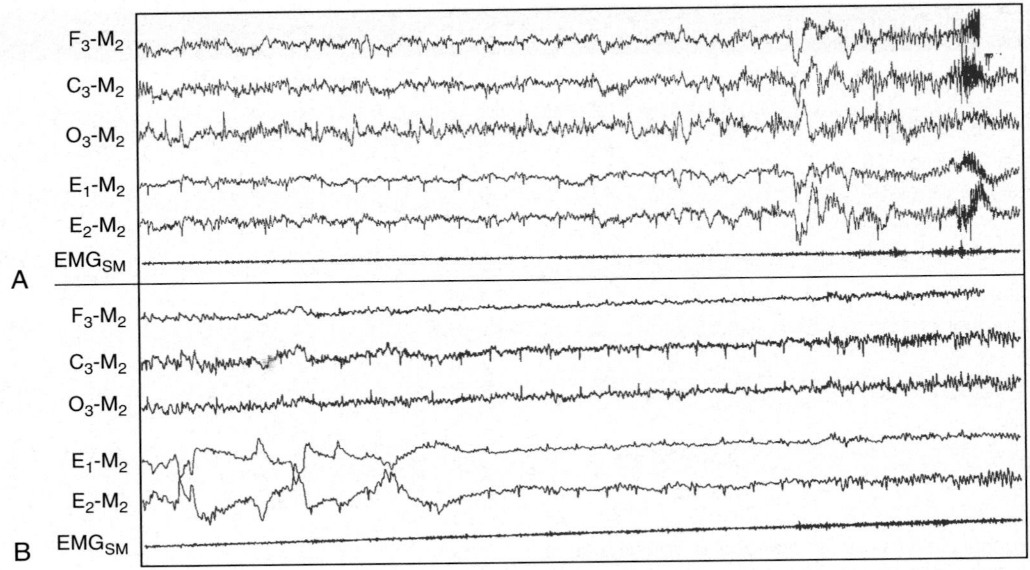

Figure 17-9.
Central nervous system (CNS) arousals from NREM (A) and REM sleep (B). C_3, left central scalp derivation; E_1, left outer canthus eye electrode location; E_2, right outer canthus eye electrode location; EMG_{SM}, surface electrode electromyogram from submentalis muscle; F_3, left frontal scalp derivation; M_2, right mastoid electrode location; O_3, left occipital scalp derivation.

would not meet AASM arousal criteria; type A2 in some cases might meet arousal criteria; and type A3 was shown to meet criteria more than 95% of the time. Sleep associated with A1 bursts was conceptualized as unstable but preserved by a descending cortical response that helps reinforce a protective thalamic gating mechanism. By contrast, if the attempt to reinforce this gate fails, an arousal or awakening occurs and an A3 burst is observed. A2 responses fall somewhere in between (Fig. 17-11).

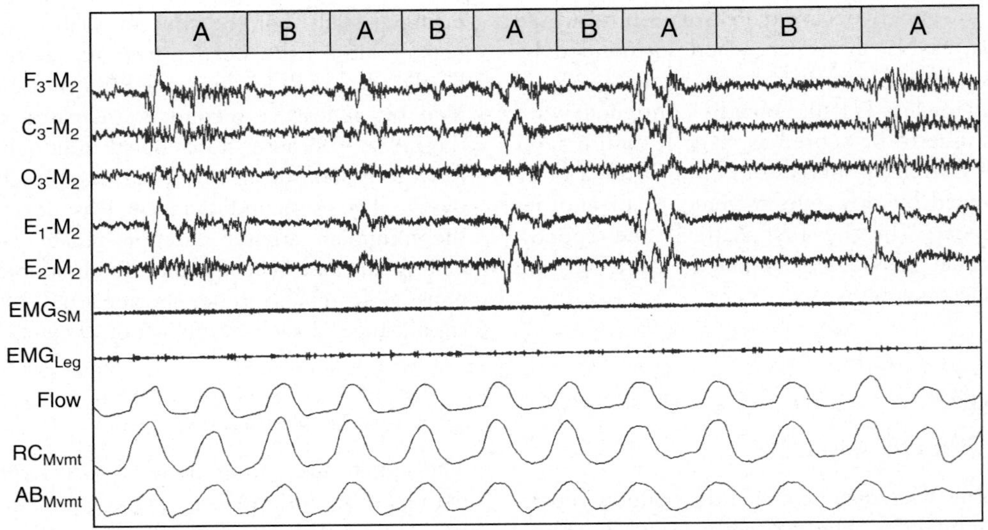

Figure 17-10.
Cyclic alternating pattern (CAP). This figure depicts PSG activity characterizing phase A (burst) and phase B (quiescent) activity. This period of CAP activity appears not to be associated with either periodic leg movements or breathing abnormalities. AB_{Mvmt}, abdominal movement measured with inductive plethysmography; C_3, left central scalp derivation; E_1, left outer canthus eye electrode location; E_2, right outer canthus eye electrode location; EMG_{Leg}, surface electrode electromyogram from left and right anterior tibialis; EMG_{SM}, surface electrode electromyogram from submentalis muscle; F_3, left frontal scalp derivation; Flow, airflow measured with nasal-nasal-oral thermistors; M_2, right mastoid electrode location; O_3, left occipital scalp derivation; RC_{Mvmt}, rib cage movement measured with inductive plethysmography.

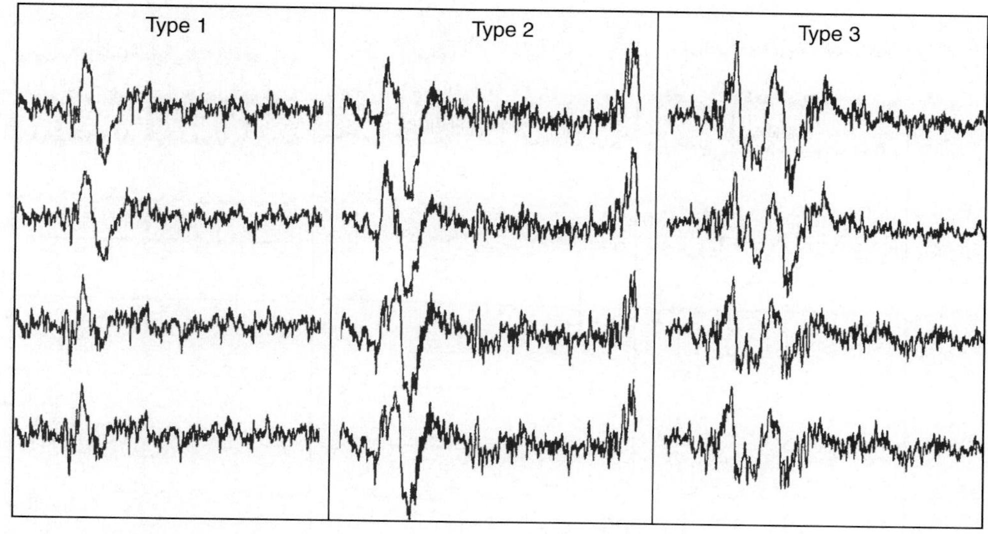

Figure 17-11.
Examples of cyclic alternating pattern A phase types 1, 2, and 3 activity. Type 1 does not appear to have EEG activity suggesting central nervous system (CNS) arousal. By contrast, type 2 activity suggests possible arousal, whereas type 3 meets AASM criteria for CNS arousal from NREM sleep.

Sleep-related Breathing Disorders

Most of the medical community now understands that sleep-related breathing disorders do not occur exclusively in hypoventilating, morbidly obese patients. An estimated 90% (or more) of all PSG studies performed on any given night are conducted to diagnose or assess treatment for sleep-disordered breathing (SDB). Ironically, recording and scoring techniques for evaluating SDB have been the least standardized part of PSG.

RECORDING TECHNIQUE

Key features needed to assess SDB include airflow, respiratory effort, blood oxygenation, and sleep disturbance. The AASM manual recommends recording the following four data channels when clinically evaluating adult patients with overnight PSG (see Table 17-1 for sampling rates and filter settings).

1. A thermal sensor at the nose and mouth to detect apnea
2. A nasal pressure transducer to detect hypopnea
3. Either an esophageal manometer or chest/abdominal inductance plethysmograph (or, alternatively, intercostal EMG) to detect respiratory effort
4. Pulse oximeter with its signal averaged over 3 seconds or less

Although end-tidal CO_2 measurement is not recommended by the AASM manual, it is also useful especially when quantifying hypoventilation. This volume contains illustrations of end-tidal CO_2 recordings. It should be noted that the 30-second, fixed epoch length specified by the AASM manual applies to sleep staging, which is a time-domain categorization. By contrast, sleep-disordered breathing parameters are mostly based on discrete, or sequences of, events. Sleep-related respiratory signals are also considerably slower than variations in EEG-EOG-EMG activity. Therefore, viewing tracings over longer-duration time frames can greatly facilitate recognition and identification of breathing patterns and events. The viewing flexibility provided by digital PSG is one of its major advantages, especially for scoring and interpreting sleep-related respiratory impairments.

DEFINITIONS AND SCORING RULES

Sleep Apnea

Conceptually, a cessation of airflow for two (or more) respiratory cycles during sleep constitutes an episode of sleep apnea. This works out to be, on average, a 10-second (or longer) halt in ventilation. Episodes can be central, obstructive, or mixed. The halt in ventilation during a central apnea is produced by cessation of inspiratory effort. An obstructive apnea results from airway occlusion as continued and even increasing inspiratory effort occurs. Finally, a mixed apnea episode is marked by an initial lack of inspiratory effort followed by an unsuccessful attempt to breathe against a closed airway.

The AASM manual defines an apnea as a 10-second (or longer) 90% (or greater) drop in the nasal/oral airflow channel's peak-to-trough amplitude that persists for at least 90% of the event's duration (Fig. 17-12).

Hypopnea

In the strictest sense, a hypopnea is merely a shallow breath and is not intrinsically pathophysiologic. However, during sleep, reduced ventilation producing significant

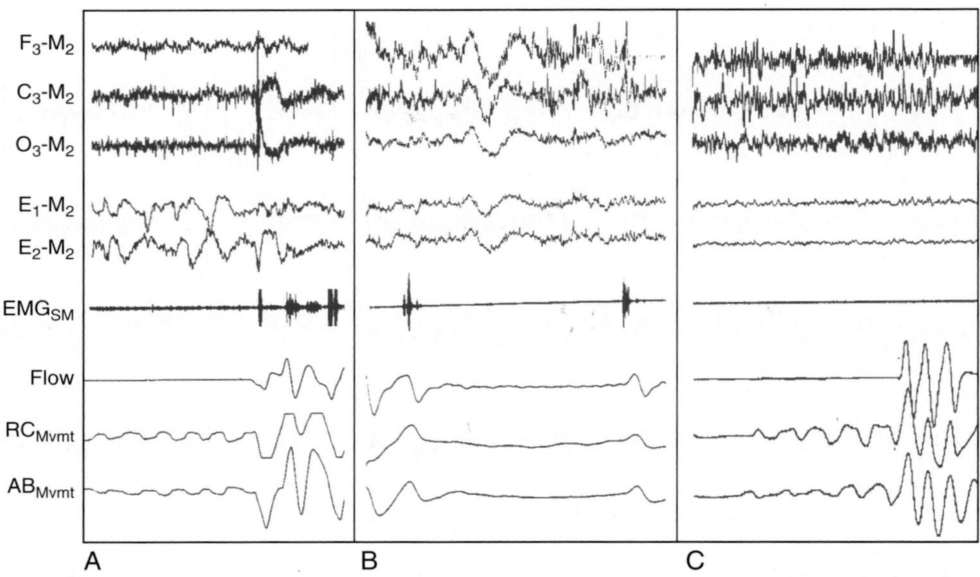

Figure 17-12.
Sleep apnea episodes: obstructive sleep apnea (**A**), central sleep apnea (**B**), and mixed sleep apnea (**C**). Note the presence of respiratory effort (rib cage and abdominal movement), notwithstanding cessation of airflow, throughout the obstructive apnea and during the latter portion of the mixed apnea. By contrast, respiratory effort is absent during the flow cessation throughout the central apnea and during the early portion of the mixed apnea. AB_{Mvmt}, abdominal movement measured with inductive plethysmography; C_3, left central scalp derivation; E_1, left outer canthus eye electrode location; E_2, right outer canthus eye electrode location; EMG_{SM}, surface electrode electromyogram from submentalis muscle; F_3, left frontal scalp derivation; Flow, airflow measured with nasal-nasal-oral thermistors; M_2, right mastoid electrode location; O_3, left occipital scalp derivation; RC_{Mvmt}, rib cage movement measured with inductive plethysmography.

oxygen desaturations can adversely affect sleep, wakefulness, and health. Also, flow limitations provoking CNS arousals, awakenings, and sleep fragmentation can undermine the sleep process. Thus, the pathophysiology lies not with the hypopnea but rather with its consequence.

The AASM manual operationalized hypopnea scoring with two different sets of rules: recommended criteria and alternative criteria. The recommended criteria for general clinical practice are basically a refinement of the Medicare definition. AASM defines hypopnea as a 10-second (or longer), 30% drop (or more) in nasal pressure signal amplitude (compared to baseline) that persists for at least 90% of the event's duration and provokes a 4% drop (or more) in oxygen saturation (Fig. 17-13). The alternative criteria stipulates a 10-second (or longer), 50% drop (or more) in nasal pressure signal amplitude (compared to baseline) that persists for at least 90% of the event duration and provokes either a 3% drop (or more) in O_2 saturation or a CNS arousal. The ambiguity of having two definitions for hypopnea has created confusion and miscommunication. It would have been preferable to create a new term for each definition—for example, "desaturating hypopnea" for events scored using the recommended criteria and "traditional hypopnea" for events meeting the alternative criteria. Actually, almost any unambiguous set of terms would do and we would be able to communicate with one another without having to review which criteria were being used (see Fig. 17-13).

Respiratory Effort–related Arousals

Respiratory effort–related arousals (RERA) traditionally were important sleep-disordered breathing events failing to meet criteria for designation as apnea or hypopnea. In that respect, they have not changed. The AASM manual criteria for scoring RERA are 10-second (or longer) increased respiratory effort that manifests as "flattening" in the nasal pressure channel that provokes a CNS arousal but does not meet apnea or hypopnea amplitude or oxygen saturation criteria. Nasal pressure recordings can alert the clinician to much more subtle respiratory events than the traditional nasal-oral thermistors. However, notwithstanding their greater sensitivity to sleep-disordered breathing events, nasal pressure recordings are compromised when sleepers "mouth breathe" due to nasal congestion, their anatomy, or both.

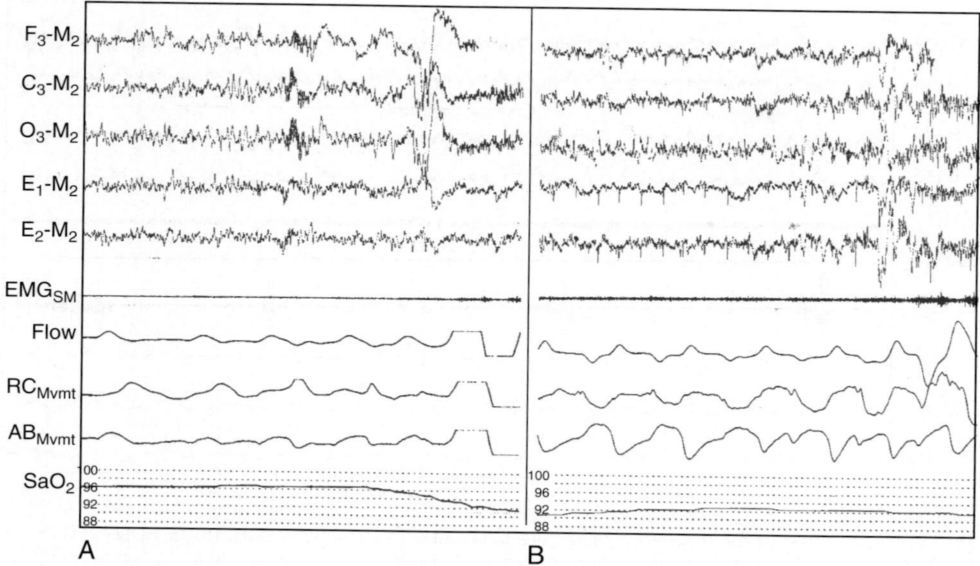

Figure 17-13.
Desaturating and traditional hypopnea episodes. A illustrates a sleep hypopnea associated with a greater than 4% oxygen desaturation (meeting Medicare criteria). B shows a sleep hypopnea terminated by a CNS arousal (meeting AASM alternate criteria). Many sleep laboratories differentiate the non-apneic respiratory event designated here as a desaturating hypopnea from the traditional hypopnea by labeling the latter as a respiratory effort—related arousal (RERA). AB_{Mvmt}, abdominal movement measured with inductive plethysmography; C_3, left central scalp derivation; E_1, left outer canthus eye electrode location; E_2, right outer canthus eye electrode location; EMG_{SM}, surface electrode electromyogram from submentalis muscle; F_3, left frontal scalp derivation; Flow, airflow measured with nasal-nasal-oral thermistors; M_2, right mastoid electrode location; O_3, left occipital scalp derivation; RC_{Mvmt}, rib cage movement measured with inductive plethysmography; SaO_2, oxygen saturation with % indicated on grid.

Movements

LEG MOVEMENT RECORDING TECHNIQUE

To record leg movements, a pair of surface electrodes is placed longitudinally at homologous sites on the belly of each leg's anterior tibialis muscle (approximately 2 to 3 cm apart). Both left and right legs should be recorded either on separate channels (greatly preferred) or combined on a single channel (see Table 17-3 for sampling rates and filter settings). The actual movement associated with periodic limb movement disorder, or PMLD, can be merely a Babinski-like extension of the great toe. However, movements may be more dramatic and involve the ankle, knee, hip, and/or upper extremities.

PERIODIC LEG MOVEMENT SCORING RULES

Periodic leg movement scoring rules have changed little since Coleman's original description. The AASM manual reasserted most of the scoring rules that were also largely endorsed by the International Restless Legs Syndrome Study Group chaired by Zucconi. The AASM manual criteria require each anterior tibialis EMG burst duration to range from 0.5 seconds to 10 seconds (inclusive) beginning when the EMG amplitude increases to 8 μvolts (minimally) above the resting level and ending when amplitude falls to within 2 μvolts of the resting level. Although an EMG recorded with surface electrodes is an uncalibratable signal, the amplitude criteria when stipulated reliably served for automated leg movement scoring. To constitute a periodic leg movement episode, there must be a sequence of four or more movements with the intermovement interval ranging from 5 to 90 seconds (inclusive). Leg movements can be unilateral or bilateral or may alternate. The leg movements occurring during sleep may be associated with CNS arousals (Fig. 17-14). Periodic leg movements occurring during wakefulness represent one of the PSG correlates of restless legs syndrome, or RLS (Fig. 17-15).

OTHER MOVEMENTS

Descriptions and criteria for other types of sleep-related movements are described in the AASM manual. These types include hypnagogic foot tremor (HFT), excessive fragmentary myoclonus, sleep bruxism, REM sleep behavior disorder, and rhythmic movement disorder. A discussion of the recording and scoring techniques for these movements is beyond the scope of this chapter. For details, see the AASM manual.

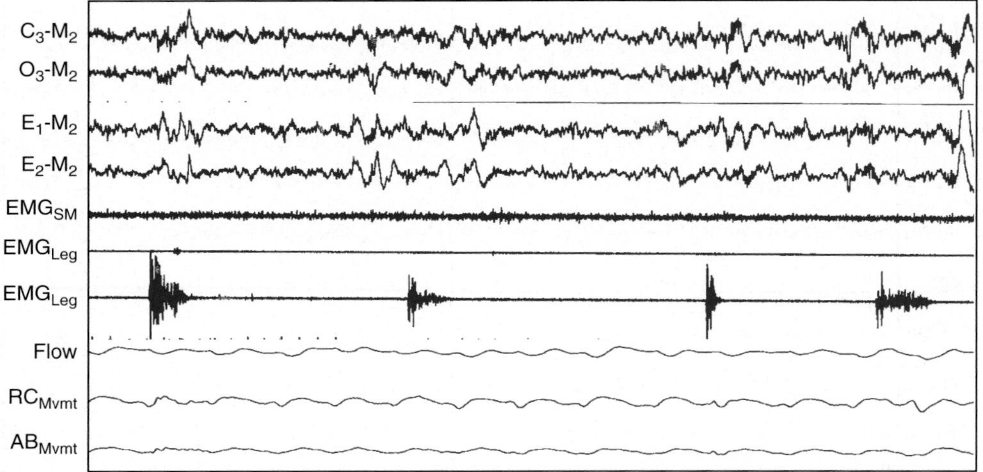

Figure 17-14.
Periodic leg movements in sleep. This figure illustrates PSG activity commonly observed on PSG recordings from individuals with periodic limb movement disorder. AB_{Mvmt}, abdominal movement measured with inductive plethysmography; C_3, left central scalp derivation; E_1, left outer canthus eye electrode location; E_2, right outer canthus eye electrode location; EMG_{Leg}, surface electrode electromyograms recorded from left and right anterior tibialis—on separate channels; EMG_{SM}, surface electrode electromyogram from submentalis muscle; Flow, airflow measured with nasal–nasal–oral thermistors; M_2, right mastoid electrode location; O_3, left occipital scalp derivation; RC_{Mvmt}, rib cage movement measured with inductive plethysmography.

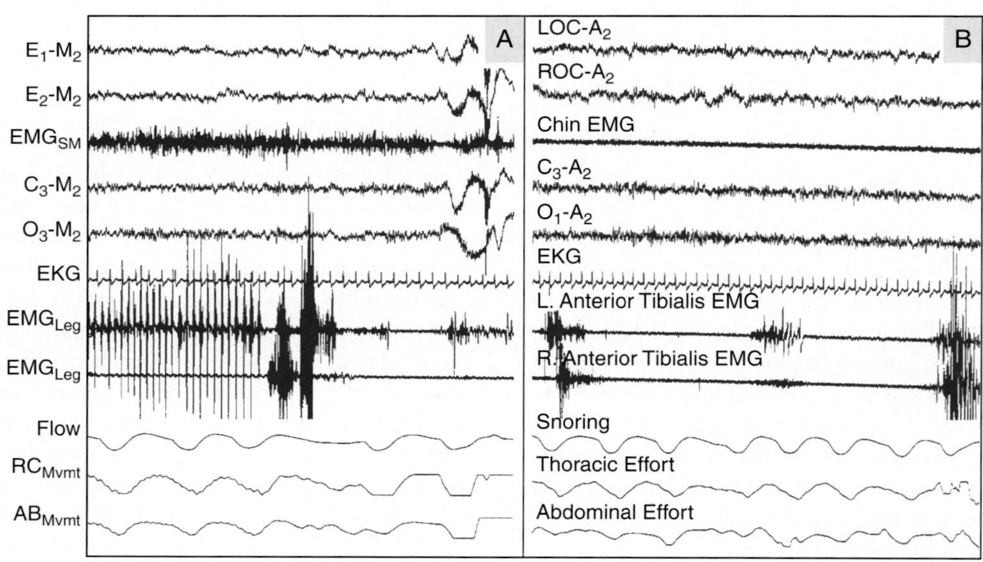

Figure 17-15.
Restless legs type I and type II activity. This figure illustrates PSG activity commonly observed on PSG recordings from individuals with restless legs syndrome. **A** illustrates very brief EMG discharges on anterior tibialis channels leading up to movements. **B** shows periodic leg movements during wakefulness. AB_{Mvmt}, abdominal movement measured with inductive plethysmography; C_3, left central scalp derivation; E_1, left outer canthus eye electrode location; E_2, right outer canthus eye electrode location; EKG, electrocardiogram; EMG_{Leg}, surface electrode electromyogram from left and right anterior tibialis; Flow, airflow measured with nasal–nasal–oral thermistors; M_2, right mastoid electrode location; O_3, left occipital scalp derivation; RC_{Mvmt}, rib cage movement measured with inductive plethysmography.

Electrocardiogram

The AASM manual recommends that cardiac rhythm be recorded during clinical PSG using a single modified electrocardiographic lead II placed on the torso aligned parallel to the right shoulder and the left hip. The criterion for adult sinus tachycardia during sleep is a sustained rate of 90 beats per minute (bpm) or higher, while bradycardia is a sustained rate below 40 bpm. Three consecutive beats with a rate above 100 bpm with a 120-msec QRS duration (or greater) meets criteria for sleep-related wide complex tachycardia. Criteria for sleep-related narrow complex tachycardia are similar except that the QRS duration must be less than 120 msec in duration. A 3-second (or greater) cardiac pause is reported as an asystole. The manual also recommends reporting other arrhythmias and ectopic beats if judged clinically significant.

Home Sleep Testing

Most clinical sleep assessments are performed to diagnose sleep-disordered breathing, titrated positive airway pressure therapy, or both. Whether home sleep testing (HST) is appropriate or helpful is a matter of heated controversy. Nevertheless, Central Medicare Services recently approved home sleep testing to diagnose sleep apnea, local coverage determination (LCD) contractors are beginning to rule that HST is "reasonable and necessary," and reimbursement codes and fee schedules are emerging. HST represents a limited test that, if used properly, may facilitate diagnosis. However, to succeed diagnostically and economically there must be (1) proper patient selection, (2) appropriate portable recorder application, (3) study interpretation by a qualified sleep specialist, (4) readily available access to laboratory PSG (when needed after a negative test or for continuing problems notwithstanding treatment), and (5) systematic follow-up (Fig. 17-16).

Only where there is a high clinical suspicion for sleep apnea should a patient be referred for HST because the test can "rule-in" but not "rule-out" sleep-disordered breathing. As an abbreviated test HST is apt to be less sensitive; therefore, it misses more subtle forms of sleep-disordered breathing events. More importantly, if the patient has a disorder other than, or in addition to, easily verified sleep apnea, it will go undetected. If symptom presentation is mixed, the patient isn't sleepy, or pretest probability is low, the patient should be referred for full laboratory assessment. Patients with symptoms suggesting other or possibly comorbid sleep disorders (e.g., sleepwalking, cataplexy, dream enactment with injury) should also be referred for

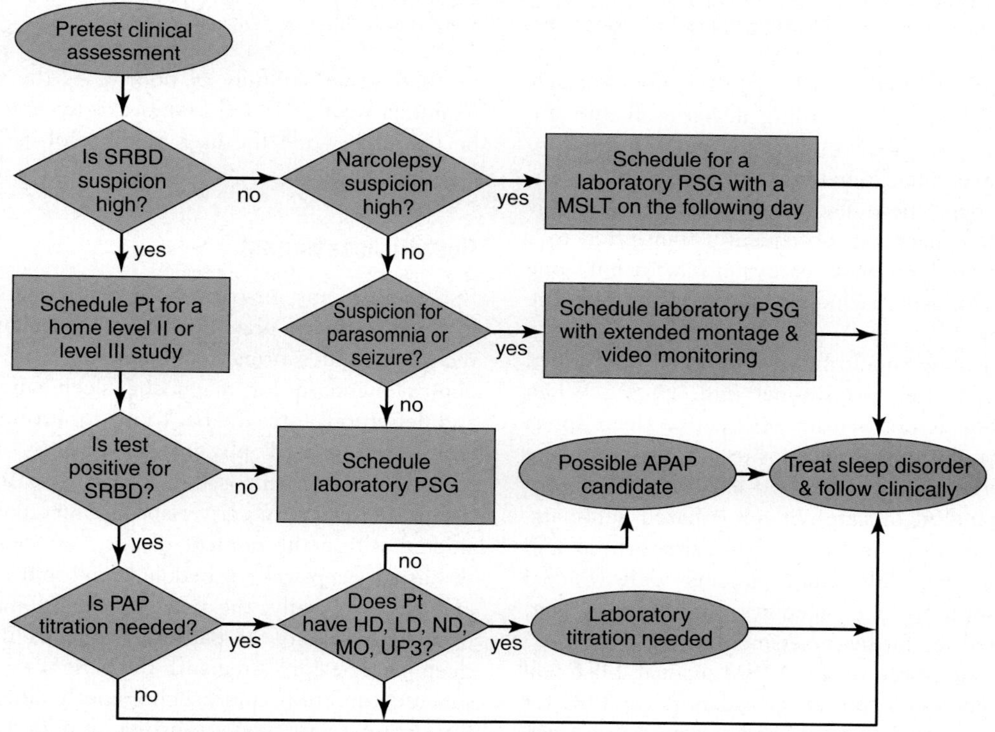

Figure 17-16.
Home sleep-testing algorithm and recording sample. This figure shows an algorithm used to perform home sleep testing with cardiopulmonary (type III) recorders. APAP, auto PAP; HD, heart disease; LD, lung disease; MO, morbid obesity; MSLT, multiple sleep latency test; ND, neurologic disease; PAP, positive airway pressure; PSG, polysomnography; Pt, patient; SRBD, sleep-related breathing disorder; UP3, uvulopalatopharyngeoplasty.

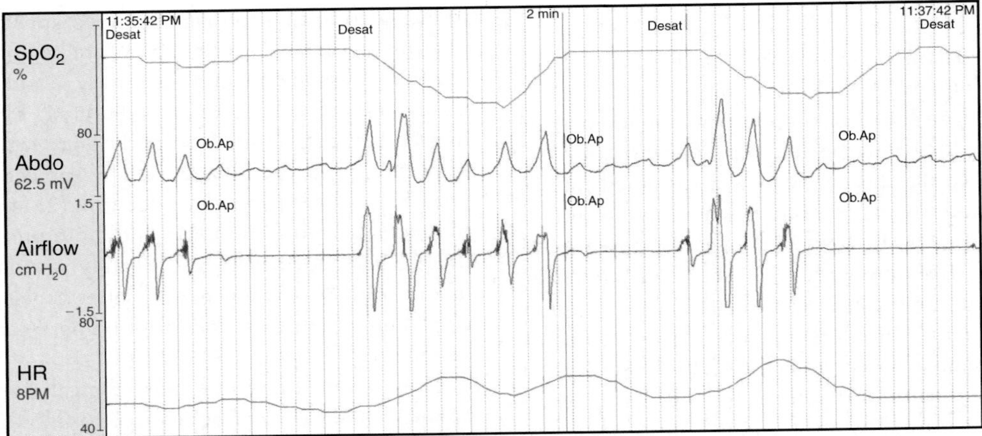

Figure 17-17.
Home sleep-testing recording sample. This figure shows a sample tracing obtained during a home sleep test on a patient with high clinical suspicion for having sleep-disordered breathing. It is an example of data obtained using home sleep-testing equipment. This is from a level III study that shows 2 minutes of data and was taken from an obese patient with classic obstructive sleep apnea syndrome by history. Thus, there was a high pretest probability of sleep apnea. A low sampling rate is evident in the SpO_2 trace as steps in the data. Notice that the airflow signal (inspiration goes up), from the measurement of nasal pressure, shows high-frequency noises that are particularly apparent at the beginning of this epoch. These represent the vibration of snoring. The patient had these types of findings as shown here during four periods of the night. Presumably, these occurred during rapid eye movement sleep. Because one does not know whether he was awake or asleep when he did not have abnormal breathing, interpretation of such a study can be difficult. Indices in such home studies are calculated on recording time. This patient's apnea index thus calculated was 14.8. In health care systems, where an apnea-hypopnea index of 15 is required to supply continuous positive airway pressure, such a result is problematic and might lead to restudy. Abdo, abdominal movement; HR, heart rate; ObAp, obstructive apnea; SpO_2, oxygen saturation.

laboratory evaluation. HST recorders are classified as levels II, III, and IV. Most HST recording devices fall into the level III category and acquire three or more respiratory channels and heart rate. Sometimes referred to as cardiopulmonary recorders, these devices are worn at home during sleep and their data are subsequently transferred to a computer for review and analysis. Systems with only one or two channels (usually including oximetry) fall into the level IV category.

The HST recording should be reviewed and interpreted by an experienced sleep practitioner (Fig. 17-17). When the portable study is positive for obstructive sleep apnea and severe enough to warrant positive airway pressure (PAP) therapy, the patient is referred for either laboratory titration (the standard of care) or home-based automatic self-adjusting PAP titration (somewhat experimental and controversial). During follow-up, patients with residual sleep-related symptoms (e.g., sleepiness, insomnia, fatigue) should be referred for further assessment.

Although not addressed in the AASM manual, HST will likely soon become as commonplace as laboratory PSG for diagnosing sleep apnea. Like cardiac Holter monitors, sleep cardiopulmonary recorders can be used to gather data from patients in whom there is a high clinical suspicion for disease. For HST to be successful, it must be embedded within an overall sleep disorders program rather than used as an isolated test. HST recorders are merely tools, which can be used either skillfully or poorly. As the Czech novelist Kunderia wrote, "A tool knows exactly how it is meant to be handled, while the user of the tool can only have an approximate idea."

Overall Assessment

PSG is an important part of the overall patient assessment in sleep medicine practice. The AASM manual focuses on recording and scoring techniques and attempts to set a clinical standard for diagnostic sleep studies. The rules and definitions form the backbone for scoring and summarizing sleep-related physiologic activity. However, this technical component is only a part of patient evaluation. Sleep continuity, integrity, and architecture must be considered within the context of age, sex, concordance with the usual sleep-wake schedule, comorbid conditions, and medication. Finally, the type, frequency, magnitude, duration, and severity of pathophysiologies detected during sleep must be correlated with the patient's symptoms, signs, somatic condition, and psychological status. Sleep evaluations can be particularly sensitive to underlying conditions inhibited by volitional or waking-stage processes. As sleep is a time when voluntary control is suspended (whether it pertains to the control of ventilation or is a defense mechanism against anxiety), sleep tests provide a unique opportunity for assessment.

SLEEP STAGE CHANGES ACROSS THE NIGHT

In normal young adults, the macroarchitectural sleep stage pattern across the night is fairly consistent (Fig. 17-18), with stage N2 occupying approximately half the total sleep time. Stage N3 may account for an eighth to a fifth of total sleep time (12.5% to 20%), with the remaining NREM stage (N1) occurring at sleep onset and during transitions (usually totaling less than 5% of sleep). REM sleep (stage R) appears every 90 to 100 minutes in distinct episodes that elongate as the night progresses, thereby loading the second half of the sleep session with the majority of time spent in this CNS organization state. In total, approximately a fifth to a quarter of sleep (20% to 25%) is spent in stage R.

Under normal circumstances, the transition from wakefulness to sleep is rapid (5 to 15 minutes) and marked by the appearance of stage N1 or N2. A healthy young adult sleeps 85% to 95% of the typical 7 to 8 hours spent in bed. Stage R typically occurs after an hour and a half. Slow-wave activity (and therefore stage N3) predominates in the first third of the night and becomes rarer toward morning awakening. Men and women differ little in sleep macroarchitecture; however, women may have slightly better preserved stage N3 with advancing age.

The above descriptions of normal sleep in the healthy young adult derive from electrophysiologic data that universally exclude results obtained during the first night in the laboratory. Sleep disturbances associated with the initial experience of sleeping in a laboratory are so well known they are called the "first night effect." These data are excluded by researchers interested in the commonalities of normal sleep who rightfully believe these are artifacts created by procedure (analogous to the uncertainty in quantum mechanics postulated by the Heisenberg principle). Ironically, first night data are routinely used in clinical practice. More appropriately, we should compare results with normative values collected from normal healthy adults sleeping in the laboratory for the first time (Table 17-4).

SLEEP STAGE CHANGES AS A FUNCTION OF AGE

Over the life span, a great many changes occur in sleep micro- and macroarchitecture. For this reason, judging sleep integrity, continuity, or composition should be against age-specific normative values. During infancy, multiple "feeding–REM sleep–NREM sleep" cycles consolidate to one major and several minor sleep episodes by the end of the first year. This further reduces to a major and a single minor sleep episode by age 4, and to the adult single major period at around age 10 years. At some time between the two milestones of 6 months and 1 year, the prevailing sleep-onset REM (or, more precisely, "active sleep") switches to the adult pattern where the transition from wakefulness to sleep is through a NREM stage. Overall, across childhood and into adulthood, total sleep time gradually decreases. Part of this is the decreasing stage N3 after adolescence; however, other stages also decline, and wakefulness within the sleep period increases. This trend continues as a function of age with N3 reduction to low levels (or even disappearing altogether) in elderly individuals. By contrast, "active sleep," the infant's equivalent of stage R, drops spectacularly from more than 50% at birth to 20% to 25% by adolescence. Then, after remaining stable for perhaps 5 decades, stage R percentage declines slightly further. Decreasing sleep duration and consolidation are often associated with sleep disturbances related to the accumulated pathologies that invariably accompany aging. However, some total sleep decline is nonspecific, or of unknown etiology. Some researchers argue that age-related deterioration of underlying physiologic sleep mechanisms is responsible. The fact remains, as we enter our senior years, we spend more time in bed but less time sleeping.

PARAMETERS, PATHOPHYSIOLOGY, AND INTERPRETATION

For summarizing a sleep study, the AASM manual provides a list of parameters for calculating, tabulating, and reporting. Some parameters are recommended and some are optional (Table 17-5). This provides an objective

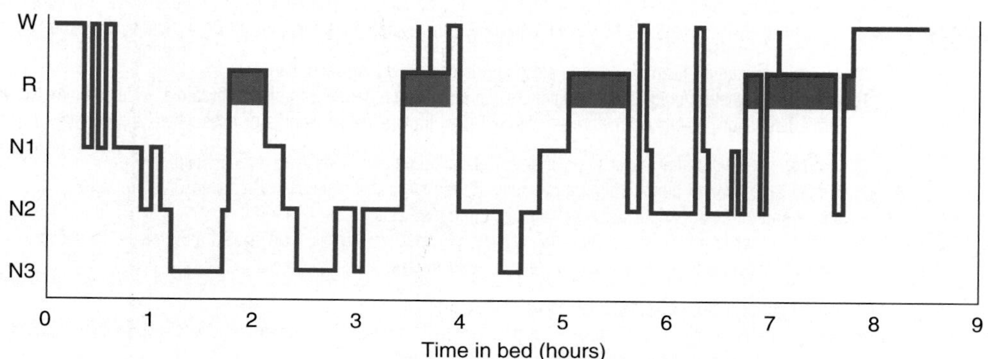

Figure 17-18.
Normal sleep macroarchitecture. This figure illustrates normal sleep stage progression for a healthy young adult. N1, sleep stage 1; N2, sleep stage 2; N3, sleep stages 3 and 4; R, rapid eye movement sleep; W, wakefulness.

Table 17-4. Normal Value Ranges* for "First Night" Laboratory Polysomnography

	AGE GROUP (NUMBER OF INDIVIDUALS)				
	20–29 Yr ($N = 44$)	30–39 Yr ($N = 23$)	40–49 Yr ($N = 49$)	50–59 Yr ($N = 41$)	≥ 60 Yr ($N = 29$)
General, sleep continuity, and integrity measures					
Time in bed (min)	361–449	335–451	355–454	342–444	353–439
Sleep latency (min)	0–25	3–24	0–28	0–20	0–30
Total sleep time (min)	285–410	269–411	275–384	268–395	237–360
Sleep efficiency index**	72–100	75–98	71–93	73–95	62–89
Latency to arising (min)	0–10	0–32	0–29	0–15	0–14
Number of awakenings	1–18	4–12	6–17	7–16	7–21
Awakenings per hour	0–3	1–2	1–3	1–3	1–3
Number of REM sleep episodes	2–4	2–4	3–5	3–5	2–5
NREM sleep stage percentages					
Stage 1 percentage of time in bed	1–7	1–6	2–9	3–9	3–10
Stage 2 percentage of time in bed	40–58	40–60	40–64	44–64	42–60
Stage 3 percentage of time in bed	12–19	11–19	4–13	3–11	2–8
Stage R percentage of time in bed	11–25	10–25	9–24	12–24	8–19

**Normal value range lower and upper bounds are calculated here as the parameter mean minus one standard deviation (SD) to the parameter mean plus one SD, respectively, with negative values replaced by zero.*

***Sleep efficiency index is the total sleep time as a percentage of time in bed.*

Table 17-5. Recommended Polysomnographic Parameters

CATEGORY	CLASS* AND DESCRIPTION
Sleep stage	**R** Clock times that PSG began and finished **R** Total duration of the recording and amount of time spent actually sleeping **R** Latencies to sleep (from lights out) and Stage R (from sleep onset) **R** Time and percent (of total sleep time) spent in each sleep stage **R** Percent time of total recording spent asleep (sleep efficiency index [SEI]) **R** Time spent awake after initial sleep onset (wake after sleep onset [WASO]) **I** Latency to persistent sleep
Arousals	**R** Number and index (number per hour of sleep) **I** Number and duration of cyclic alternating pattern (CAP) episodes
Respiration	**R** Number of each type of apnea (i.e., central, mixed, obstructive) and hypopnea **R** Number of all apnea and hypopnea combined **R** Apnea, hypopnea, and apnea-hypopnea indices (number per hour of sleep) **R** Mean and minimum oxygen saturation percentages **R** Indication of whether Cheyne Stokes breathing pattern occurred **O** Indication of whether hypoventilation was observed **O** Number and index (number per hour of sleep) of respiratory effort–related arousals (RERAs) **O** Number and index of 3% (or more) or 4% (or more) oxygen desaturations **I** During positive airway pressure titration; optimal pressure; time at optimal pressure; whether stage R occurred during time at optimal pressure; indices for apnea, apnea/hypopnea, and apnea/hypopnea/RERA at optimal pressure
Heart rhythm	**R** Mean and maximum heart rate during sleep and maximum during recording **R** Indication of whether bradycardia, asystole, sinus tachycardia, narrow complex tachycardia, wide complex tachycardia, atrial fibrillation, or other arrhythmias occurred (and provide pause lengths or rates where appropriate)
Movement	**R** Number and index (number per hour of sleep) of periodic limb movements during sleep **R** Number and index of periodic limb movements during sleep that were associated with CNS arousal **I** Number and index of periodic limb movements during wakefulness **I** Indication of whether bruxism, restless leg activity, rhythmic movement, REM-related movements, fragmentary myoclonus, or other types of movements occurred during sleep or wakefulness
Other	**R** Clinical correlates of pathophysiologies and diagnosis **R** Other EEG abnormalities (e.g., spikes, sharps, excessive or diminished waveform activity, hypersynchronous delta, alpha-delta sleep) **R** Heart rhythm abnormalities (see above) **R** Behavioral observations **O** Sleep histogram

**Classification by AASM as recommended (R), Optional (O), or not mentioned but considered important and recommended in other guidelines (I).*

technique for assessing sleep disturbances and instability. Indexed measures are useful to control for differences in recording, or in sleep duration that occurs across nights or, more importantly, between individuals. For example, the number of leg-movement-related arousals per hour better characterizes activity level than does the overall number of leg-movement-related arousals.

PSG interpretation must proceed from context. Important contexts include (1) sleep schedule and napping pattern, (2) symptoms, (3) comorbid illnesses and conditions, and (4) medications, alcohol, and recreational substances. Sample forms useful for such assessments are included as Figures 17-19 to 17-22. The screening questionnaire includes a check-box version of the Epworth Sleepiness Scale, whose validation study was presented at the Helsinki World Sleep Apnea Congress in 2003. It also inquires about overall sleep disturbances and collects information concerning sleep schedule and napping from which

Sleep Center Screening Questionnaire

Patient name Date

EPWORTH SLEEPINESS SCALE

How LIKELY are you to DOZE off or FALL ASLEEP in the following situations, in contrast to feeling just tired? This refers to your usual way of life in recent times. Even if you have not done some of these things recently, try to work out how they would have affected you. Please check one box per line.

---CHANCE OF DOZING OFF---

never	slight	moderate	high	
☐	☐	☐	☐	sitting and reading
☐	☐	☐	☐	watching TV
☐	☐	☐	☐	sitting, inactive in a public place (example, a theater or a meeting)
☐	☐	☐	☐	as a passenger in a car for an hour without a break
☐	☐	☐	☐	lying down to rest in the afternoon when circumstances permit
☐	☐	☐	☐	sitting and talking to someone
☐	☐	☐	☐	sitting quietly after lunch without alcohol
☐	☐	☐	☐	in a car, while stopped for a few minutes in traffic

BRIEF SLEEP SYMPTOM CHECKLIST *(please check the boxes that best describe you)*

never	rarely	frequently	always	
☐	☐	☐	☐	I snore loudly
☐	☐	☐	☐	I awaken gasping or choking for breath
☐	☐	☐	☐	I awaken in the morning unrefreshed
☐	☐	☐	☐	I have problems falling asleep or staying asleep (insomnia)
☐	☐	☐	☐	My sleep is very restless
☐	☐	☐	☐	My sleep is disturbed by unusual behaviors (for example: nightmares, sleepwalking, dream enactments, tongue biting, bedwetting... etc.)
☐	☐	☐	☐	I fall asleep while driving
☐	☐	☐	☐	I've been told that I stop breathing in my sleep (told by ______________________)

SLEEP SCHEDULE *(please provide the following information)*

What time do you go to bed on WEEKDAYS? ____ AM or PM Do you nap? [yes] [no]
What time do you get up on WEEKDAYS? ____ AM or PM How often do you nap? ____ times per week
What time do you go to bed on WEEKENDS? ____ AM or PM How long are the naps? ________ minutes
What time do you get up on WEEKENDS? ____ AM or PM Do you awaken refreshed? [yes] [no]
Are you a shift worker? [yes] [no] If yes, what kind of shift do you work? ______________________

Figure 17-19.
Sleep clinic screening questionnaire. Sample of a self-administered questionnaire form used to assess sleepiness (using the Epworth Sleepiness Scale developed by Dr. Murray Johns), sleep schedule, napping, and general symptoms of sleep disorders.

Sleep Problems Checklist

Patient name ________________________ Date ____________

What problem causes you to seek our help and how does it affect your life? ____________

____

____

CHECK the box for each problem you CURRENTLY HAVE.

- ☐ loud snoring with frequent awakenings
- ☐ crawling feelings in legs when trying to sleep
- ☐ leg-kicking during sleep
- ☐ leg cramps in sleep
- ☐ trouble falling asleep at night
- ☐ trouble staying asleep at night
- ☐ racing thoughts when trying to sleep
- ☐ increased muscle tension when trying to sleep
- ☐ fear of being unable to sleep
- ☐ laying in bed worrying when trying to sleep
- ☐ waking too early in the morning
- ☐ sleep talking
- ☐ sweating a lot at night
- ☐ waking up with reflux (and/or heartburn)
- ☐ waking up to urinate 2 or more times nightly
- ☐ nightmares
- ☐ teethgrinding during sleep
- ☐ morning headaches
- ☐ morning dry mouth
- ☐ sleepwalking
- ☐ tongue biting in sleep
- ☐ bedwetting
- ☐ acting out dreams
- ☐ uncontrollable daytime sleep attacks
- ☐ falling asleep unexpectedly
- ☐ falling asleep at work
- ☐ falling asleep at school
- ☐ I use sleeping pills to help me sleep
- ☐ I use alcohol to help me sleep
- ☐ pain interfering with sleep

  Where is the pain? ____________

For each symptom, please CHECK the boxes that BEST DESCRIBE YOU.

never	rarely	sometimes	usually	always	
☐	☐	☐	☐	☐	When falling asleep, I feel paralyzed (unable to move)
☐	☐	☐	☐	☐	I feel unable to move (paralyzed) after a nap
☐	☐	☐	☐	☐	I have dream-like images (hallucinations) when I awaken in the morning even though I know I am not asleep
☐	☐	☐	☐	☐	I see dream-like images (hallucinations) either just before or just after a daytime nap, yet I am sure I am awake when they happen
☐	☐	☐	☐	☐	I am often unable to move (paralyzed) when I am waking up in the morning
☐	☐	☐	☐	☐	I get "weak knees" when I laugh
☐	☐	☐	☐	☐	I get sudden muscular weakness (or even brief periods of paralysis, being unable to move) when laughing, angry, or in situations of strong emotion

Figure 17-20.
Sleep problems checklist. Sample of a self-administered questionnaire form used in the sleep medicine clinic to determine chief complaint, the presence or absence of common symptoms associated with sleep disorders, and severity of complaints constituting narcolepsy's symptom tetrad other than sleepiness (i.e., cataplexy, sleep paralysis, and hypnagogia).

Sleep Center Health and Family Questionnaire

Patient name ______________________ Date ____________

1. How would you rate your current general health?

☐ very poor ☐ poor ☐ average ☐ good ☐ very good

2. Check (√) if you now have or in the past had the following:

Diabetes	☐ now	☐ past	Anemia	☐ now	☐ past
High blood pressure	☐ now	☐ past	Peptic ulcers	☐ now	☐ past
Stroke	☐ now	☐ past	Acid reflux (heartburn)	☐ now	☐ past
Heart disease or CHF	☐ now	☐ past	Kidney disease	☐ now	☐ past
Heart attack	☐ now	☐ past	Thyroid disease	☐ now	☐ past
Angina	☐ now	☐ past	Arthritis	☐ now	☐ past
Emphysema or COPD	☐ now	☐ past	Back pain	☐ now	☐ past
Asthma	☐ now	☐ past	Head trauma	☐ now	☐ past
Tuberculosis	☐ now	☐ past	Severe headaches	☐ now	☐ past
Other lung disease	☐ now	☐ past	Epilepsy (seizures)	☐ now	☐ past
Nasal allergies	☐ now	☐ past	Passing-out spells (fainting)	☐ now	☐ past
Runny or blocked nose	☐ now	☐ past	Depression	☐ now	☐ past
Hormonal problem	☐ now	☐ past	Anxiety disorder	☐ now	☐ past
Urological problem	☐ now	☐ past	Problems with alcohol	☐ now	☐ past
Prostate disease	☐ now	☐ past	Problems with drugs	☐ now	☐ past

3. Please list hospitalizations. Please give the reasons for each hospitalization and the dates (as best you can remember).

REASONS FOR HOSPITALIZATION	DATE

4. Please give important details about your medical conditions.

____

____

____

____

Figure 17-21.
Sleep center health and family questionnaire. Sample of a self-administered questionnaire form used in the sleep medicine clinic to collect information about an individual's comorbid health conditions; hospitalizations; caffeine, alcohol, and nicotine use; marital status; occupation; and general family health status.

(Continued)

5. List your current average for each category below.

_______ hours worked per day
_______ days worked per week
_______ days of vacation per year
_______ number of cigarettes smoked per day
_______ other tobacco used per day (pipefuls or cigars)
_______ cups of regular coffee per day
_______ cups of tea per day
_______ glasses of cola or other caffeinated beverages per day
_______ cans of beer per day (12 oz.)
_______ glasses of wine per day (3–4 oz.)
_______ alcoholic drinks per day (1–2 oz. straight or mixed)

6. If you smoke or used to smoke...
   What is the most you ever smoked? _______ If you quit, how long ago did you quit? _______

7. What is your current relationship status?
   ☐ single ☐ married ☐ divorced ☐ widowed ☐ separated ☐ living with someone

8. How many times have you been married? _______

9. What is your occupation? _______________________________________

FAMILY INFORMATION

1. Is your **father** living? ☐ yes ☐ no If yes, how old is he? _______
   If no, at what age did he die? _______ What caused his death? _______________________
   What was your father's major occupation? _______________________________
2. Is your **mother** living? ☐ yes ☐ no If yes, how old is she? _______
   If no, at what age did she die? _______ What caused her death? _______________________
   What was your mother's major occupation? _______________________________
3. Do any of your **brothers and sisters** (if applicable) have any major diseases or sleep disorders?
   If yes, please describe: _______________________________________
   ____
   ____
   ____

Figure 17-21, cont'd

one can deduce (1) whether the sleep schedule is adequate, (2) whether the patient is "fasting" and "binging" on sleep, and (3) whether the patient phase delays, phase advances, or remains regular. The symptom checklist is straightforward and patients can affirm any sleep problems they may be experiencing. Some of the symptoms are strong markers for particular sleep disorders while others are nonspecific. Furthermore, some symptoms serve to alert the sleep specialist reviewing the PSG to pay special attention to distinct electrophysiologic phenomena. If a patient bites his tongue during sleep, extra careful scrutiny of the tracing for spikes, phantom spikes, and sharp waves would be prudent. Or if a patient endorses "dream enactment with injury," the polysomnographer would sharpen her or his focus on REM-related movements as a correlate of possible REM behavior disorder. The bottom section of the questionnaire specifically addresses the tetrad of symptoms associated with narcolepsy (i.e., sleep paralysis, hypnagogia, and cataplexy). Sleep-relevant comorbid conditions are listed on the sleep clinic health problems checklist so that patients can easily affirm active or past history of each infirmity. In addition to the instruments used here as examples, many sleep clinics administer a depression screening test (e.g., Beck Depression Inventory or Zung Depression Scale) and the International Restless Legs Screening Test.

In sleep medicine, few diagnostic criteria are quantitatively codified numerically. Pathophysiologies are mainly correlates. The disease process can be an upstream or downstream effect, or it can be only indirectly related. In the case of sleep apnea, however, cutting scores have been established. For Medicare to diagnose sleep apnea and qualify a patient for positive airway pressure therapy, the

Sleep Center Medication Questionnaire

Patient name ______________________ Date ______________

We need to know what drugs, vitamins, and herbal substances you have taken in the past 6 months. Please complete the form below. Check your medicine cabinet and your medical records for drugs. Think back about the health problems you have had and the medicines you took for them.

Name of drug, vitamin, or herbal substance used	Dose	# of pills	Taken for how long?	Taken for what problem?	Still taking?	
					Yes	No

Figure 17-22.
Sleep center medication log. Sample of a self-administered questionnaire form used in the sleep medicine clinic to collect information about medication and substance use.

apnea-hypopnea index (AHI) must be 5 (or more) for patients with symptoms or relevant comorbidities. However, for patients who are neither sleepy nor have any significant, potentially related comorbid medical conditions, the AHI must reach 15 (or more). Note that the AHI must be calculated using the "recommended" definition for hypopnea, which we designate as a "desaturating hypopnea." AASM criteria are similar but use the respiratory disturbance index (RDI) rather than the AHI in the decision paradigm.

The *multiple sleep latency test* is used to document sleepiness and supplies information helping support a diagnosis of narcolepsy. Usually the patient is given the opportunity to nap for up to 20 minutes, at 2-hour intervals, during the daytime. The mean sleep latency is calculated, and the naps during which REM sleep occurs is determined. A mean sleep latency less than 5 minutes is considered pathologic sleepiness and values greater than 10 are considered normal, with values in-between a gray zone. A diagnosis of narcolepsy is supported when two or more naps contain REM sleep.

Summary

The AASM manual represents an initial attempt to establish recording and scoring criteria for nearly the full range of PSG parameters, including sleep stages, arousal scoring, respiratory events, cardiac events, and movement activity. This chapter summarizes and illustrates the critical features and essence of the manual's content. Clearly there is room to grow. However, the manual's compilation of methods and technique guidelines into a single source, underwritten and endorsed by the major clinical professional society, represents an aggressive first step toward standardizing the field.

SELECTED READINGS

Bonnet M, Carley D, Carskadon M, et al: ASDA Report. EEG arousals: Scoring rules and examples. Sleep 15:173–184, 1992.

Coleman RM: Periodic movements in sleep (nocturnal myoclonus) and restless legs syndrome. In: Guilleminault C (ed): Sleeping and Waking Disorders: Indications and Techniques. Menlo Park, CA: Addison-Wesley, 1982, pp. 267–295.

Hirshkowitz M, Moore CA, Hamilton CR, et al: Polysomnography of adults and elderly: Sleep architecture, respiration, and leg movements. J Clin Neurophysiol 9:56–62, 1992.

Iber C, Ancoli-Israel S, Chesson A, Quan SF, for the American Academy of Sleep Medicine: The AASM Manual for the Scoring of Sleep and Associated Events: Rules, Terminology and Technical Specifications. Westchester, Ill: American Academy of Sleep Medicine, 2007.

Loomis AL, Harvey N, Hobart GA: Cerebral states during sleep, as studied by human brain potentials. J Exp Psychol 21:127–144, 1937.

Rechtschaffen A, Kales A: A manual of standardized terminology, techniques and scoring system for sleep stages in human subjects. NIH Publication No. 204. Washington, DC: U.S. Government Printing Office, 1968.

Terzano MG, Parrino L, Smerieri A, et al: Atlas, rules, and recording technique for scoring of cyclic alternating pattern (CAP) in human sleep. Sleep Med 3:187–199, 2002.

Zucconi M, Ferri R, Allen R, et al: The official World Association of Sleep Medicine (WASM) standards for recording and scoring periodic leg movements in sleep (PLMS) and wakefulness (PLMW). Developed in collaboration with a task force from the International Restless Legs Syndrome Study Group (IRLSSG). Sleep Med 7:175–183, 2006.

CHAPTER 18

GALLERY OF POLYSOMNOGRAPHIC RECORDINGS

Max Hirshkowitz and Meir Kryger

This is a catalog of the multimedia content of the Atlas, which can be accessed on the Web at www.expertconsult.com. It is recommended that the reader use an up-to-date computer with a high-resolution display and audio with high-speed Internet access. This website includes all the sleep recodings printed in this volume and many others. Chapter 19 is a catalog of patient interview videos that are available on the website. Chapter 20 is a catalogue of videos of patients obtained during polysomnography.

Obstructive Sleep Apnea

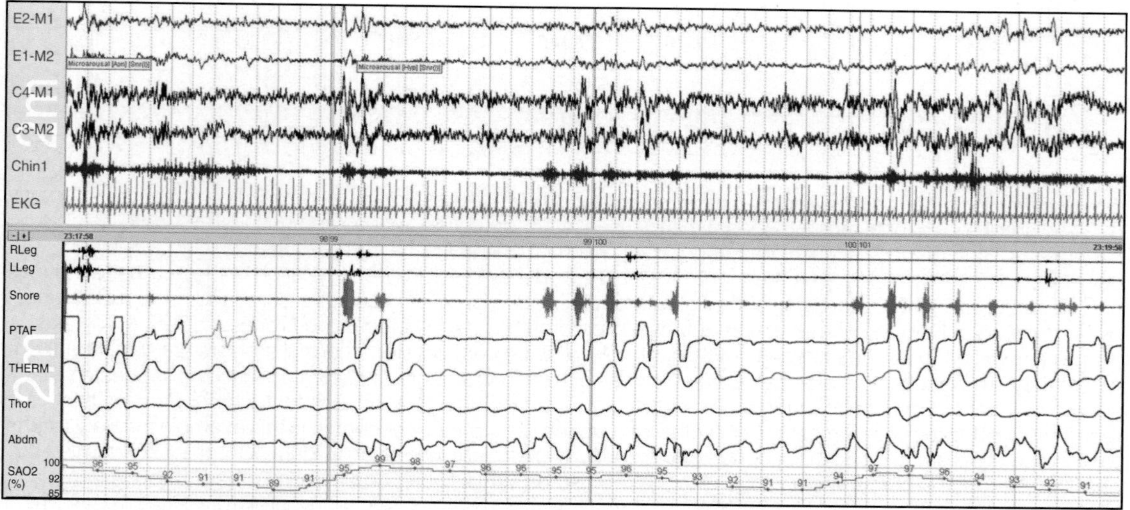

Figure 18-1.
Obstructive sleep apnea. In obstructive sleep apnea, in spite of thoracic and abdominal efforts, there is a cessation of airflow. In this example, airflow is being monitored by the use of the thermocouple (THERM) and nasal pressure (PTAF, for nasal pressure airflow). It is recommended by the *American Academy of Sleep Medicine Scoring Manual* (see chapter 11.2, page 168; chapter 17, page 269) that apnea be scored when there is a 90% or more reduction in the peak thermal sensor (or the alternate sensor, nasal air pressure) excursion for more than 10 seconds. The same manual suggests that hypopnea be scored when nasal pressure signal excursions (or their alternates, calibrated or uncalibrated inductance plethysmography) drop by more than 30%. In this example, the scoring technician has labeled the first event a hypopnea, and the next two events apneas. In reality, there is little physiologic difference between hypopneas and apneas, and, indeed, more hypoxemia was present with the hypopneic episode. The reader is encouraged to look at all the data: in this example, the snoring channels, the chin EMG, which is also detecting snoring, and the EEG channels, which show the arousals linked to the abnormal respiratory events. The reader is also encouraged to use epoch lengths (not always the recommended 30 s) that best enhance the interpretation and understanding of the patient.

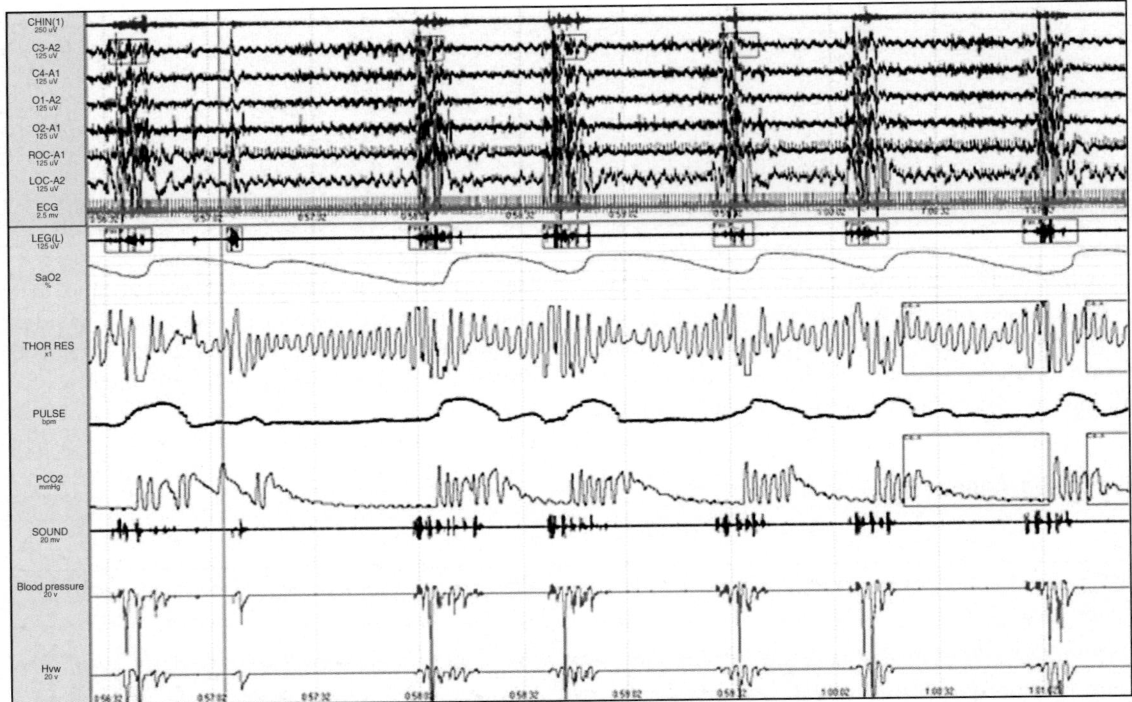

Figure 18-2.
Obstructive sleep apnea. The importance of understanding cardiorespiratory sensors. The American Academy of Sleep Medicine manual recommends a thermal sensor for detecting apneas and nasal pressure to detect hypopneas. Both of these sensors have significant potential limitations. Nasal pressure results in absent or decreased airflow in patients who are mouth breathers, and may result in overestimation of the number of apneas and the length of individual events. In this figure oronasal end-tidal pCO_2, nasal pressure, and nasal airflow are being monitored. Notice that many more unobstructed breaths are detected using oronasal pCO_2. pCO_2 lags pressure by 5 to 10 seconds because of the technology of the capnometer. Thermal sensors are dependent on where they are placed in the airstream, are nonlinear with airflow, and are uncalibrated, and it is suggested that a square root transformation be made on the signal to prevent reporting hypopneas that are not present. It is recommended that pulse oximetry be collected with signal averaging of 3 seconds. In this example the SaO_2 starts to increase rapidly within 5 to 10 seconds of the onset of breathing, whereas in Figure 18-1 the SaO_2 lagged by about 30 seconds. There a finger probe was used, whereas in this figure, and in many others in this volume, a rapidly responding ear oximeter is used. Notice that this patient has a classic tachycardia/bradycardia pattern, which corresponds very closely to the episodes of obstructive apnea. The pulse rate is usually derived directly from the calculation of the R-R interval of the EKG, and is a fast-responding accurate signal. Thus, it is important to understand phase differences between channels.

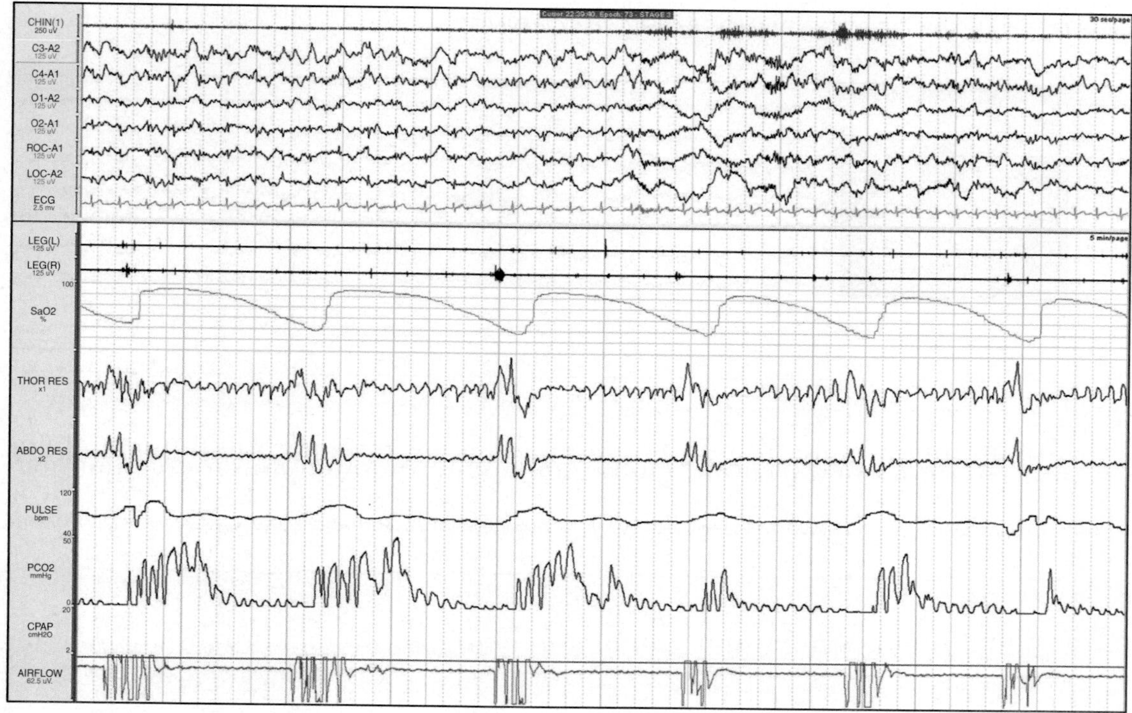

Figure 18-3.
Obstructive sleep apnea. This 47-year-old former boxer, who had his nose broken multiple times, had severe sleep apnea. The minimal channels required to differentiate obstructive from central apnea are SaO_2, breathing effort (thoracic and/or abdominal), and oronasal airflow. A calibrated, rapidly responding, end-tidal CO_2 analyzer monitoring oral and nasal airflow and the presence of hypoventilation is superior to a thermistor or thermocouple, which merely detects the presence or absence of airflow. Notice that the end-tidal CO_2 has detected more breaths than the pressure transducer (labeled *airflow*) in this patient who does a great deal of mouth breathing. For examining sleep, the ideal epoch length is 30 seconds, and for examining breathing during sleep, the ideal epoch length is 2 to 5 minutes, although these may vary somewhat from patient to patient. In this example, the top window is 30 sec; the bottom is 5 min.

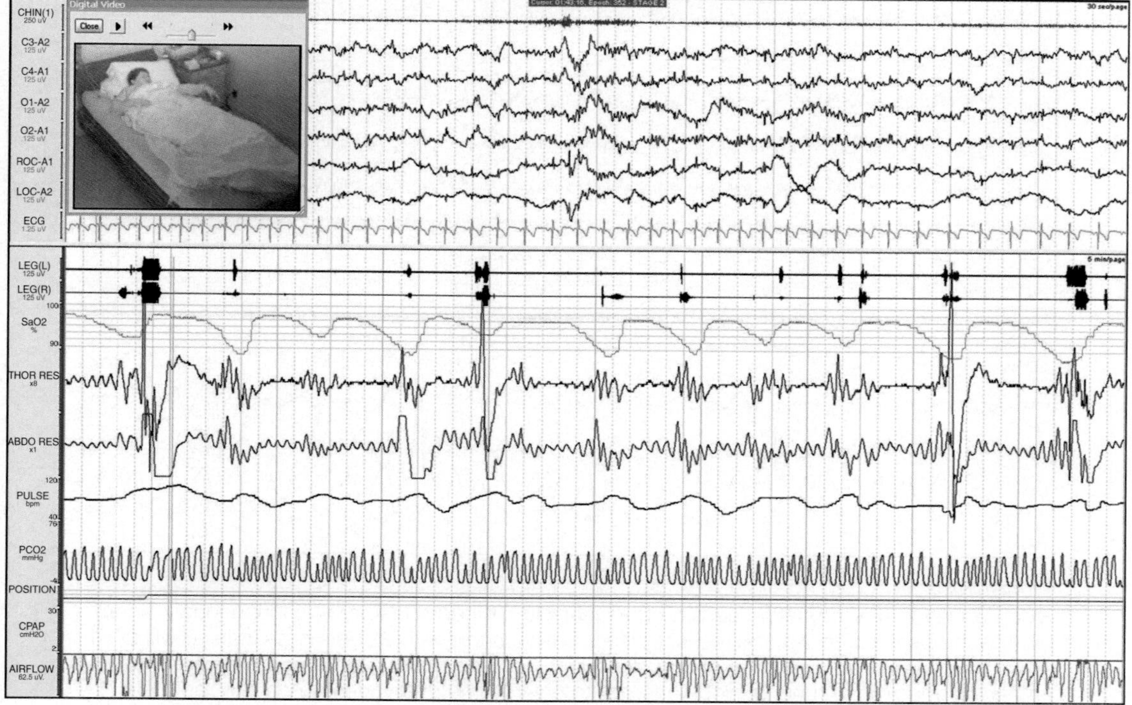

Figure 18-4.
Sleep apnea in a child. This 12-year-old boy had been snoring since birth. He was modestly overweight, had headaches and a history of awakening with shortness of breath, and was a restless sleeper. His preferred sleeping position was on his stomach. Here he is sleeping on his back and has obstructive sleep apnea (see Video 22, chapter 20). It is not unusual for children with sleep apnea to assume positions that minimize airway obstruction.

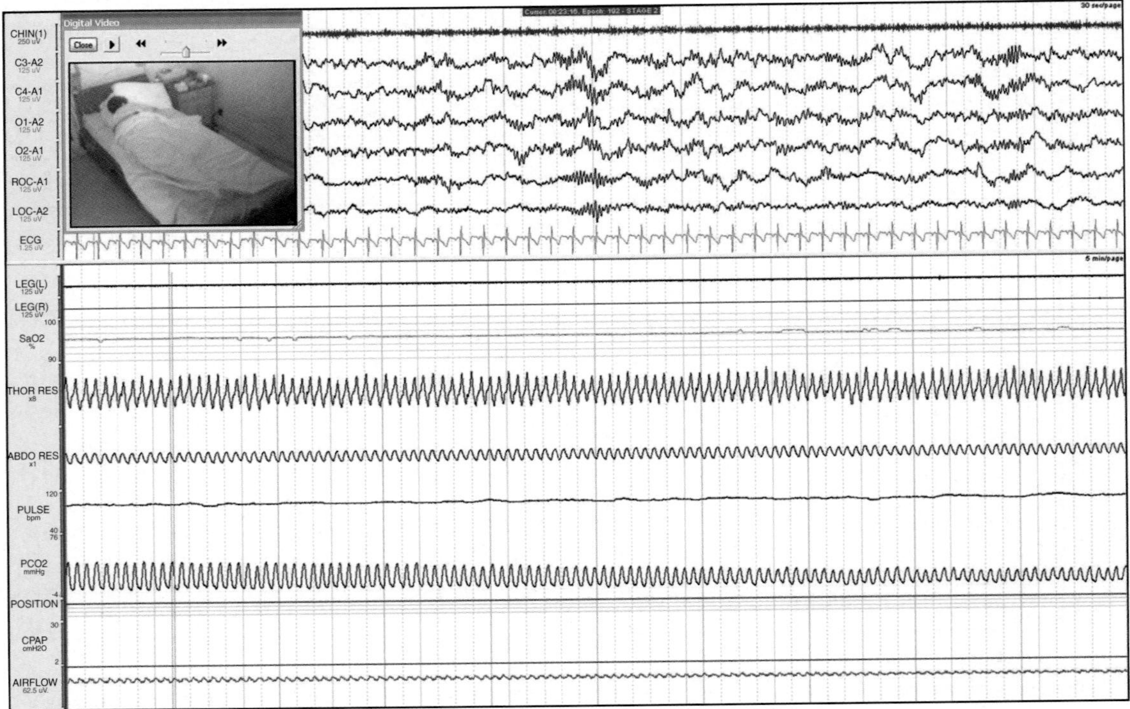

Figure 18-5.
Sleep apnea in the same patient as in Figure 18-4. Here the patient is sleeping mostly on his stomach. The apnea has resolved entirely. This child had enlarged tonsils and adenoids that were surgically removed, resulting in the resolution of the sleep apnea.

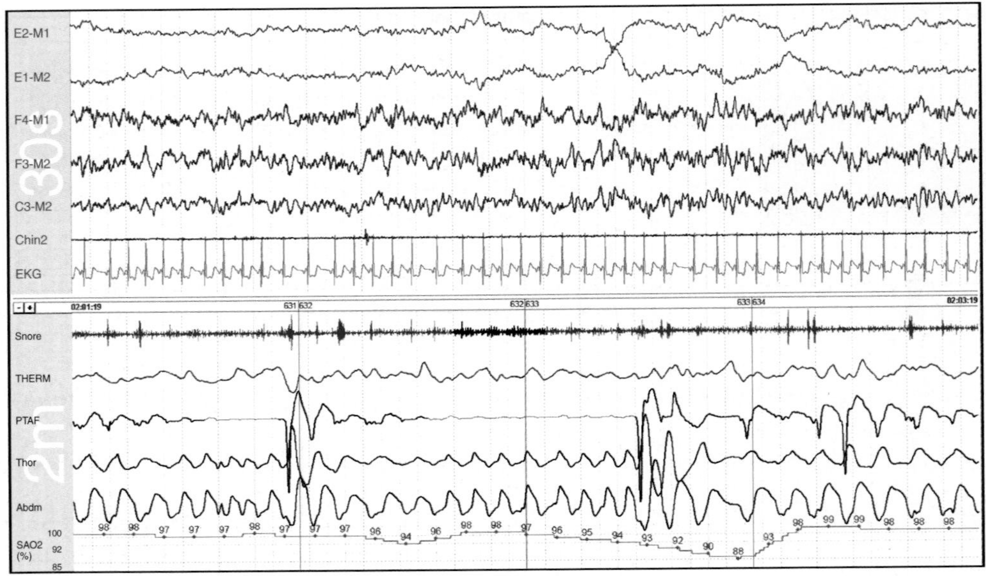

Figure 18-6.
Sleep apnea in a retrognathic child. This 7-year-old girl had a history of snoring loudly since birth, with observed apnea and restless sleep. She was thin with a body mass index (BMI) of 21. The patient assumed a posture during sleep in which she thrust her lower jaw forward and arched her neck in an unconscious attempt to enlarge the pharyngeal airway. In rapid eye movement sleep, the patient had at times quite long episodes of apnea, as shown in this figure. Note the thoracic/abdominal paradox when the apnea "breaks."

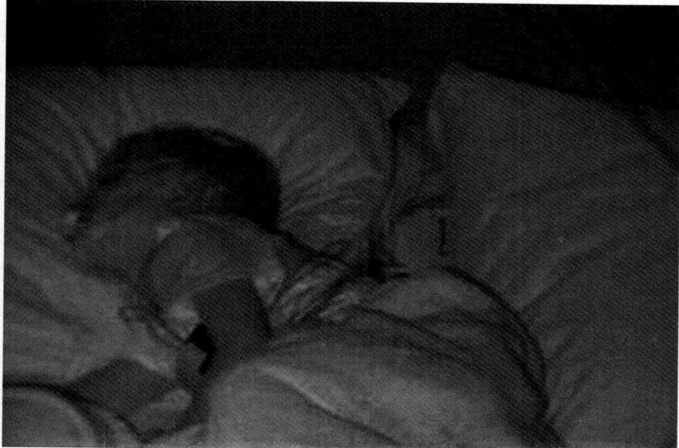

Figure 18-7.
Retrognathic child with sleep apnea. This 5-year-old boy slept with his lower jaw thrust forward in an attempt to enlarge the pharyngeal airway. He had a history of snoring, witnessed apnea, waking up gasping, and shortness of breath. He snored 62% of the night, and had an apnea-hypopnea index of 2.4, which is above the threshold of 1 required for the diagnosis of pediatric sleep apnea.

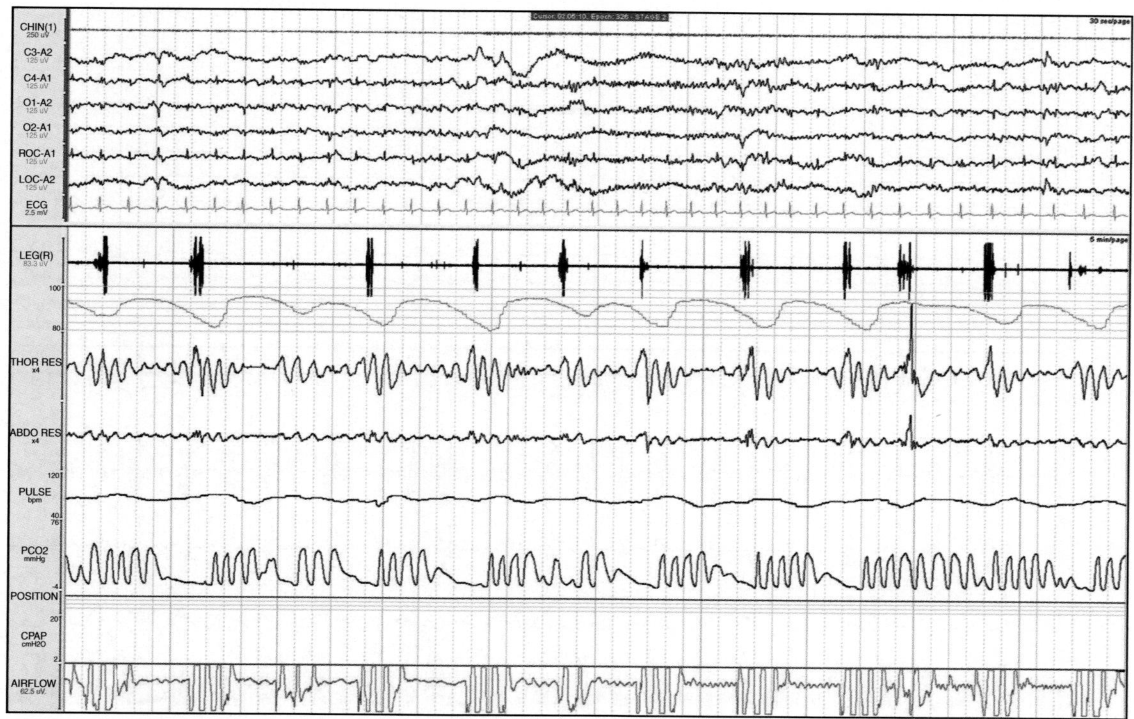

Figure 18-8.
Obstructive sleep apnea with activity in the leg channels. Monitoring leg movements is very useful in patients with sleep apnea. Here, leg movements are detected with every apneic episode. The movement generally occurs at the time of the greatest thoracic respiratory effort. Are these periodic limb movements, or are they merely movements linked to respiratory effort? These movements do meet the criteria for periodic movements in sleep and should be scored as such, as this is what the data show. However, does this patient have one or two diagnoses?

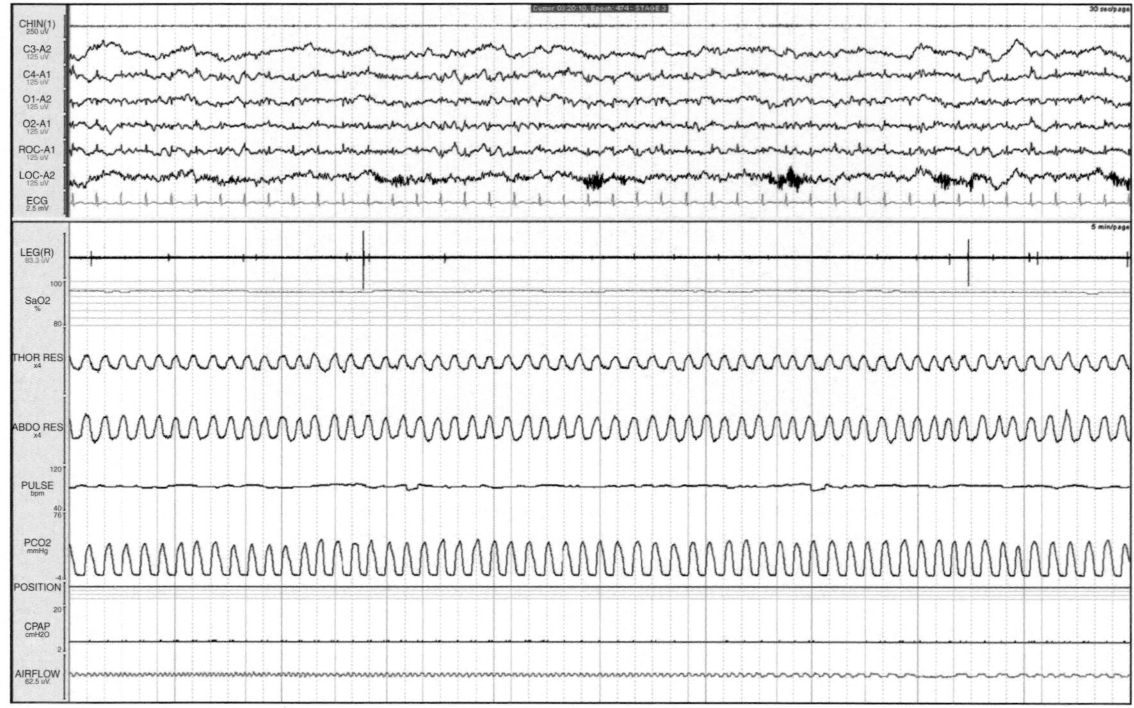

Figure 18-9.
Obstructive sleep apnea with activity in the leg channels on CPAP. These data are from the same patient as in Figure 18-8 but later on in the night. On CPAP, the leg movements have resolved entirely. Thus, the movements were linked to the abnormal breathing pattern, and this patient does not have periodic limb movements in sleep.

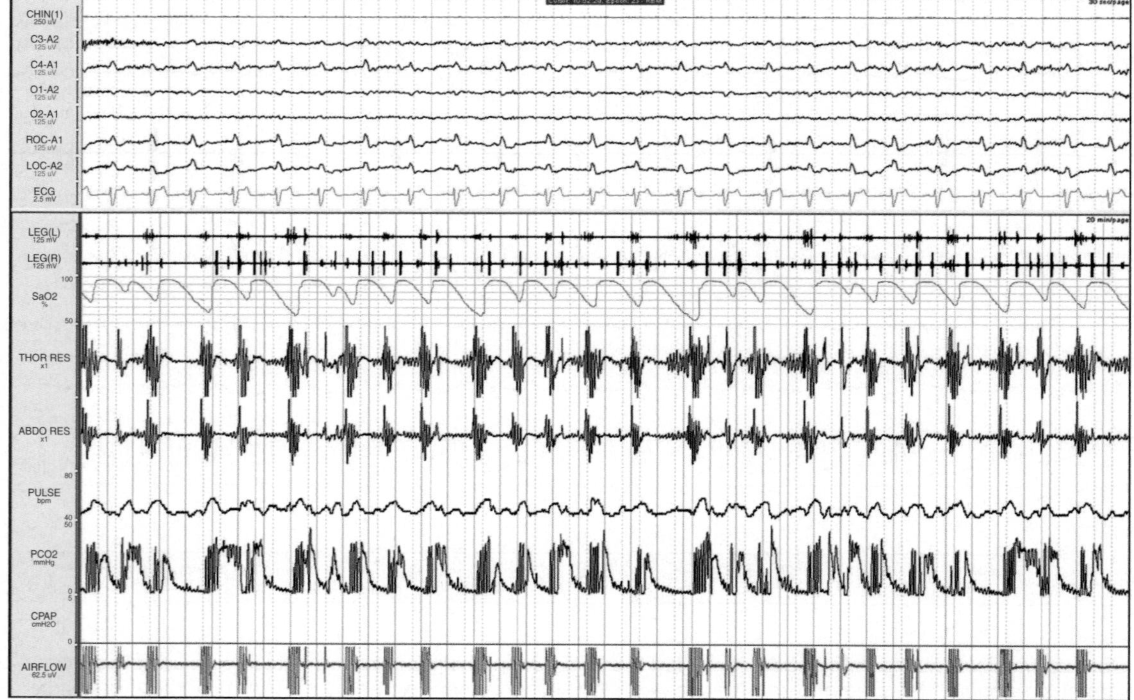

Figure 18-10.
Mixed sleep apnea with leg activity. This is an example from another patient who had leg movements and severe sleep apnea. The leg movements are not as periodic or regular as in the previous example. Are the movements simply a reflection of the breathing efforts? One clue is that the heart rate, measured by the pulse, shows oscillations that are not always linked to the abnormal breathing patterns.

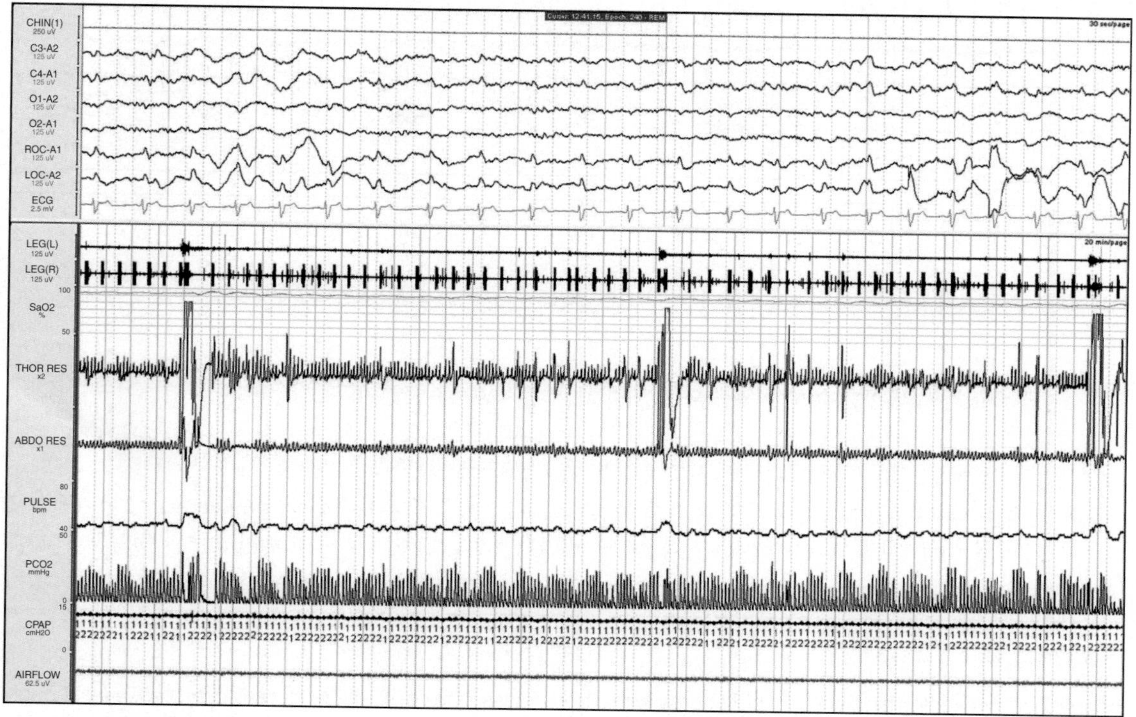

Figure 18-11.
Mixed sleep apnea with activity in the leg channels on CPAP. The apnea has resolved and the leg movements continue at a very high rate. This patient has both sleep apnea and periodic limb movements in sleep.

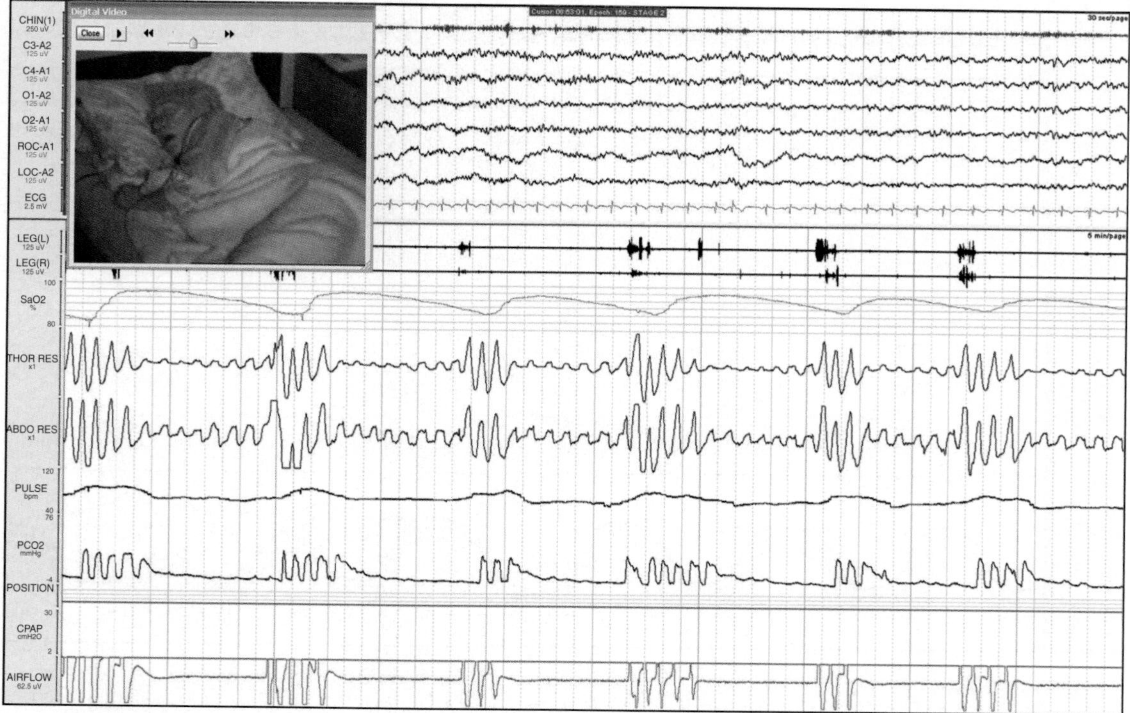

Figure 18-12.
Obstructive sleep apnea with acromegaly. Examination of synchronized visual video is extremely helpful in further understanding the physiologic abnormalities present. In this patient, it was apparent that she slept with her mouth wide open and moved her jaw forward in order to reestablish breathing (see chapter 20).

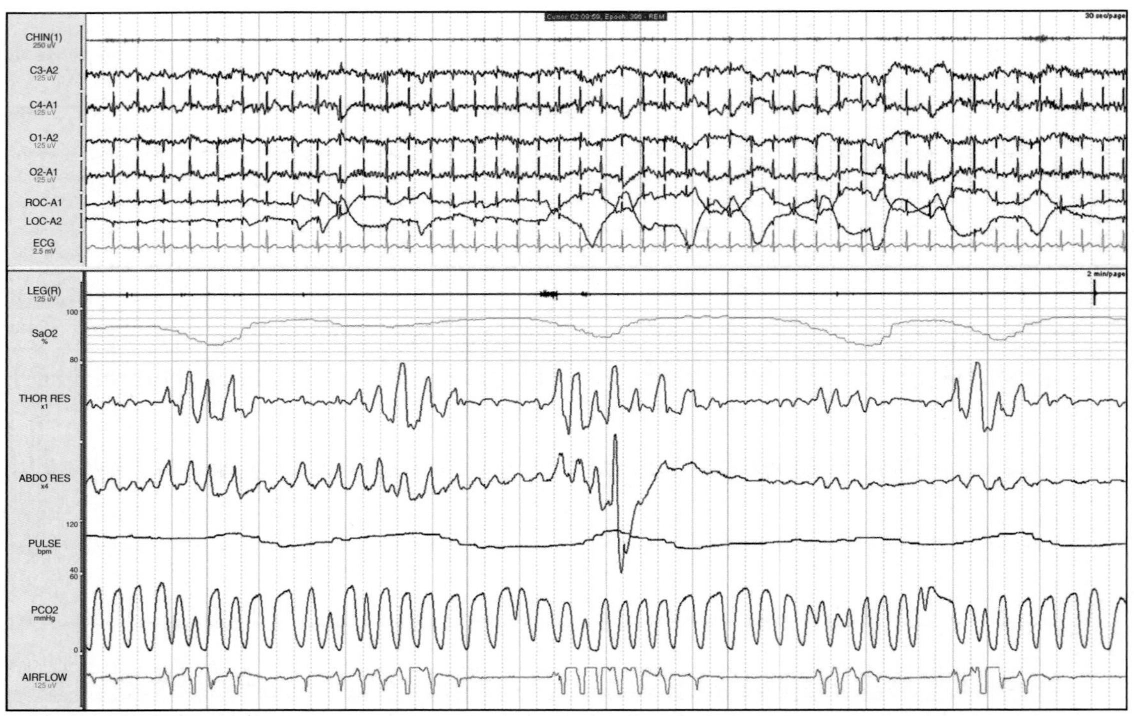

Figure 18-13.
OSA or hypoventilation? The patient is a 31-year-old gentleman with a history of snoring, severe nocturnal headaches awakening him, and morbid obesity with a body mass index of 49. REM sleep is detected, even though all the EEG channels show a great deal of EKG artifact. The nasal pressure channel suggests that the events are simply episodes of obstructive apnea. The pCO_2 channel shows breaths occurring throughout the 2-minute epoch in the lower window. Hypoventilation is suggested because of the high end-tidal pCO_2 being recorded. Using current data acquisition systems, one can drill down and examine individual breaths in great detail (see Fig. 18-14).

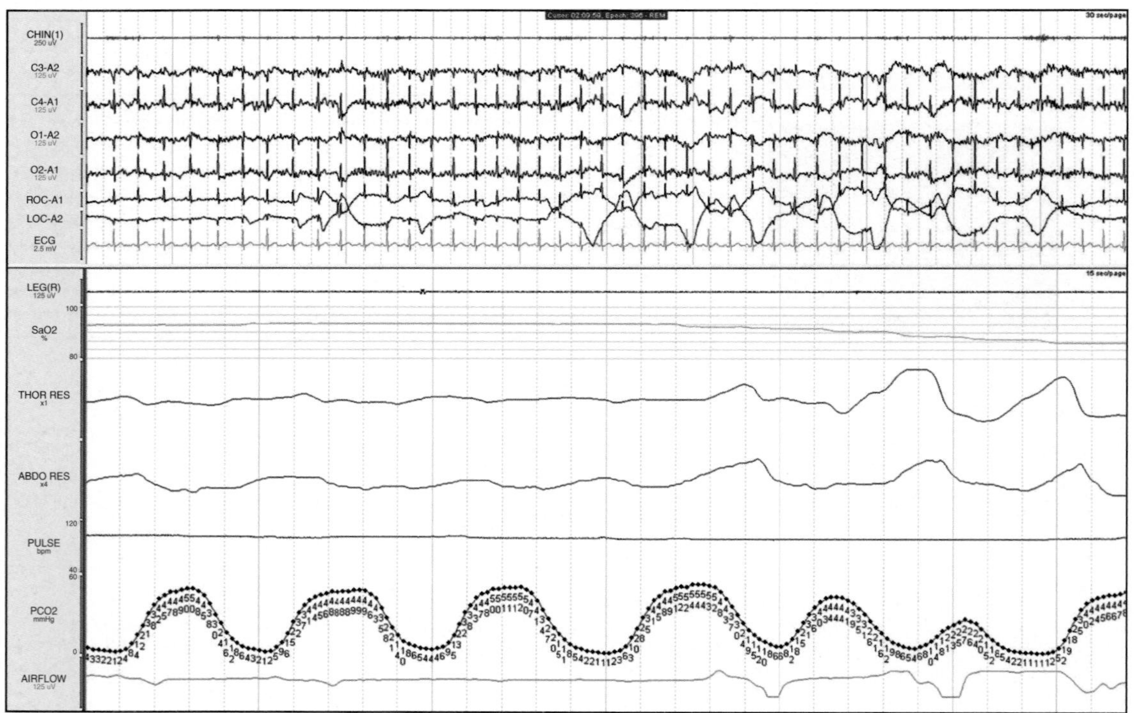

Figure 18-14.
OSA or hypoventilation? The bottom window is now a 15-second epoch. CO_2 is being detected with each of the small breaths, and breathing frequency is about 26 breaths per minute. The digital system can include data points collected throughout on the CO_2 channel. The highest end-tidal pCO_2 noted here is 54 mmHg. There are two reasons why this number underestimates the true pCO_2: oronasal sampling will entrain some air, diluting the airstream, and the patient has a rapid, shallow breathing pattern, which will not result in a true measurement of alveolar pCO_2. Thus, interpreting all the data leads to the conclusion that the main problem is hypoventilation. Some health care systems require such documentation in order to provide the patient with a mechanical ventilator or a bilevel airway pressure device.

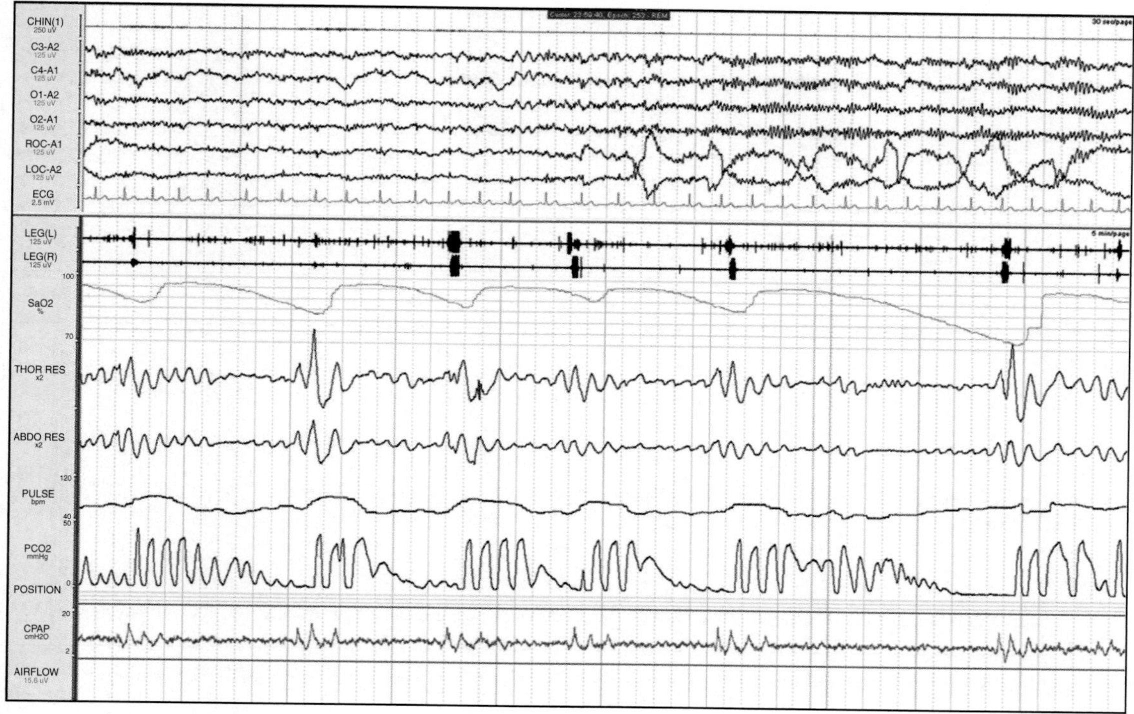

Figure 18-15.
Obstructive sleep apnea. The importance of sleep stage recording. In this example, the patient has five episodes of oxygen desaturation followed by a much longer episode of apnea, and much greater oxygen desaturation. The top window is 30 seconds, while the bottom is five minutes. The top and bottom windows are synchronized by the vertical orange lines in both windows. In the middle of the upper window, the patient has gone into REM sleep with sawtooth waves immediately followed by REMs. Sleep apnea is generally more severe in REM sleep.

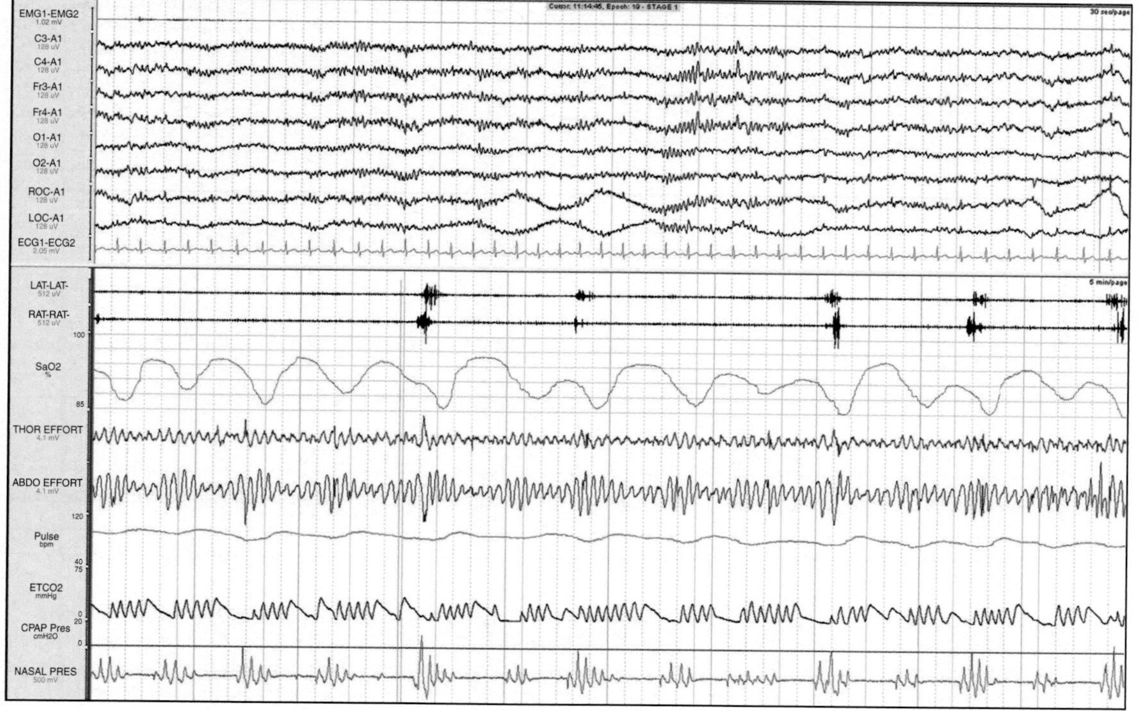

Figure 18-16.
Awake and asleep obstructive apnea. Sleep laboratories often ignore data obtained during wakefulness. These data are from a 49-year-old female who for 3 years had the perception that she stops breathing during wakefulness. In addition, there is a history of snoring and very severe sleepiness with an Epworth sleepiness score of 24. Here the patient is awake but drowsy (notice the slow eye movements).

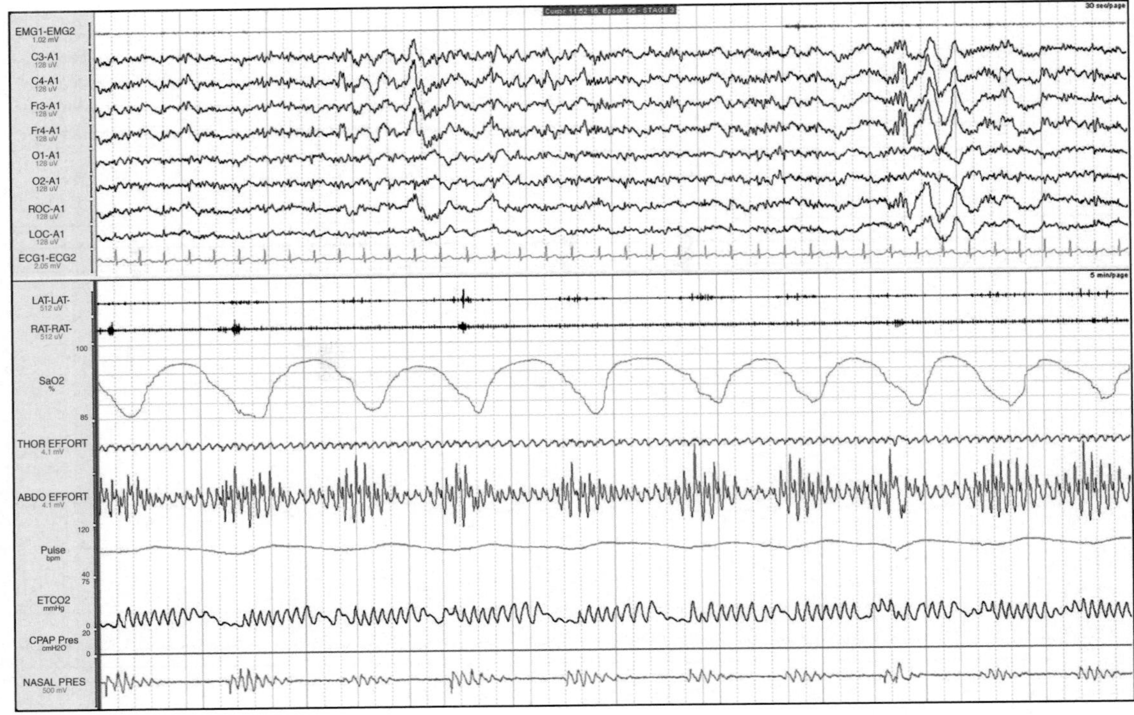

Figure 18-17.
Awake and asleep obstructive apnea. Same patient as in Figure 18-16. Here the patient is in NREM sleep. The abnormal breathing pattern continues.

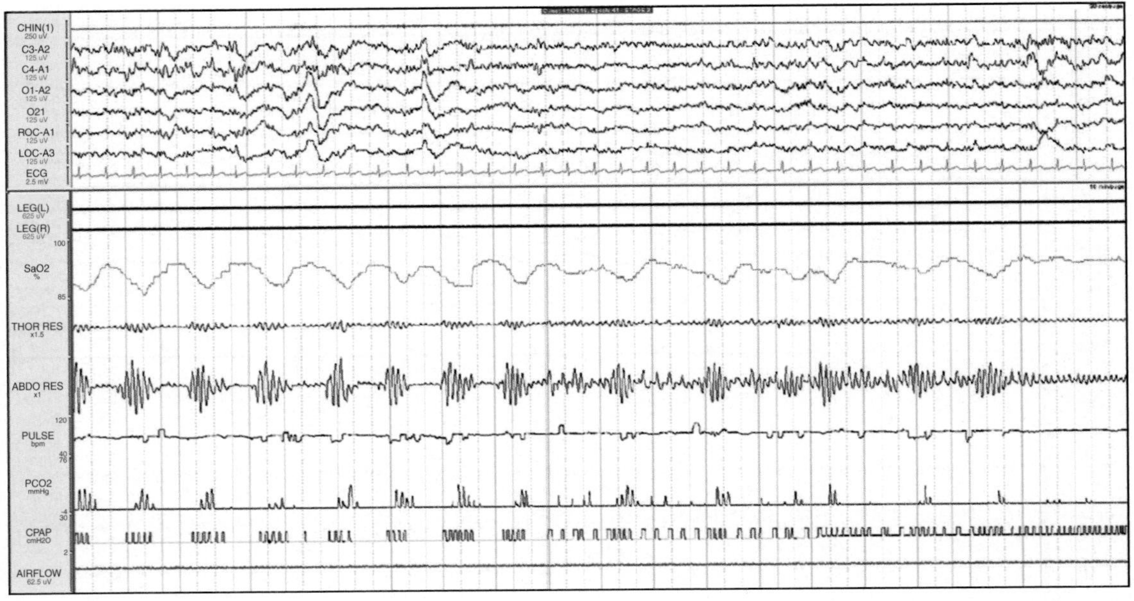

Figure 18-18.
Awake and asleep obstructive apnea. Same patient as in Figures 18-16 and 18-17. CPAP treatment was ineffective; the patient was then treated with bilevel pressure in a spontaneous mode. Notice in the channel labeled CPAP that there are clusters of 4 to 5 square waves representing the pressure generated by the bilevel machine in response to patient effort, but the apnea episodes continue. In fact, the patient now has central apneas. At the vertical orange line in the middle of the bottom window, backup rate is added to the bilevel system. By the end of the epoch, both the breathing pattern and SaO_2 have normalized.

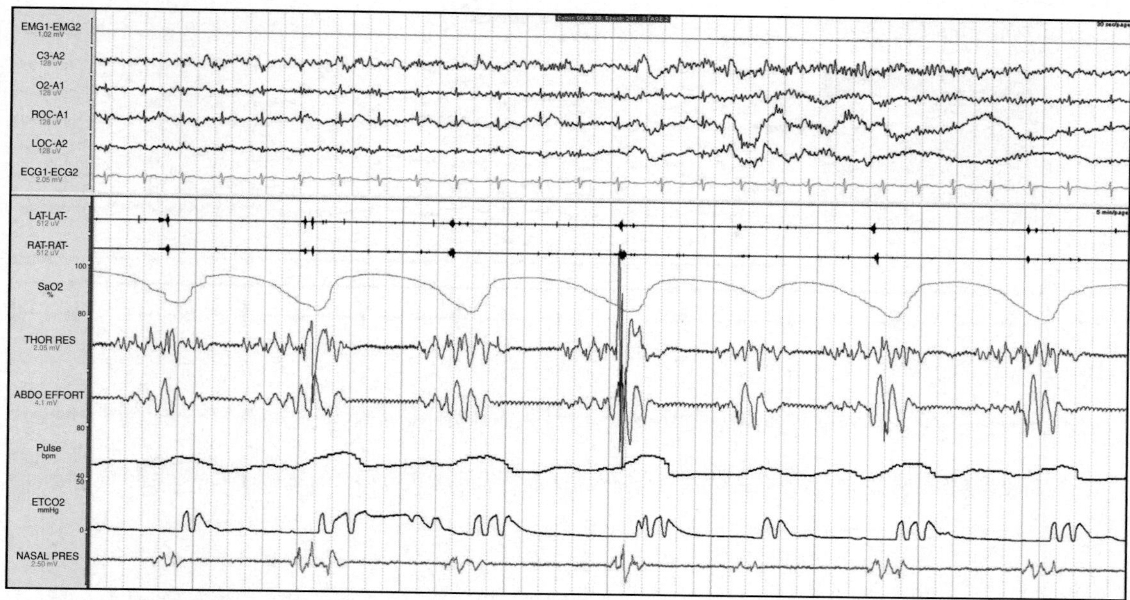

Figure 18-19.
Mixed apnea. Mixed apnea usually begins with a central apnea (absent thoracic and abdominal effort), followed by obstructive apnea, as documented by efforts to breathe in the absence of airflow. Physiologically, the changes with mixed apneas are almost identical to the changes in obstructive apnea (oxygen desaturations, increases in heart rate, arousals). Such patients may respond extremely well to CPAP, or they may develop pure central apneas on CPAP. These data are from a 50-year-old male who began to snore at age 16 after suffering a broken nose playing hockey. Nasal obstruction related to the fracture was never treated. He responded well to CPAP.

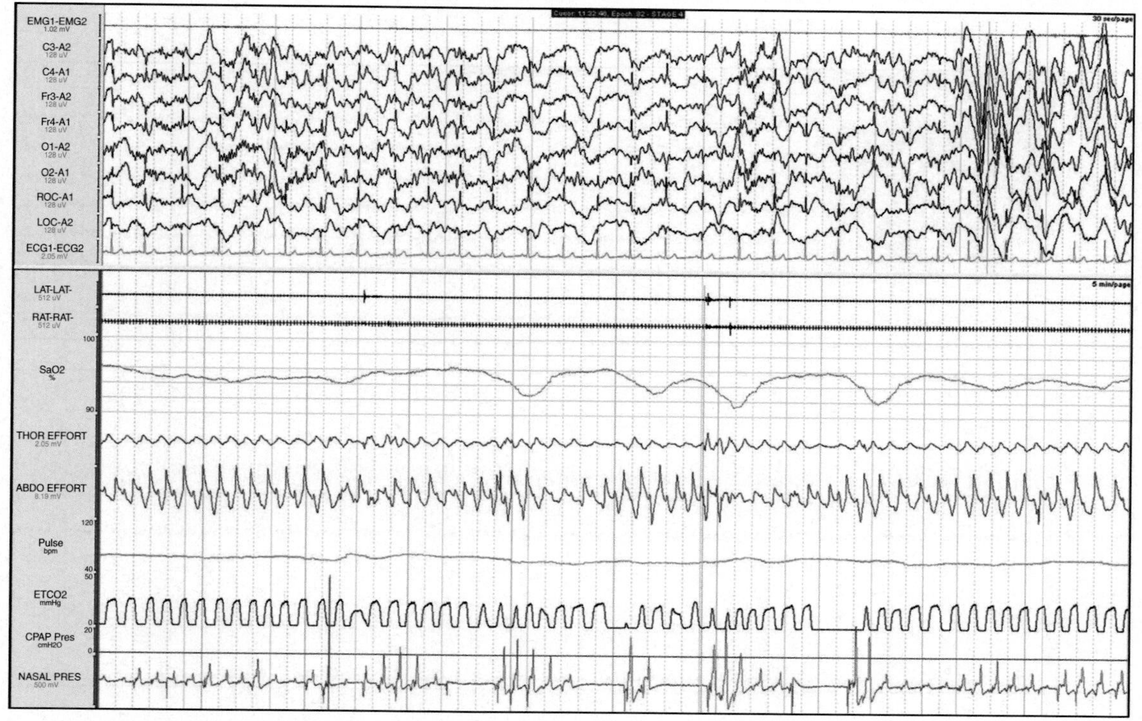

Figure 18-20.
Obstructive apnea in a patient with Down syndrome. Physical examination showed an enlarged tongue. In this fragment, the range of SaO_2 is between 90% and 100%. Thus, the drops in SaO_2 are quite small. Even though the findings might be considered not physiologically severe, the patient had severe sleepiness caused by the abnormal breathing pattern.

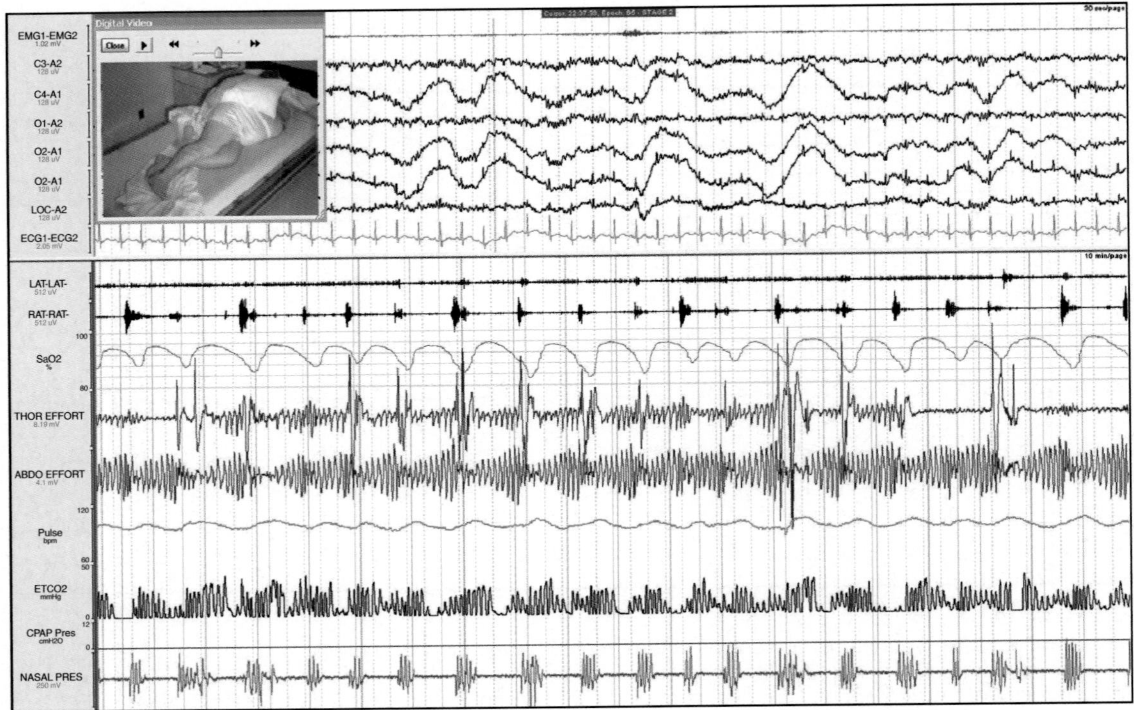

Figure 18-21.
OSA and periodic limb movements. This female patient had both severe apnea and severe periodic limb movements. Examining the synchronized digital video is very useful with such patients because one can see and hear the episodes of obstruction and the often vigorous movements. She moved a great deal during sleep, sweated, and kicked off her bedclothes. Notice the very large-amplitude low-frequency oscillation in the three channels that include the A1 electrode, representing sweat artifact.

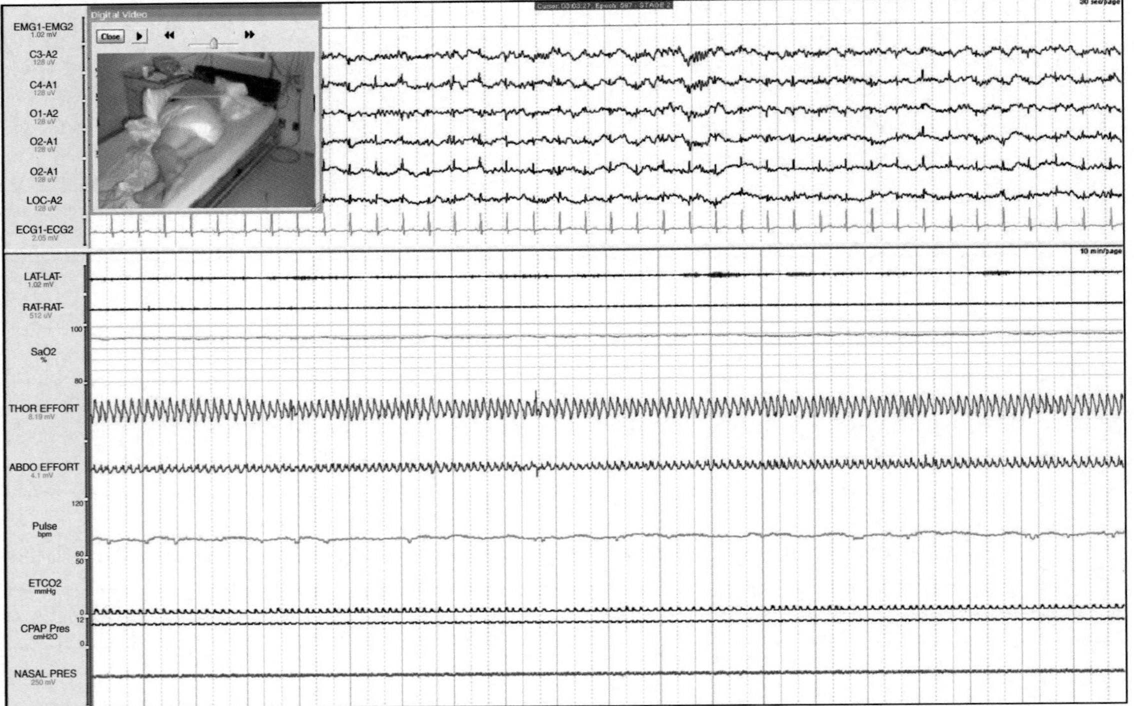

Figure 18-22.
Obstructive sleep apnea and periodic limb movements. Same patient as in Figure 18-21. The patient is now on CPAP. Her breathing has become entirely normal, the leg movements have ceased, and the sweat artifact has gone.

Upper Airway Resistance Syndrome

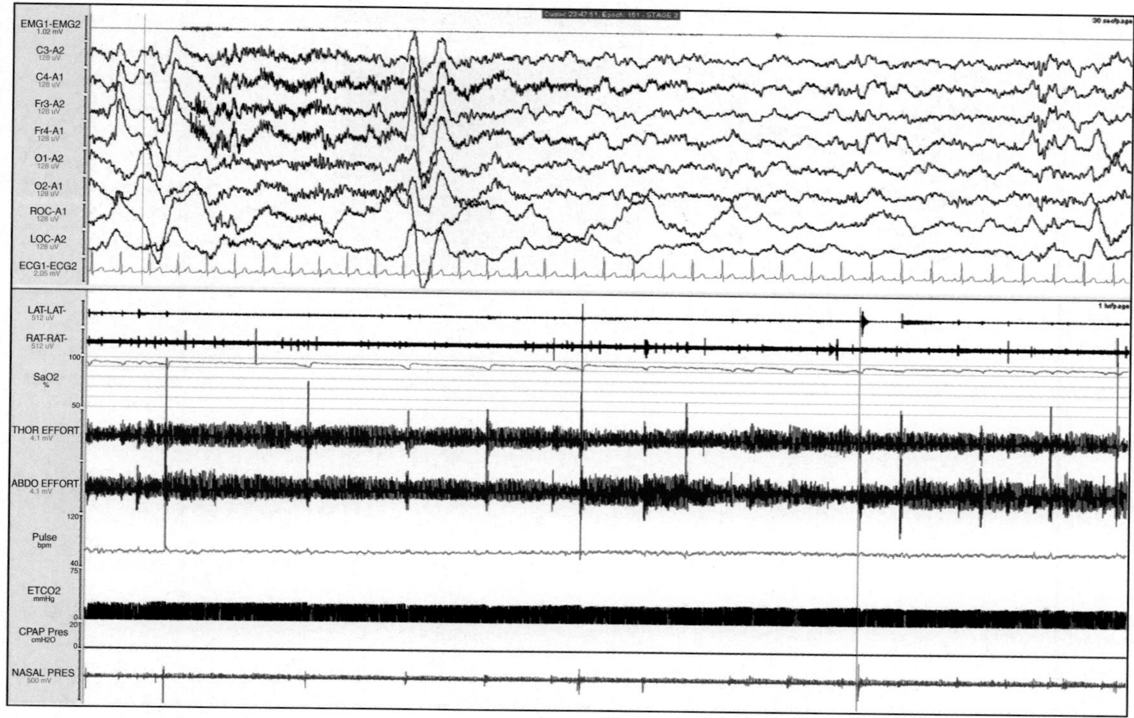

Figure 18-23.

Upper airway resistance syndrome (UARS). The first clue that there is a sleep breathing abnormality becomes evident when examining the breathing variables in time compression (the bottom window is 20 minutes). The SaO_2 signal is "ragged" and tiny deflections are associated with sudden increased excursion in thoracic and abdominal effort, and an arousal in EEG (note in the top and bottom windows the red vertical lines which are synchronized). Figures 18-24 and 18-25 show additional information when drilling down on the data.

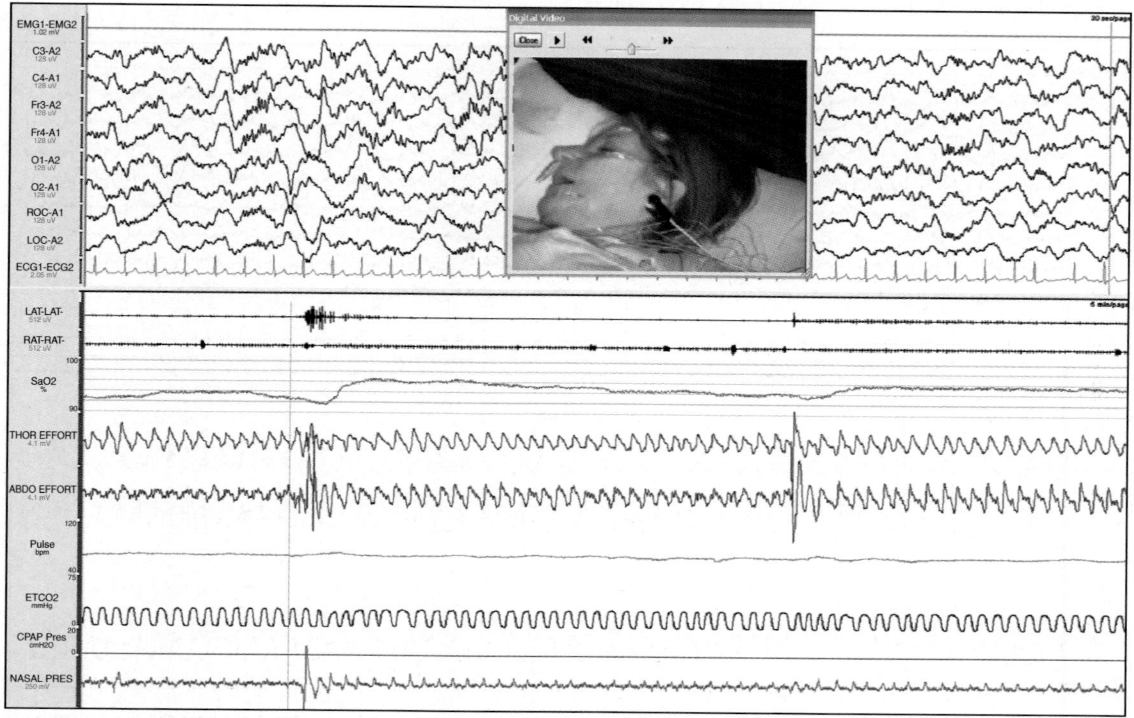

Figure 18-24.

UARS. Drilling down on the previous PSG fragment (Fig. 18-23). The upper window is 30 sec; the lower window is 5 min. The gain of the SaO_2 signal has been increased; the scale is 90% to 100%. The synchronized digital video shows that the mouth is open and the patient is snoring quietly. The synchronizing vertical orange lines show that we are one breath away from an event. The drop in SaO_2 is only 2%. The nasal pressure changes are small; the oronasal end-tidal CO_2 measurement shows continuous breathing. Figure 18-25 shows a moment one breath later.

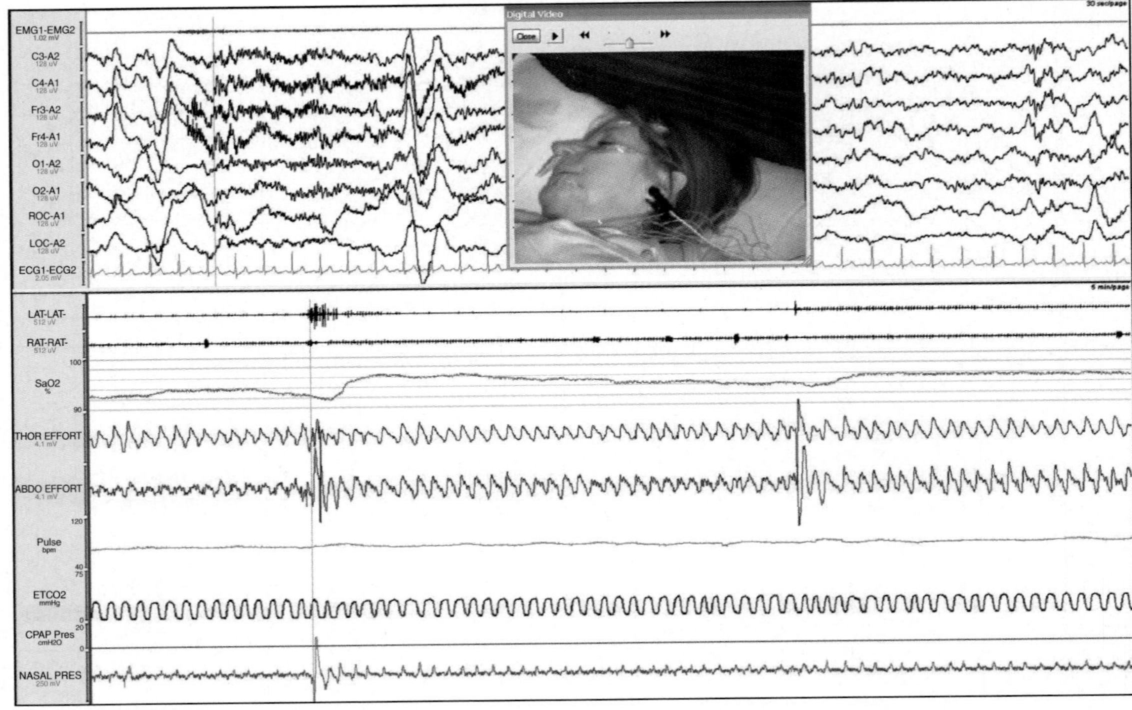

Figure 18-25.
UARS. Same patient as in Figure 18-24, one breath later. The patient has closed her mouth and is now breathing via her nose (see the nasal pressure change). This is followed by an increase in SaO_2. On the video she is heard to snort and then turn her head. The red vertical lines which synchronize the top and bottom windows show that this is associated with an arousal on EEG. This is a respiratory-related arousal (RERA). The nasal pressure transducer was not giving the information needed to properly characterize the event. Whereas some experts claim that the nasal pressure transducer is adequate for scoring hypopneas because, in part, they believe mouth breathing is a rare event, in our experience mouth breathing is a very common finding.

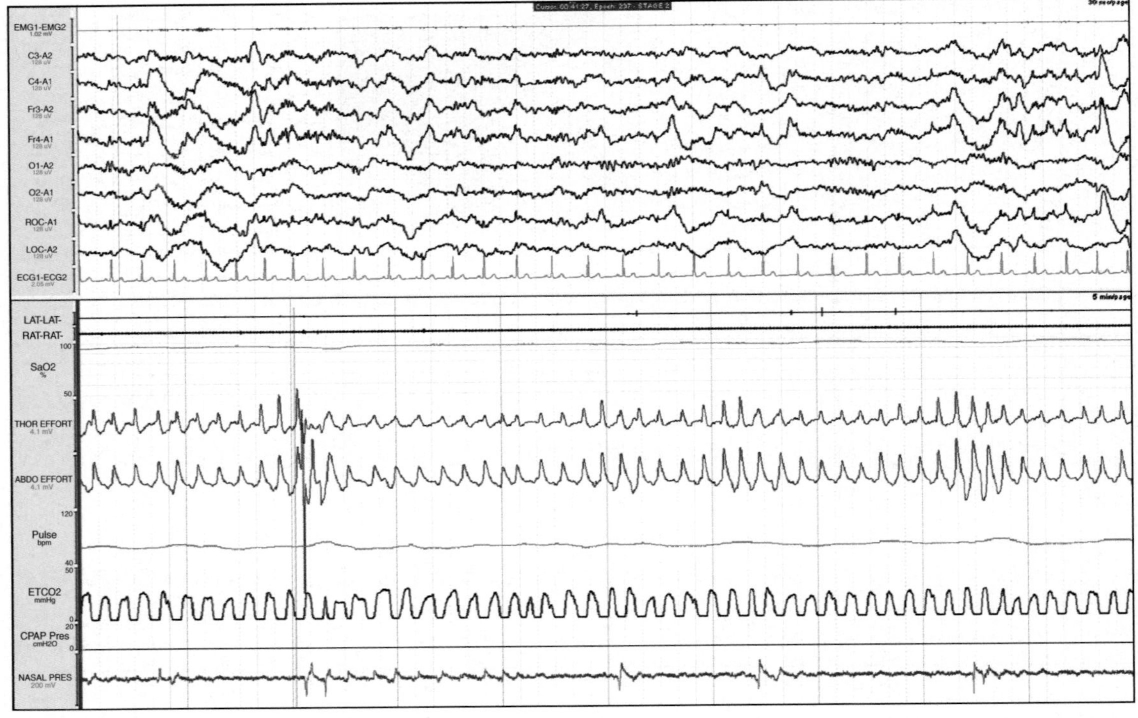

Figure 18-26.
UARS. The lower window is 5 minutes. There are small reductions in SaO_2 that reverse when there are increases in the nasal pressure signal. Here the synchronizing vertical lines precede a K-complex and a speeding up of the EEG. This is a respiratory effort–related arousal, or RERA.

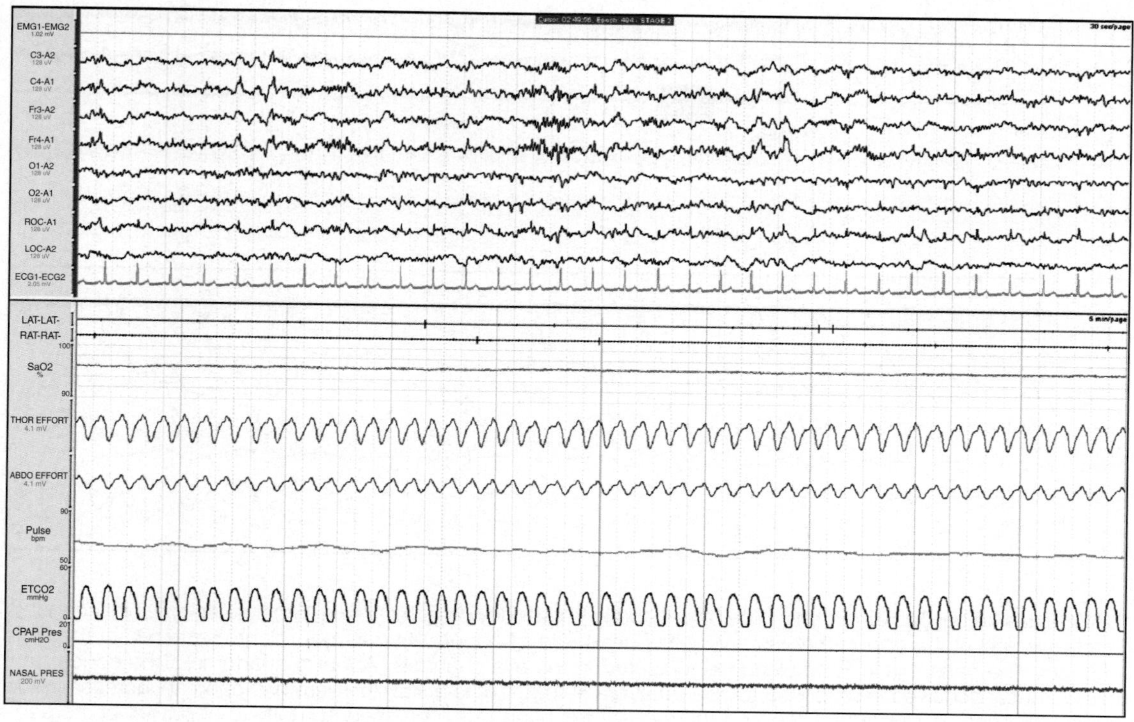

Figure 18-27.
UARS. Same patient as in Figure 18-26. The SaO_2 is rock-steady, as is the breathing pattern. There was a huge amount of REM in the second part of the night when the patient was on CPAP (not shown here).

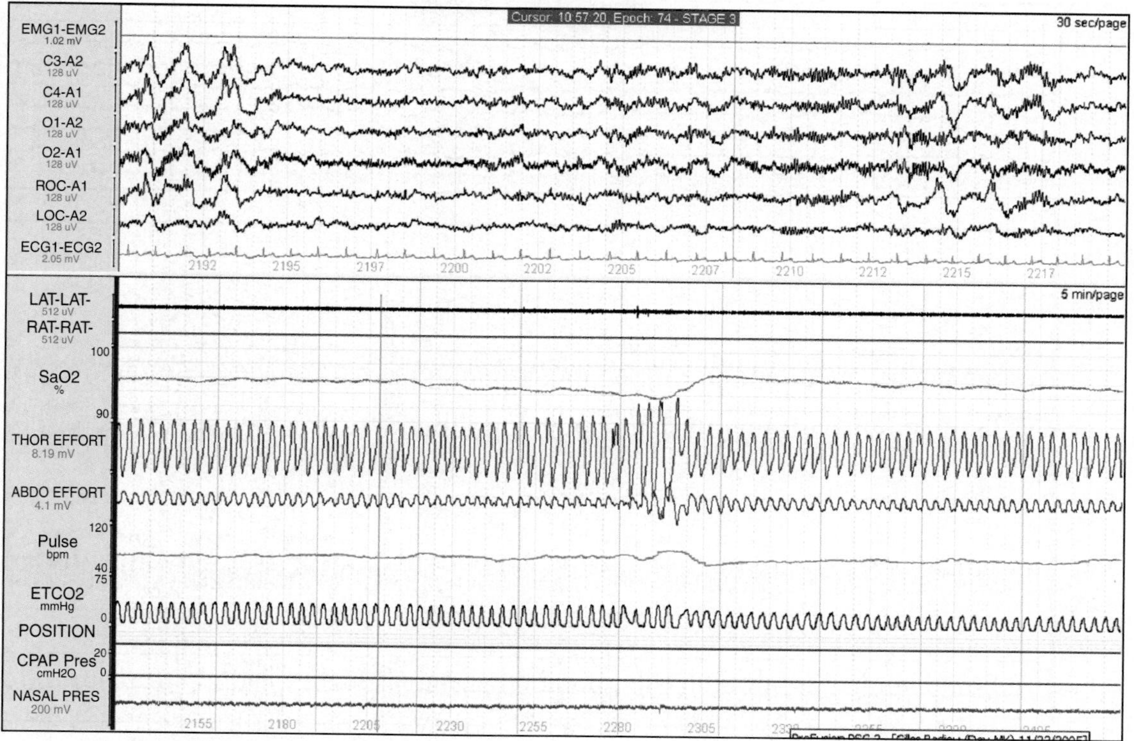

Figure 18-28.
Prolonged obstructive hypoventilation. In some patients who are continuous heavy snorers one sometimes sees a progressive slow reduction in SaO_2 associated with a progressive increase in effort, followed by a snort, and then an increase in SaO_2. In this example, the change in SaO_2 is only about 3%. The patient is mouth breathing entirely, and the nasal pressure trace is completely flat and not helpful. This would be scored as a respiratory effort–related arousal.

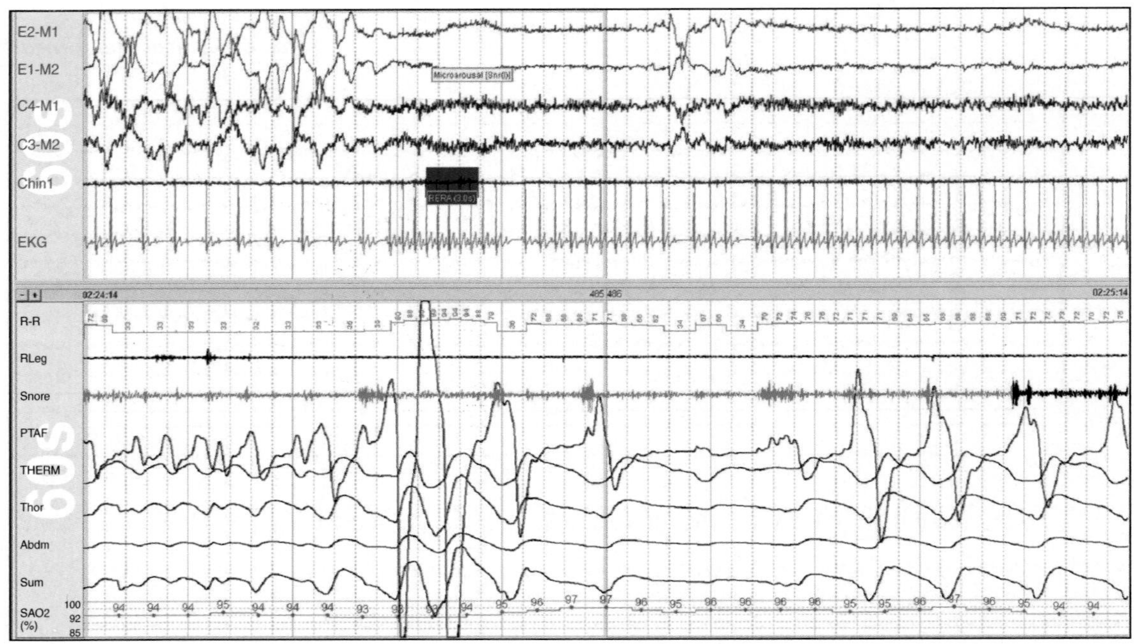

Figure 18-29.
UARS causing cardiac arrhythmia. The upper and lower windows each show a 1-minute epoch. Notice that in the beginning of the epoch there is a very low heart rate of about 33 beats per minute recorded in the R-R channel. The patient is in REM sleep, as indicated in the eye channels. About a quarter into the epoch, a microarousal occurred in response to abnormal breathing. This is a RERA. There has been an increase in the snoring channel at this time. Following the arousal the heart rate increased abruptly to about 94 beats per minute. When the heart rate was low the EKG indicated that a 2:1 Mobitz 2°AV block was present. There were two P waves for each conducted beat. This was presumably caused by increased parasympathetic activity, which in turn was caused by the increase in the patient's respiratory effort when the upper airway was obstructed. See Figures 18-70 to 73 for more details about heart blocks.

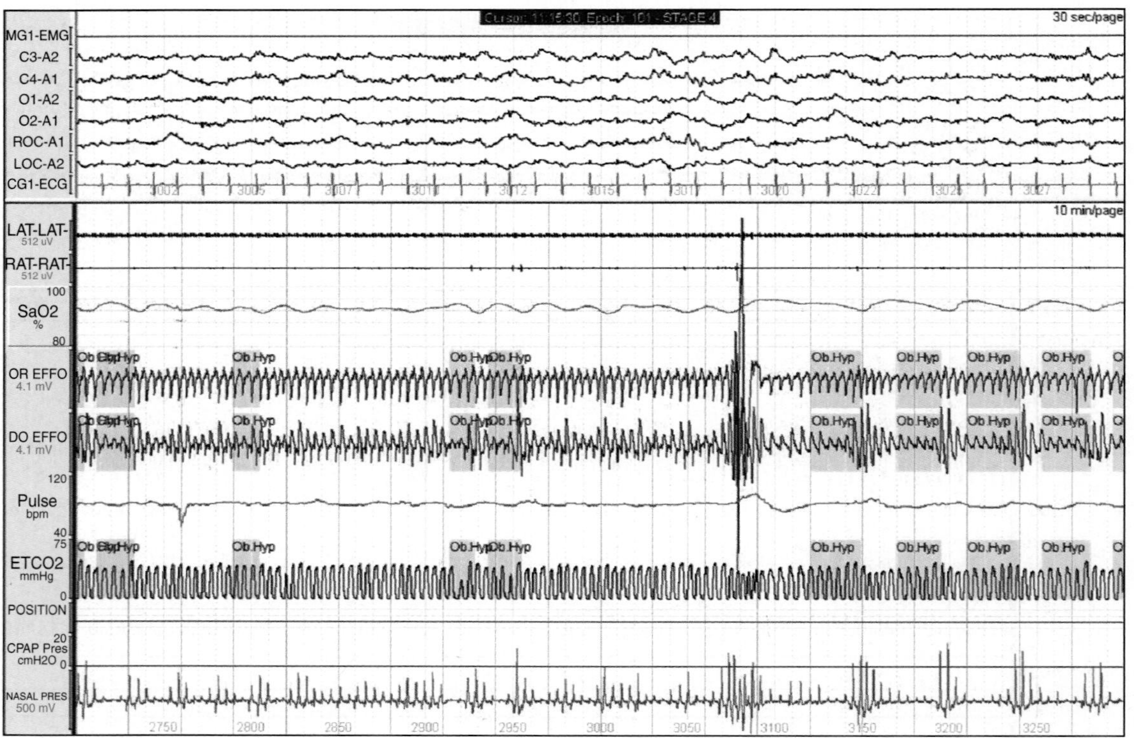

Figure 18-30.
UARS or obstructive hypopneas? The lower window is 10 min. There are small oscillations in SaO_2 associated with changes in nasal pressure, but note that there is little change in the oronasal pCO_2 trace. This suggests that the patient is mouth breathing during each event, thereby causing the reduction in SaO_2. One could infer that these are hypopneas. The patient is a 54-year-old male with a body mass index of 31 and a 20-year history of snoring, more recently observed apnea, and sleepiness. His apnea-hypopnea index (AHI) was 52.3. On CPAP, his AHI decreased to 7.9. Interpretation of a study should include consideration of all available data. The final diagnosis was severe obstructive sleep apnea syndrome.

Central Sleep Apnea

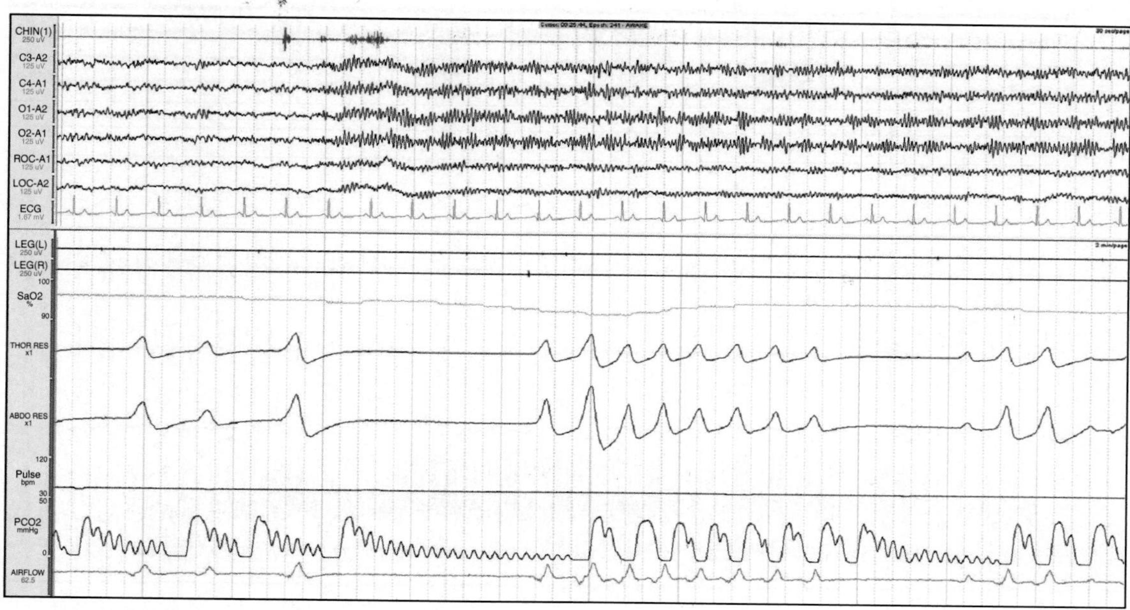

Figure 18-31.
Idiopathic central sleep apnea. The term *central apnea* refers to a cessation of breathing in excess of 10 seconds with markedly reduced or absent effort to breathe. Central apnea may occur during wakefulness, as in this example. This is a 71-year-old patient who had central apnea recorded during both wakefulness and sleep but without a known etiology. Note the absence of effort in both the thoracic and abdominal effort channels. The longest episode of apnea is almost 30 seconds. Note the cardiogenic oscillations in the CO_2 trace. Although the patient is awake throughout, there are fluctuating levels of alpha activity in the EEG channels. The patient's overall breathing rate, in this example, is only seven breaths per minute. The top window is 30 sec; the bottom, 2 min. Similar findings occur in some patients using opioid medications. This patient responded well to low CPAP.

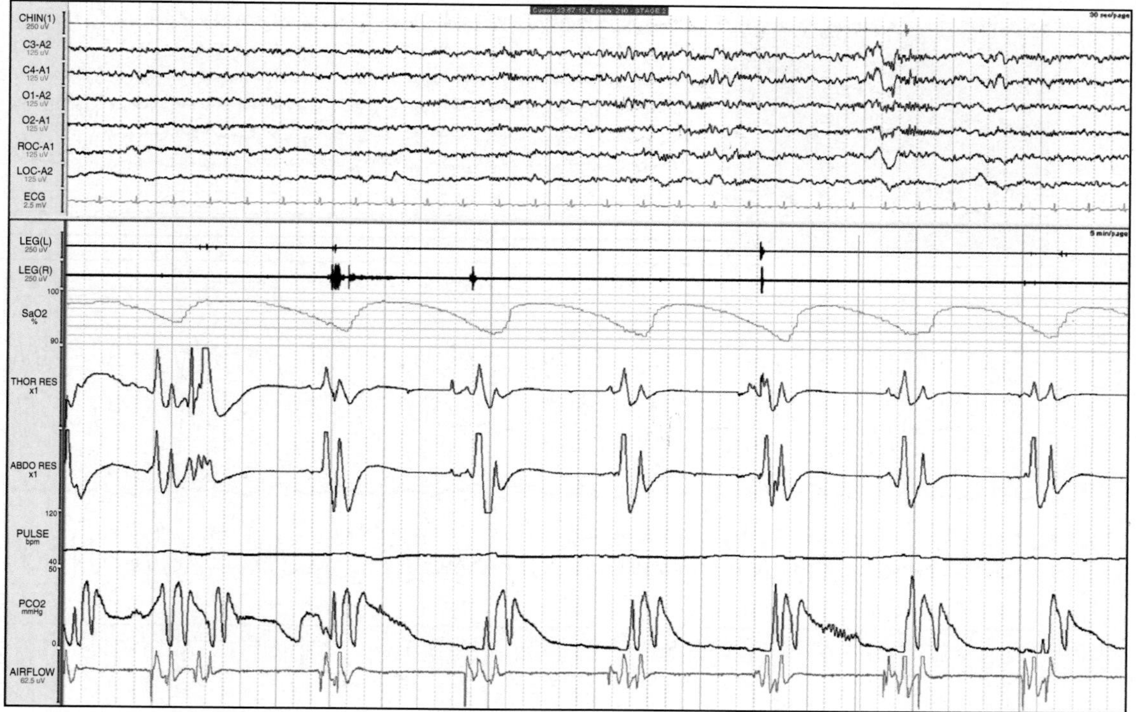

Figure 18-32.
Central apnea related to opiate. These data are from a 44-year-old soldier treated for severe nerve pain related to an ankle injury. He had had snoring, severe sleepiness, and witnessed apnea for 2 to 3 years. He was treated with morphine for pain. He had a breathing frequency of only four or five breaths per minute and repetitive cycles of two to three breaths, followed by central apneic episodes. The bottom window is 5 min. It is likely that this pattern is related to the morphine. The patient also had central apneas during wakefulness.

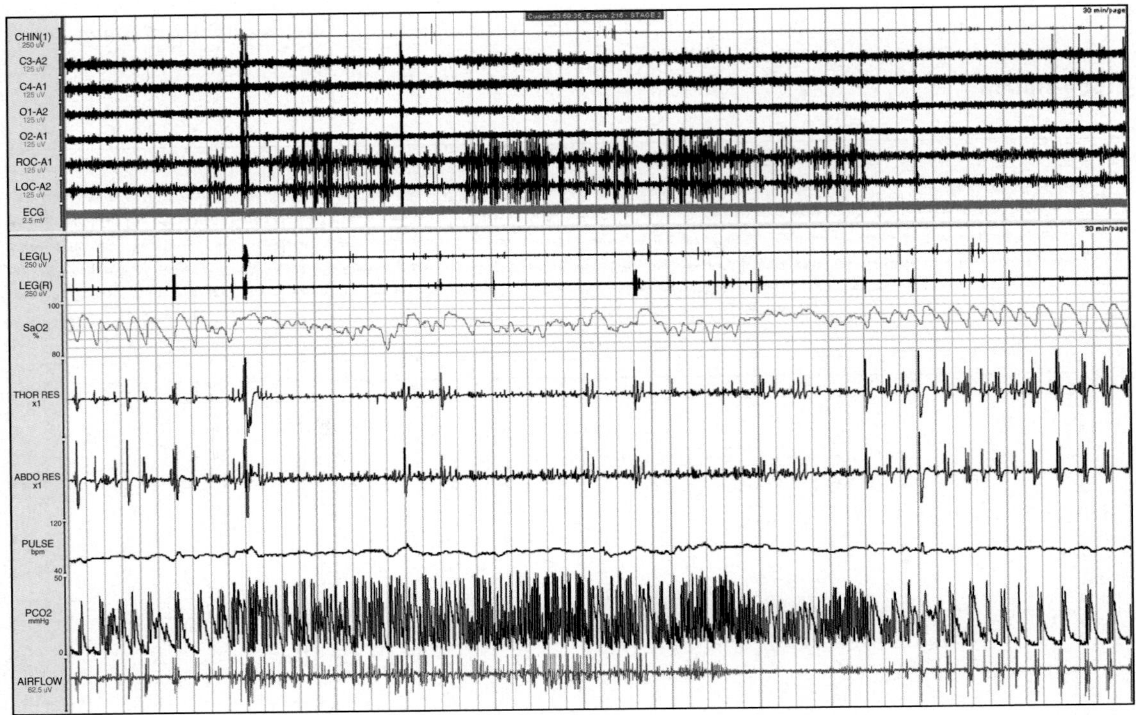

Figure 18-33.
Central apnea related to opiate. The top and bottom windows each show a 30-min epoch. REMs occur when there are large, dense deflections in the two EOG channels. Notice that the patient's breathing pattern actually changes during REM and there is much less periodicity in the breathing pattern and the SaO_2. When the patient emerges from REM sleep at the end of this epoch, the abnormal breathing pattern seen in Figure 18-32 returns. The central apneic episodes in NREM sleep are likely being maintained by the ventilatory chemical control system, which is depressed by morphine. When the patient goes into REM sleep, REM processes override the ventilatory control system.

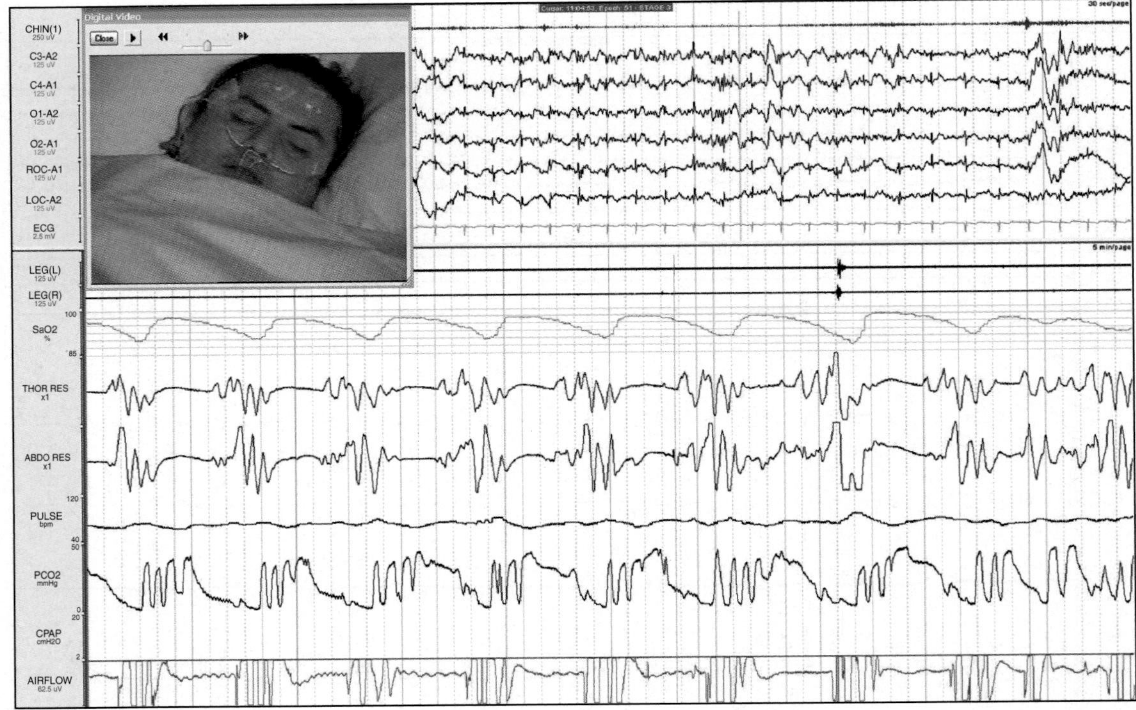

Figure 18-34.
Idiopathic central sleep apnea. Use of the term *idiopathic central sleep apnea* means that the patient has central apnea, but without any known cause. This male patient is 30 years old and presented with severe daytime sleepiness, snoring, and nocturnal headaches. There are episodes of central apnea (reduced or absent thoracic and abdominal efforts) and oxygen desaturations. Note that each cluster of breaths is made up of only four to five breaths. The apnea episodes are about 20 seconds long. The top window is 30 sec; the bottom, 5 min. Because of his snoring history, he was first tested on CPAP (see Fig. 18-35).

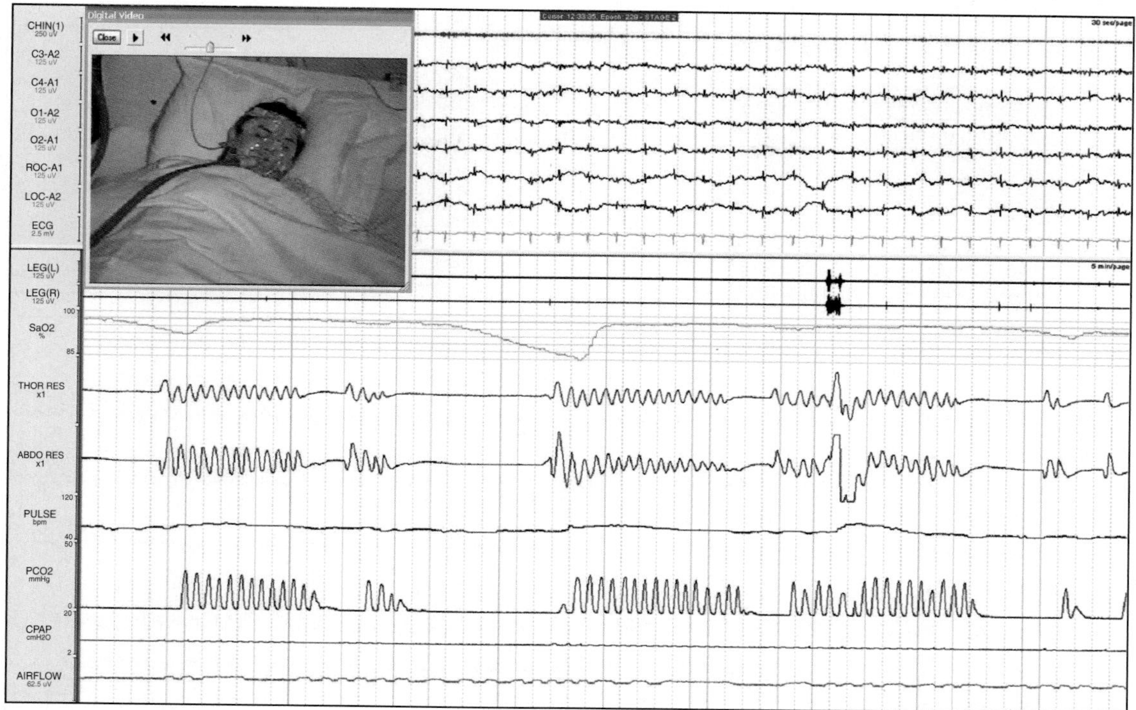

Figure 18-35.
Idiopathic central sleep apnea on CPAP. Same patient as in Figure 18-34. On CPAP shown here there was a marked worsening of the patient's apneic episodes to about 40 seconds long. *Complex sleep apnea* is a term recently introduced that implies that ventilatory instability in some patients leads to episodes of central apnea. Operationally, this is defined as patients developing central sleep apnea with positive pressure therapy. By that definition, some might conclude that this patient had a variant of complex sleep apnea. However, defining a disease based on the response to treatment is problematic, and many do not believe that this is an independent entity. Thus, although his history suggested OSA, simply having put him on CPAP without monitoring or without first determining apnea type would have placed him at increased risk. In the sleep laboratory setting one could proceed to the next step, testing on a bilevel device, shown in Figure 18-36.

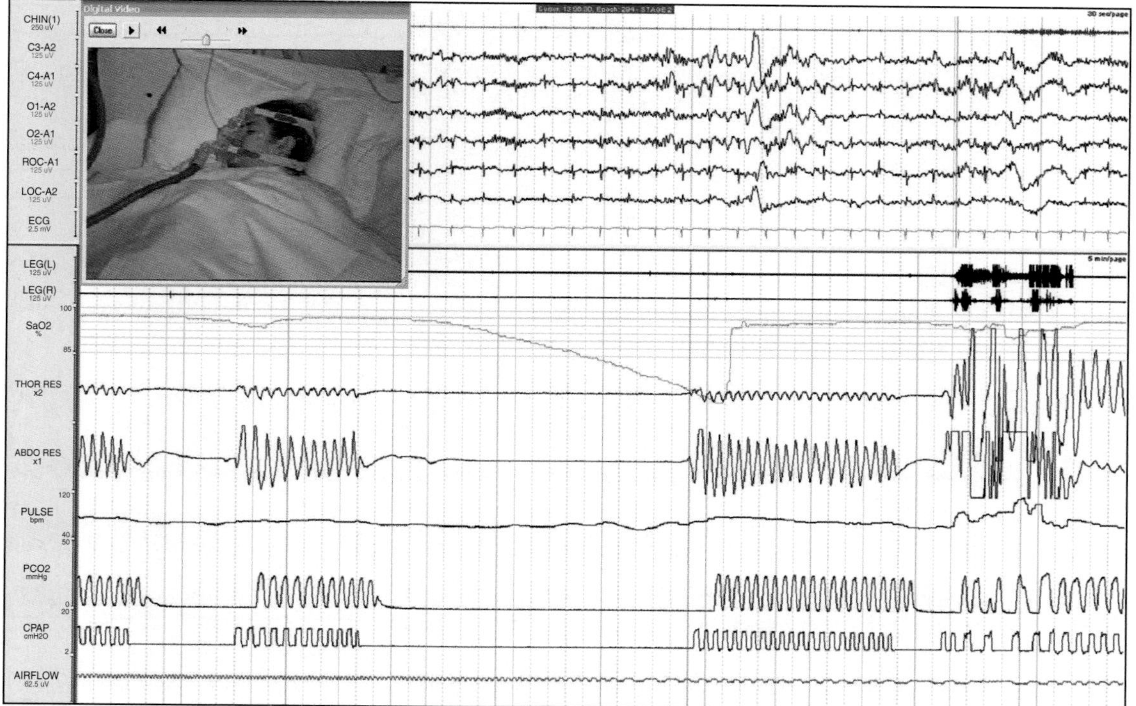

Figure 18-36.
Idiopathic central sleep apnea on bilevel pressure. Same patient as in Figure 18-35. There was a further marked lengthening of his apneic episodes to about 100 seconds. Clearly this approach was not going to be effective, and rather than proceeding to bilevel positive airway pressure with a time backup, we started this patient on adaptive servo-ventilation, shown in Figure 18-37.

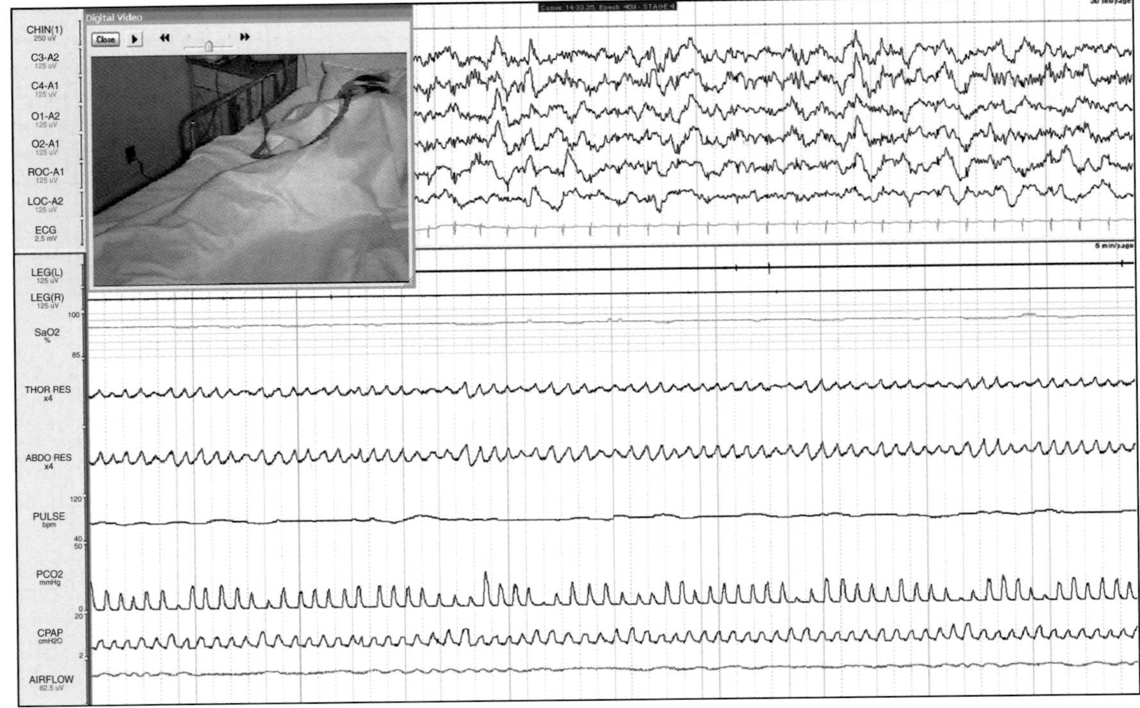

Figure 18-37.
Idiopathic central sleep apnea on adaptive servo-ventilation. This type of airway pressure support calculates the patient's minute ventilation and takes into account his or her breathing pattern. It compensates by adding additional support during episodes of apnea and less support during hyperpnea. The patient's episodes of central apnea were resolved by this treatment, and he was sent home on it.

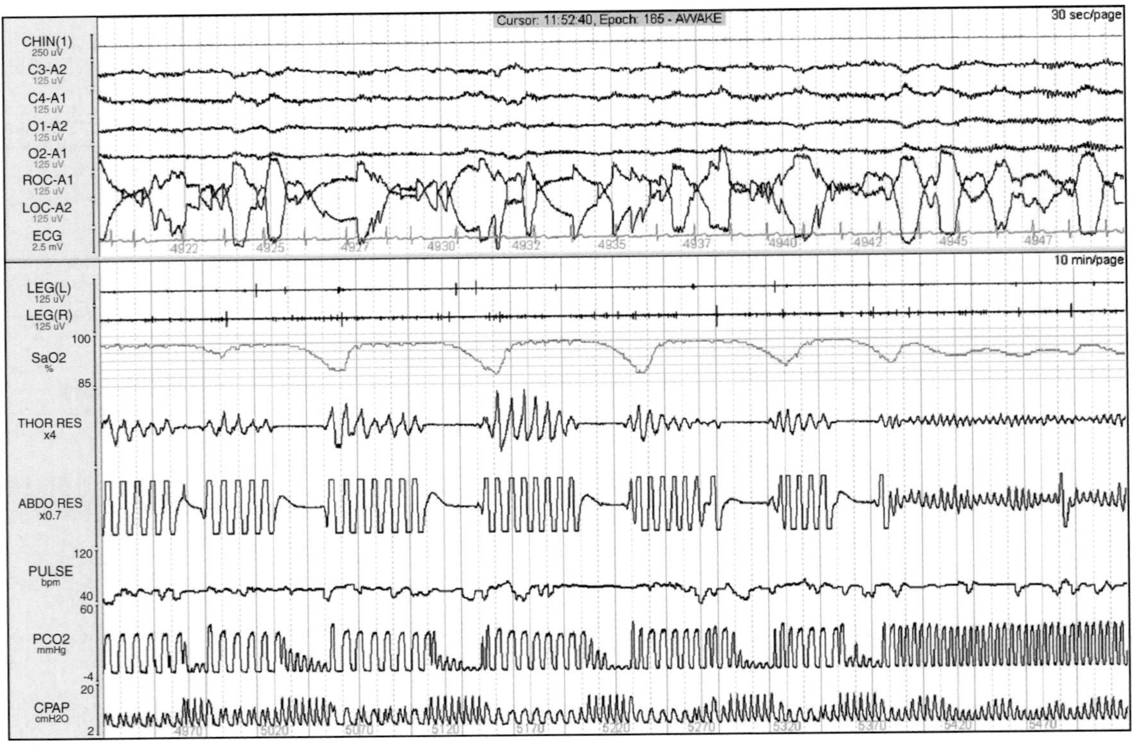

Figure 18-38.
Idiopathic central sleep apnea: treatment with adaptive servo-ventilation. This 55-year-old male presented with cognitive impairment and sleepiness but no snoring. He was found to have episodes of central apnea and had worsening episodes on CPAP, had no response to oxygen, and was then tested on adaptive servo-ventilation. The top window is 30 sec; the bottom window, 10 min. The channel labeled "CPAP" shows the pressure output of the adaptive servo-ventilation device. Notice that when the patient is apneic, the device produces the most pressure. By the end of the epoch, the patient's breathing pattern is normalizing, as is his SaO_2. Figure 18-39 shows a more prolonged response.

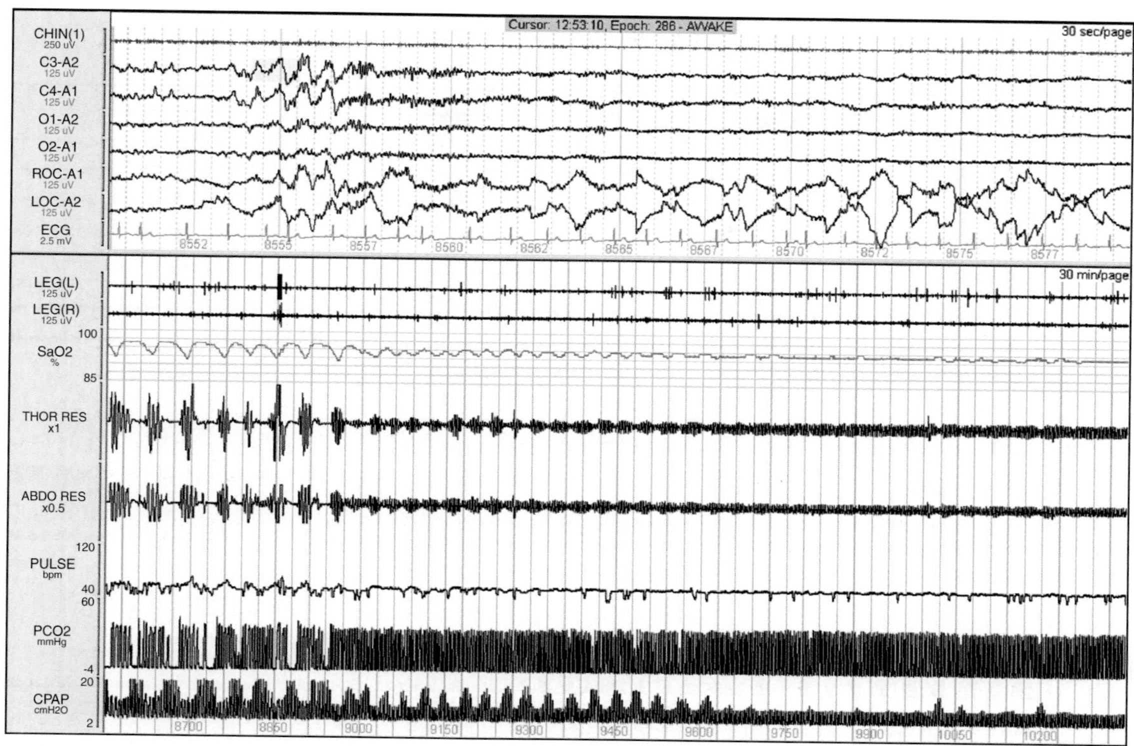

Figure 18-39.
Idiopathic central apnea: treatment with adaptive servo-ventilation. Same patient as in Figure 18-38, showing 30 minutes in the lower window. Notice that after about 7 minutes all the data show signs of normalizing, except that the adaptive servo-ventilator is still showing periodic changes in pressure support. By the end of the epoch, everything has normalized, including the output of the adaptive servo-ventilator, which is now steady.

Mixed and Complex Sleep Apnea

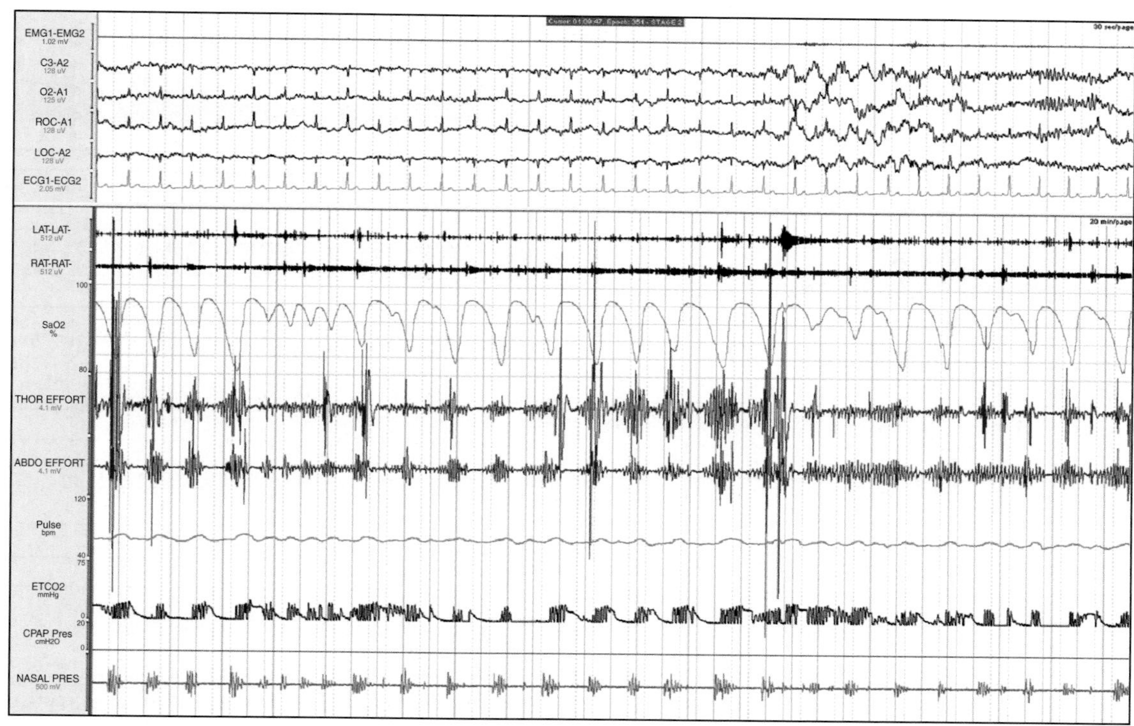

Figure 18-40.
Mixed apnea, becoming complex sleep apnea. This 63-year-old male has a history of a recent coronary artery bypass graft, daytime sleepiness, snoring, and observed sleep apnea. The top window is 30 seconds; the bottom, 20 minutes. Examination of the thoracic and abdominal respiratory effort channels revealed that several of the more than 20 apnea episodes shown here had evidence of a central component (absent or decreased effort) followed by efforts. These are episodes of mixed apnea. Figure 18-41 shows the response to treatment.

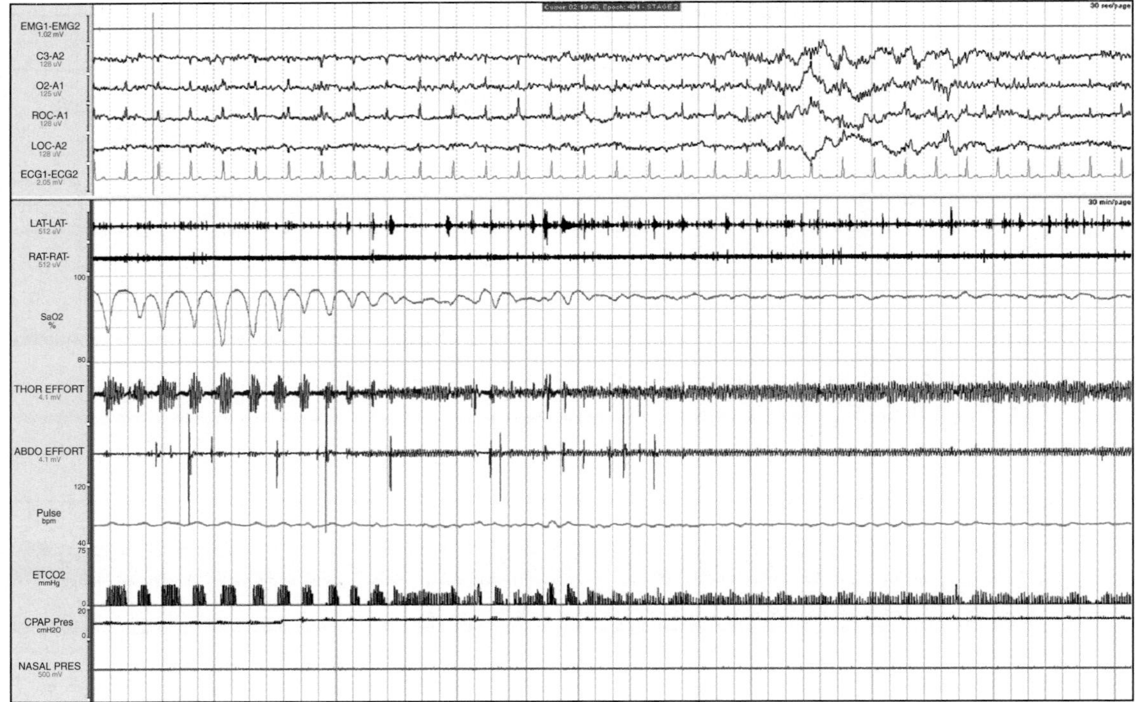

Figure 18-41.
Mixed apnea becoming complex sleep apnea. Same patient as in Figure 18-40. The first treatment that was tried was continuous positive airway pressure (CPAP), which caused the mixed apneas to become central apneas. The patient even had episodes of central apnea while he was awake. At about the vertical orange line in the bottom window, oxygen was added to the CPAP system and the episodes of central apnea resolved entirely.

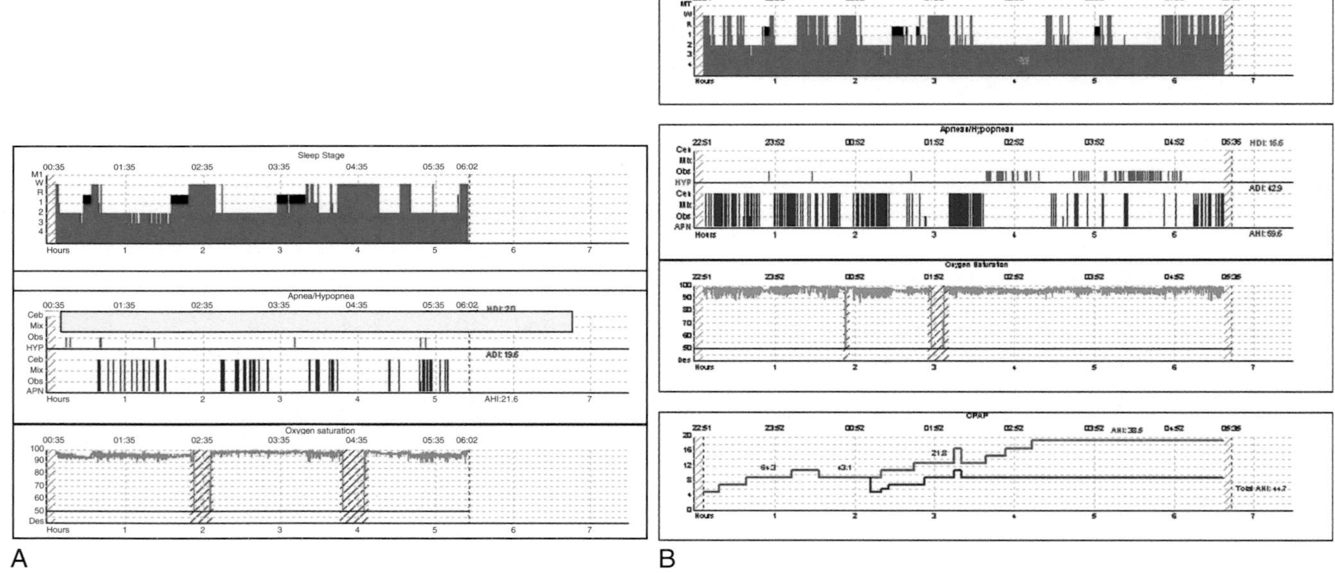

Figure 18-42.
Sleep apnea worsening with treatment. This is another variant of complex apnea. A is a hypnogram of a patient being treated with opiates for pain. He had central sleep apnea with an apnea index of 19. B is a hypnogram of the patient while he was being titrated, first on continuous positive airway pressure, then on bilevel, ending with bilevel and a backup rate. The treatments worsened his sleep breathing findings and sleep structure. There is a tendency for some technicians to "chase their tails," increasing ventilatory support, which only worsens the problem.

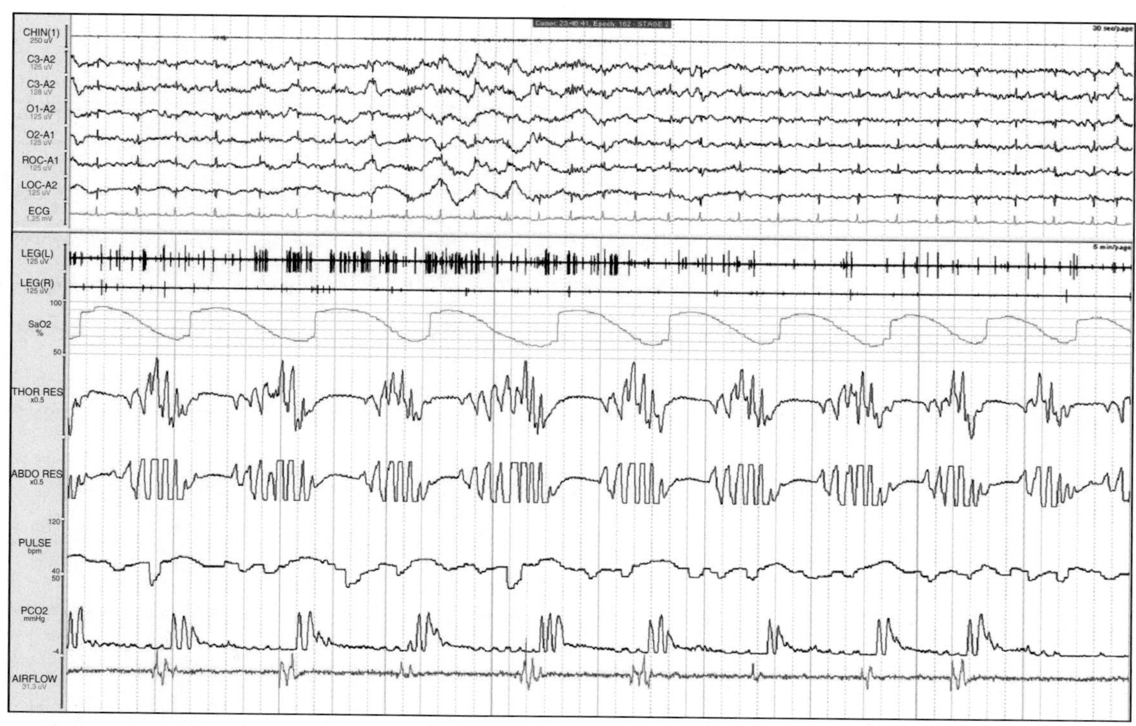

Figure 18-43.
Mixed apnea in a patient with idiopathic pulmonary fibrosis. This patient had very rapid and severe oxygen desaturations likely related to low lung volumes.

Heart Failure

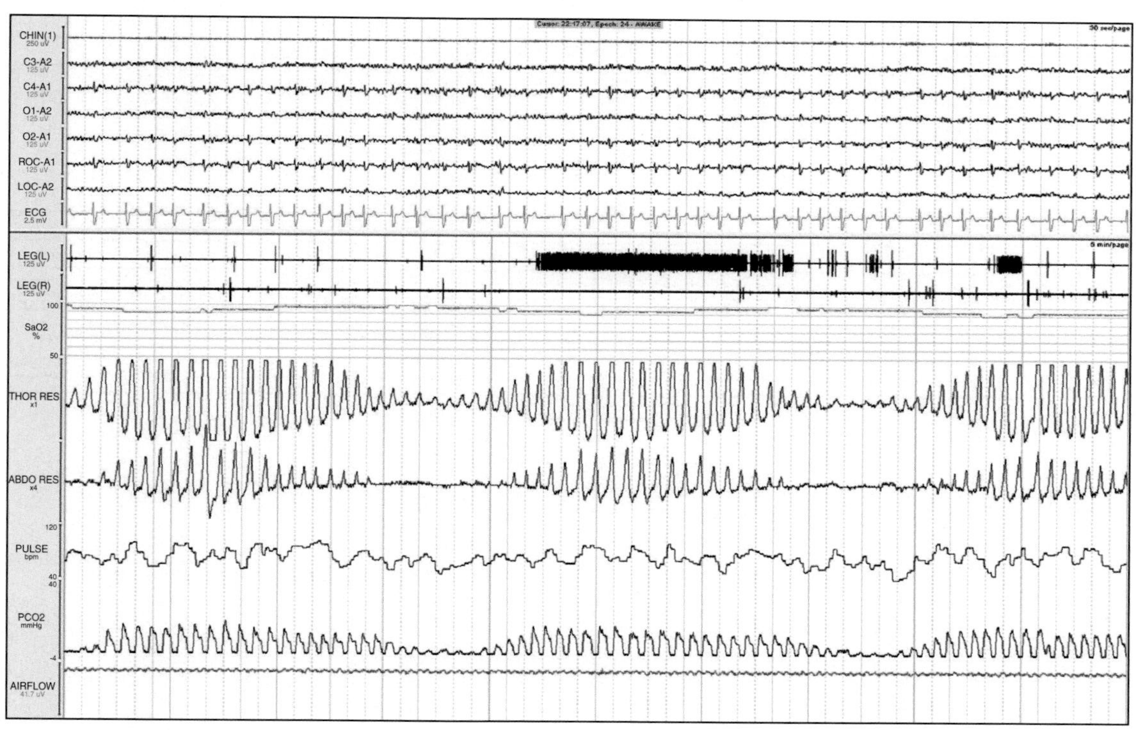

Figure 18-44.
Congestive heart failure (CHF) with awake Cheyne Stokes breathing. Sleep-onset insomnia and paroxysmal nocturnal dyspnea are common in CHF and were present in this patient. The epoch in the upper window is 30 seconds; in the bottom window, 5 minutes. The patient was wide awake. Notice the classic periodic breathing (Cheyne Stokes) with a waxing and waning of ventilation with a large number of breaths in each cycle. In other forms of Cheyne Stokes breathing (e.g., those of high altitude), the number of breaths in each periodic breathing cycle is much smaller. As the patient begins to doze off, the episodes of apnea or hypopnea may lead to an arousal, which may prevent the patient from achieving sleep. Notice the lack of deflections in the nasal pressure trace. The patient was short of breath, hyperventilating (the end-tidal pCO_2 was low; oronasal CO_2 was being monitored), and breathing via his mouth.

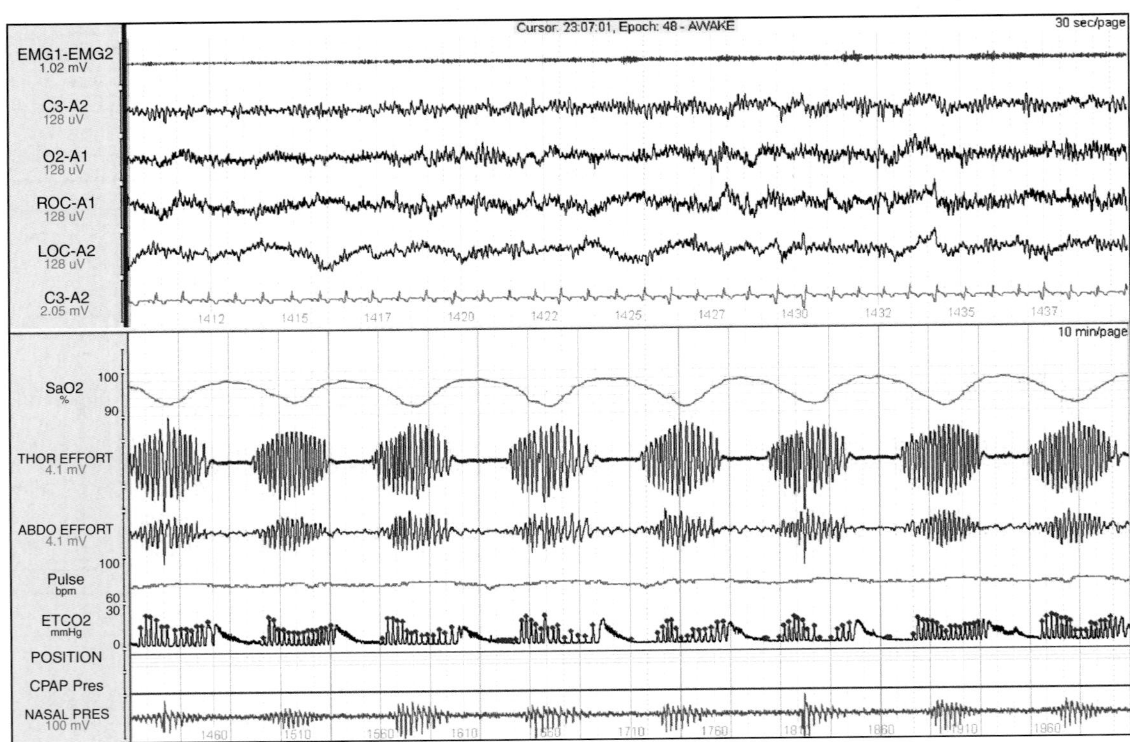

Figure 18-45.
CHF with awake Cheyne Stokes breathing. The top window is 30 seconds and the bottom window is 10 minutes. Notice the almost monotonous regularity of the periodic breathing pattern. Three or more cycles of periodic breathing are scored as Cheyne Stokes breathing. Here, the patient was wide awake and had significant episodes of hypoxemia. Hypocapnia was present. Careful examination of the end-tidal pCO_2 trace during apnea indicated that it was thicker than normal. This was because there were oscillations in the trace. The cause of such oscillations is shown in the next figure (Fig. 18-46).

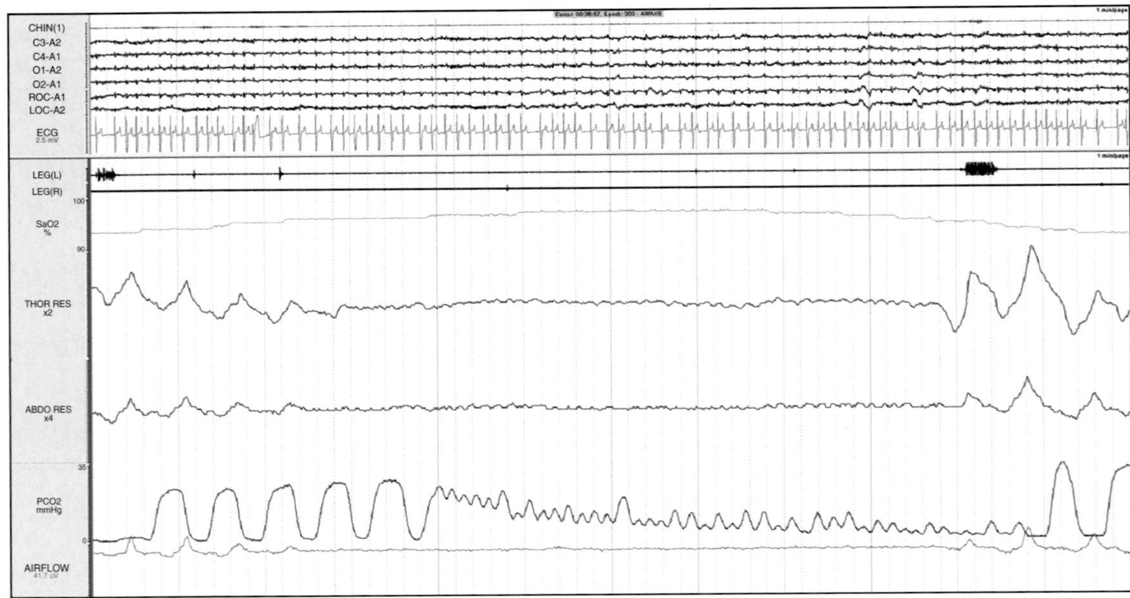

Figure 18-46.
CHF with awake Cheyne Stokes breathing with cardiogenic oscillations. Same patient as in Figure 18-45. Both top and bottom windows are 1-minute epochs. Examination of the pCO_2 trace shows that when the patient is apneic, there are high-frequency oscillations in CO_2 that correspond to the heartbeat. These oscillations occur because the beating heart results in tiny puffs of airflow with CO_2, which are detected by the CO_2 analyzer. This proves that the upper airways are patent.

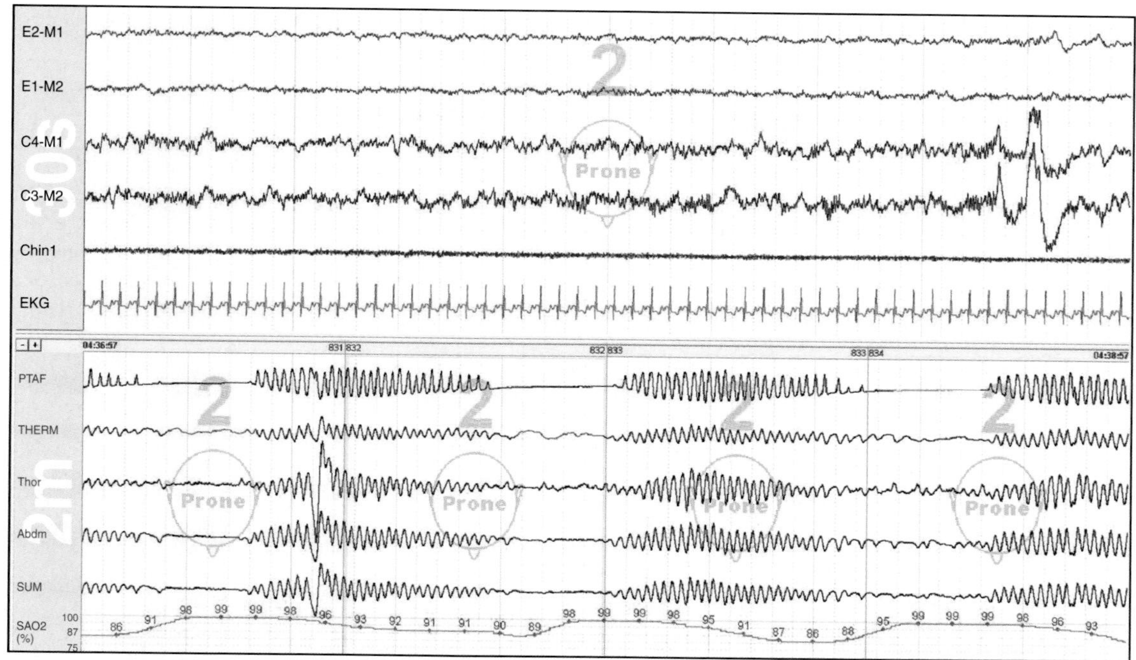

Figure 18-47.
CHF in a 9-year-old child. This patient had a history of rheumatic fever, Sydenham chorea, mitral regurgitation, pulmonary hypertension, and CHF. The sleep study was done prior to her having mitral valve replacement. The patient is in stage N2 sleep. She has Cheyne Stokes breathing with a large number of breaths per cycle, which is typical in CHF. There was evidence of crescendo increase in depth of breathing, followed by a decrease. Notice the significant oscillations in oxygen saturation. Her apnea-hypopnea index was 66.

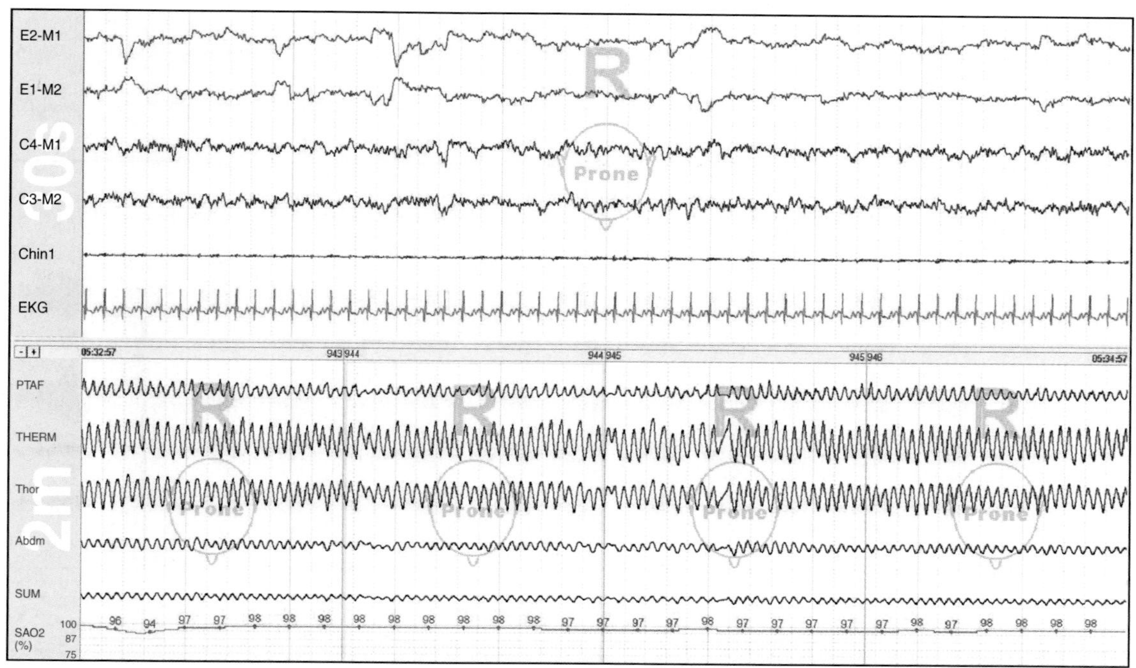

Figure 18-48.
CHF in a 9-year-old child. Same patient as in Figure 18-47. Here, the patient is in REM sleep, and the Cheyne Stokes breathing pattern has normalized. This finding, in which breathing pattern improves in REM sleep, is common in patients with CHF, and has also been described in the Cheyne Stokes breathing of high altitude.

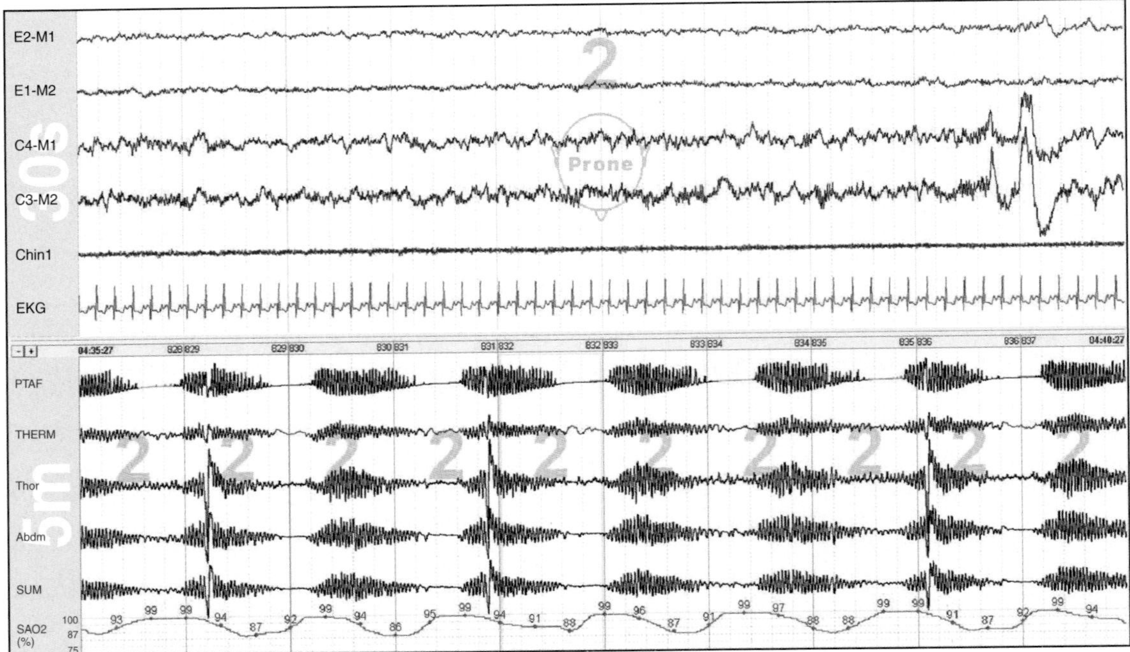

Figure 18-49.
CHF in a 9-year-old child. Same patient as in Figure 18-47. Although Cheyne Stokes respiration is sometimes described as a breathing instability, in fact, the pattern can be extremely stable for very long periods of time. Notice the almost monotonous regularity of the breathing pattern and oscillations in oxygen saturation over 5 minutes.

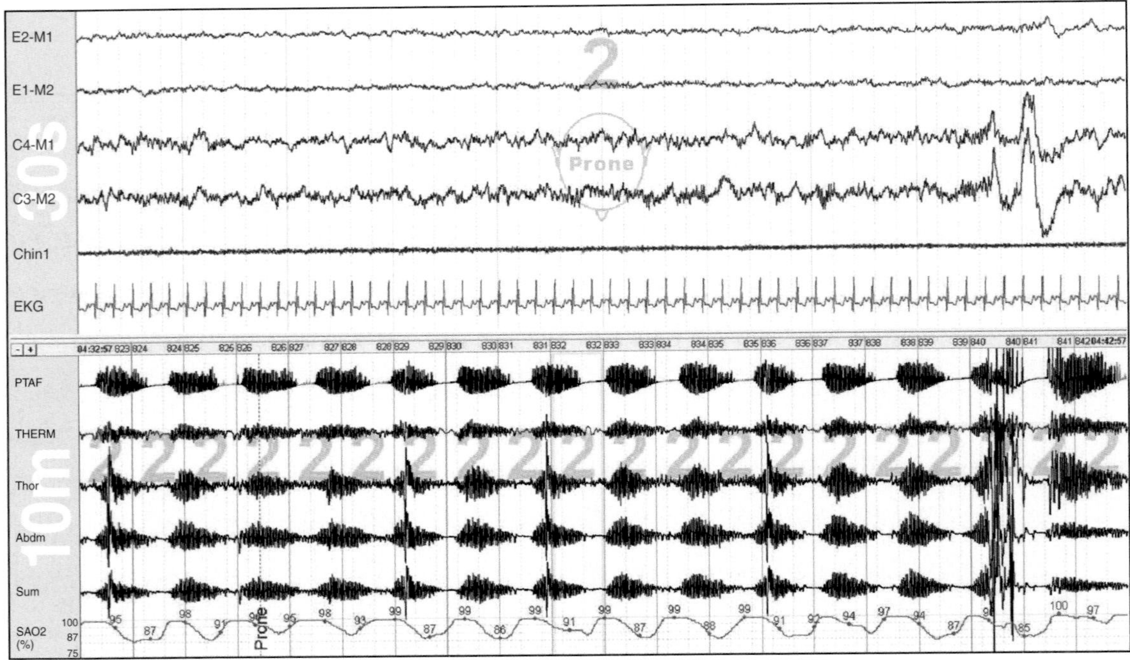

Figure 18-50.
CHF in a 9-year-old child. Same patient as in Figure 18-47. The breathing pattern persists during this entire 10-minute epoch. There were 13 central apnea episodes over the 10 minutes. Her NREM apnea index was about 100. The patient was subsequently assessed on CPAP in preparation for her cardiac surgery. Her apnea-hypopnea index on a pressure of 6 cm H_2O was 5. The patient used CPAP at home in preparation for surgery and perioperatively. After mitral valve replacement the patient's breathing pattern normalized and she was asymptomatic with respect to sleep.

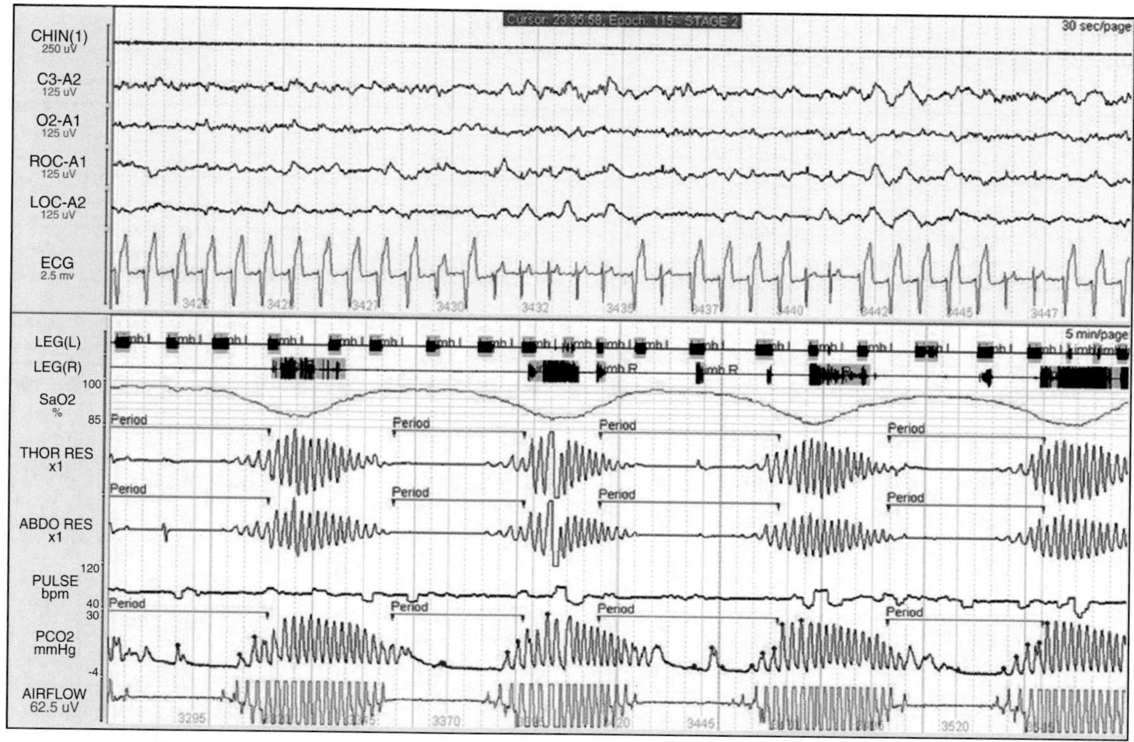

Figure 18-51.

CHF. This patient has well-developed Cheyne Stokes breathing with periodic crescendo increases in efforts to breathe, followed by decrescendo reductions in effort, resulting in the typical diamond-shaped pattern seen in the bottom 5-min window. The nadir SaO_2 occurs during the peak of hyperpnea. A rapidly responding ear oximeter is being used. This type of breathing pattern may resolve while the patient is in REM sleep. The periodic breathing cycles may occur in the absence of arousals, suggesting that they are maintained by chemical control of breathing, which is blunted in REM sleep. This is one of the few conditions in which abnormal breathing patterns may improve in REM sleep. The EKG shows two types of beats: narrow complex ventricular beats, which reflect the patient's underlying atrial fibrillation, and wide complex beats initiated by a cardiac pacemaker. The pacing pulses that are extremely short are missed entirely by the data acquisition system. The patient also had significant periodic limb movements, a common finding in heart failure.

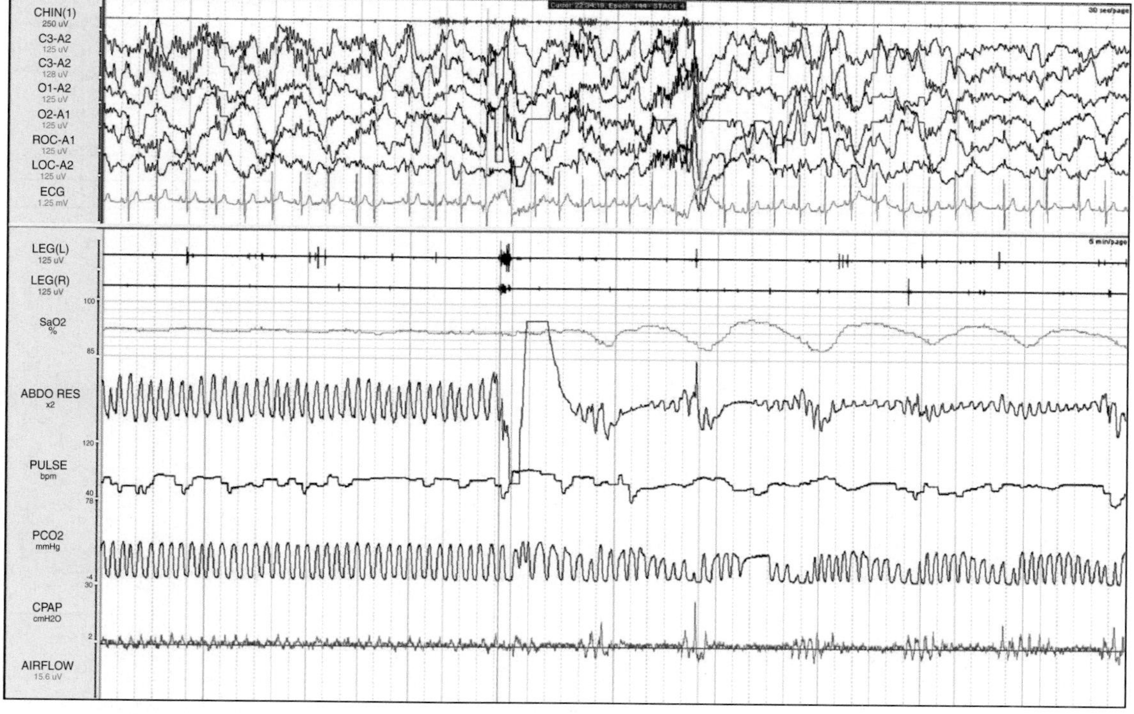

Figure 18-52.

Periodic breathing in CHF being initiated by a big breath. Patients with CHF do not have periodic breathing the entire night. It was shown many years ago that breathing in such patients could be stable, and then an event such as a loud noise could result in temporary hyperventilation, in turn causing the instability leading to Cheyne Stokes breathing as shown here. At the orange vertical line, the patient takes a very big breath, which is soon followed by oscillations in his SaO_2.

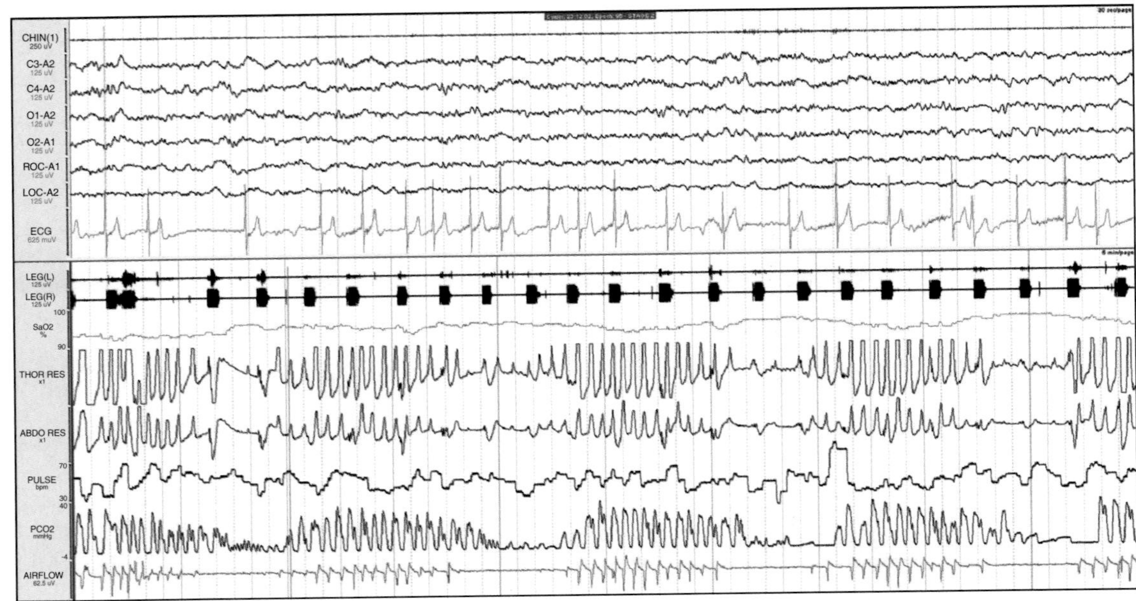

Figure 18-53.
CHF with multiple abnormalities. This 75-year-old patient had myocardial infarction and mitral valve replacement. The eye is first drawn to the periodic leg movements. Other abnormalities include an underlying periodicity in the breathing pattern, the heart rate is grossly irregular, and the ear oximeter SaO_2 trace is ragged. The latter is likely related to the poor perfusion through his ear caused by low cardiac output. Perhaps the last thing that is noticed is the most important: the patient had about 3 seconds between RR intervals between the second and third heartbeat of this epoch. The top window is 30 sec; the bottom window, 5 min. Figure 18-54 shows the effect of treatment.

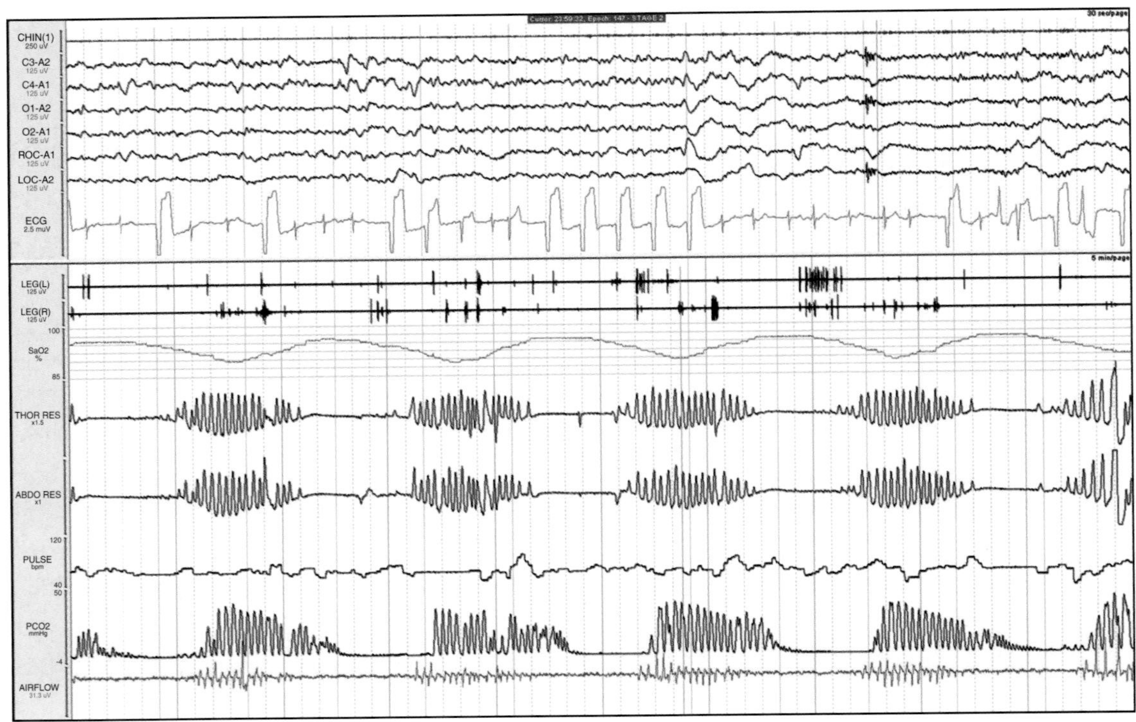

Figure 18-54.
CHF with multiple abnormalities. Same patient as in Figure 18-53, 13 days later. The heart rate is not as variable, the Cheyne Stokes breathing pattern is more developed, and the SaO_2 shows a clean oscillating signal with the nadir SaO_2 occurring during the peak of hyperpnea. This is from a fast-responding ear oximeter. However, the EKG looks worse. The top window is 30 sec; the bottom window, 5 min. Figure 18-55 drills down on the bottom window.

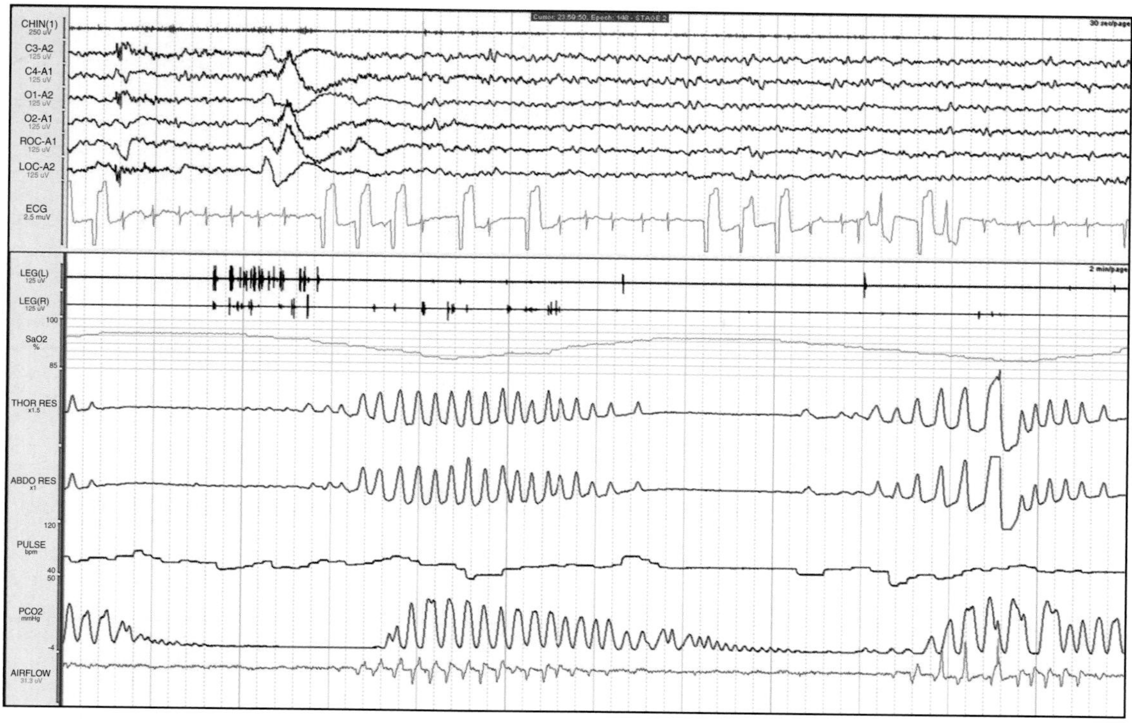

Figure 18-55.
CHF with multiple abnormalities. Same patient as in Figure 18-53. Another fragment from the same night. The bottom window is now 2 minutes. Cardiogenic oscillations are now clearly visible in the CO_2 channel following the hyperpneic breaths in the middle of the epoch. The abnormal cardiac beats were initially scored as ventricular tachycardia. Indeed, the abnormal heartbeats are wide complex, and could be ventricular tachycardia or a low junctional rhythm (see Figs. 18-75 and 18-79). However, the pulse channel shows after the middle of the epoch an absolutely rock-steady pulse rate. The abnormal beats, on careful inspection, occur initially after a slightly increased time between beats. In fact, a cardiac pacemaker had been placed in the patient, and the pacing pulses were missed entirely because of the sampling rate of the EKG. The abnormal beats are paced beats.

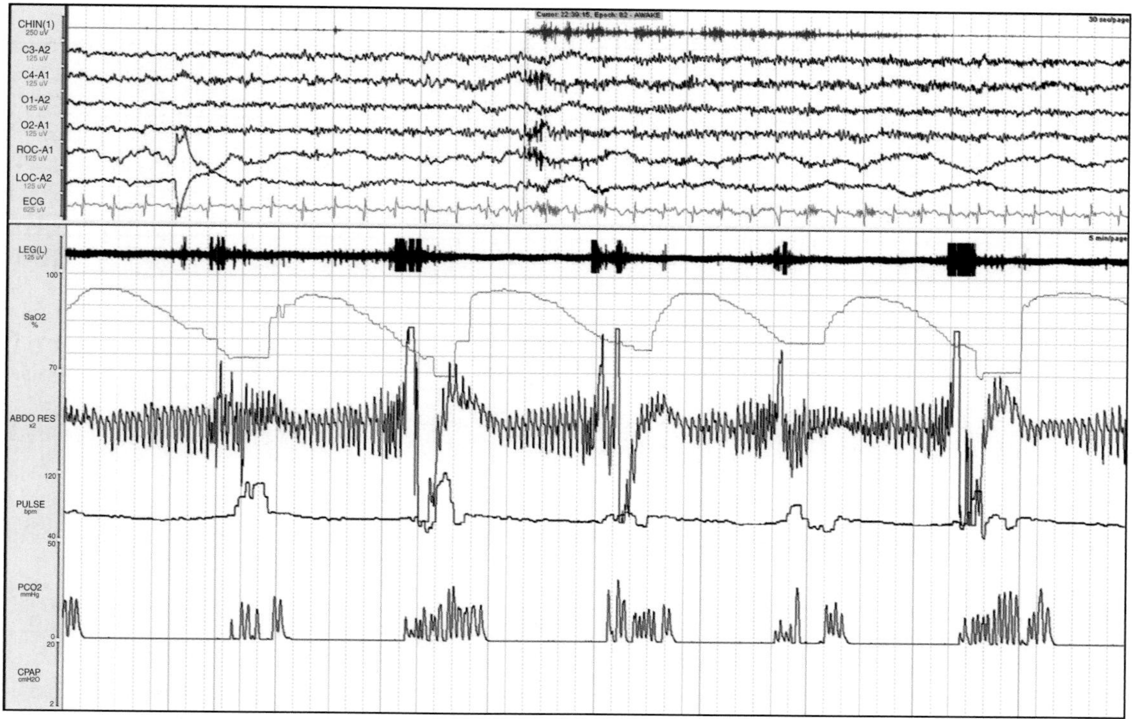

Figure 18-56.
Acute heart failure and OSA. The top window is 30 seconds; the bottom window is 5 minutes. At the time of this PSG, the patient was awake, had severe oxygen desaturations, and was in florid pulmonary edema caused by acute left ventricular failure (see Video 46, chapter 20). The patient had a few unobstructed breaths, followed by shallow breaths, and then had evidence of obstructive apnea with large efforts but no airflow. Nadir SaO_2 was long after breathing resumed. A fast-response ear oximeter was used. Because of heart failure, there was a long heart-to-ear circulation time. He was unable to achieve persistent sleep without ventilatory support (see Fig. 18-57).

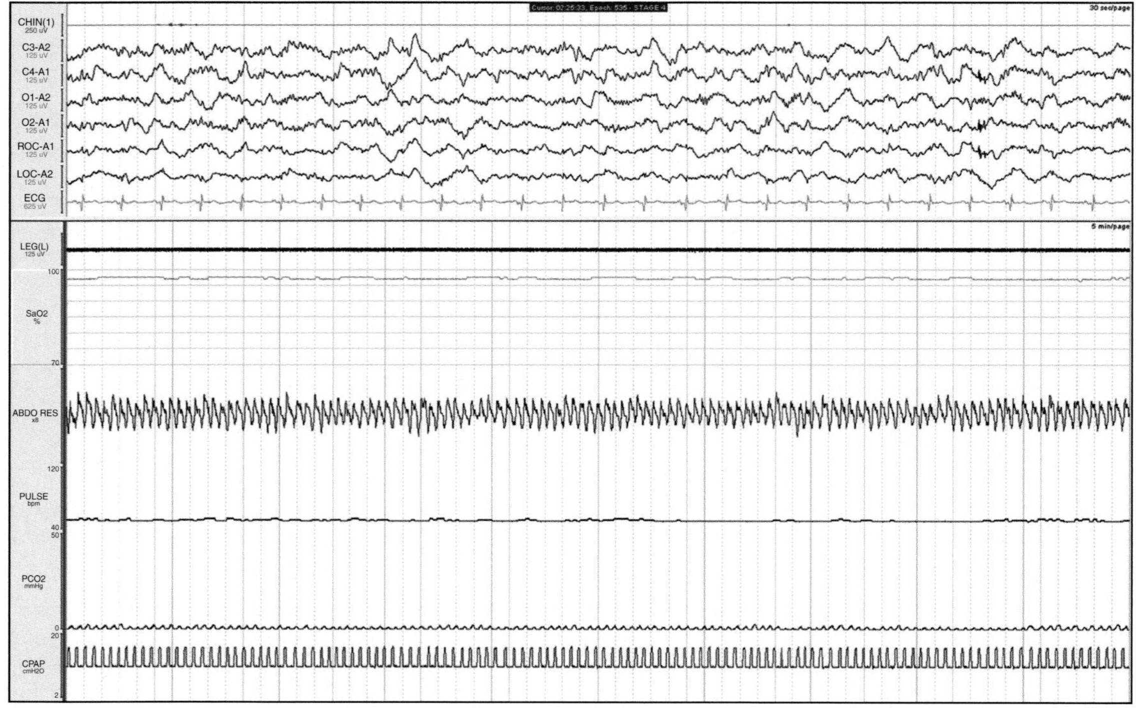

Figure 18-57.
Acute heart failure and OSA on ventilatory support. Same patient as in Figure 18-56. Notice the regular deflections in the bilevel pressure CPAP channel. Both a high inspiratory pressure and a high expiratory pressure were used. That the pressure waves generated by the bilevel machine show clocklike regularity indicates that a timed backup rate was used. The apnea is completely resolved, hypoxemia is no longer present, and the patient is in slow-wave sleep.

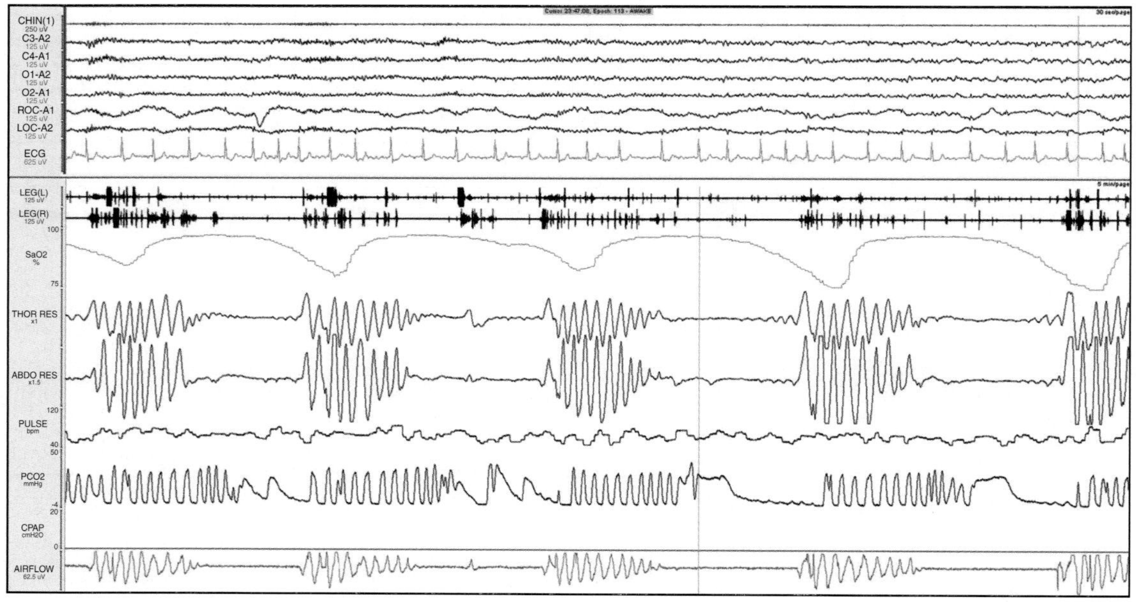

Figure 18-58.
CHF and apnea during wakefulness. This figure and Figures 18-59 through 18-61 are from a 61-year-old male with a 30-year snoring history, 5 years of apnea observed by his wife, and, at the time of this PSG, nightly paroxysmal nocturnal dyspnea, documented atrial fibrillation, and mild CHF. The top 30-second window shows that the patient was awake. The bottom 5-minute window shows that the patient had Cheyne Stokes breathing. The patient also had atrial fibrillation; notice the regularly irregular variation in the heart rate in the pulse channel and the lack of developed P waves in the EKG. Awake Cheyne Stokes breathing is common in heart failure.

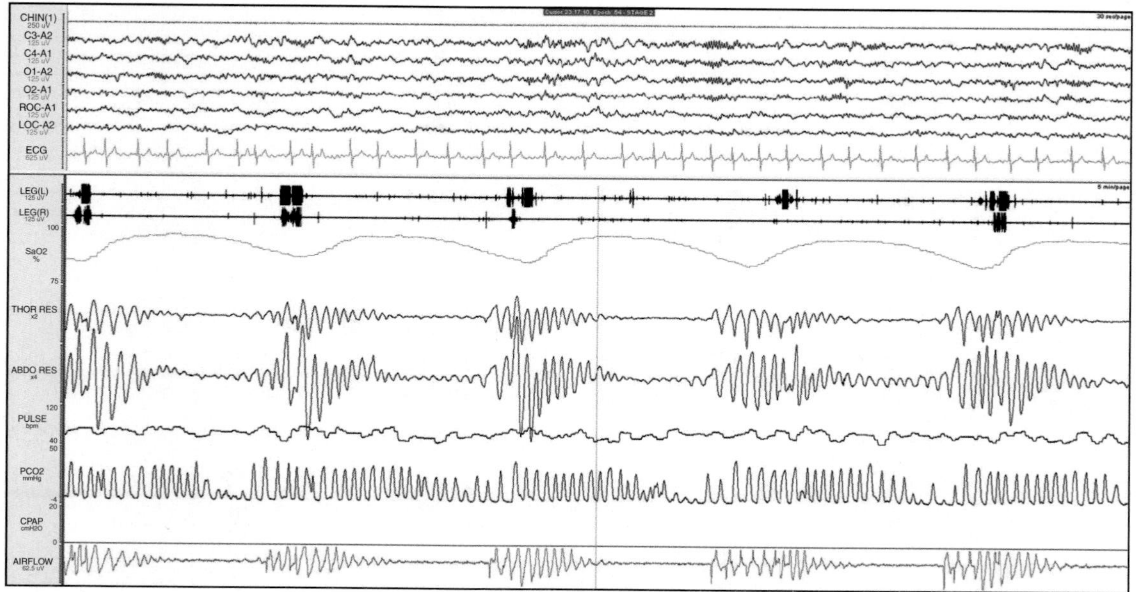

Figure 18-59.
Heart failure and apnea during sleep. Same patient as in Figure 18-58. The patient now has features of both Cheyne Stokes respiration and obstructive apnea. Note that in the abdominal effort channel there are at times efforts to breathe that are not accompanied by airflow, as noted in the bottom channel. During these times the CO_2 channel shows some expiratory airflow. The CO_2 channel detects expiratory air that is rich in CO_2.

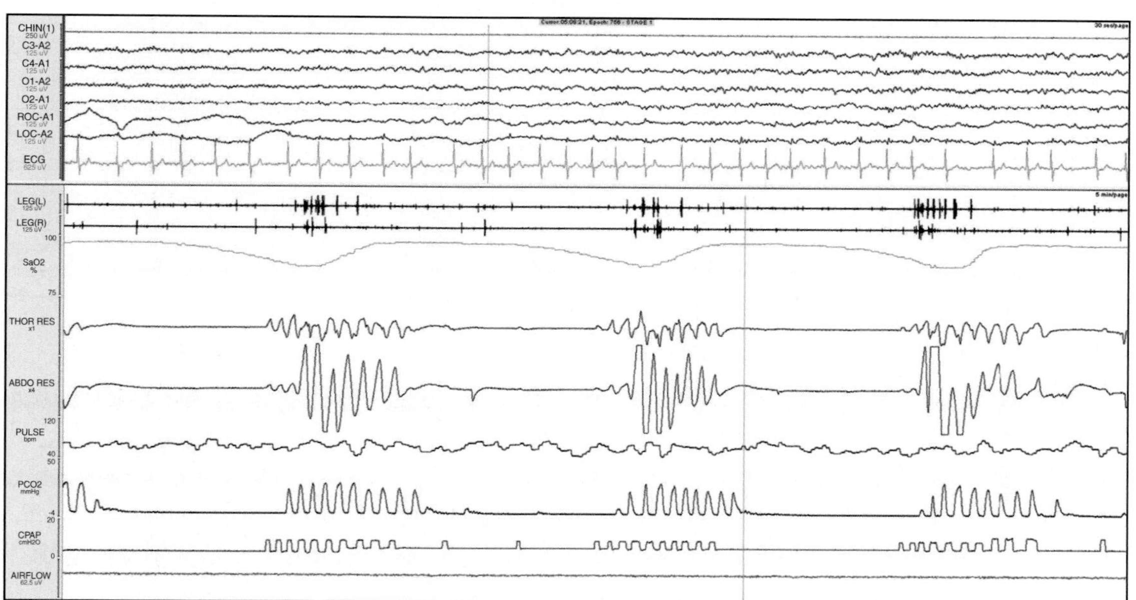

Figure 18-60.
Heart failure and obstructive apnea on bilevel pressure. Notice in the CPAP channel that there are deflections with flattened peaks. The patient is on a bilevel machine in spontaneous mode. This has no effect on his breathing pattern. The patient is awake and was unable to achieve persistent sleep. Figure 18-61 shows the effect of raising pressures and changing the patient to fixed-pressure CPAP.

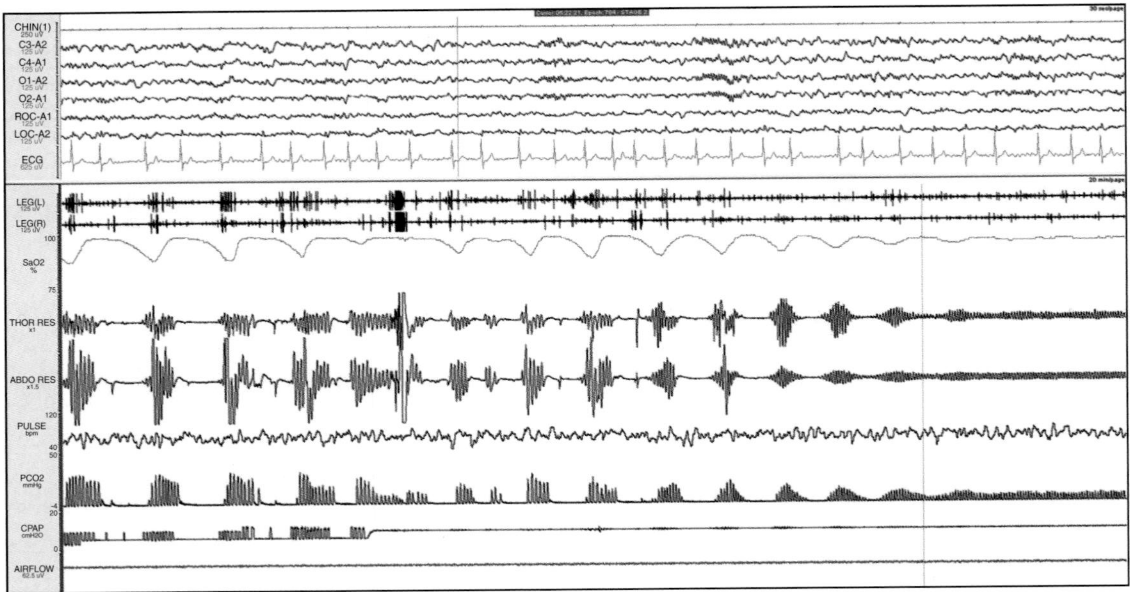

Figure 18-61.
CHF and OSA on CPAP. Same patient as in Figure 18-60. The bottom window now shows 20 minutes of data, during which time attempts were made to titrate the patient on bilevel pressure. Then, about a third of the way into the 20-minute epoch, the patient was switched to fixed pressure. Within about 10 minutes the patient achieved sleep and shortly thereafter his breathing pattern and oxygenation normalized. By the end of this epoch he was in stage N2. Most of the time titrations in patients with CHF and OSA are complicated and involve trial and error since it is difficult to predict how a patient will respond to a specific treatment. Because of this it is inappropriate to ever attempt unattended home titration in a patient with heart failure.

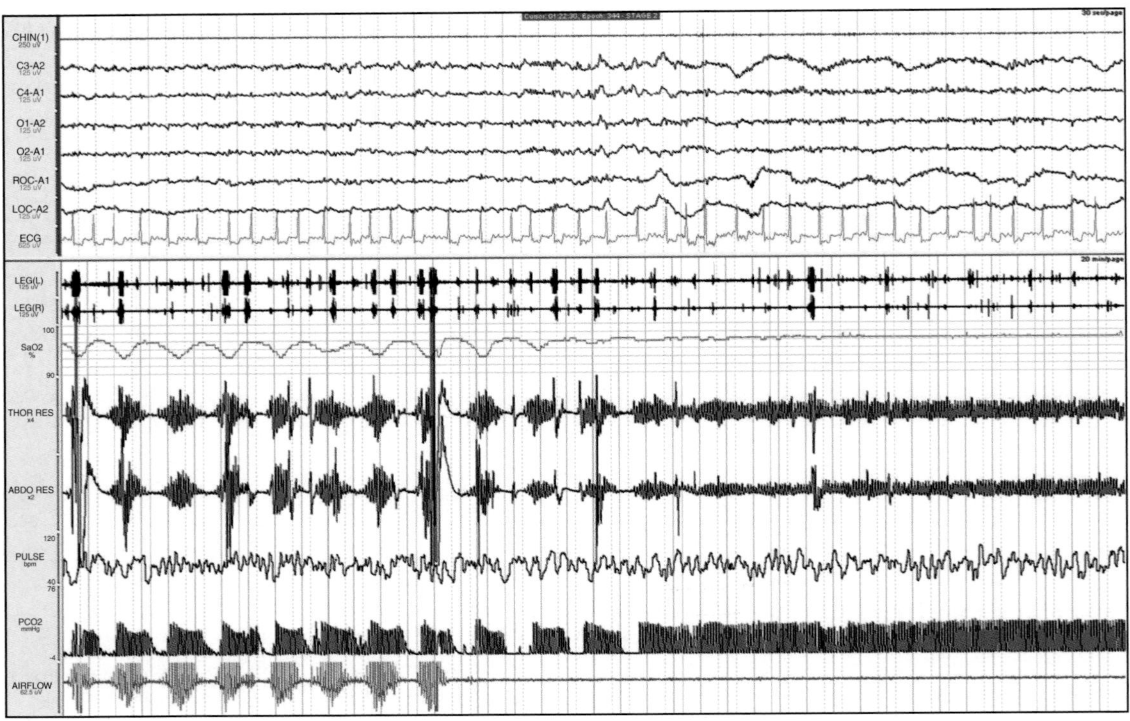

Figure 18-62.
CHF, periodic breathing, and the effect of oxygen. The top window is 30 seconds; the bottom window is 20 minutes. At the beginning of the 20-minute epoch, it is apparent that the patient has a Cheyne Stokes breathing pattern, a chaotic heart rate consistent with atrial fibrillation, and 2% to 4% oscillations in SaO_2. The SaO_2 does not go below 90%. The patient was started on oxygen (airflow deflections in the bottom channel ceased). Within 4 to 5 minutes the breathing pattern becomes regular and the SaO_2 is rock steady. For reasons not entirely clear, even though significant hypoxemia was not detected, the patient responded to O_2 administration.

Cardiac Rhythm Abnormalities

In sleep laboratories one often sees cardiac arrhythmias related to the blood gas and autonomic nervous system changes that are seen in sleep pathology, such as sleep apnea, arrhythmias related to primary heart disease, or a combination of both. Understanding the genesis of arrhythmias will facilitate interpretation of the abnormal rhythm.

Because maintaining a heartbeat is so critical, if one pacemaker fails others take over, but at a lower intrinsic rate. The main pacemaker is the sinoatrial node that normally drives a heart at rates that vary between 60 and 100 beats per minute. If the node fails, other atrial foci take over the pacemaker function and drive the heart at rates between 60 and 80 beats per minute. If atrial foci fail, then tissues at the atrioventricular junction take over and drive the heart at rates that vary between 40 and 60 beats per minute. If the junctional pacemakers fail, then tissue in the ventricles with pacemaking properties will fire, driving the heart at a rate between 20 and 40 beats per minute. The function and rate of these pacemakers can be affected by changes in the autonomic nervous system, the levels of catecholamines, blood gases, and myocardial pathology.

Most arrhythmias seen in the sleep disorders center fall under one of four general categories: irregular rhythms, escape rhythms, premature beats, and tachyarrhythmias. Most commonly seen are atrial fibrillation (AF) and premature ventricular contractions (PVCs).

The optimal epoch length for evaluating cardiac rhythm abnormalities varies according to the type of abnormality and the abnormality's relation to other sleep findings. Frequently the rhythm is best evaluated when different epoch lengths for the EKG and the sleep breathing data are used.

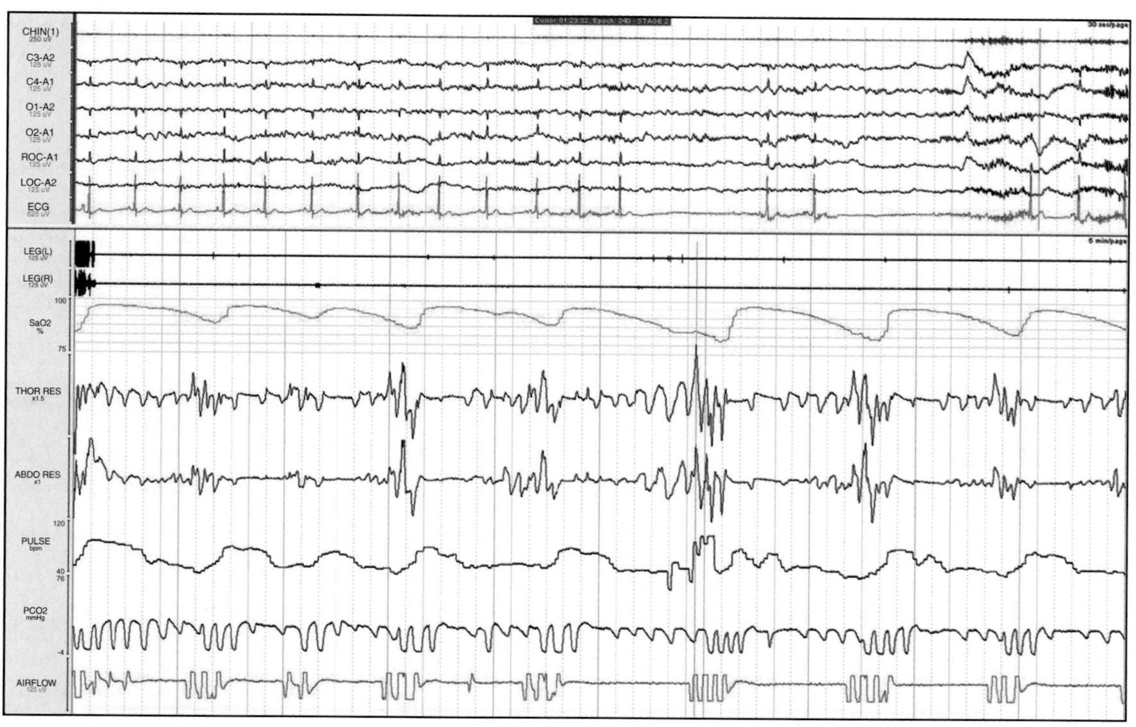

Figure 18-63.
Sinus arrest and junctional escape rhythm in sleep apnea. A bradycardia/tachycardia pattern has long been recognized in patients with sleep apnea. This pattern is easily appreciated when the heart rate is examined, as in the pulse channel shown here. Such a pattern is usually present when the patient has an underlying sinus rhythm that responds to the autonomic nervous system changes associated with the apneic episodes. In this example, the patient developed sinus arrest toward the end of an apneic episode. The configuration of the P waves has changed in the preceding heartbeats. Note that there is an EKG artifact in the EEG that accurately reflects QRS complexes. This is a junctional rhythm because the QRS complex is narrow and similar to the QRS complexes before the sinus arrest. The top window is 30 sec; the bottom, 5 min.

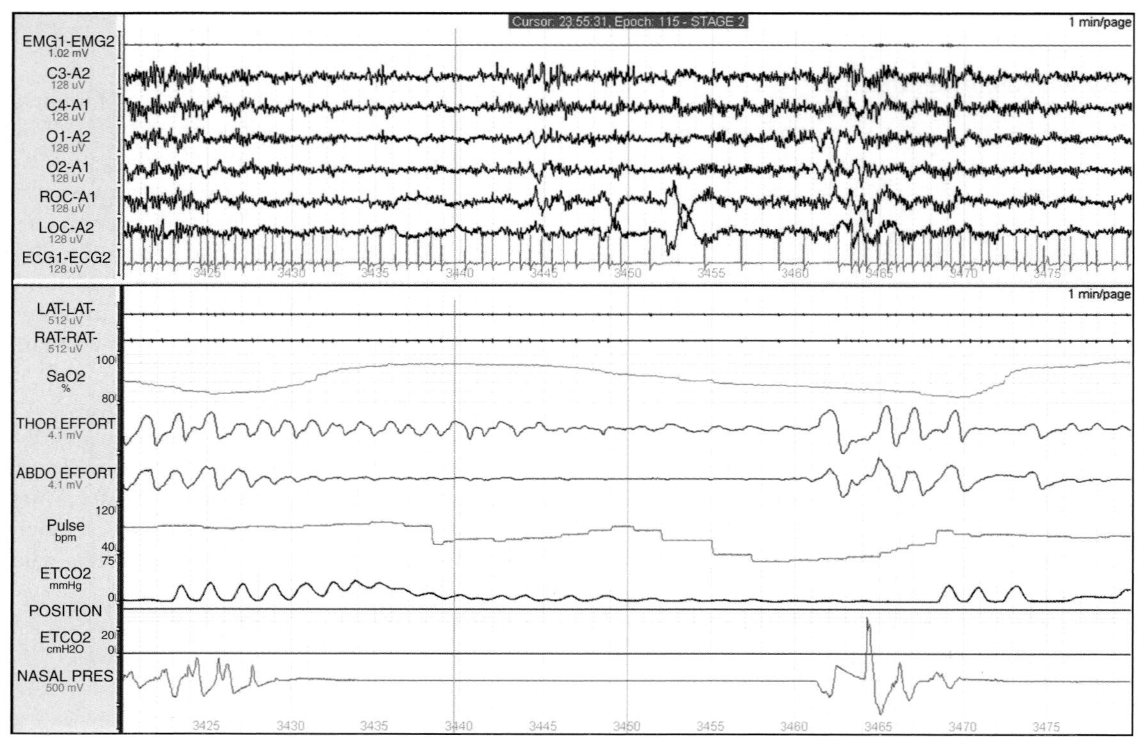

Figure 18-64.
Atrial fibrillation in OSA. AF is a common finding in sleep apnea patients. In some cases, in a sleep apnea patient who normally has a sinus rhythm, it begins during sleep. Here, one sees the classic findings of absent P waves and disorganized electrical activity preceding the QRS waves. There is extreme slowing of the cardiac rate, which occurs toward the end of an apneic episode. The slowing is due to increased parasympathetic activity. The top and bottom windows are each 1 min.

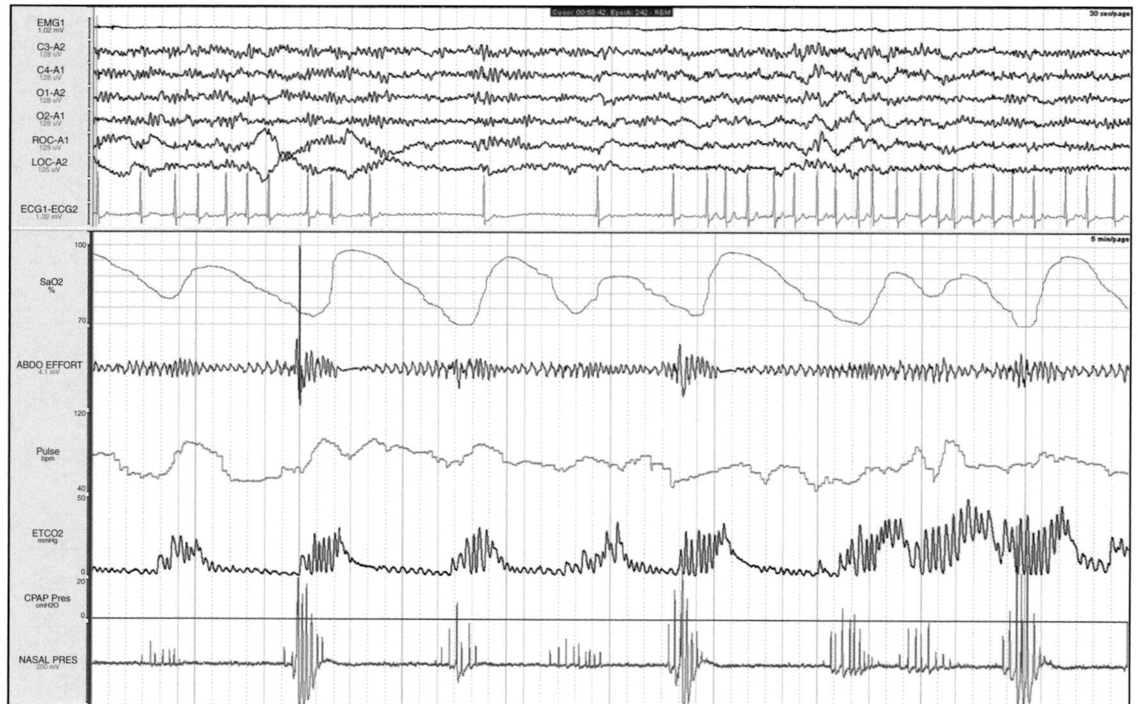

Figure 18-65.
AF in OSA. Here, there is AF and failure of the atrial foci to generate a heartbeat, resulting in junctional escape as evidenced by a narrow QRS. The longest R-R interval here is more than 3 seconds, or a rate of 20 beats per minute. This suggests either disease or suppression of the junction, as the intrinsic rate is generally between 40 and 60 beats per minute. Parasympathetic activity related to the effort to breathe has suppressed atrial and junctional pacemaking tissues. This patient had OSA and coronary artery disease. The top window is 30 sec; the bottom is 5 min.

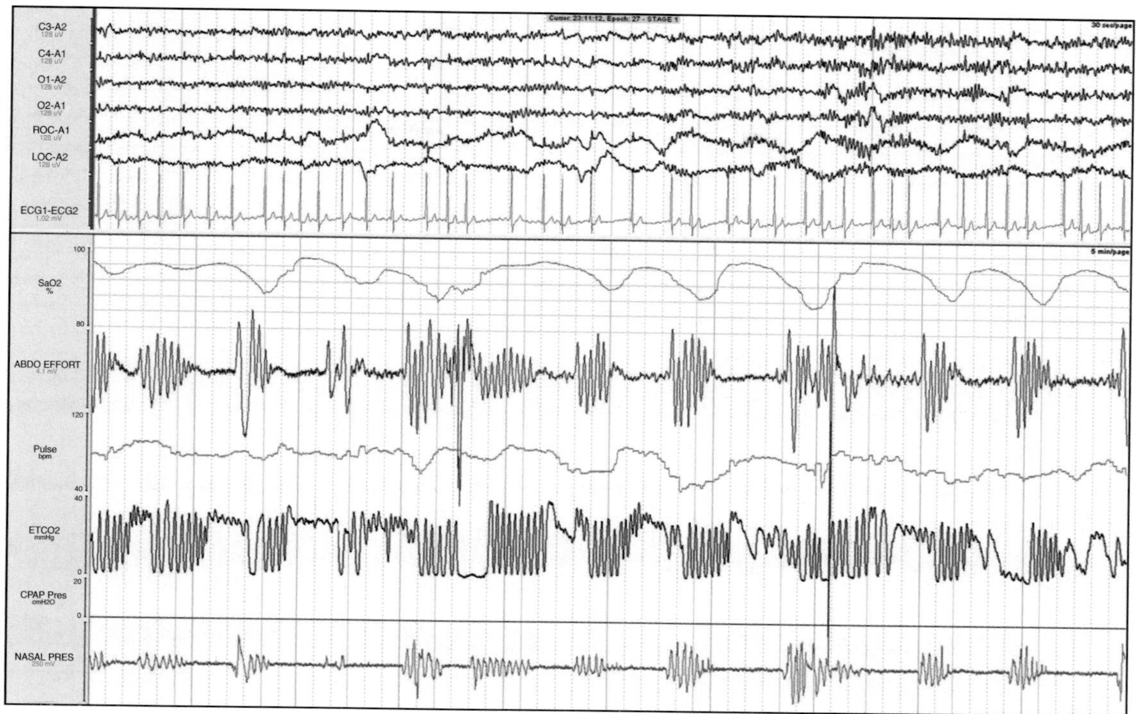

Figure 18-66.
AF in an awake patient with Cheyne Stokes breathing due to heart failure. There are no well-developed P waves, and the ventricular rate is irregular. Such patients may have severe sleep-onset insomnia. The top window is 1 min; the bottom is 5 min.

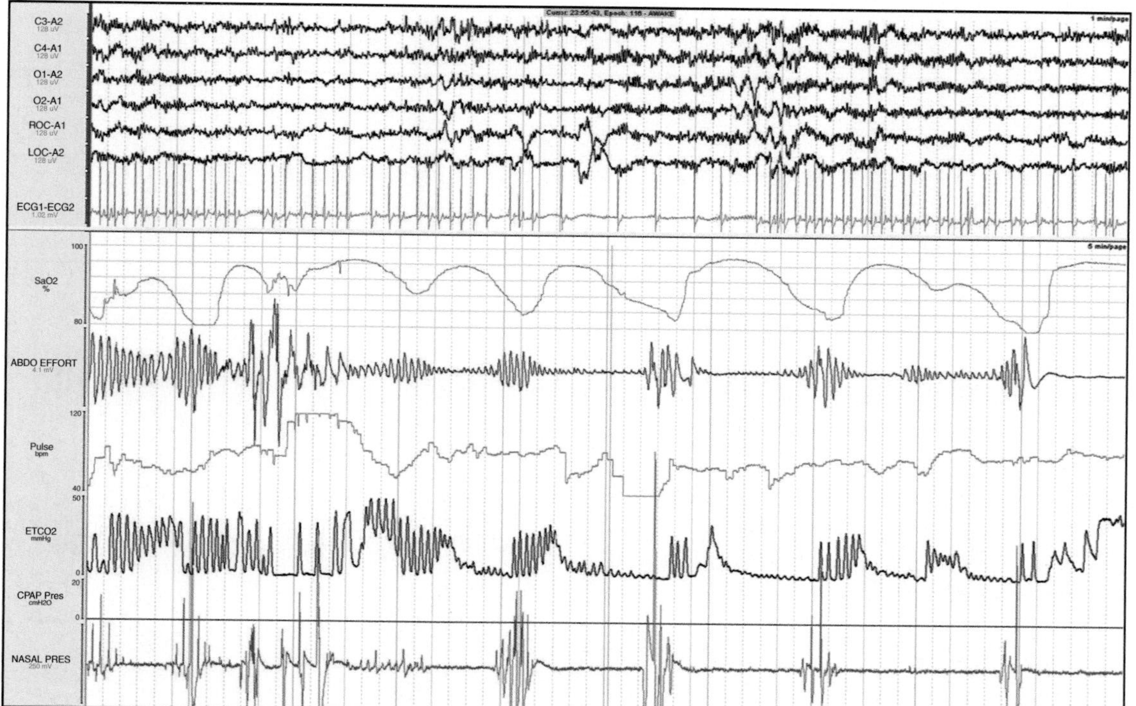

Figure 18-67.
AF in an awake patient with Cheyne Stokes breathing due to CHF. Same patient as in Figure 18-66, but later during the night. There are no well-developed P waves, and the ventricular rate is irregular. There is a sudden slowing of the heart rate to less than 40 beats per minute (notice the flat line at 40 beats on the pulse trace), occuring during a central apneic episode with significant hypoxemia. This is followed by a tachycardia during which the heart rate is about 100 beats per minute but still irregular. The top window is 1 min; and the bottom window is 5 min.

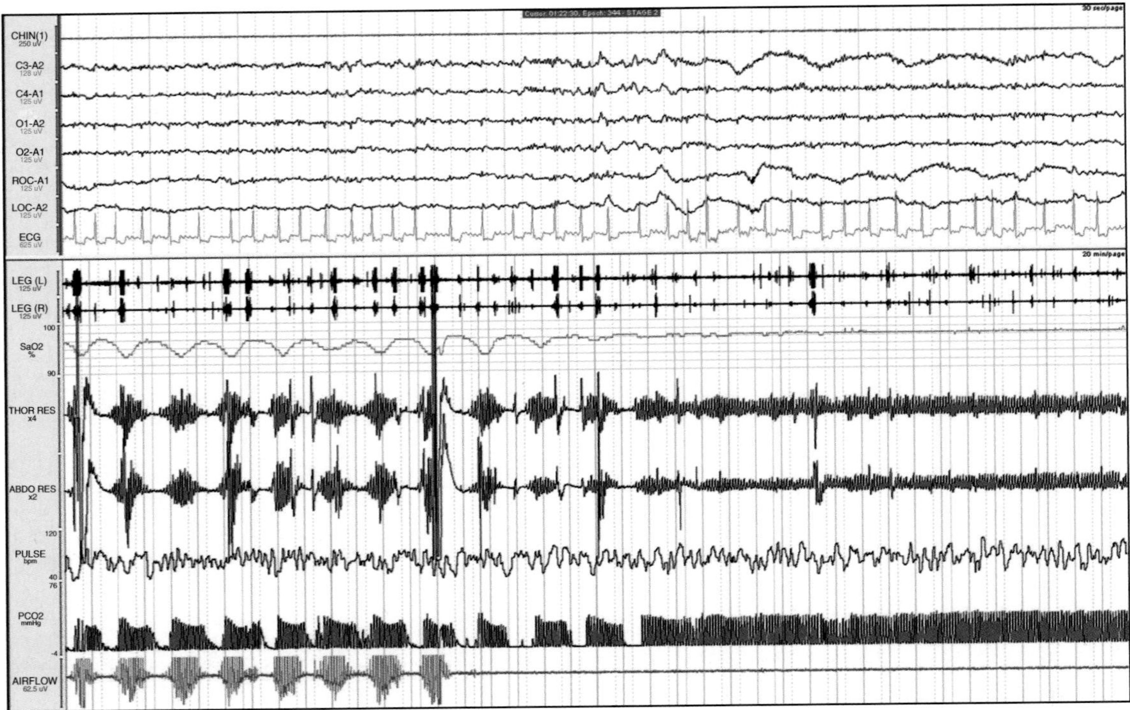

Figure 18-68.
Irregular rhythm: AF in a patient with CHF and Cheyne Stokes breathing. This figure is identical to 18-12. The pulse is the first clue that atrial fibrillation is present. The pulse rate is regularly irregular (actually it is random), and the patient appears to have a movement disorder. Most of the brisker movements occur during a peak of hyperpnea. At the vertical orange line the patient is given oxygen. Within a minute the breathing becomes more regular, there is a reduction in the leg movements, and SaO_2 normalizes. There is no effect on the cardiac rhythm. The top window is 30 sec; the bottom is 20 min.

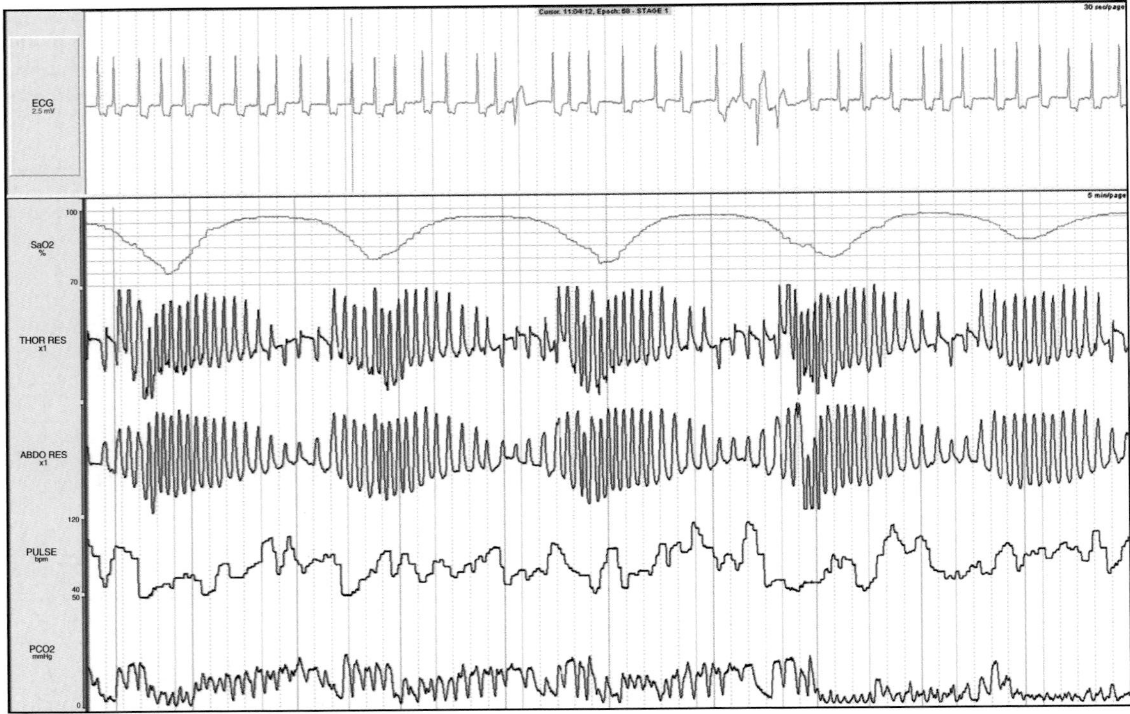

Figure 18-69.
Irregular rhythm and escape beats with severe heart failure. The pulse channel indicates a chaotic rhythm. Atrial fibrillation is present. Occasionally the patient has narrow, complex escape beats, most likely arising from the atrioventricular junction. Modern PSG systems have flexibility in what channels to examine, at different gains and differing epoch lengths. The top window is 30 sec; the bottom is 5 min.

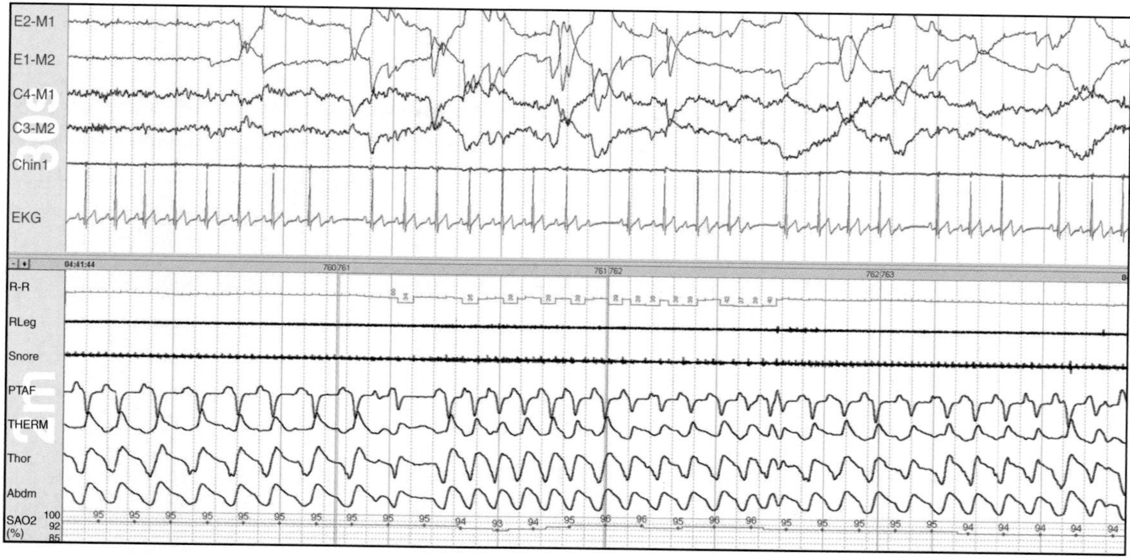

Figure 18-70.
Heart blocks. Heart blocks interfere with the conduction of depolarization waves, resulting in missed beats. This can occur at the sinoatrial (SA) node, at the atrioventricular (AV) node, or within the Purkinje fibers. SA blocks and AV blocks are frequently seen in sleep studies. Bundle branch blocks and hemiblocks, which occur below the AV junction, are less frequently seen. With sinus block, the SA node fails to depolarize, resulting in an absent P wave, leading to missed beats. There are three types of AV blocks called 1°, 2°, and 3° (first-degree, second-degree, and third-degree) blocks. A first-degree block is simply a prolongation of the PR interval to greater than 0.2 seconds. Here there are missed beats. To appreciate why the beats are missed it is necessary to "drill down." The top window is 30 sec.

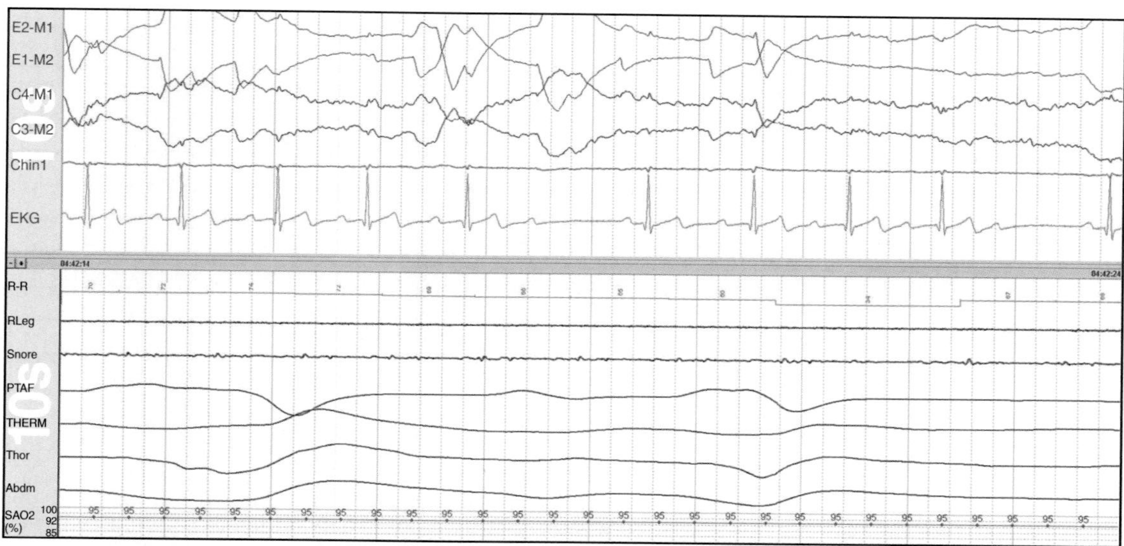

Figure 18-71.
Wenckebach 2° AV block. This is a 10-sec epoch of the PSG fragment in Figure 18-70. In this heart block, there is a gradual lengthening of the PR intervals. Compare the PR interval from the last conducted beat toward the middle of the epoch with the PR interval at the beginning of the epoch and you will note that it is much longer. It is believed that in this type of AV block, the nonconducted P wave is blocked entirely in the AV node, possibly as a result of increased parasympathetic activity. In this example, the patient is in REM sleep, and possibly there has been a surge of parasympathetic tone.

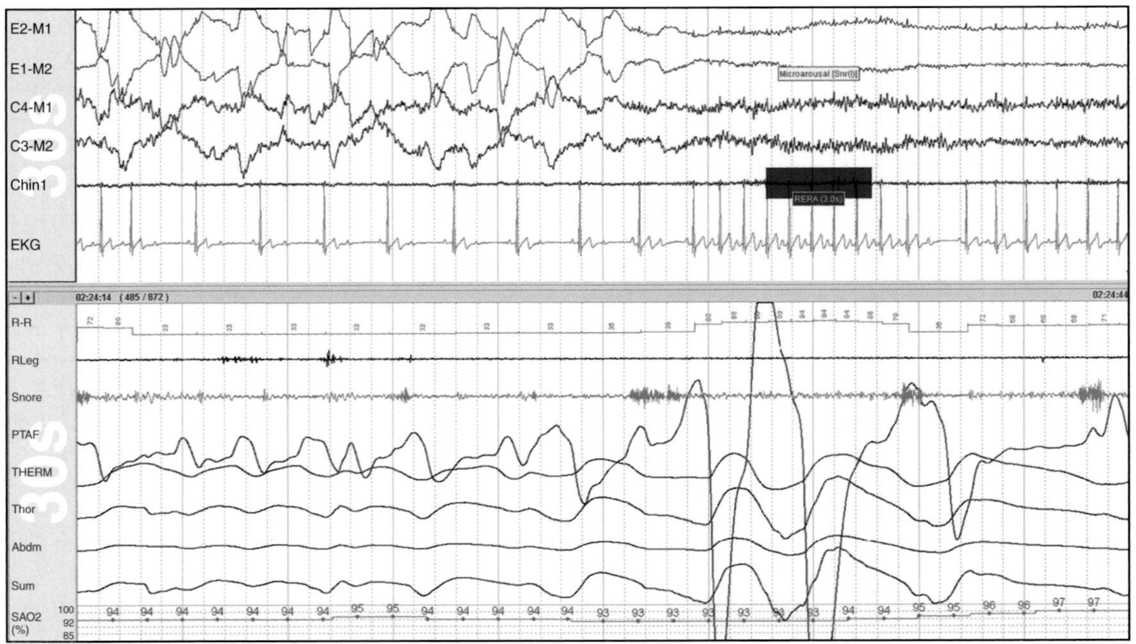

Figure 18-72.
Mobitz 2° AV block. In the Mobitz 2° AV block, there are one or more blocked P waves followed by a conducted ventricular beat. In this example there are two P waves to each QRS in the beginning of the epoch. This is called a Mobitz 2:1 AV block. In a 3:1 block there are three P waves to each conducted QRS. This type of block occurs in the lower part of the AV node, or His bundle, or in the right or left bundle branches. If it occurs in the bundle branches, the QRS will be wider.

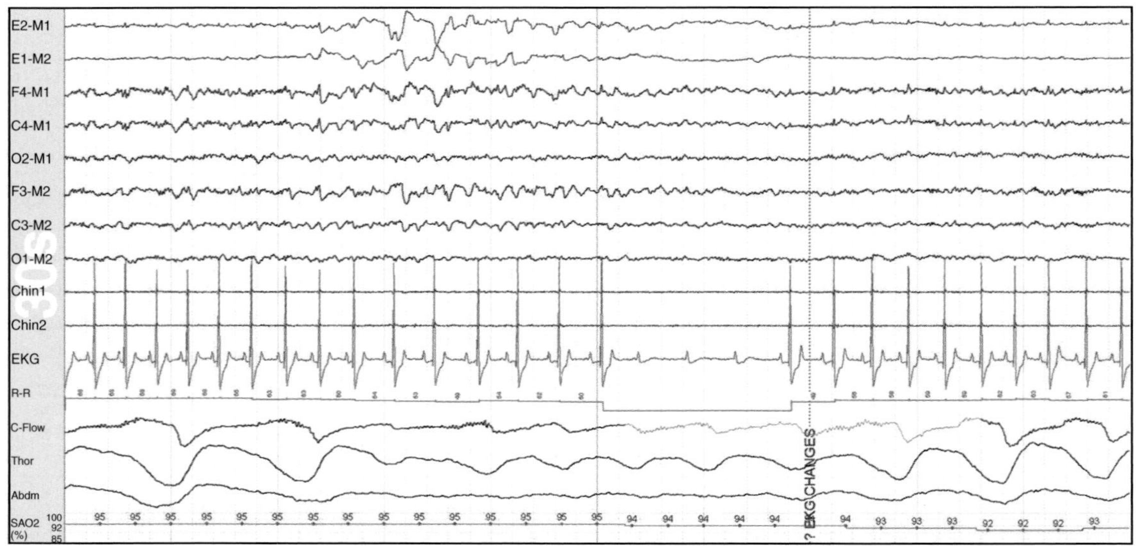

Figure 18-73.
3° heart block. SA node–generated P waves are not followed by an escape rhythm. The three P waves that are not conducted are identical to the ones that are conducted before and after the cardiac pause. This patient had sleep apnea, but in this PSG fragment there is no apnea or hypoxemia. These episodes might be related to REM sleep. Note the eye movements in the EOG channels and the sawtooth waves on EEG. Findings such as these should lead to cardiology assessment since the patient might require a pacemaker.

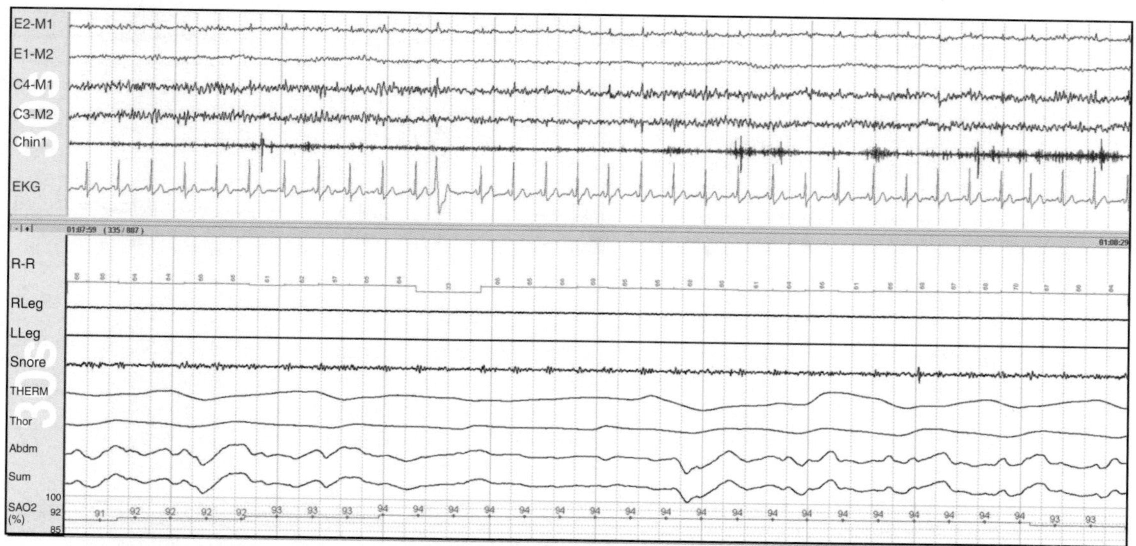

Figure 18-74.
Premature ventricular contraction (PVC). PVC arises from an irritable focus in the ventricle that depolarizes. The depolarization wave travels to the remainder of that ventricle, and then the opposite ventricle, producing a large and wide ventricular complex, as seen in this example. It is likely that the sinoatrial node depolarizes, but the P wave is usually lost in the PVC's QRS and arrives at the ventricle when it is refractory. Thus, a conducted beat is missed, but the following P wave is conducted, resulting in a compensatory pause.

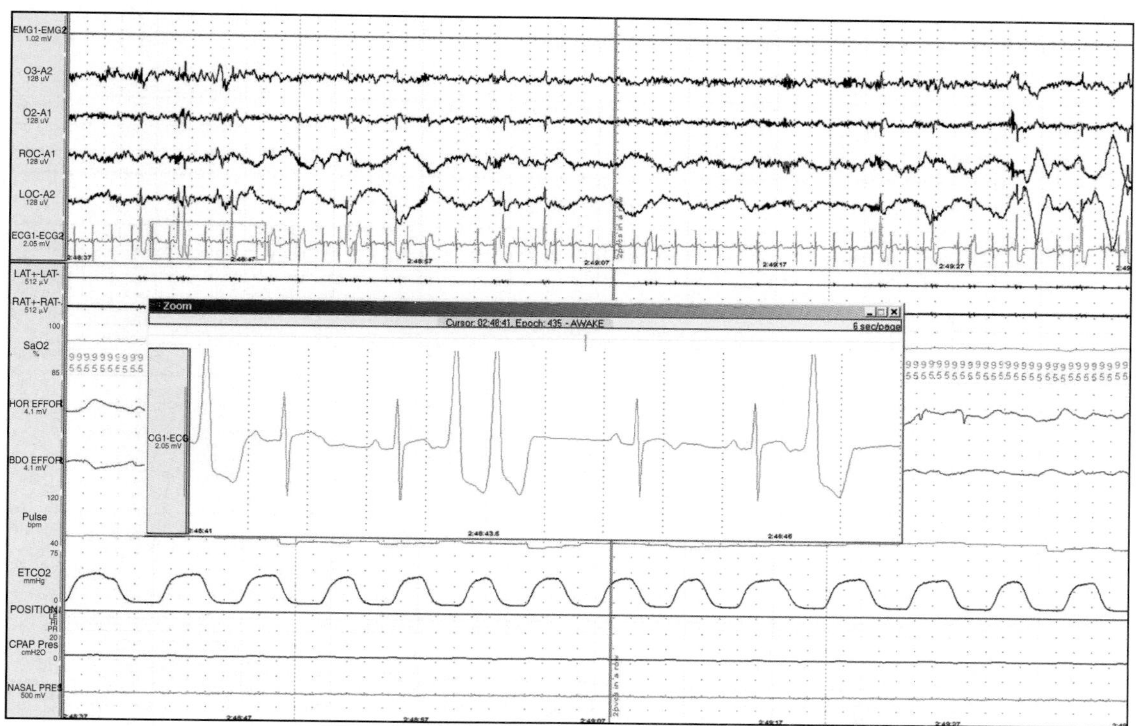

Figure 18-75.
Premature ventricular contractions (PVCs). The underlying rhythm is sinus. The abnormal beats are early and wide complex and at times are followed by a compensatory pause. One can with some data acquisition systems drill down. The middle window shows a 6-second epoch corresponding to the beats surrounded by the box on the EKG trace of the PSG. This allows one to better characterize the rhythm abnormality. More than six PVCs per minute should cause concern. Two PVCs in a row are called *couplets*; three are called *triplets*. When there are more than three, the event is called *ventricular tachycardia*.

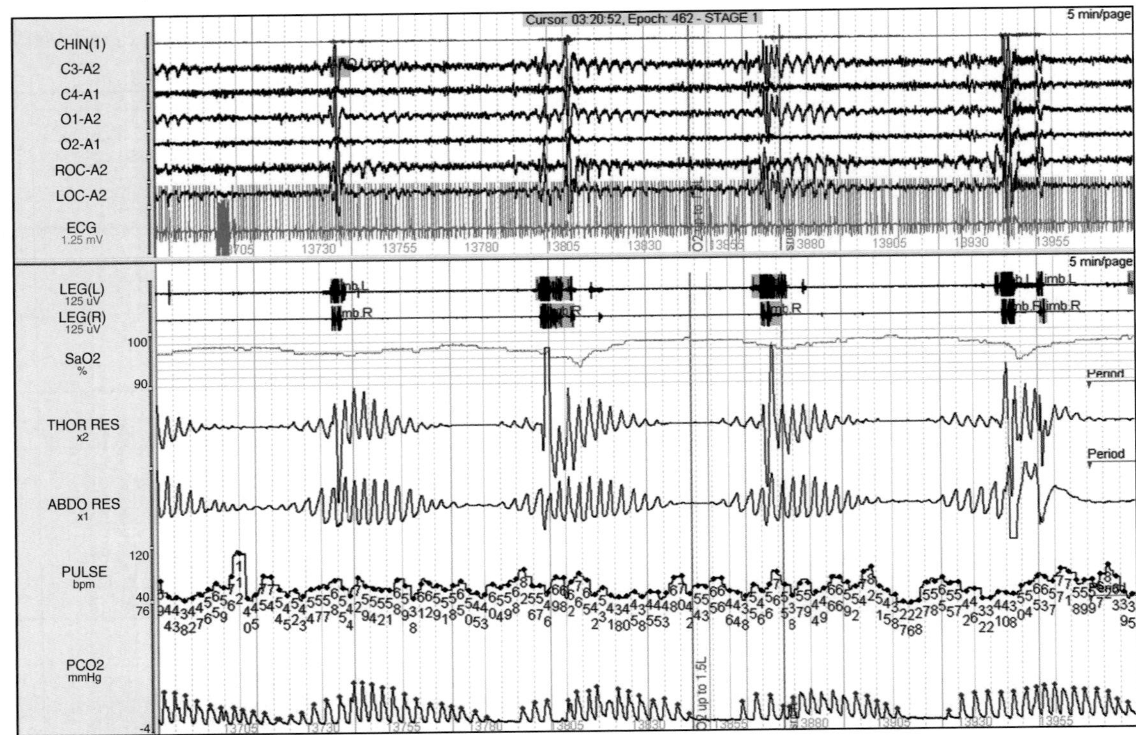

Figure 18-76.
Tachycardia in CHF and Cheyne Stokes breathing. Although it is counterintuitive, examining a long epoch gives an overall impression of the overall rhythm, and one's eye is immediately drawn to differences from the underlying pattern. Here, the top and bottom windows are both 5 min. On examining the EKG, the overall impression is that the underlying rhythm is regularly irregular. A narrow, dense band on the EKG at the beginning of the epoch corresponds to an increased heart rate detected in the pulse channel. Once a suspected abnormality is detected, one can change the epoch length to examine it in more detail. Figure 18-77 shows details of the beginning of the epoch.

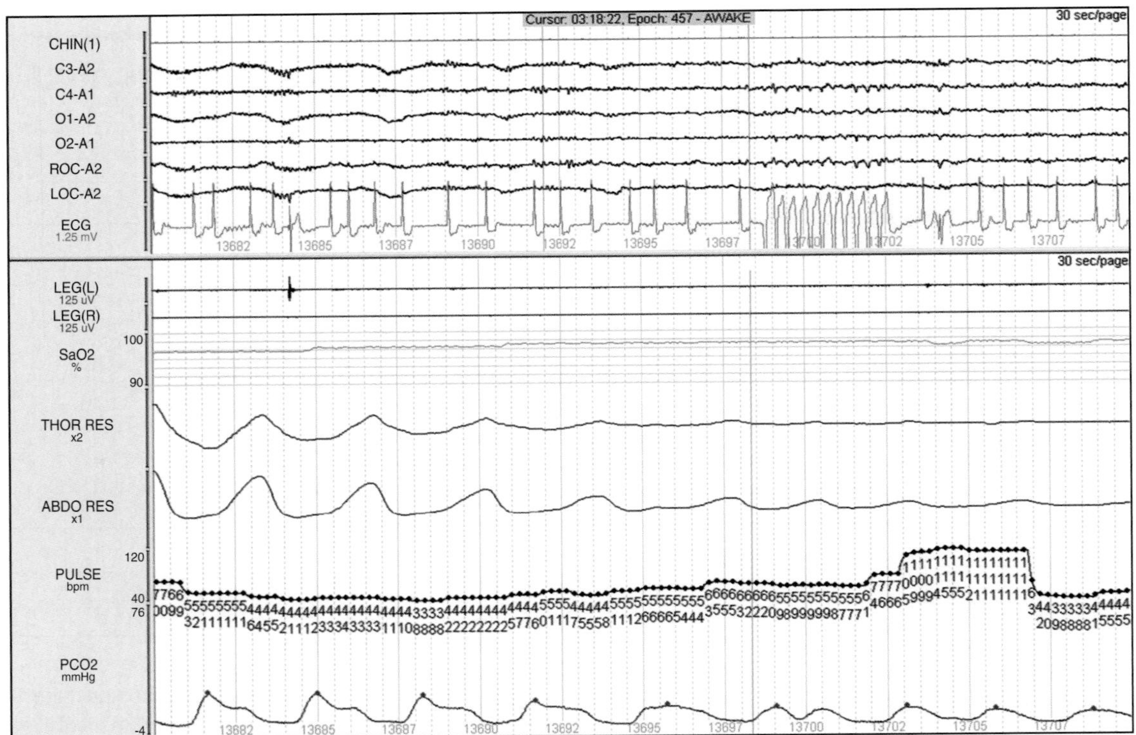

Figure 18-77.
Ventricular tachycardia. At this epoch length (top and bottom are 30 sec) one can more easily see the configuration of the abnormal beats. This epoch length allows one to manually calculate the rate from the EKG. In fact, the rate is actually about 160 beats per minute, not the 109 to 115 indicated on the pulse channel. In this example the rate on the recording is obtained from the output of an oximeter, not from the R-R interval of the EKG, and not all the beats were detected.

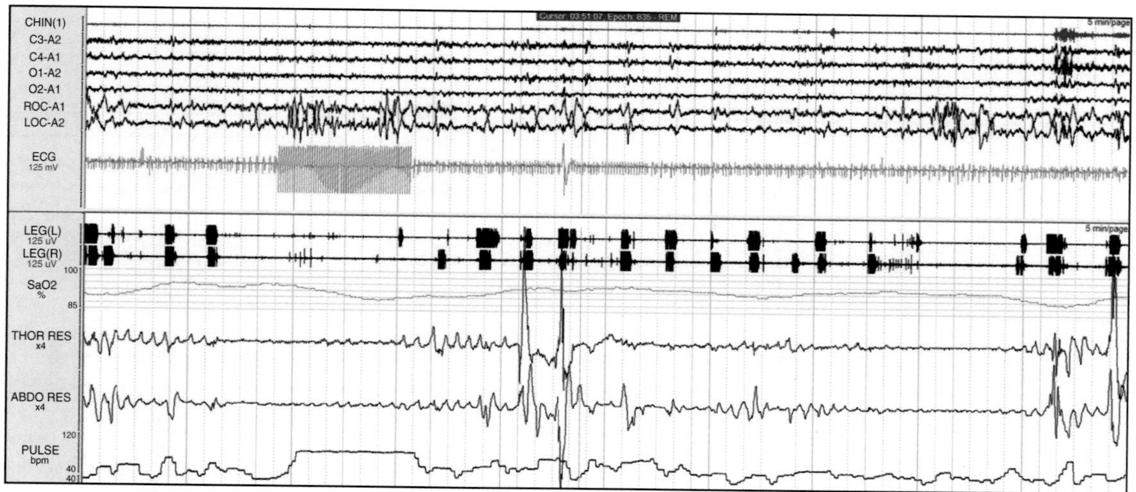

Figure 18-78.
Tachycardia. Through scanning by 5-minute epochs we detected an unusual pattern that suggested a tachycardia on the EKG about a minute into the epoch. The pulse rate was 120 at this time, and REMs are apparent on the eye channels. At the same time, there is a reduction in the number of leg movements. This patient had severe sleep apnea and a movement disorder. In Figure 18-79 we examine a shorter epoch length, wherein the data are shown in greater resolution.

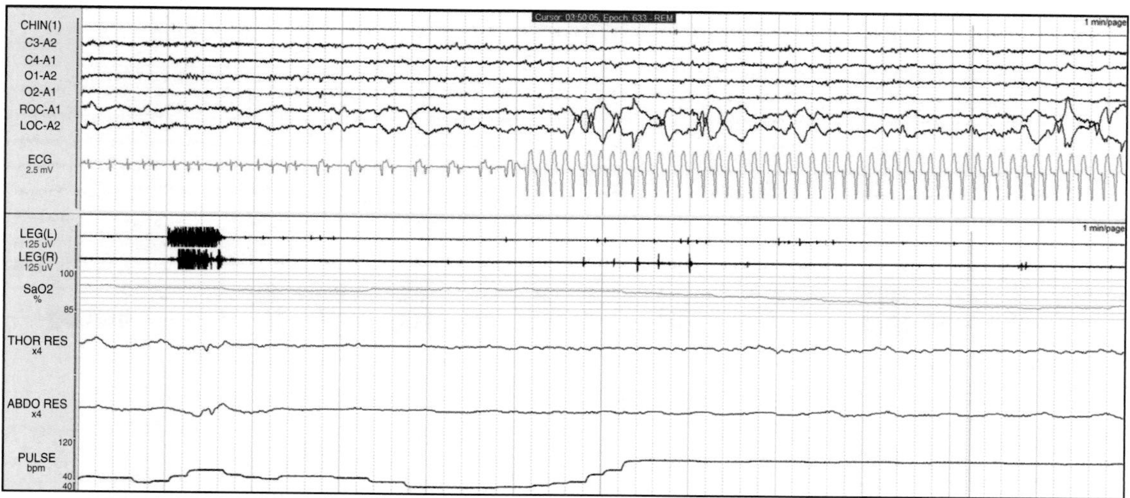

Figure 18-79.
Ventricular tachycardia. The beginning of the epoch shows an irregular pattern without well-developed P waves—atrial fibrillation. This is followed by what appears to be a mirror image of bigeminy. Instead of a normal beat alternating with a wide, complex premature ventricular contraction (PVC), the narrow complex beat follows the wide complex beat. This suggests that the wide complex beat is leading to retrograde conduction, in turn leading to the narrow complex beat. These wide complex beats are likely junctional beats. A wide complex beat falls on a T wave leading to a run of sustained ventricular tachycardia. The rate is 90 beats and rock steady (see the pulse channel). A ventricular contraction on a T wave should alert staff to the possibility of impending ventricular fibrillation. It is likely that surges in sympathetic activity occurring during REM sleep are playing a role in the genesis of the tachycardia.

Neurologic Diseases

MOVEMENT DISORDERS

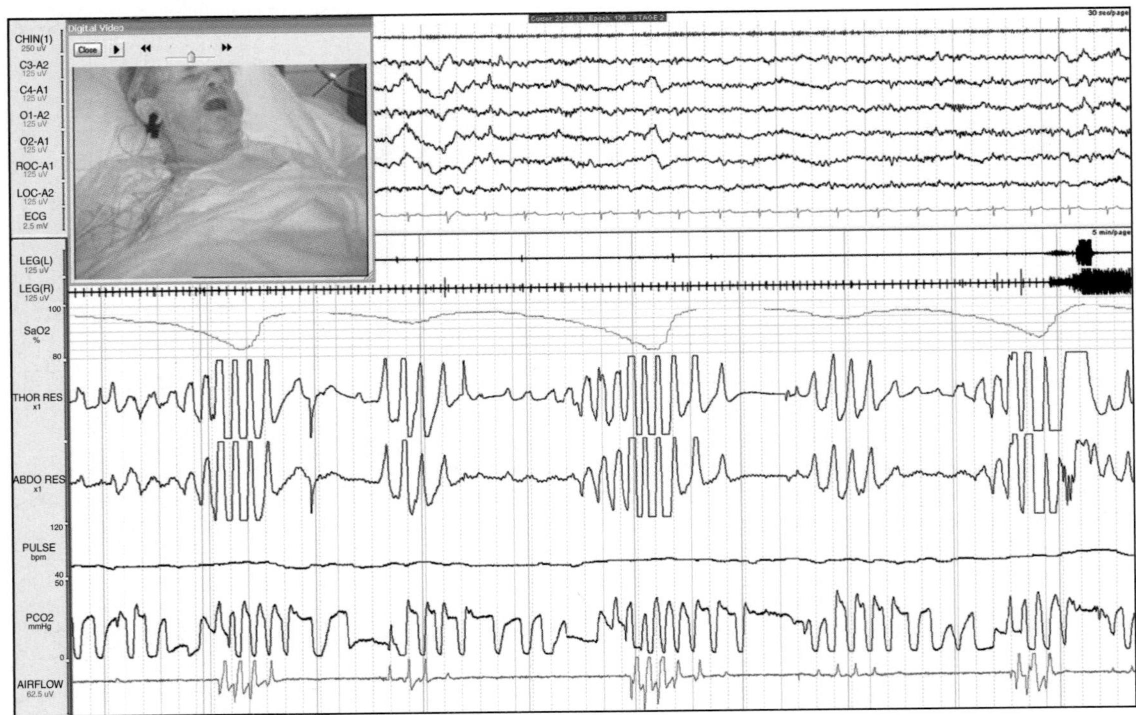

Figure 18-80.
Parkinson's disease. This patient had sleep apnea. His mouth is wide open. The nasal pressure channel overestimates the length of the apneas, which are more accurately detected by oronasal CO_2. The top window is 30 sec; the bottom is 5 min.

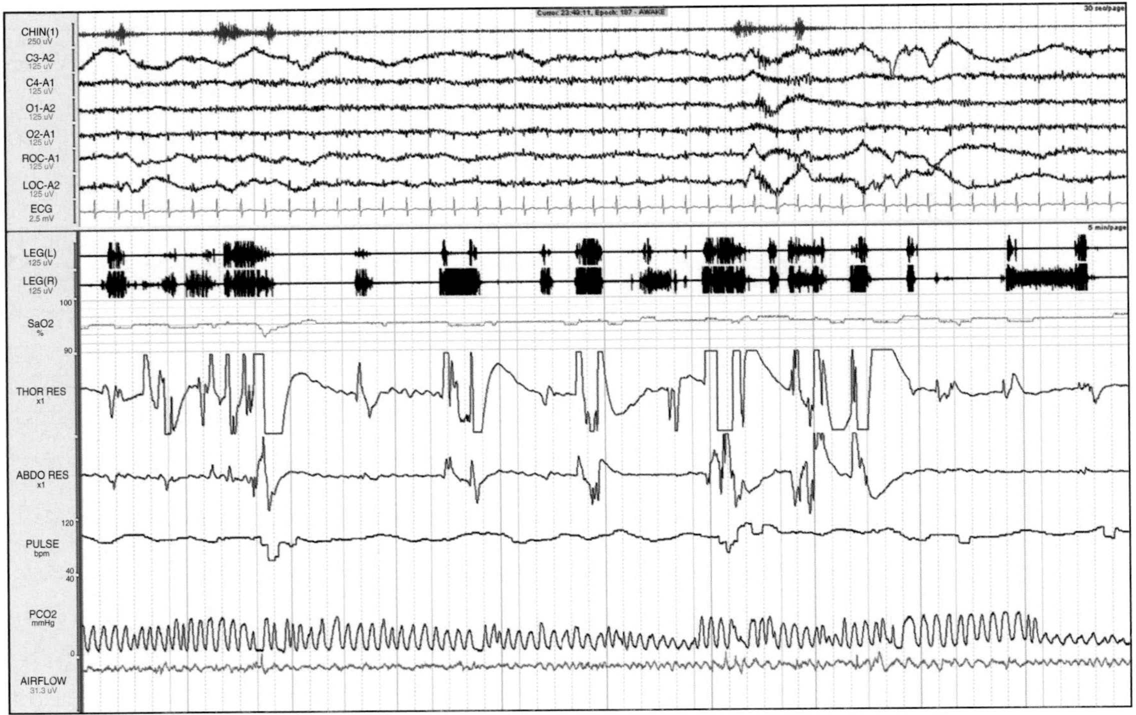

Figure 18-81.
Restless legs syndrome. Sleep latency was prolonged. During the time she was trying to fall asleep, the patient was extremely fidgety, had difficulty staying still, and demonstrated continuous movements in her legs. The movements caused artifacts in the abdominal and thoracic effort channels. The top window is 30 sec; the bottom is 5 min.

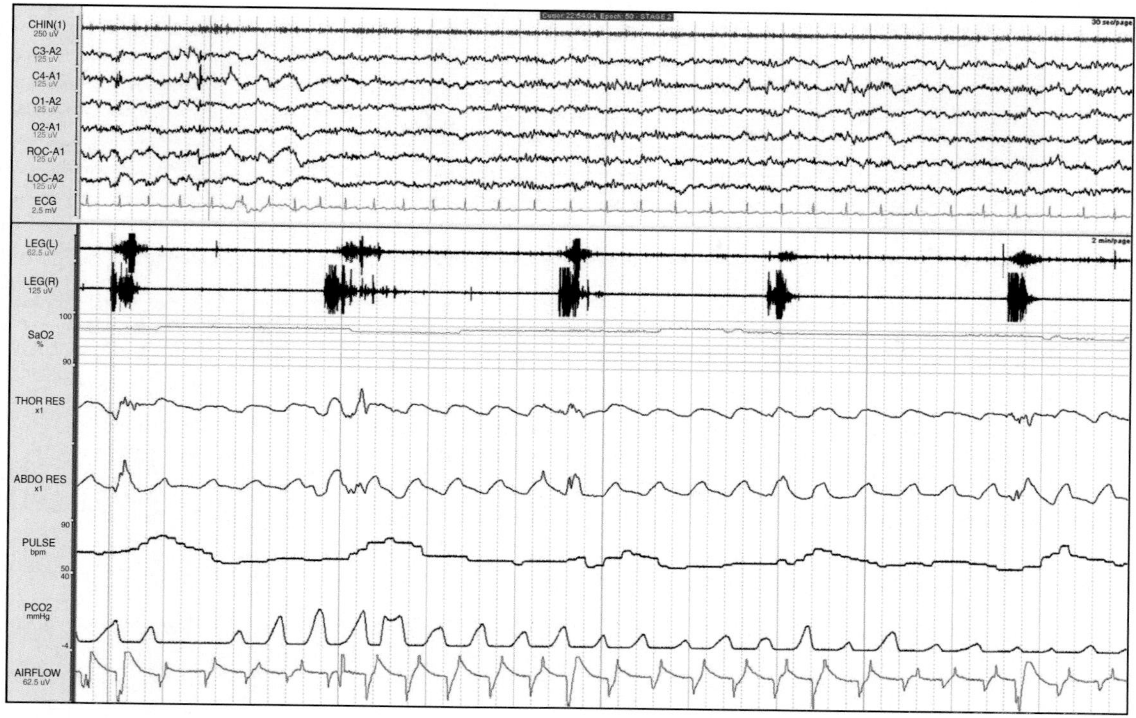

Figure 18-82.
Periodic limb movements in sleep (PLMS). Notice that the movements are followed by increases in heart rate, presumably caused by increased sympathetic tone. This patient was a lifelong vegetarian who had reduced iron stores. The top window is 30 sec; the bottom is 2 min.

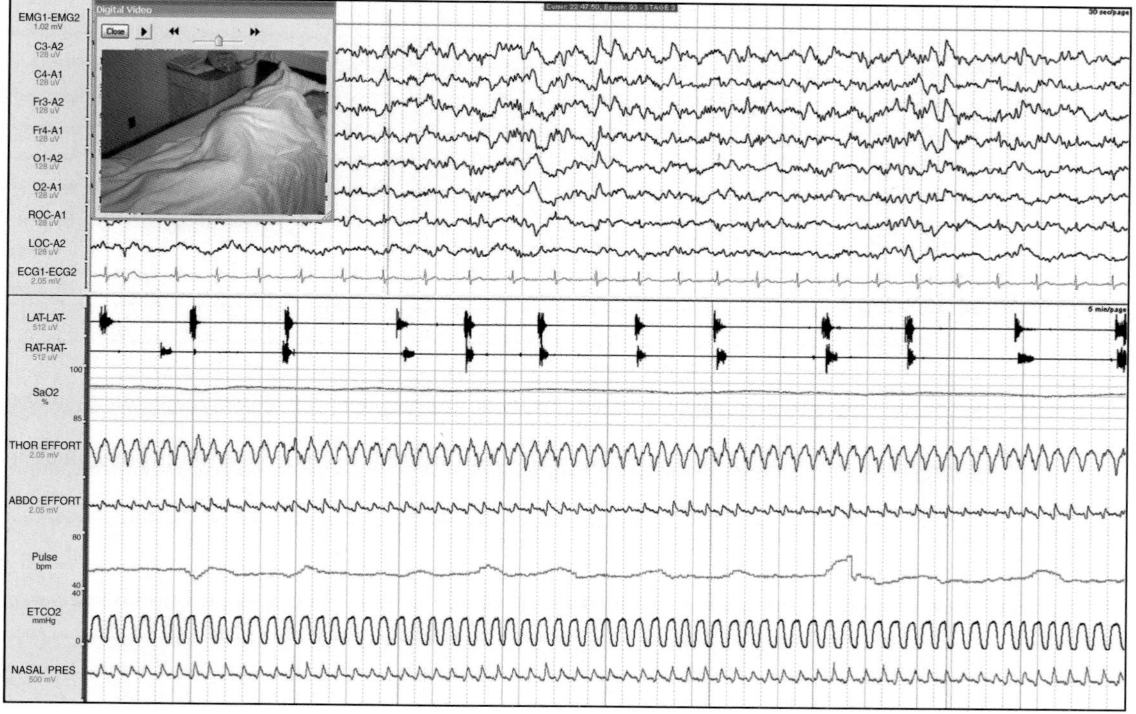

Figure 18-83.
Periodic limb movements in sleep (PLMS). The patient, lying on his side, had typical findings of PLMS. There are small synchronous increases in heart rate. The top window is 30 sec; the bottom is 5 min.

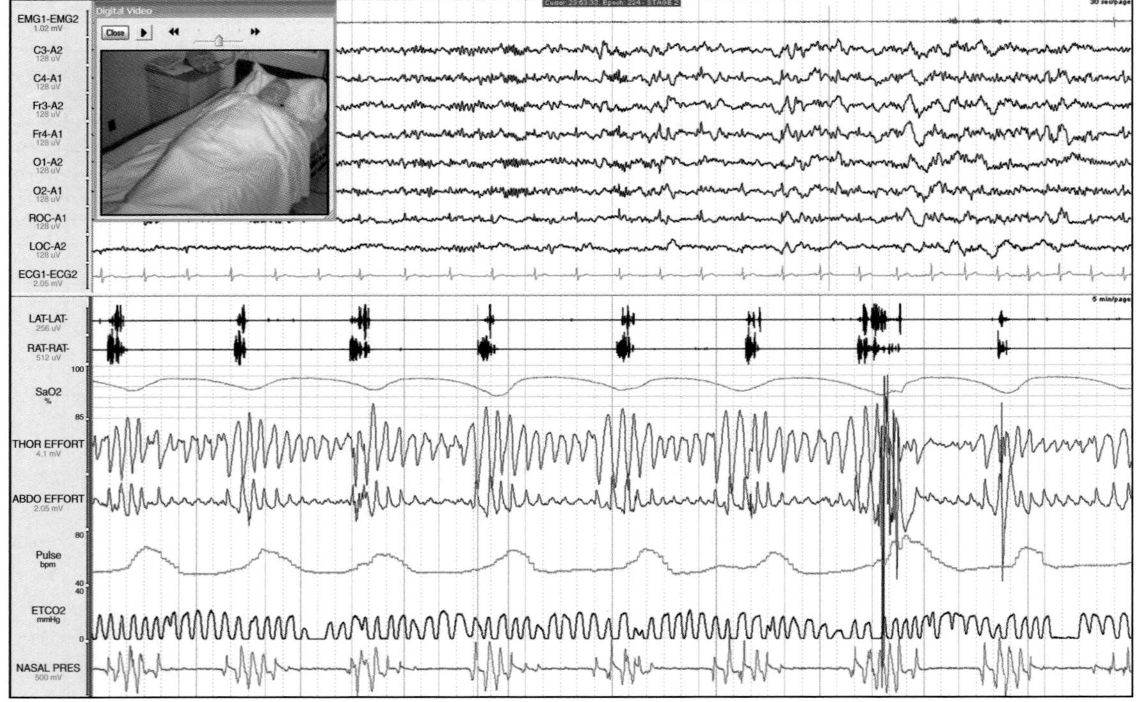

Figure 18-84.
Periodic limb movements in sleep (PLMS). The patient, sleeping on his back, had a sleep breathing disorder. Limb movements are now synchronized with the peak of hyperpnea. The top window is 30 sec; the bottom is 5 min.

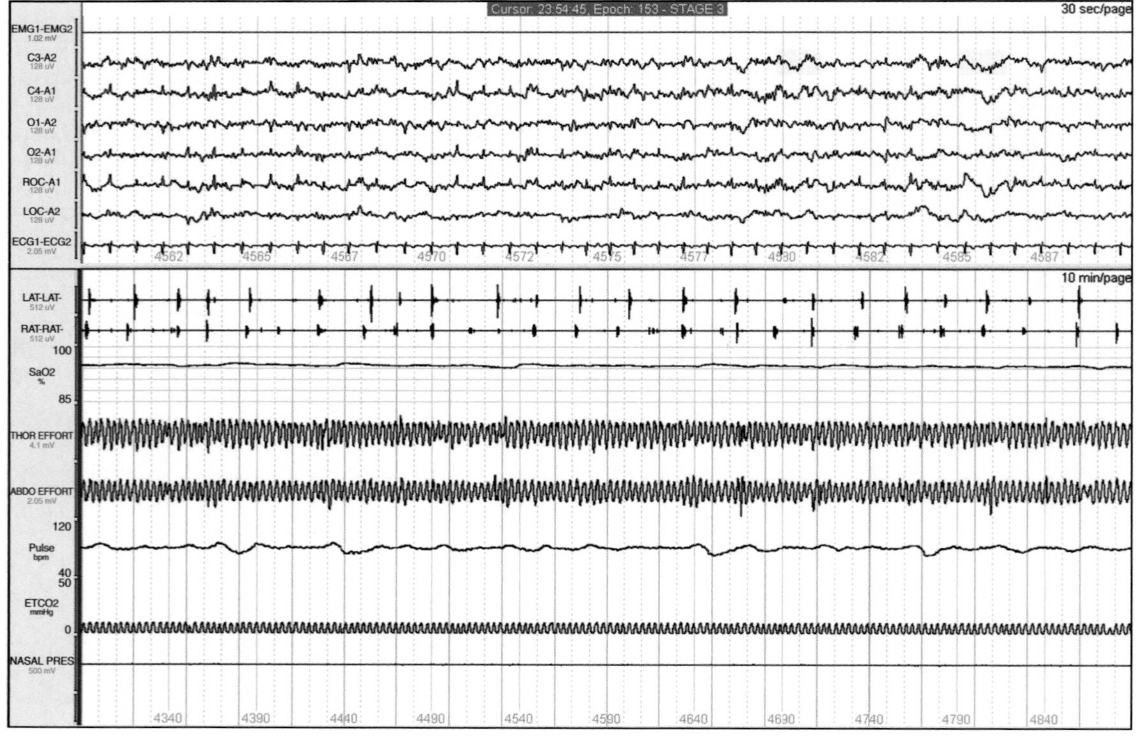

Figure 18-85.
Calf cramp. This patient had a history of severe leg cramps that awakened him. He had severe periodic limb movements in sleep (PLMS) with a PLMS index of about 150. The top window is 30 sec; the bottom is 10 min.

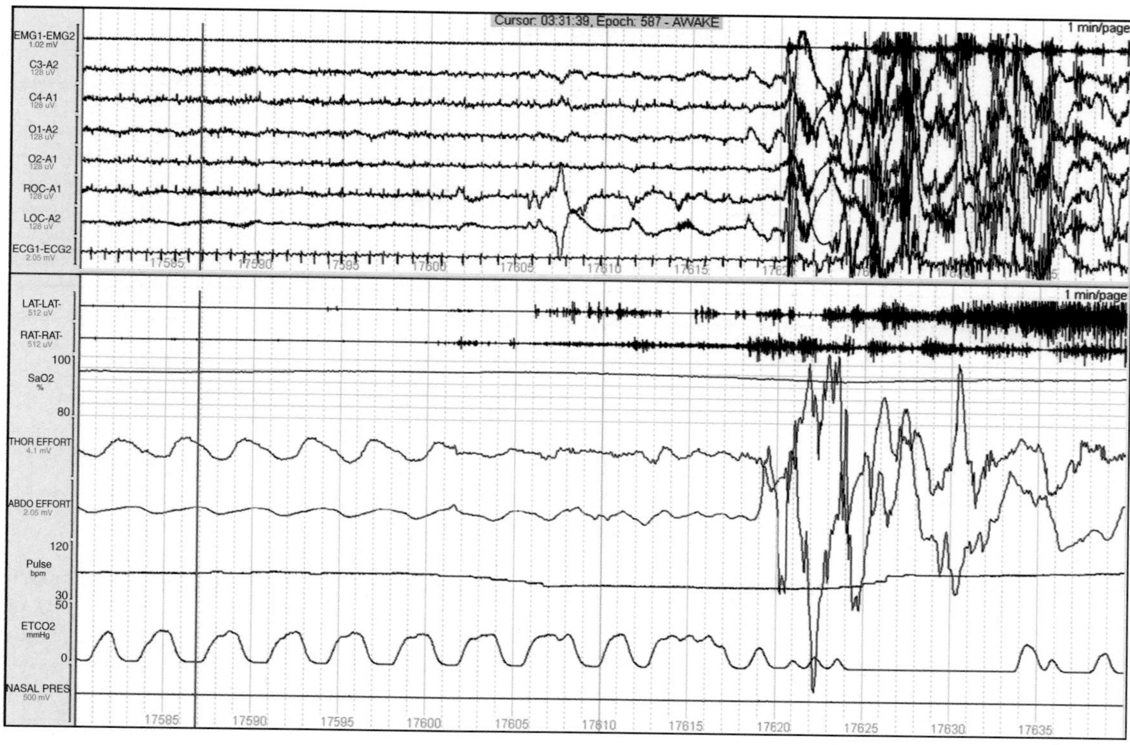

Figure 18-86.
Same patient as in Figure 18-85. At the beginning of the 1-minute epoch, the patient was in REM sleep. Activity in the legs was noticeable beginning in the middle of the epoch. Within about 10 seconds of the first leg movement activity, the patient awakened abruptly with a painful cramp. The synchronized video shows a sudden, very high-speed movement, resembling a kick, just before awakening.

GENETIC DISORDERS

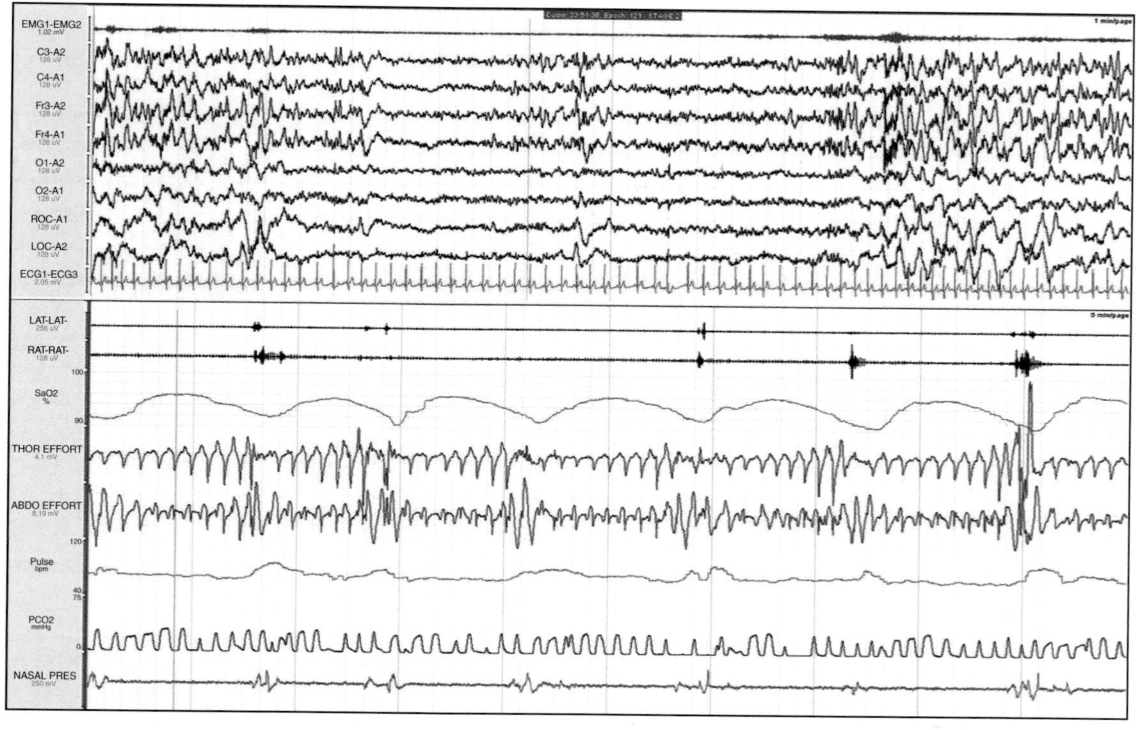

Figure 18-87.
Becker's muscular dystrophy. The 35-year-old patient had muscular dystrophy of the Becker's type, diagnosed at age 13. At age 15, he started snoring and developed daytime sleepiness. This PSG fragment shows sleep apnea. There is a discrepancy between nasal pressure and oronasal CO_2 because the patient often breathed through his mouth. The top window is 1 min; the bottom is 5 min.

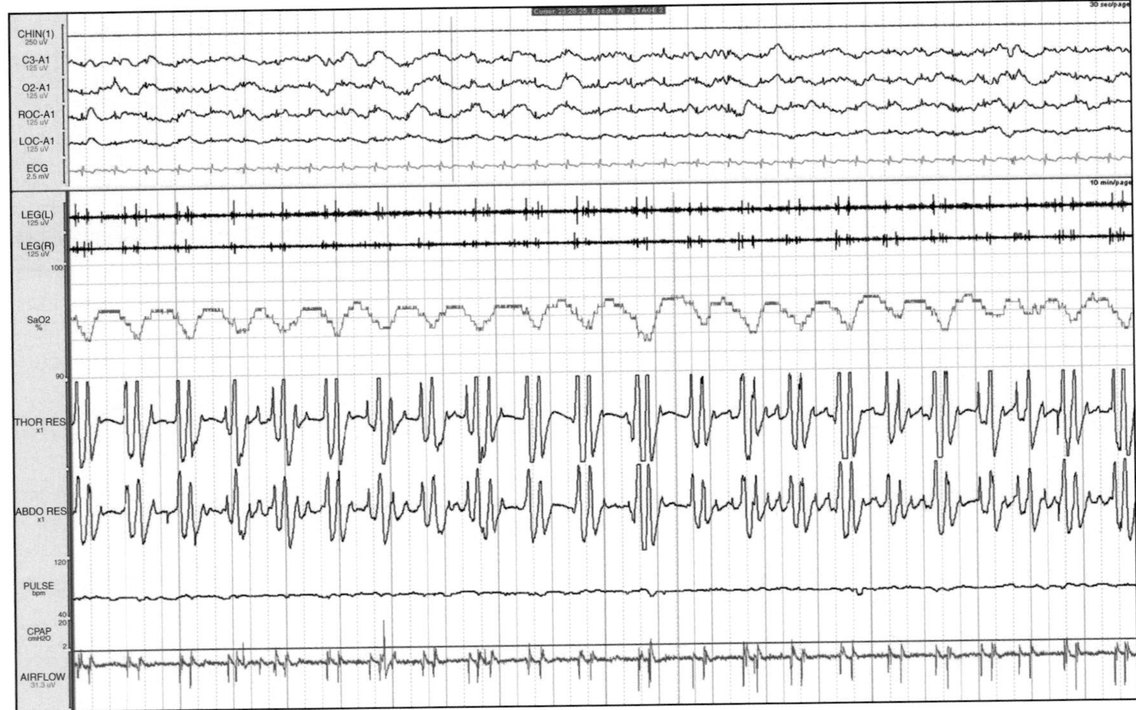

Figure 18-88.
Retinitis pigmentosa. These data are from a 75-year-old male with blindness due to retinitis pigmentosa, a 20-year history of severe daytime sleepiness and a history of snoring, observed apnea, and restlessness in his legs. The patient also had white fingernails. The breathing abnormality shown, a variant of Cheyne Stokes breathing, was also present during wakefulness. The patient responded well to adaptive servo-ventilation with an end-expiratory pressure of 10 cm H_2O. The top window is 30 sec; the bottom is 10 min.

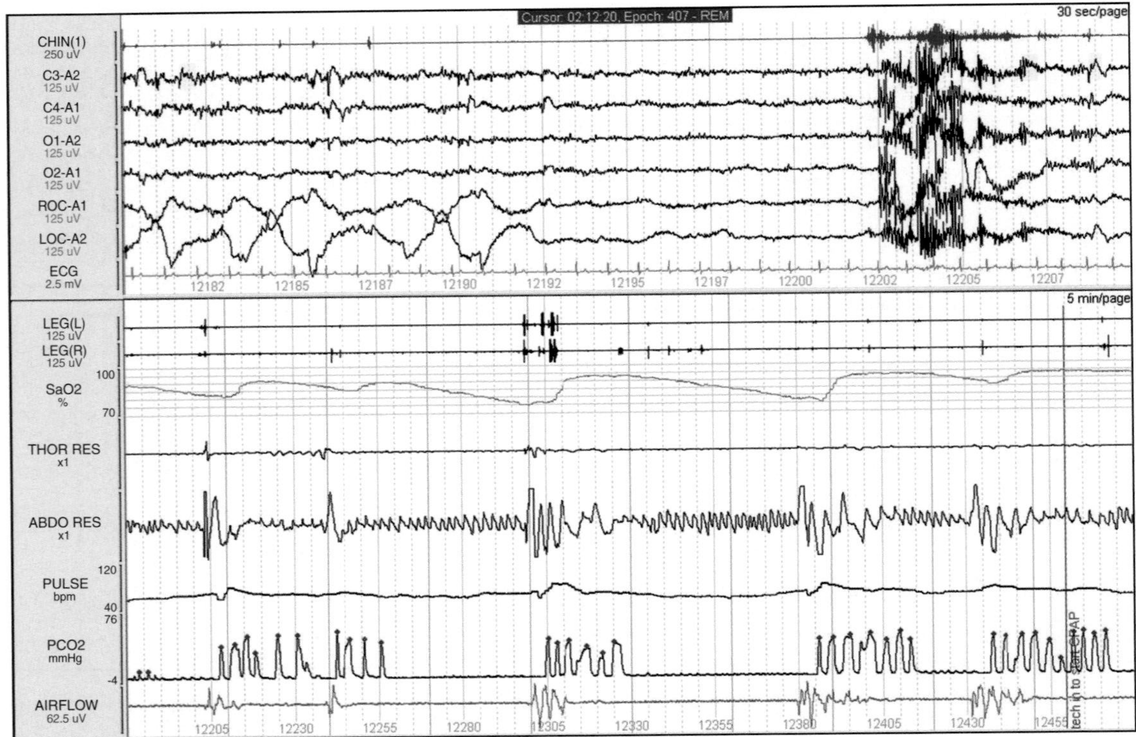

Figure 18-89.
Huntington disease. This 60-year-old female had continuous choreoathetotic movements during wakefulness that decreased during sleep. She had no breathing abnormalities in NREM sleep. During REM sleep (shown here) she had very long episodes of obstructive apnea.

STROKE

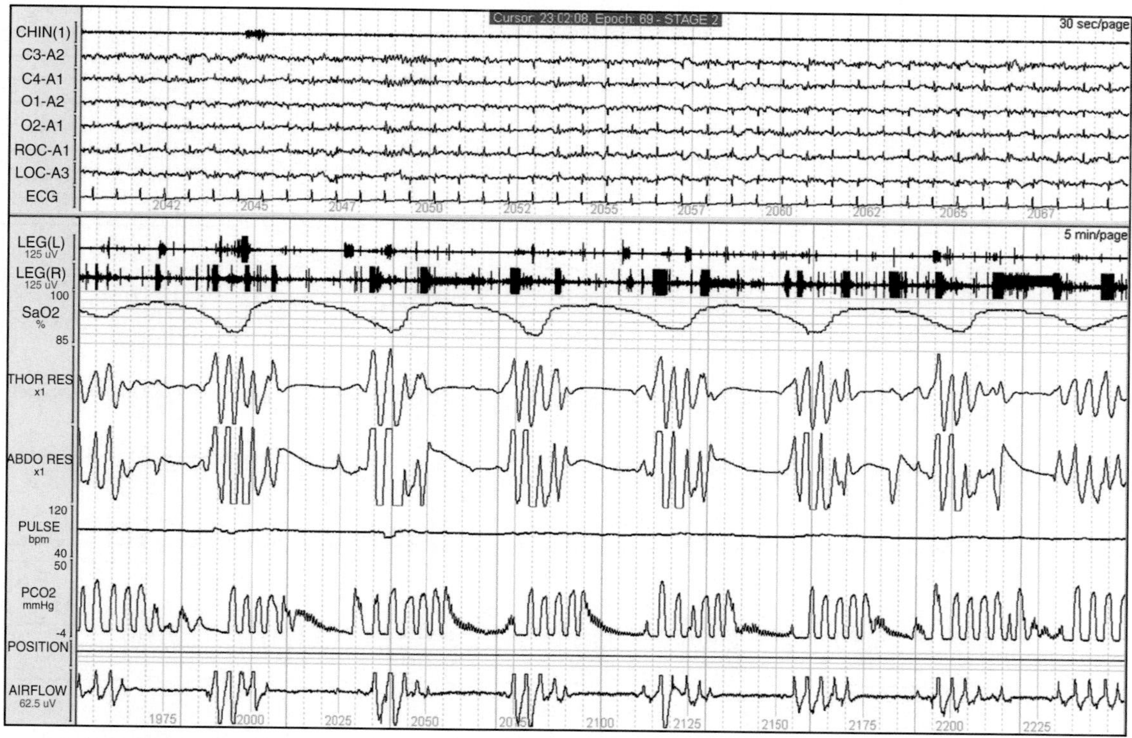

Figure 18-90.
Stroke. This PSG is of a 54-year-old male who developed excessive daytime sleepiness, snoring, and episodes of observed apnea during sleep after a stroke at age 51. There was also a history of excessive movements during sleep. The patient has central apnea with cardiogenic oscillations evident in the CO_2 trace. The top window is 30 sec; the bottom is 5 min.

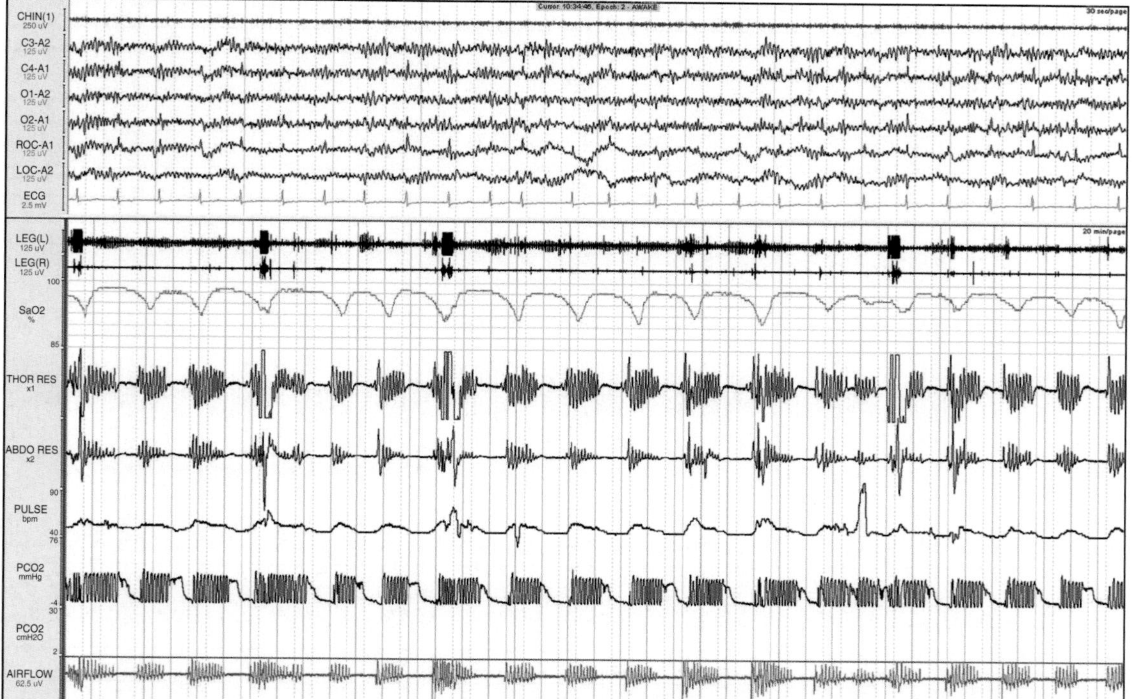

Figure 18-91.
Awake central apnea in stroke. These data are from an 81-year-old woman with insomnia that began 3 years earlier following a stroke that resulted in right-sided weakness and some impairment of speech. The patient had central apnea the entire night and never achieved persistent sleep. The top window is 30 sec; the bottom is 20 min.

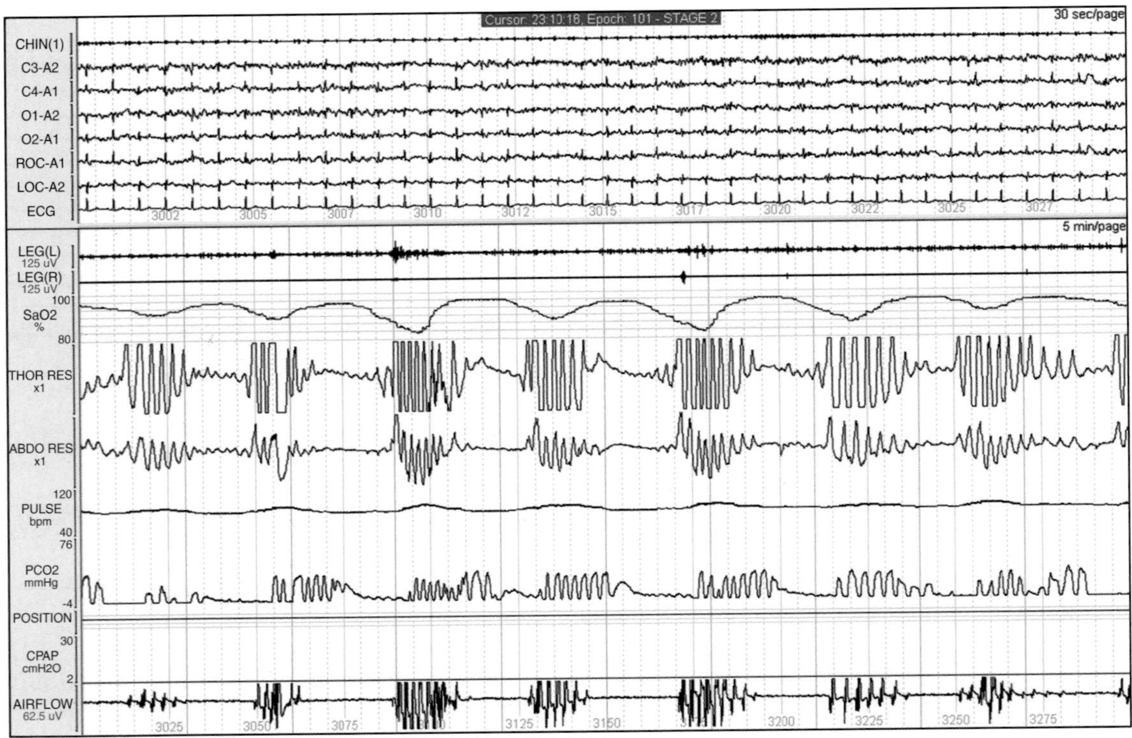

Figure 18-92.
Central sleep apnea in stroke. These data are from a 72-year-old male who had daytime sleepiness that began after a stroke. His wife also witnessed apneas during his sleep. The patient had a periodic breathing pattern, a variant of Cheyne Stokes, during both sleep (as shown here) and wakefulness. The top window is 30 sec; the bottom is 20 min.

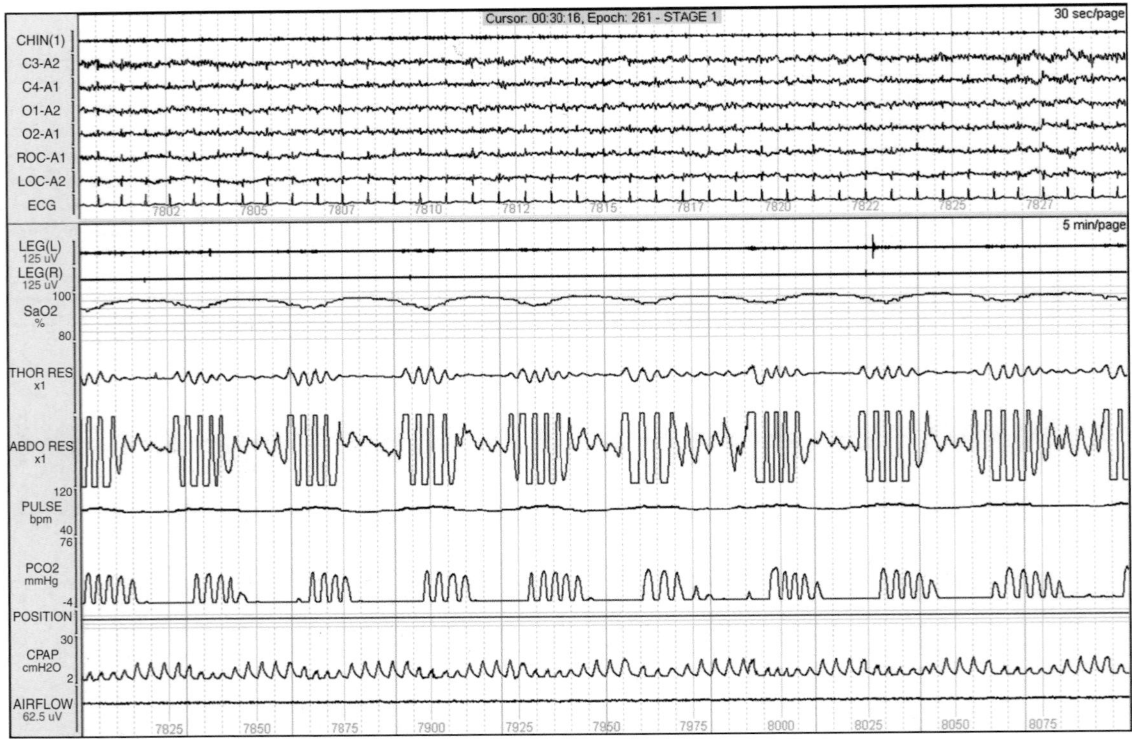

Figure 18-93.
Central sleep apnea in stroke. Same patient as in Figure 18-92. Here, later in the night, the patient was assessed on an adaptive servo-ventilation (ASV) system. The CPAP channel shows increases in pressure generated by the servo-ventilator when the patient became apneic. Figure 18-94 shows the 20 minutes of transition onto ASV. The top window is 30 sec; the bottom is 5 min.

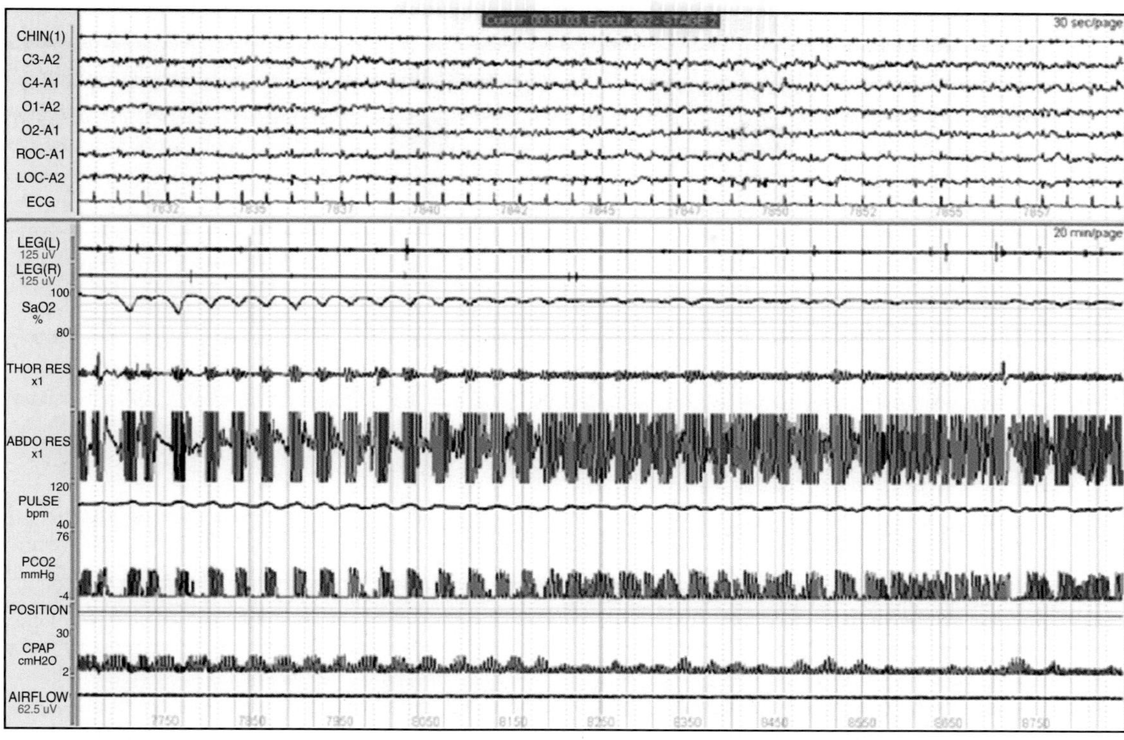

Figure 18-94.
Central sleep apnea in stroke. Same patient as in Figure 18-92. The bottom window shows 20 minutes of data on adaptive servo-ventilation (ASV). There is a gradual normalization of SaO_2 and reduction of periodic breathing as ASV entrains and normalizes the breathing pattern. There was dramatic improvement in symptoms on home use of ASV.

NARCOLEPSY

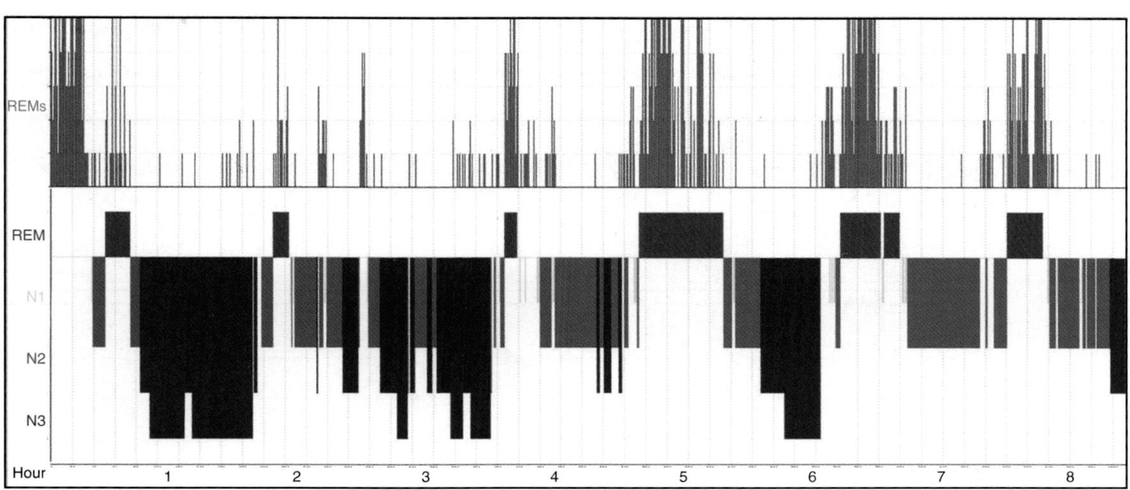

Figure 18-95.
Narcolepsy. This is a sleep histogram from a 15-year-old female complaining of sleepiness with an Epworth sleepiness score of 19. The top part of the histogram shows the presence of REMs; the bottom part, sleep stages. N3 is made up of stage 3 (shorter blue bands) and stage 4 (longer blue bands). The first episode of REM sleep occurred 6.5 minutes after lights out. The multiple sleep latency test done the next day was terminated after three naps during which the patient was in REM sleep. The mean sleep latency was 6 minutes.

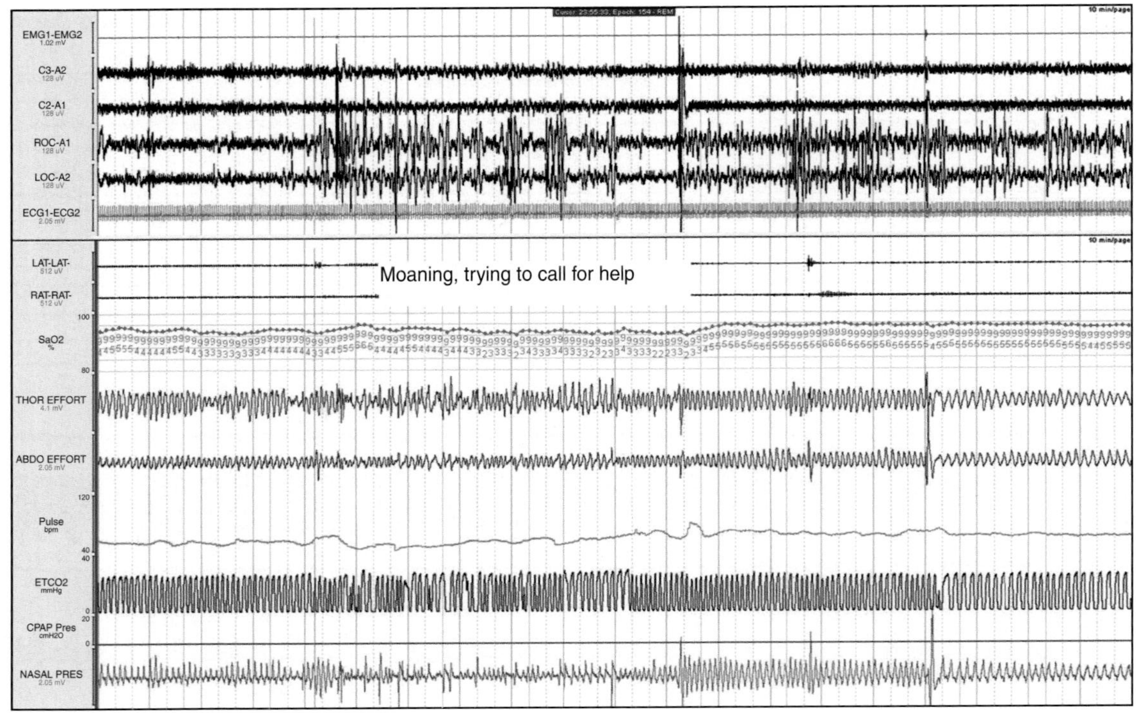

Figure 18-96.
Sleep paralysis. This 10-minute PSG epoch is from a 49-year-old female with a 15-year history of sleep paralysis. Notice the notation of moaning during the REMs. The patient stated that she was awake, but paralyzed, and was trying to call for help by making moaning noises. This patient did not have any other features of narcolepsy.

REM SLEEP BEHAVIOR DISORDER

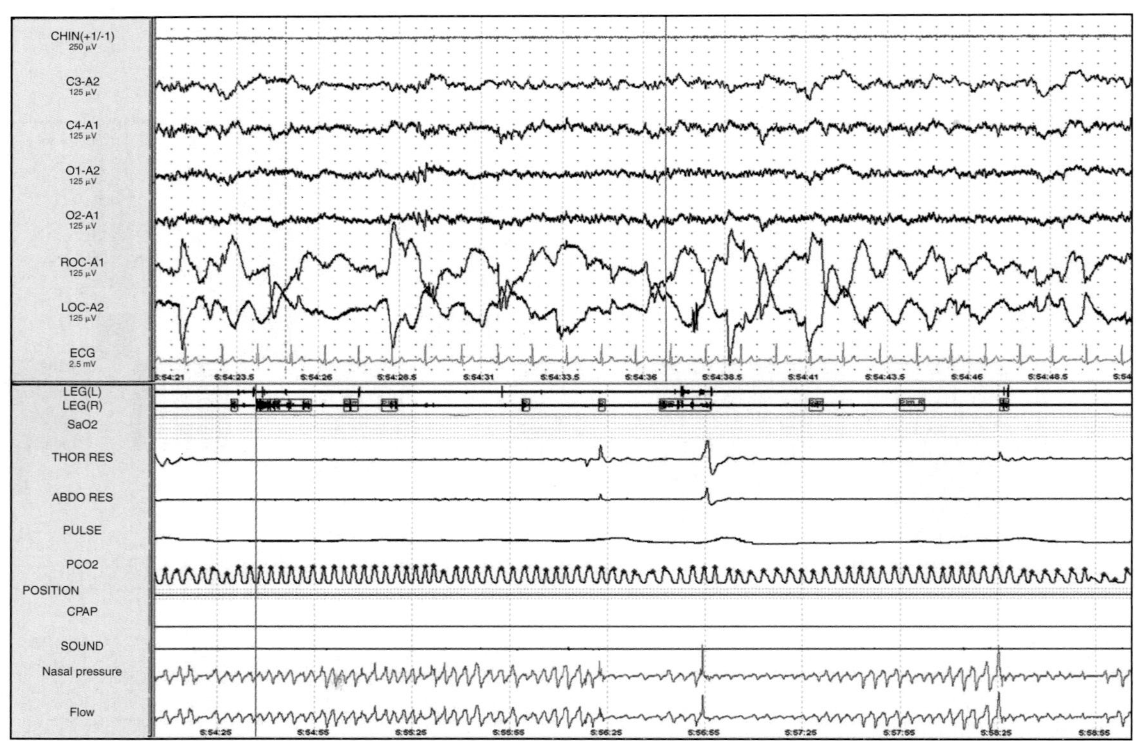

Figure 18-97.
REM sleep behavior disorder. From a woman with a long history of reacting to dream content in which she was being attacked (see Video 15, chapter 19). The patient is in REM sleep and has movements noted in her legs. The blue vertical lines synchronize the top and bottom windows. The top window is 30 sec; the bottom is 5 min.

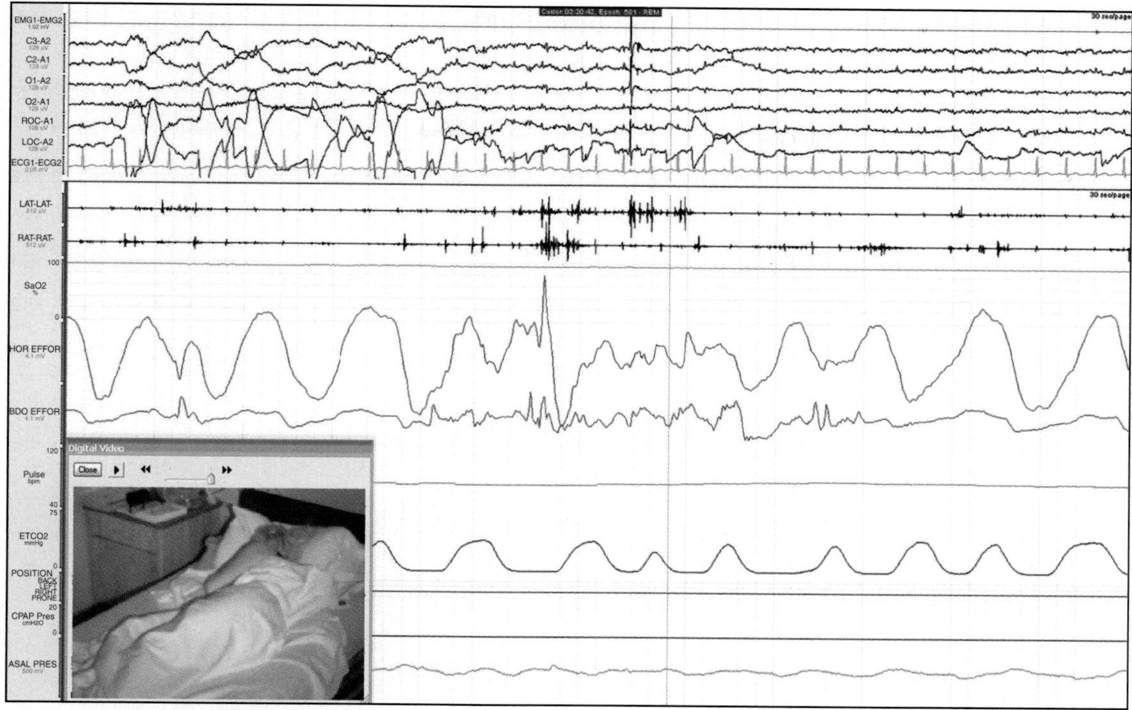

Figure 18-98.
REM sleep behavior disorder. From a 53-year-old woman with a long history of reacting to dream content. Four to five nights a week she strikes out during dreams about "a bad man who is deformed and ugly" who might be attacking her. On examination of synchronized digital video during this episode of REM sleep one could see that the patient was moving her right hand (see Video 61, chapter 20).

SEIZURES

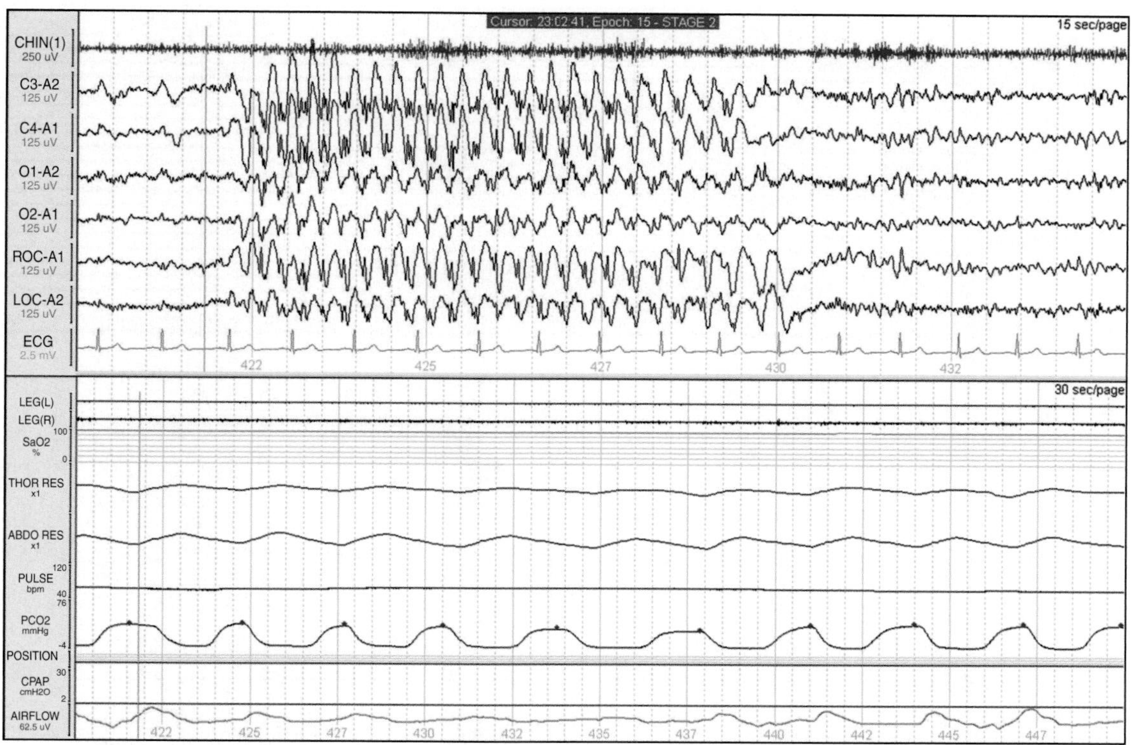

Figure 18-99.
Seizure disorder. The seizure activity lasting about 5 sec in this epoch is not associated with any other recorded abnormality. The top window is 15 sec; the bottom is 30 sec.

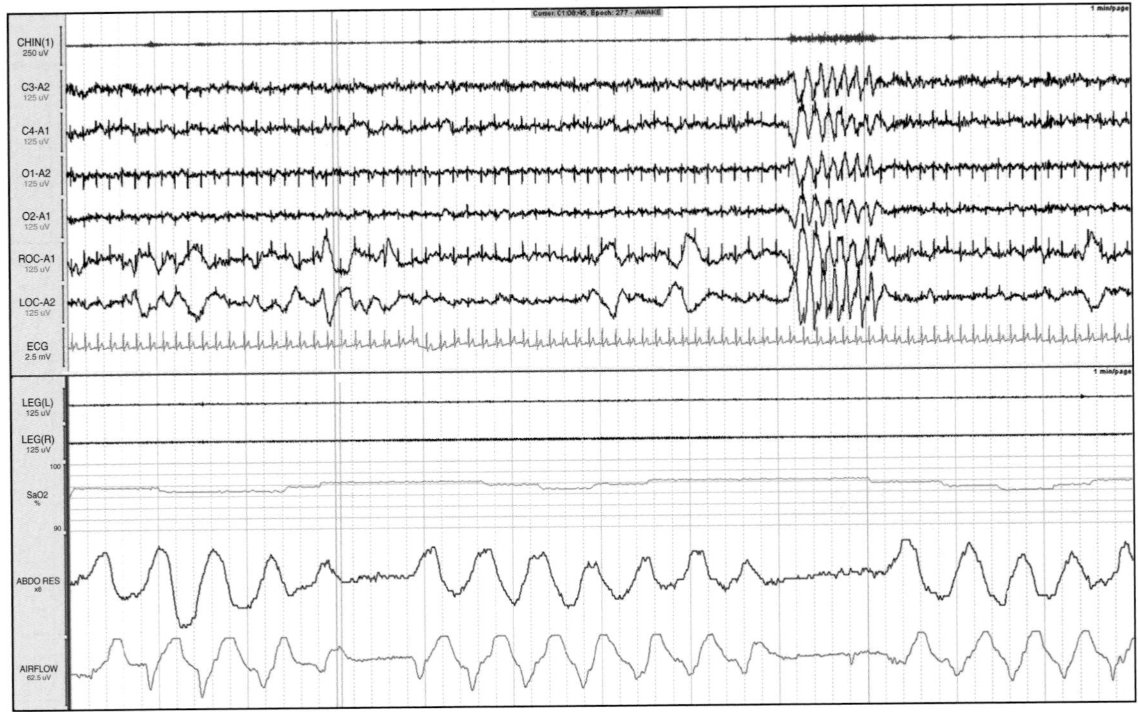

Figure 18-100.
Seizure disorder. The first episode of central apnea is not associated with apparent seizure activity. The second one is. The top and bottom windows are 1 min.

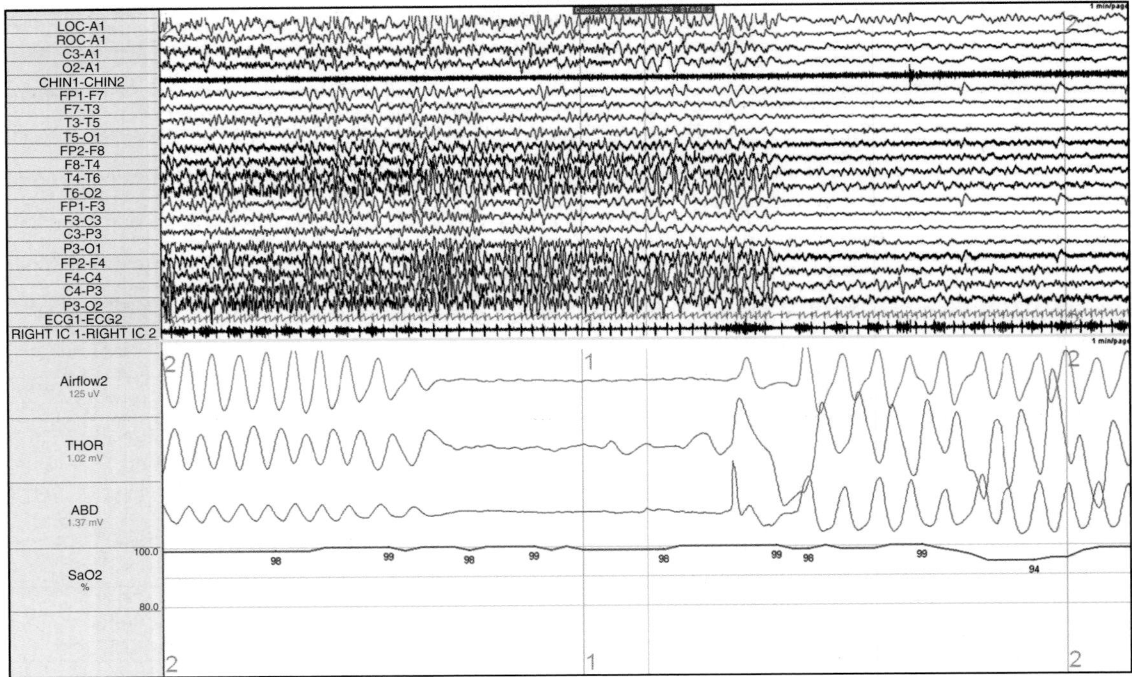

Figure 18-101.
Seizure disorder. Central apneic episode associated with significant oxygen desaturation is the sole manifestation of the seizure. The true nature of the event (a right-sided seizure) would not be evident without a full seizure montage. Blue EEG traces refer to left side, black to right side. The top and bottom windows are 1 min. (Courtesy of M. Mahowald.)

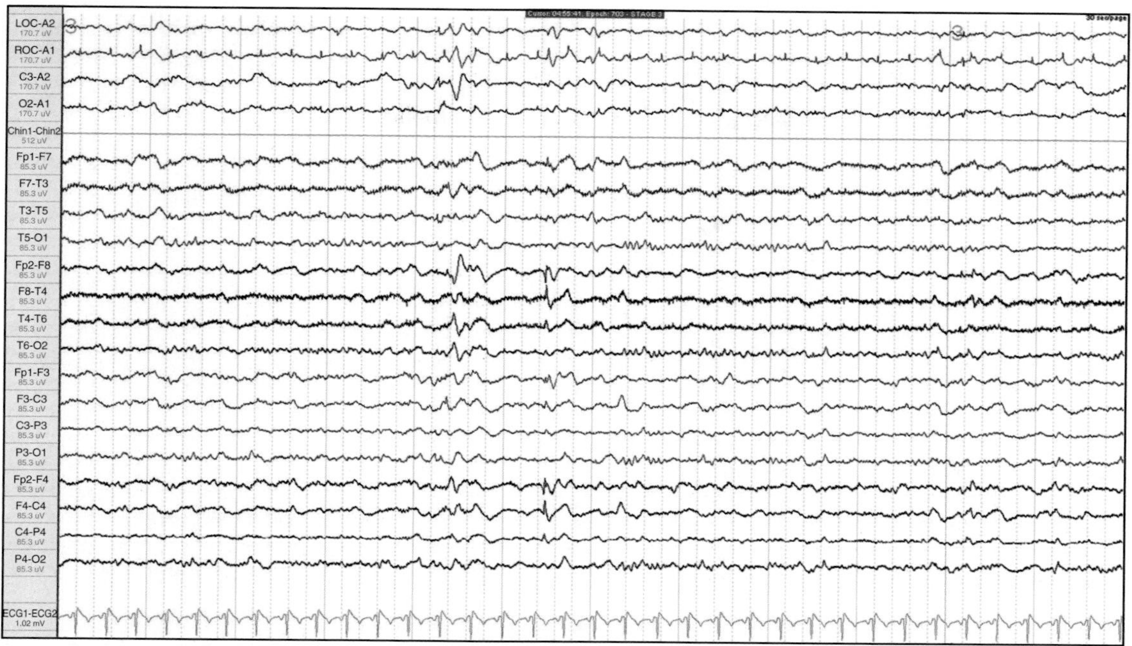

Figure 18-102.
Seizure disorder. Rare, very localized spikes over the right anterior temporal region in a patient with nocturnal seizures. Only a few such spikes occurred during the entire study, underscoring the necessity of personally reviewing each epoch when looking for evidence of spikes. This activity could not have been identified the conventional sleep stage scoring montage. The window is 30 sec. (Contributed by M. Mahowald.)

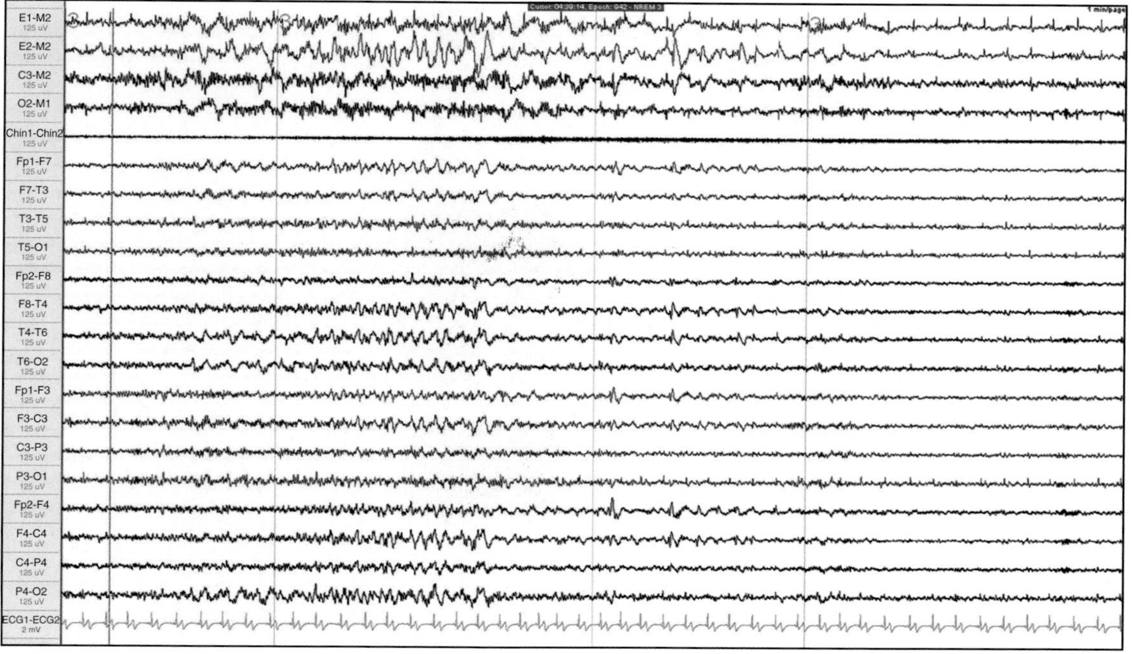

Figure 18-103.
Seizure disorder. This is an example of an electrical seizure emanating from the right hemisphere followed by isolated spikes over the same region. There are no clinical correlates of this electrical seizure. This could not be identified on the sleep scoring montage. The tendency is often for the technicians to "mark" only clinically obvious events–which are often nothing but movement artifact. The true nature of the events is only identified by finding subclinical electrical seizure activity such as on this epoch. (Contributed by M. Mahowald.)

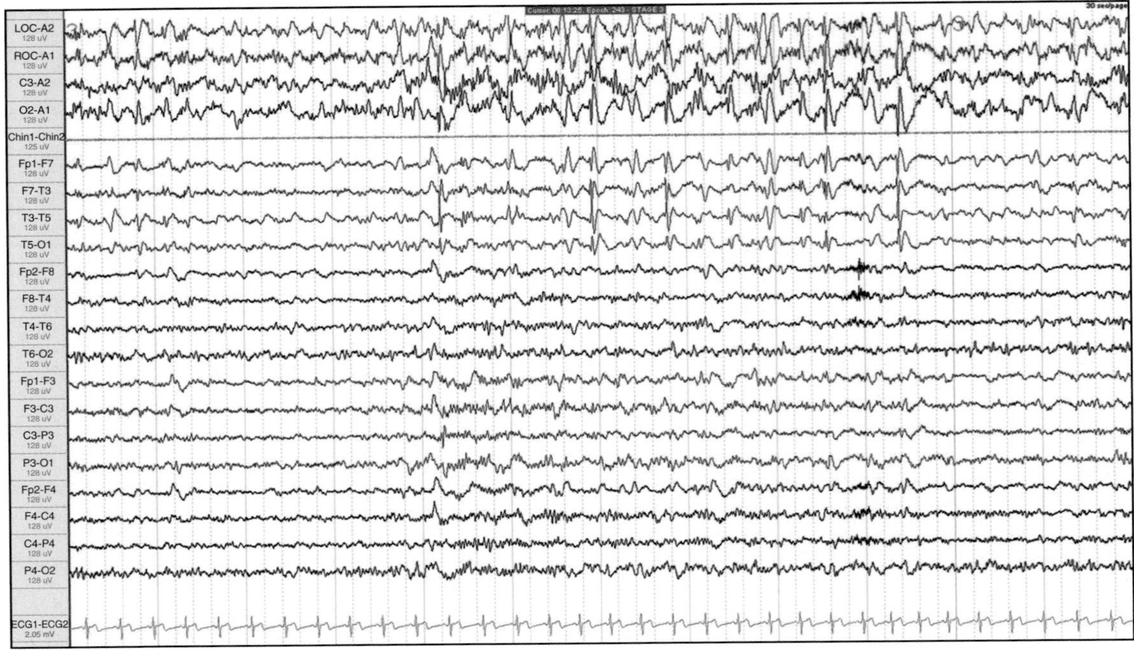

Figure 18-104.
Seizure disorder. Very periodic spikes emanating from the left midtemporal region (without clinical correlates). Localization would not be possible on the conventional sleep scoring montage. The window is 30 sec. (Courtesy of M. Mahowald.)

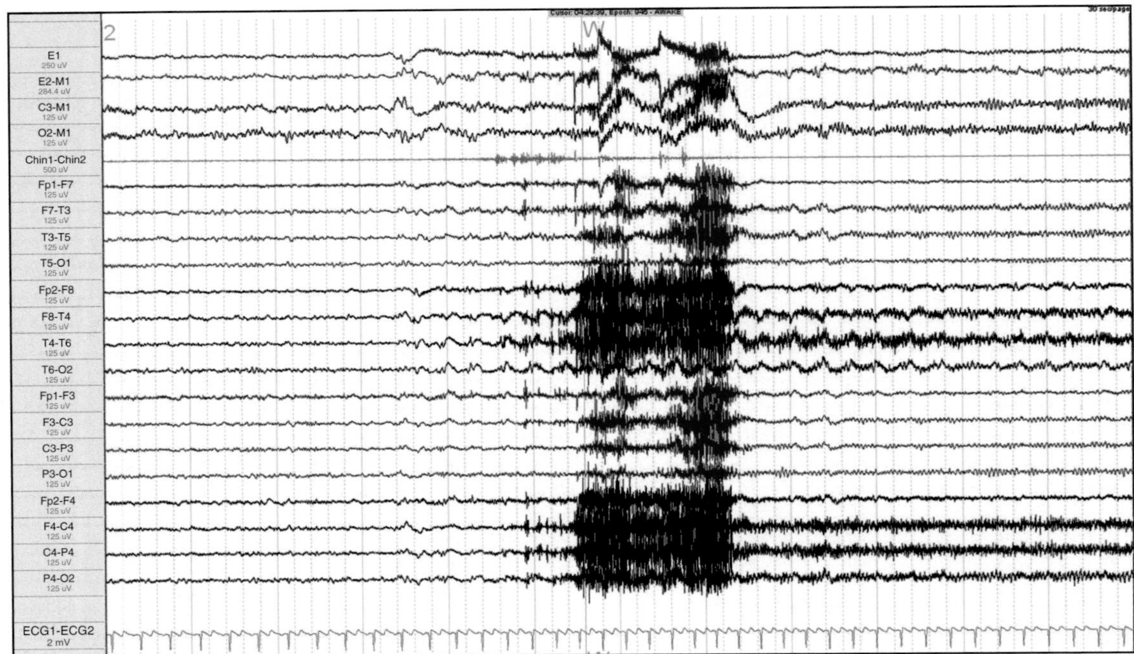

Figure 18-105.
Seizure disorder. On the conventional sleep scoring montage, this would appear to be a simple, nonspecific arousal. The EEG montage reveals periodic spikes from the right midtemporal region culminating in an arousal followed by residual postictal slowing over the same region. This "arousal" was actually the sole clinical manifestation of a focal temporal lobe epileptic discharge. (These may occur hundreds of times a night, resulting in frequent arousals [sleep fragmentation] presenting as excessive daytime sleepiness.) For this reason, it is prudent to employ a full seizure montage in all patients with a history of seizures and the complaint of excessive daytime sleepiness. If these arousals are associated with extremity movements, an erroneous diagnosis of PLMS might be made. The window is 30 sec. (Courtesy of M. Mahowald.)

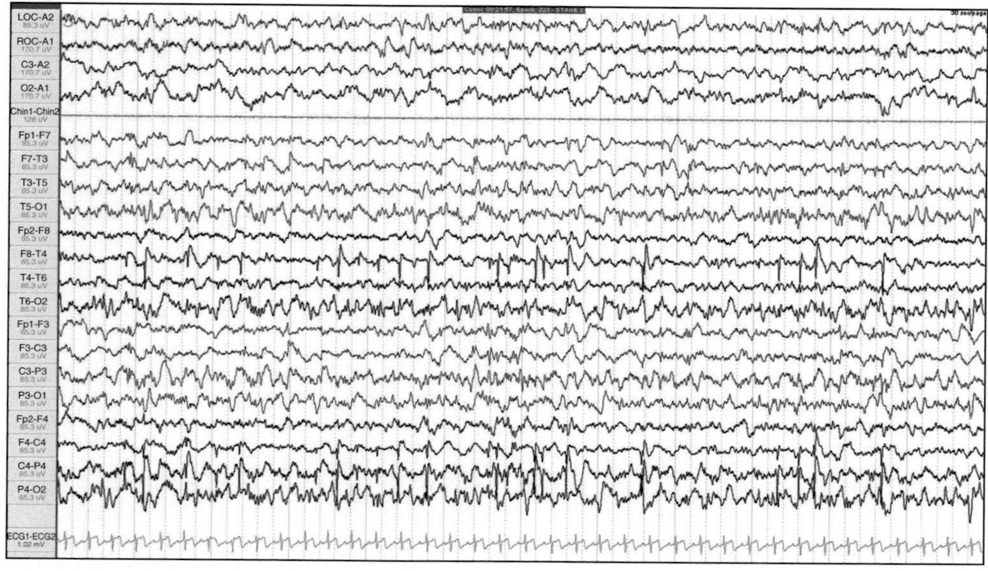

Figure 18-106.
Seizure disorder. These spikes are characteristic of "Rolandic" spikes (seen in benign Rolandic epilepsy). The spikes are most prominent over the central and midtemporal regions. They are often only present during NREM sleep, when they may become very active. Clinically, there may be twitching of the mouth on the contralateral side with or without drooling. Occasionally these usually trivial seizures will generalize. The prognosis is generally very good, with a natural history of spontaneous resolution over time, hence the name "benign Rolandic epilepsy." Epoch length is 15 seconds. (Courtesy of M. Mahowald.)

HEAD TRAUMA

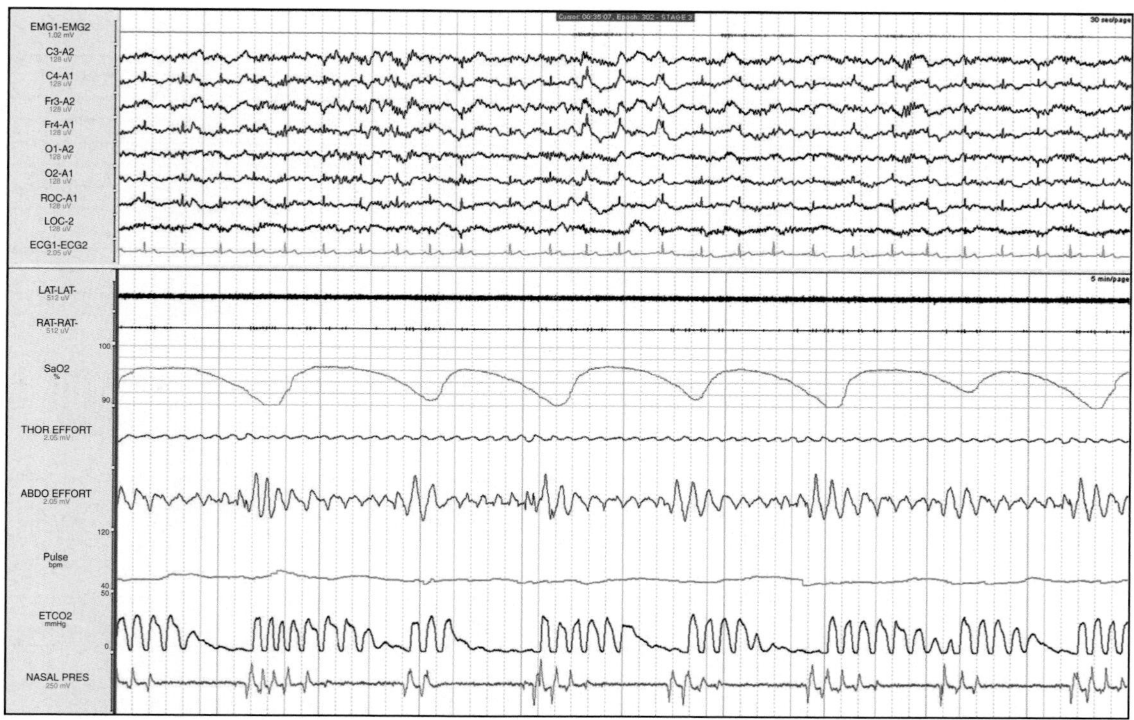

Figure 18-107.
Head trauma in NREM sleep. As a result of head trauma and fractures of his jaw and facial structures, this 57-year-old patient spent 3 years in the hospital for rehabilitation. He had a periodic breathing pattern, but there was no history of snoring. During the sleep study, one could not hear this patient breathe.

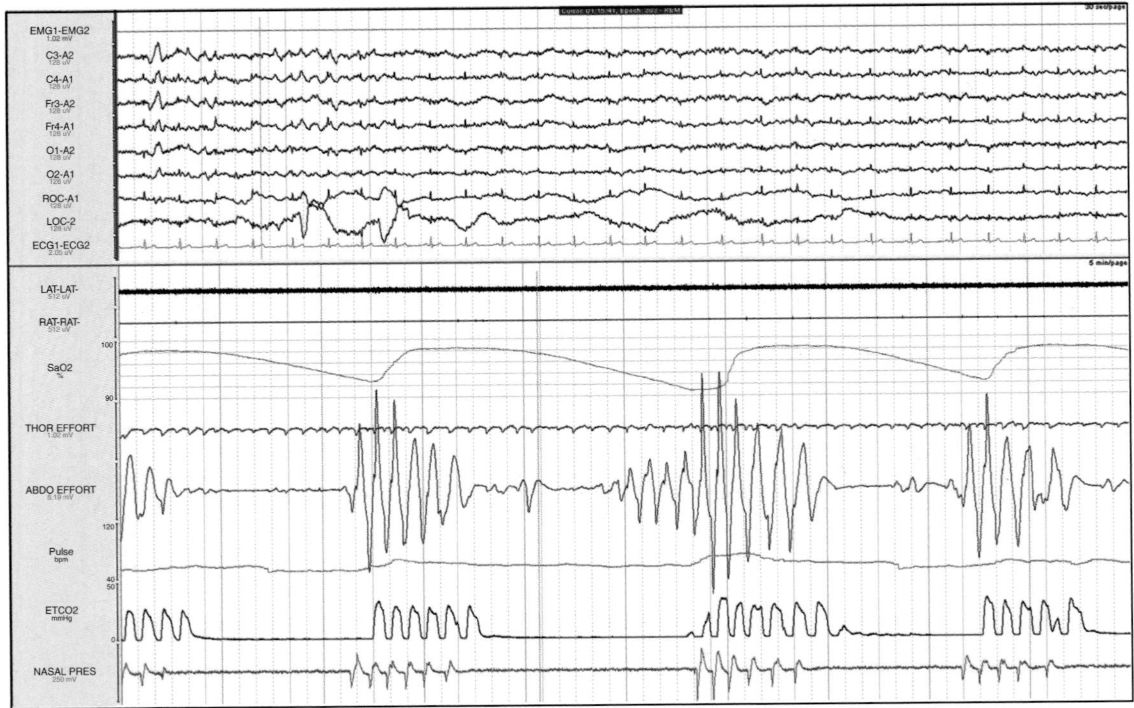

Figure 18-108.
Head trauma in REM sleep. Same patient as in Figure 18-107. The breathing pattern now has the configuration of Cheyne Stokes breathing, with long central apneic episodes. The patient had an underlying breathing pattern that was slow. During the 5-minute epoch seen in the lower window, he had fewer than 30 breaths. The top window is 30 sec; the bottom is 5 min.

Multiple Sclerosis

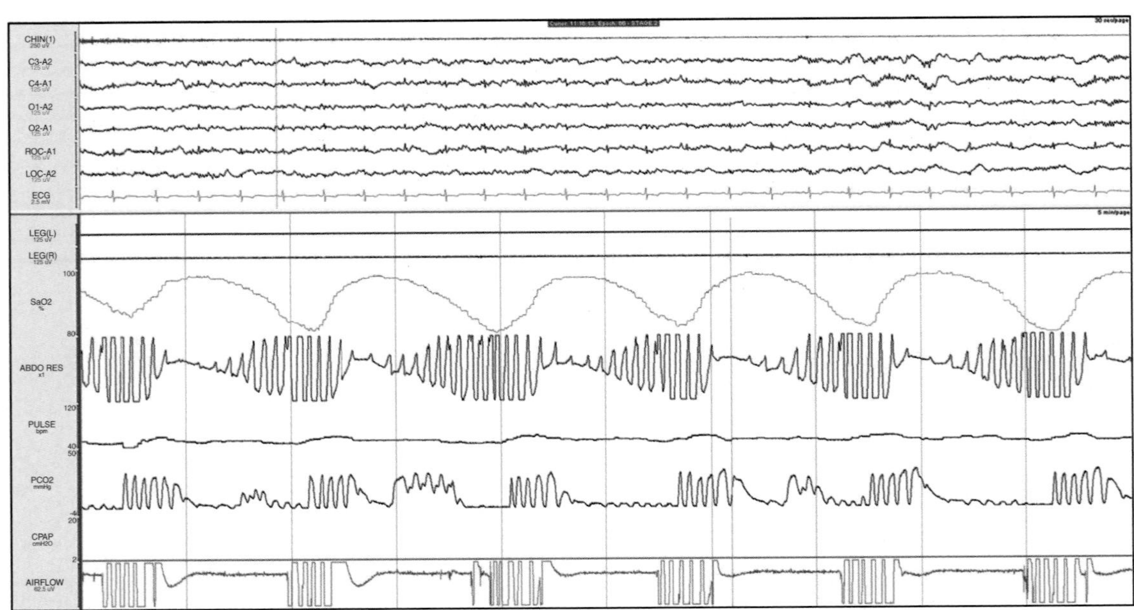

Figure 18-109.
Multiple sclerosis. This PSG fragment is taken from a 56-year-old male with a 5-year history of multiple sclerosis. The main symptom was severe daytime sleepiness. He had put on between 50 and 60 pounds since the diagnosis of multiple sclerosis. During wakefulness, the patient had central apnea; during sleep, shown here, the patient demonstrated mixed apnea episodes. The top window is 30 sec; the bottom is 5 min.

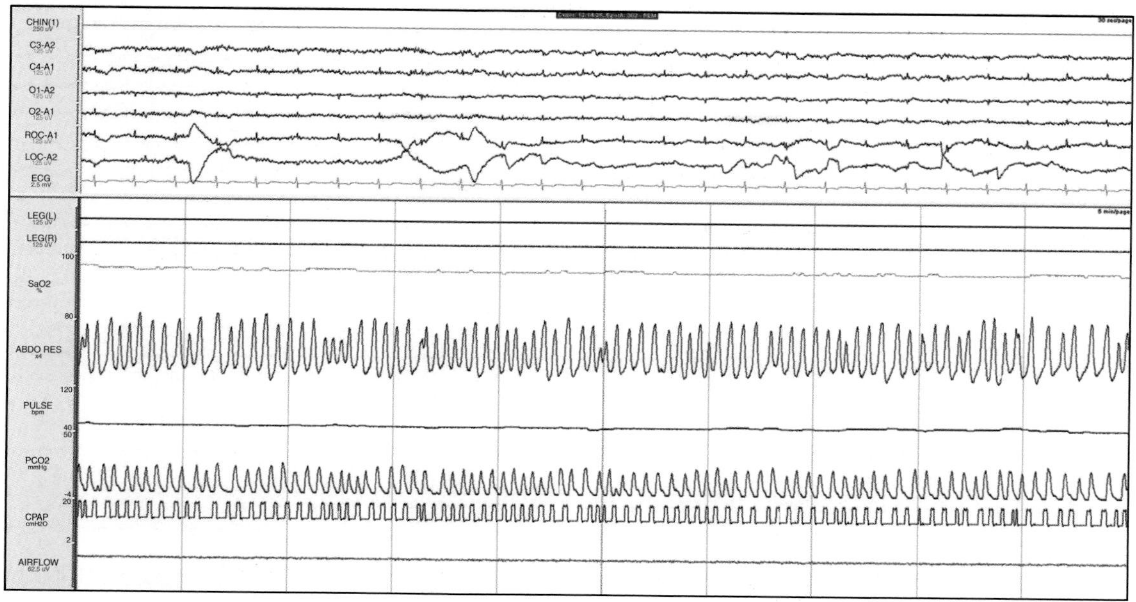

Figure 18-110.
Multiple sclerosis. Same patient as in Figure 18-109. The patient, now in REM sleep, was treated with a bilevel device, which led to resolution of his mixed apneas. He had a great deal of REM sleep on starting bilevel treatment. The top window is 30 sec; the bottom is 5 min.

Artifacts in Sleep Recordings

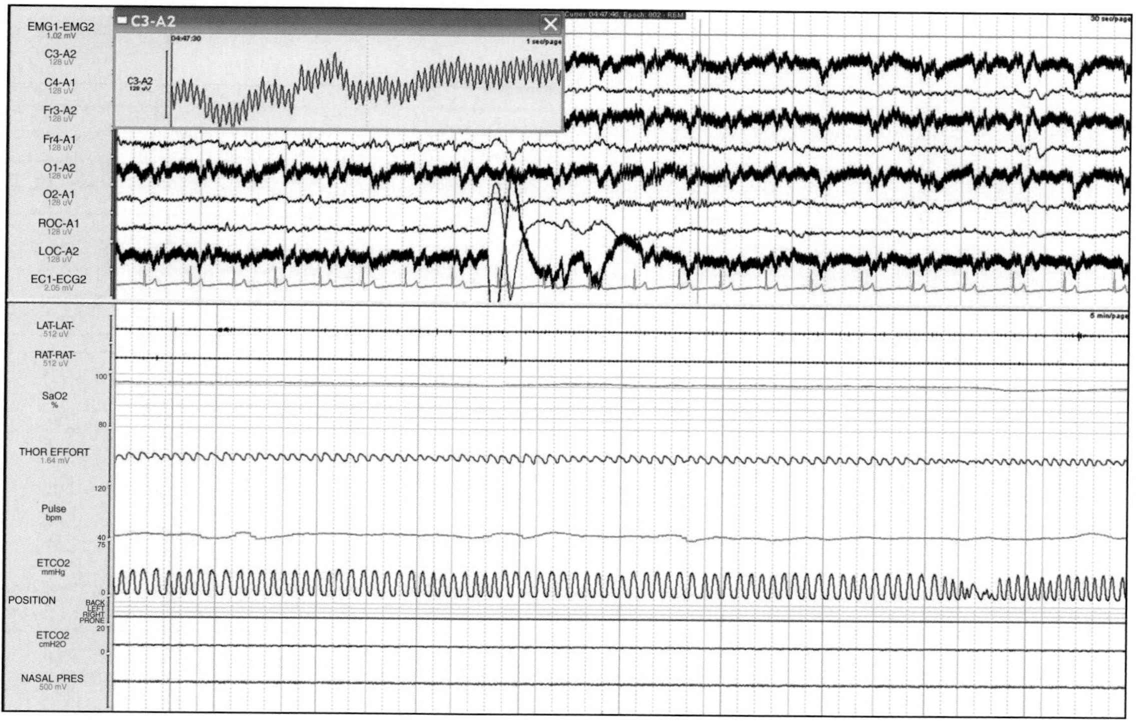

Figure 18-111.
60 Hz interference. Note the obvious broad band of black that appears in four of the channels. Modern data acquisition systems allow the frequency analysis (visual or numerical) of channels. The inset, which shows 1 second of one of the channels, clearly shows that there is an underlying 60 Hz wave in the channel. This is 60-cycle electrical interference. Lead A2 is the cause, because that artifact was found in all the channels that include this lead. Figure 18-112 shows ways of dealing with such noise. The top window is 30 sec.

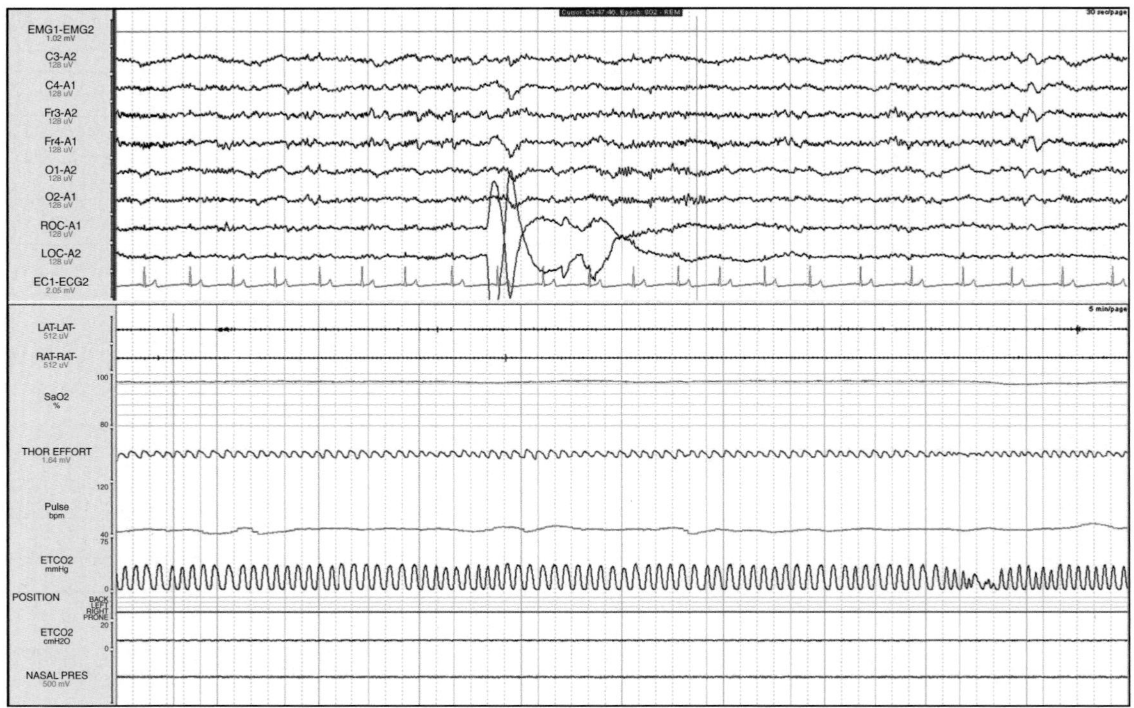

Figure 18-112.
60 Hz interference corrected. This is the same epoch as in Figure 18-111, except that the montage has been modified so that the A1 lead is used instead of lead A2. Digital filters can also be used to remove 60 Hz noise.

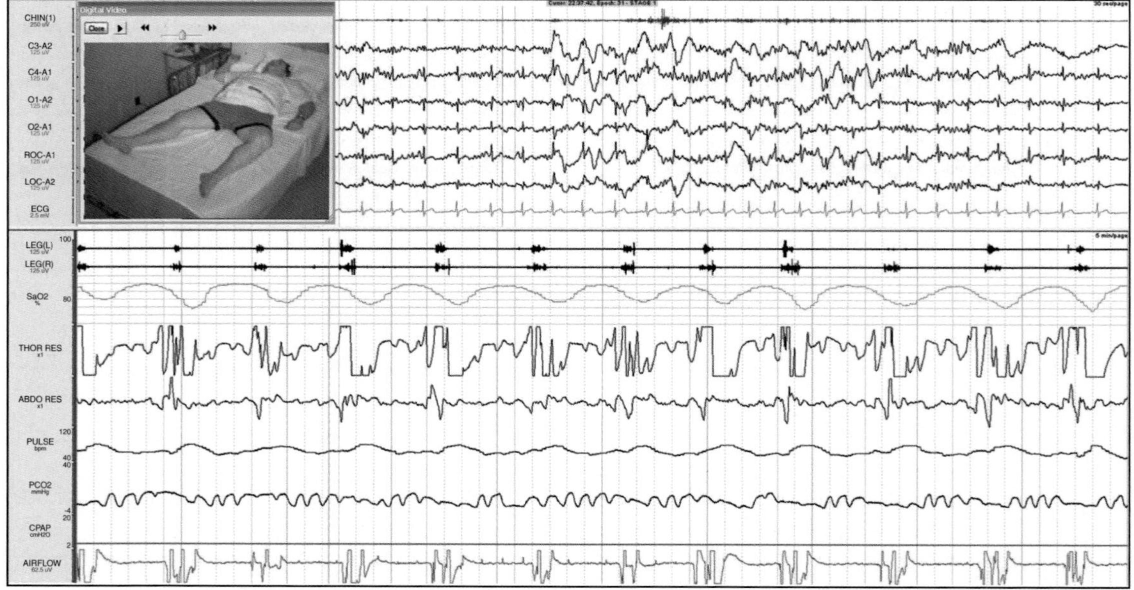

Figure 18-113.
Artifacts affecting EEG and respiratory channels. What is the main finding in this epoch? Is it leg movements or sleep apnea? There is an EKG artifact in all the EEG channels. That sometimes makes scoring for sleep stage difficult. In the bottom window there is an artifact affecting both the thoracic and abdominal respiration channels. The leg movements and breathing are very closely linked; leg movements occur precisely during the peak of respiratory effort. Many would interpret this as the apneas causing the movements. This is a situation in which examining the synchronized video is helpful. The orange vertical lines synchronize the upper (30 sec) and lower (5 min) windows.

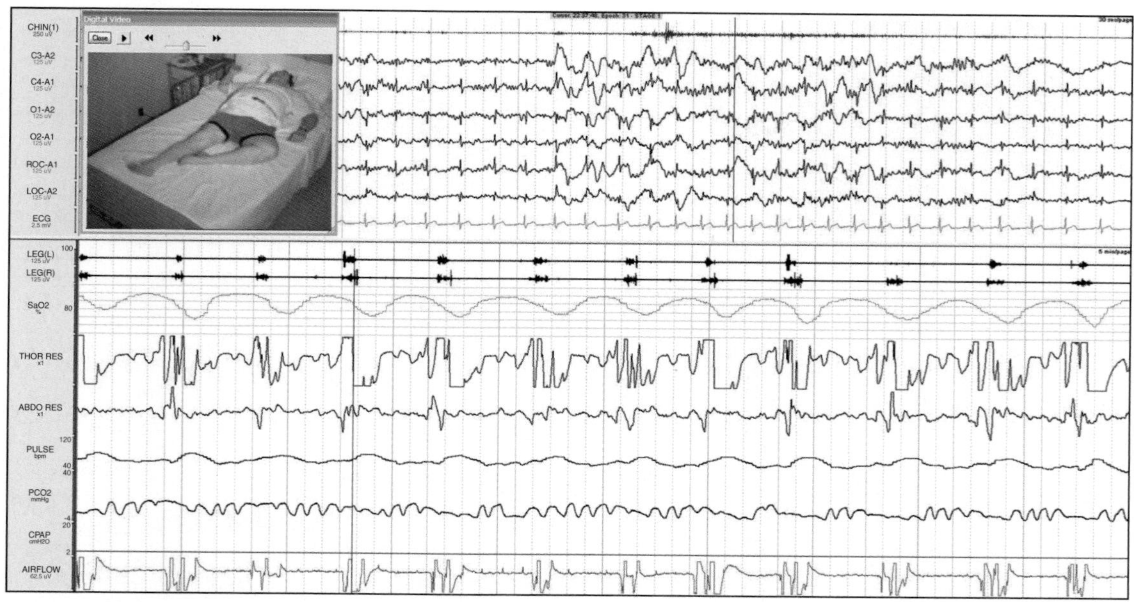

Figure 18-114.
Artifacts affecting EEG and respiratory channels. The vertical orange lines have moved forward about 5.5 seconds. An arousal has occurred in the EEG channels. There has been a dramatic movement of the legs evident in the synchronized digital video. The question still remains whether the apneas are causing the movements. The answer comes in the fragment shown in Figure 18-115, after the patient has been placed on CPAP.

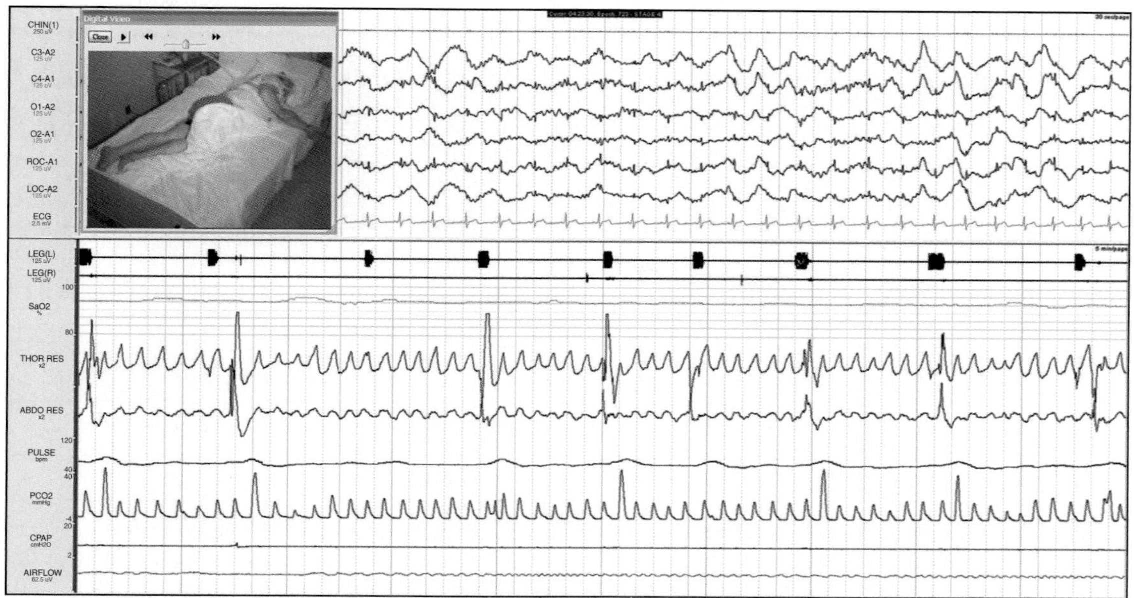

Figure 18-115.
Artifacts affecting EEG and respiratory channels. With the above patient placed on CPAP, the apneas have been abolished, but the movements remain. Notice that they still cause an artifact in the thoracic and abdominal channels. Notice also that each twitch is associated with a reproducible increase in heart rate, suggesting that subcortical arousals are recurring. The nasal pressure channel reflects the pressure being delivered by the CPAP machine. The patient is in stage N3.

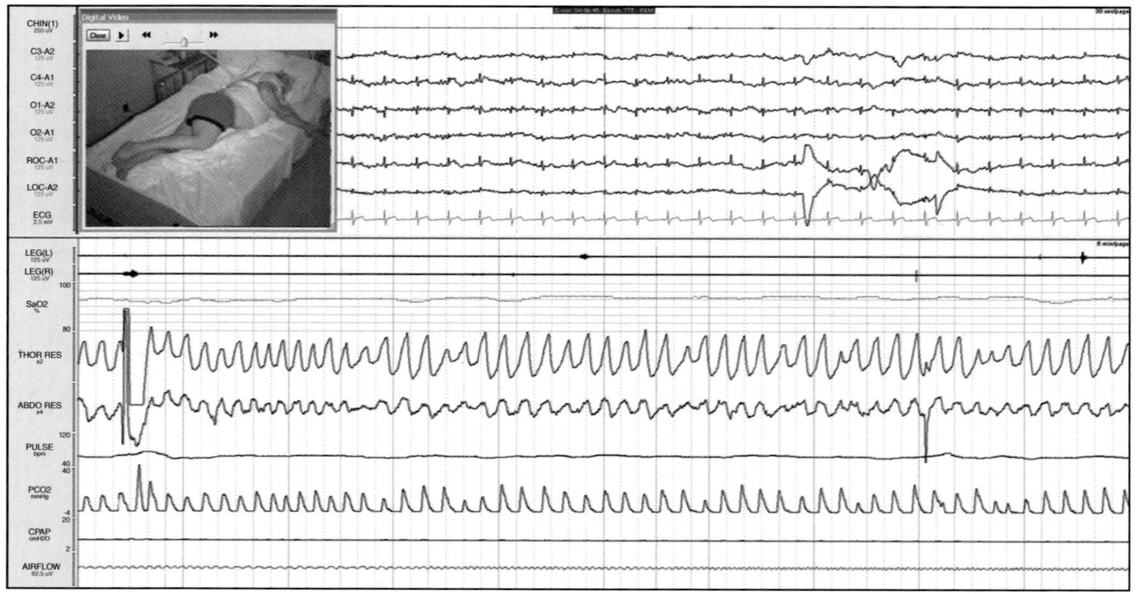

Figure 18-116.
Artifacts affecting EEG and respiratory channels. The patient is now in REM sleep. There has been a dramatic decrease in both the leg movements and the artifacts in the thoracic and abdominal channels. The EEG still contains EKG artifact. Notice the regular movements in the two eye channels. This patient has both obstructive sleep apnea and periodic limb movements in sleep.

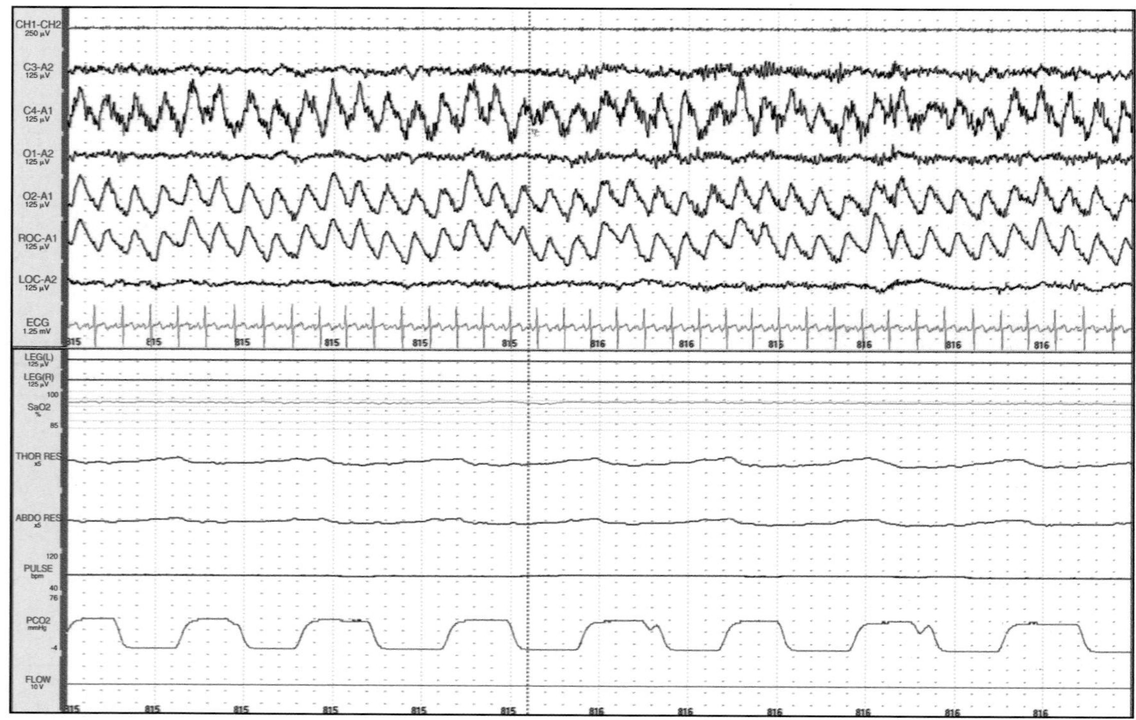

Figure 18-117.
Cardiac artifact in EEG. There are two types of cardiac artifacts that may be observed in the EEG. One is caused by the transmission of electrical waves from the EKG to the EEG (seen in Fig. 18-116), whereas the other is related to, or caused by, a beating heart. Here, three of the EEG channels have a high-amplitude sinusoidal wave embedded in them. These waves are exactly synchronous with the heartbeat. In addition, examination reveals that the three channels have something in common, that is, an A1 electrode as one of the pair. Figure 18-118 shows how this is remedied. Both windows are 30 sec.

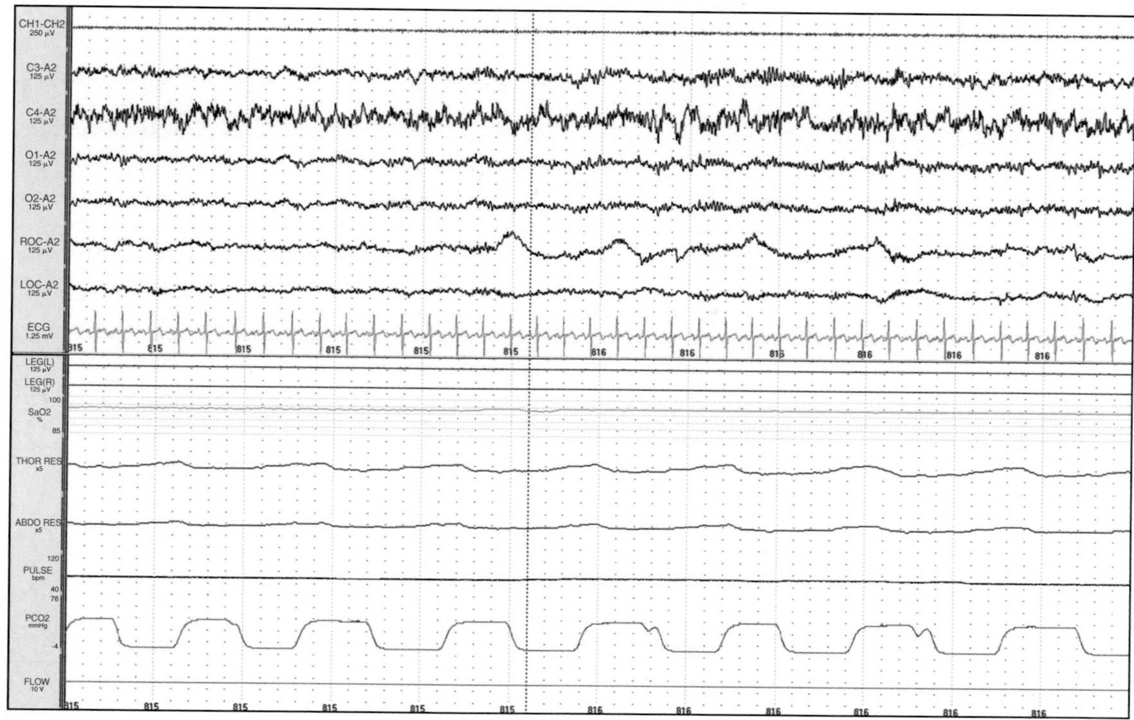

Figure 18-118.
Cardiac artifact in EEG rectified. This is the same epoch as shown in Figure 18-117. Modern computer systems allow the user to digitally re-reference electrode pairs. By removing A1 from the montage and using A2 instead, the problem has been solved. Presumably the original artifact was caused by motion that affected the A1 electrode. This is a 30-sec epoch.

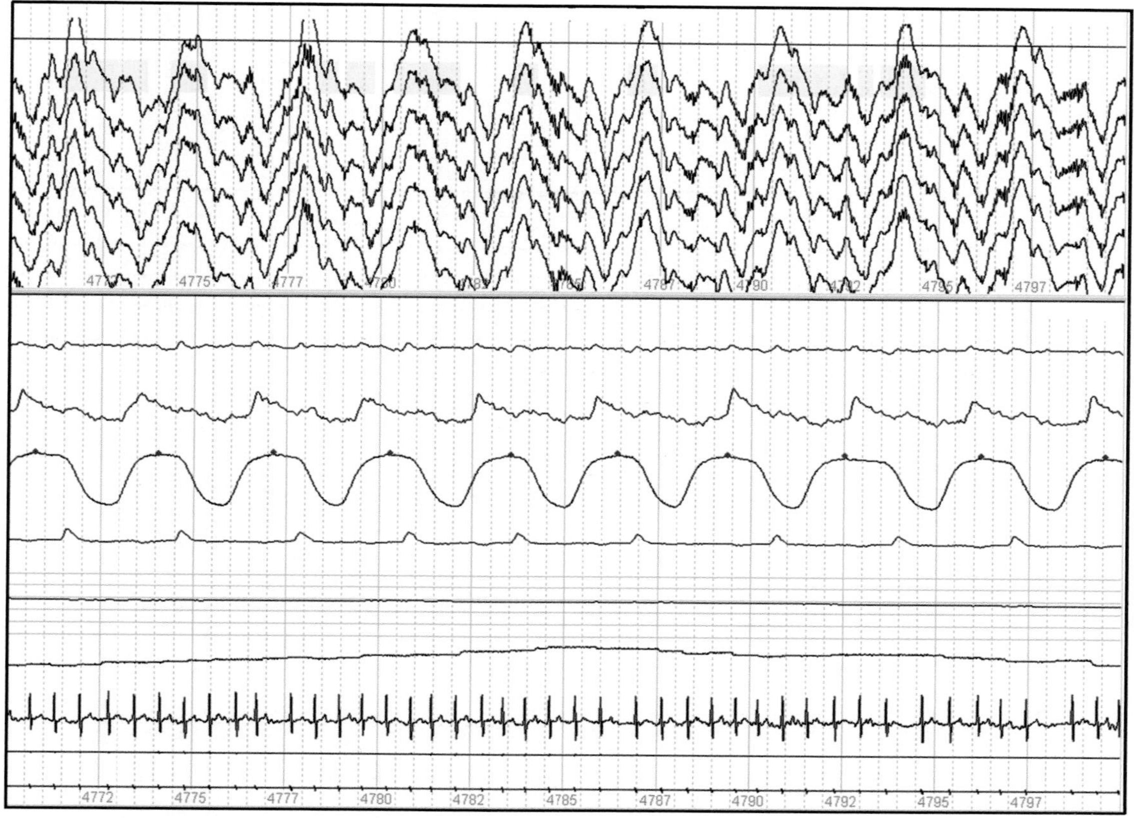

Figure 18-119.
When an artifact helps make a diagnosis. Here, there is a very high-amplitude, low-frequency wave superimposed on all the EEG channels. Clearly the high-amplitude deflections are synchronous with breathing. The technician might call this a sweat artifact, but it is really a breathing artifact in a sweaty patient. This patient did indeed have severe night sweats, and the EKG showed atrial fibrillation. Based on the clues presented in this PSG fragment, the patient was evaluated for hyperthyroidism, and the diagnosis was confirmed. This is a 30-sec epoch.

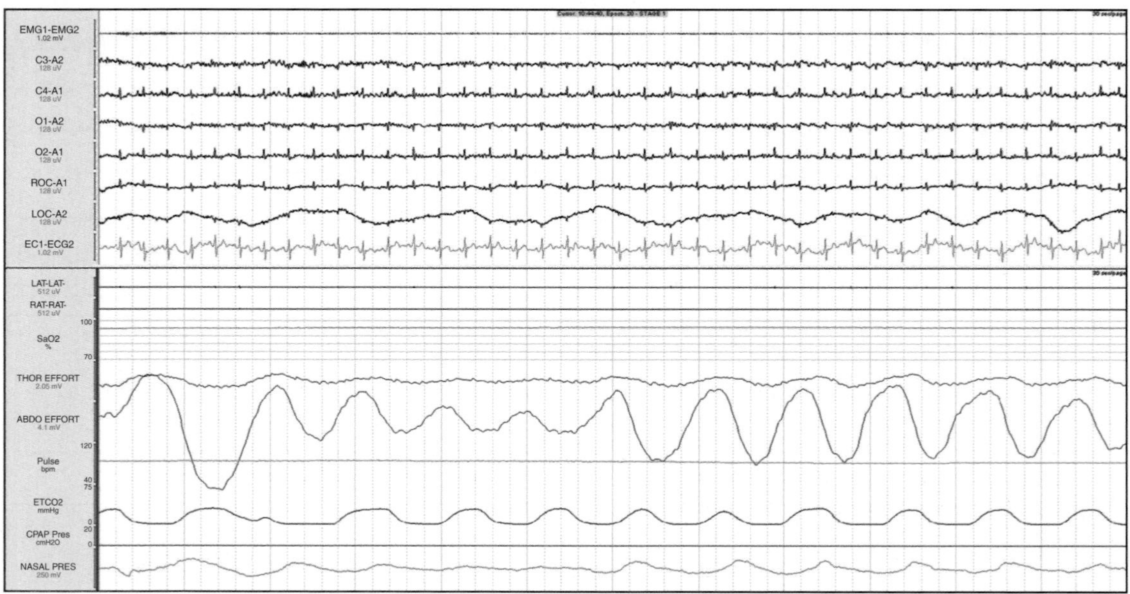

Figure 18-120.
Eye channel artifacts. Scoring technicians most often have no contact with the patient whose study they are scoring. Nighttime technicians are often too busy to evaluate findings that are abnormal and therefore may attribute them to artifact. Here, at the beginning of the night, there was a low-frequency oscillation in the left eye channel that was dismissed as probably a breathing artifact.

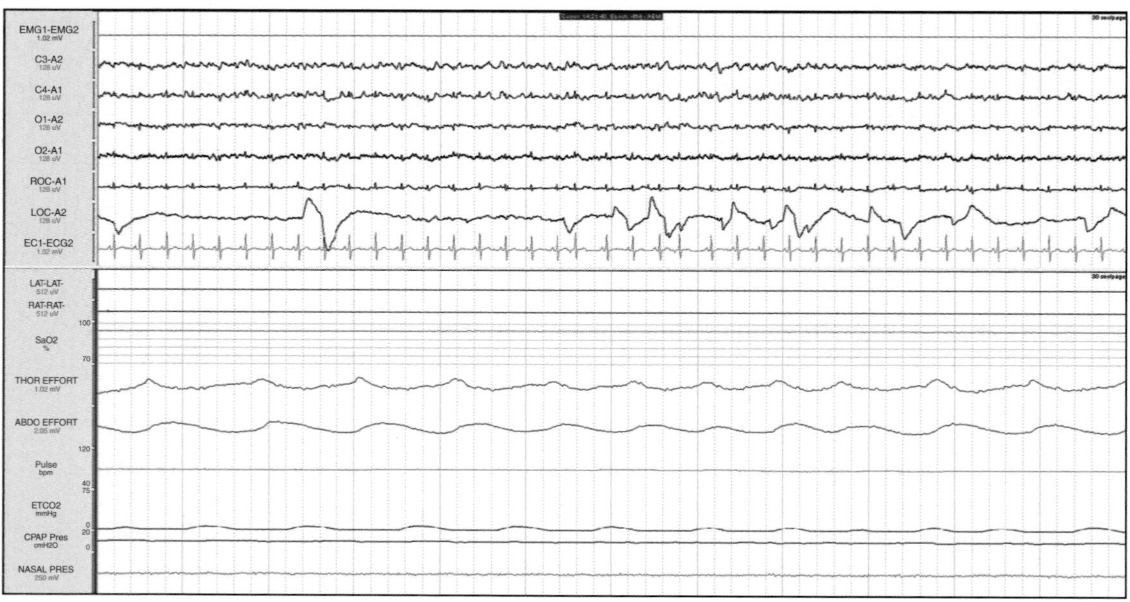

Figure 18-121.
Eye channel artifacts. Originally the patient was scored as having no REM sleep. The eye movements in the left eye channel were interpreted as being artifacts. The clinician who evaluated the patient later that morning examined the patient's extraocular movements, shown in Figure 18-122.

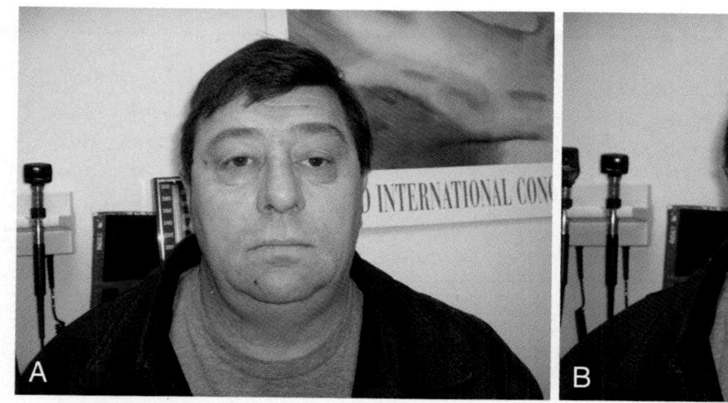
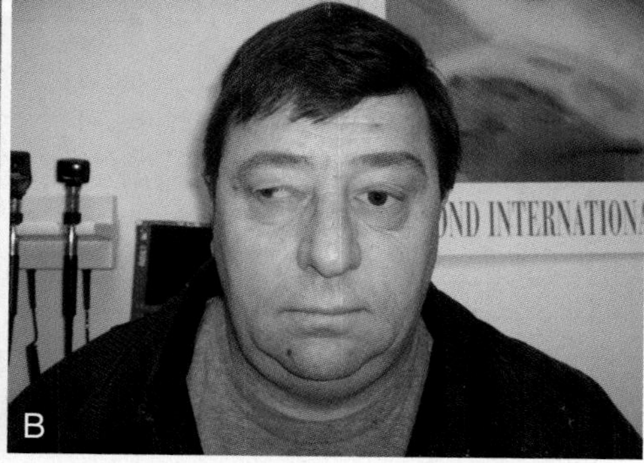

Figure 18-122.
Eye channel artifacts. **A,** When the patient looked straight ahead, everything seemed normal. **B,** When he was asked to look to his right, only his right eye moved. What is going on, and how did this affect the eye channels the previous night? The patient had a left glass eye. What the EOG channel was detecting was only the movements of the right eye. Figure 18-121 actually does show REM sleep. The night technician had also mixed up the right and left eye channels and was actually recording movements of the right eye.

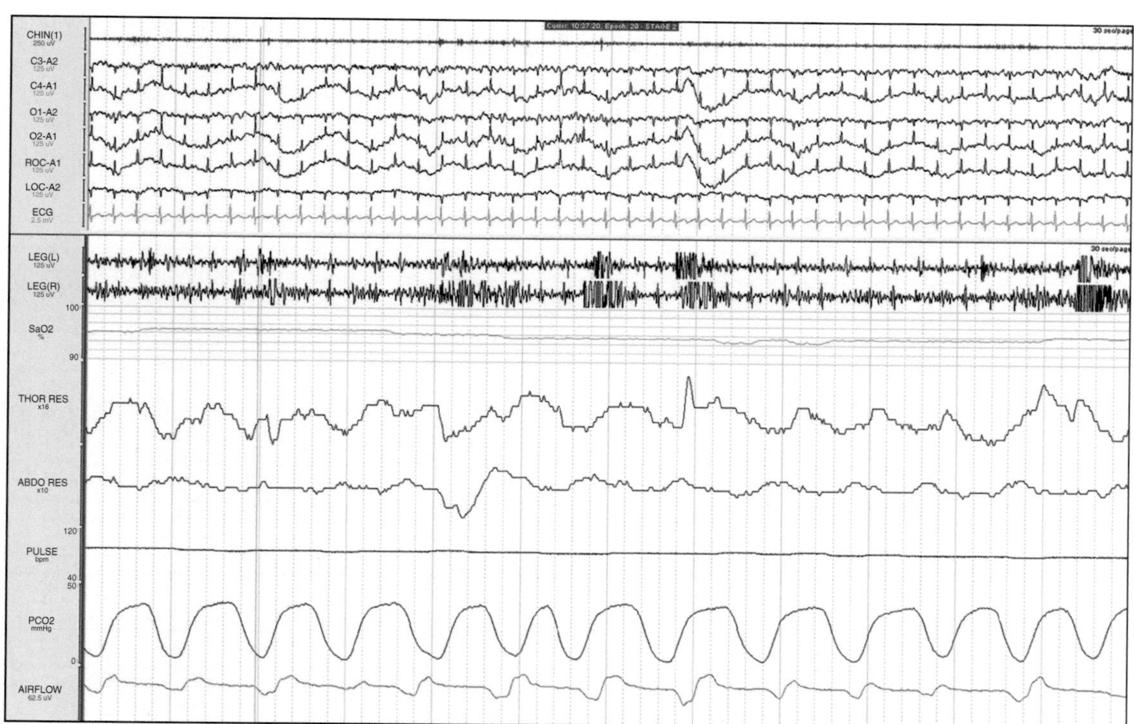

Figure 18-123.
Recording artifact in both leg channels. An artifact-free leg movement recording could not be attained in this patient. She had massive peripheral edema related to right heart failure. There was probably 2 cm of edema fluid between the recording electrode and the anterior tibialis muscle. The EMG channels were not recording EMG but were recording electrical noise.

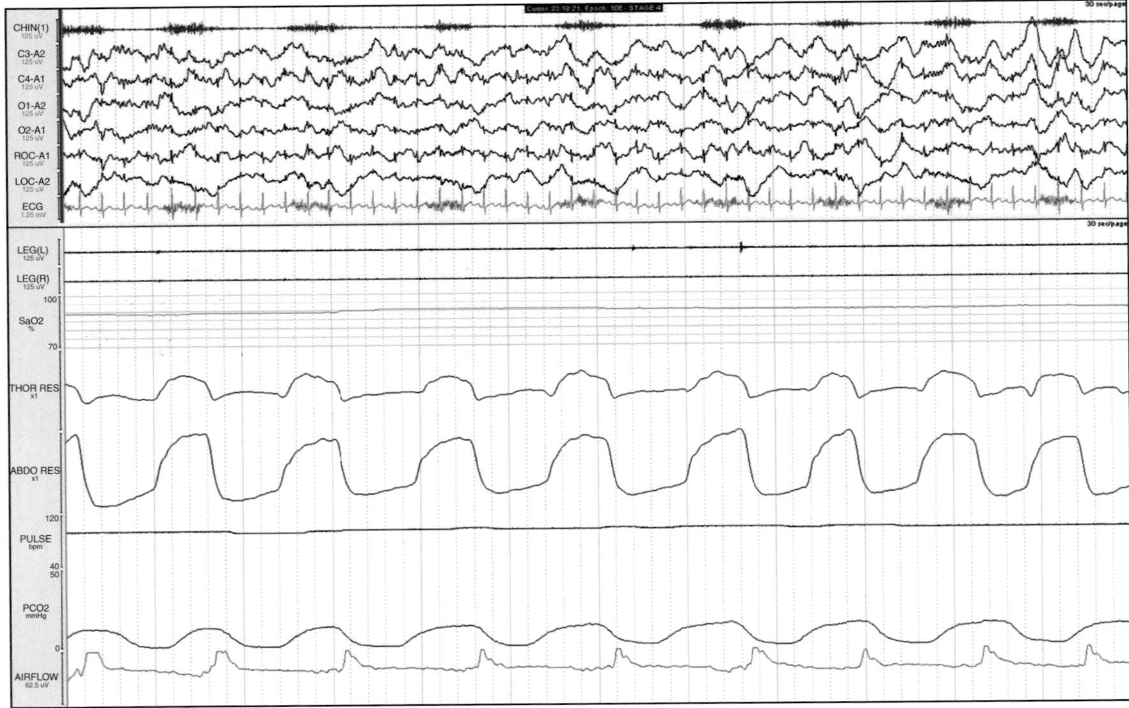

Figure 18-124.
Periodic artifact in the chin EMG and in the EKG. High-frequency noise is present with regular periodicity in both the chin EMG and EKG. The noise is clearly linked to the patient's breathing and is actually being caused by snoring. The top and bottom windows are 30 sec.

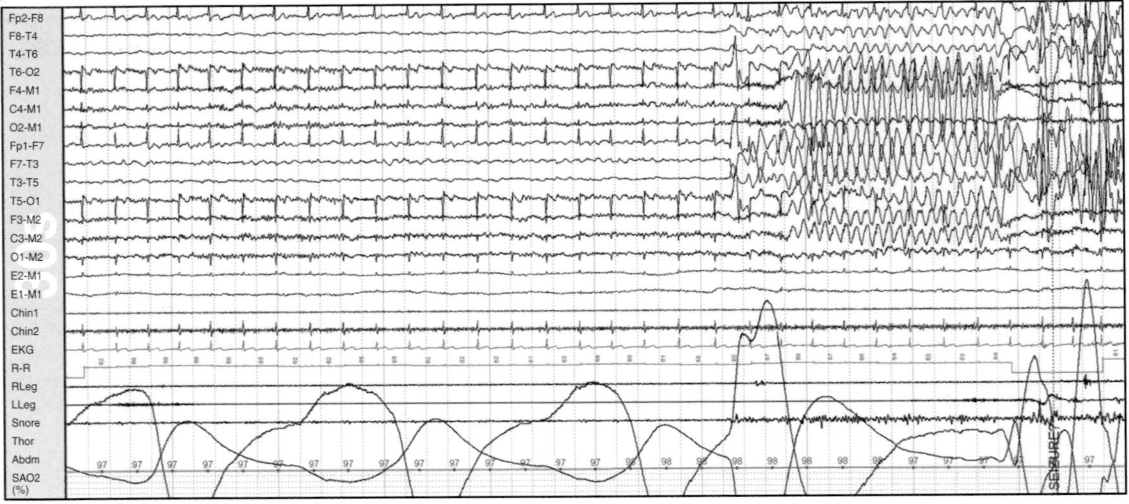

Figure 18-125.
A seizure? The scoring technician, on observing the high-amplitude activity and EEG channels at the end of this epoch, scored the event as a seizure. Synchronized digital video showed that the patient was simply scratching himself at this time. One should always view the synchronized digital video when such a finding is made. Notice also the EKG artifact in most of the EEG channels. This is a 30-sec epoch.

GALLERY OF PATIENT INTERVIEW VIDEOS

CHAPTER 19

Meir Kryger

The video clips referred to here are of interviews of patients with sleep disorders and can be seen on the Web at www.expertconsult.com.

Sleep-related Breathing Disorders

AN 8-YEAR-OLD WITH SLEEP APNEA (VIDEO 1)

This 8-year-old has a strong family history of sleep apnea and is being treated with continuous positive airway pressure (CPAP). He had cardiovascular complications of apnea.

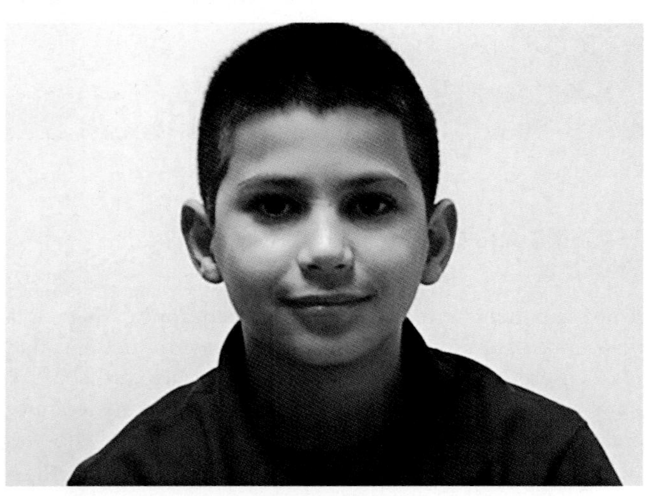

AN 82-YEAR-OLD WOMAN WITH SLEEP APNEA (VIDEO 2)

This woman, aged 82, had been on CPAP for 13 years.

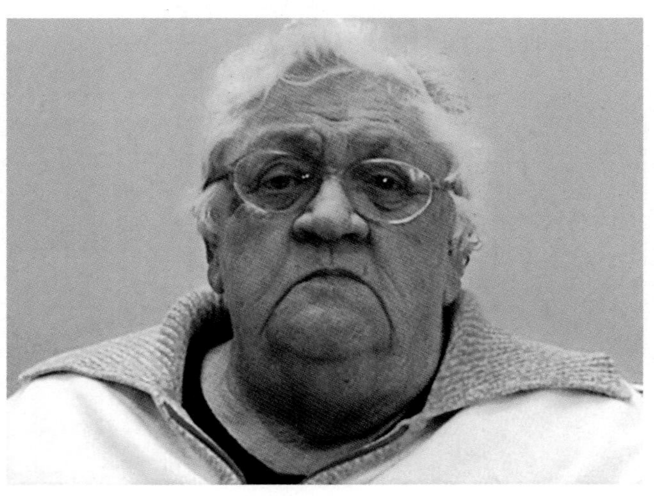

A 43-YEAR-OLD WOMAN WITH DOWN SYNDROME (VIDEO 3)

This woman with Down syndrome had sleep apnea.

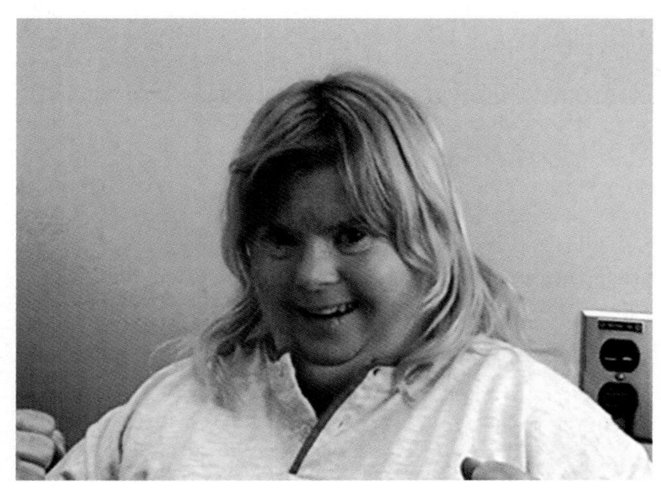

APNEA WITH CARDIOVASCULAR COMORBIDITIES (VIDEO 4)

This patient had heart failure and treatment-resistant hypertension that resolved with treatment.

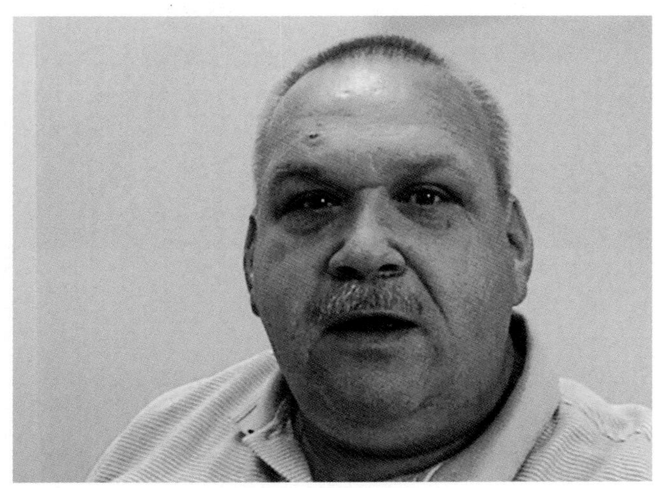

APNEA PRESENTING AS RESTLESS SLEEP (VIDEO 5)

This patient had as his main complaint restless sleep and frequent awakenings. He also had difficulty in walking due to osteoarthritis caused by his weight.

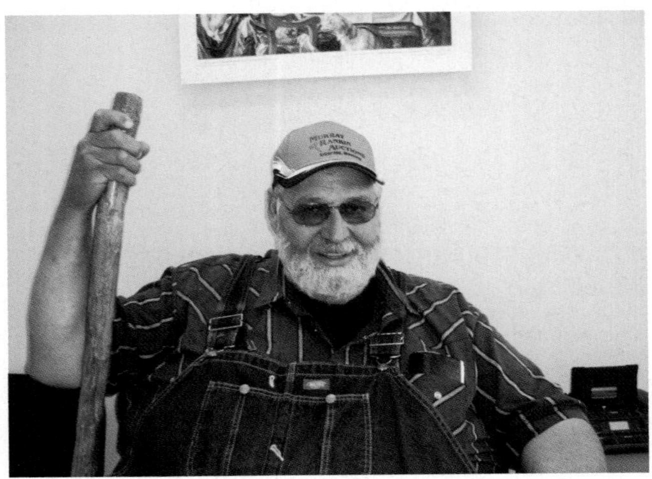

EXPLAINING THE RESULTS (VIDEO 7)

It is extremely important that the patient understand the results of the sleep test. An effective way of accomplishing that is to show the patient the actual study and the synchronized digital video. This is often a "teachable moment" that not only can have a great effect on the patient but also is likely to improve CPAP compliance and motivate the patient to deal with comorbidities.

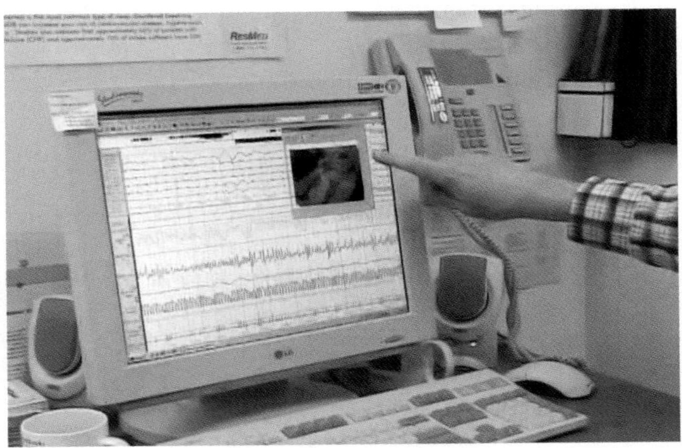

APNEA IN A TRUCK DRIVER (VIDEO 6)

Sleepiness can be particularly dangerous in a truck driver. The patient recounts some near misses while he was driving a truck.

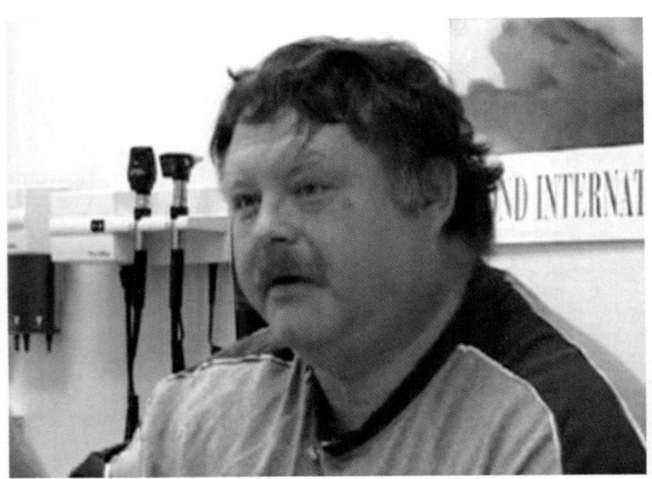

TEACHING AND CPAP MASK FITTING (VIDEO 8)

Once a patient is diagnosed with sleep apnea, there is a very important aspect of management to consider and that is to ensure proper teaching about and fitting of the CPAP mask. If unsuccessful, the patient may become noncompliant and not benefit from treatment. This patient who was being taught about her mask was apprehensive.

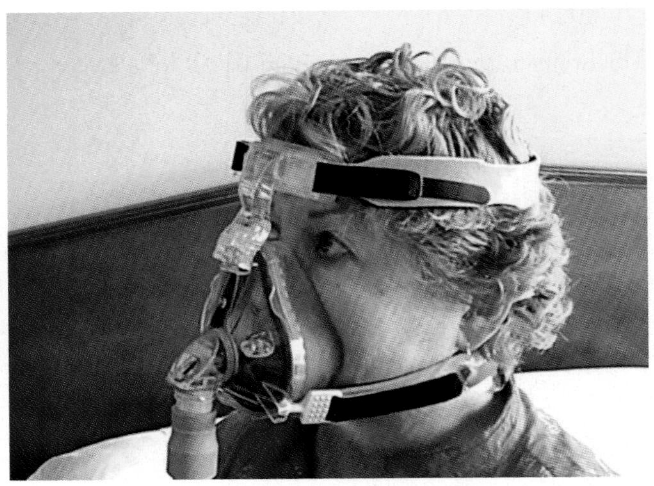

Neurologic and Other Disorders

UNDIAGNOSED NARCOLEPSY PATIENT WITH CATAPLEXY (VIDEO 9)

This young woman was evaluated for the first time and found to have narcolepsy and prominent cataplexy symptoms.

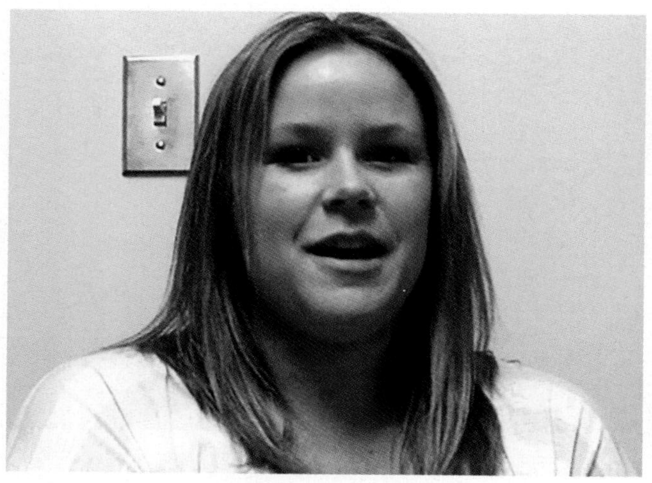

THIRTY-FIVE YEARS OF UNDIAGNOSED NARCOLEPSY (VIDEO 10)

Patients with classic narcolepsy frequently go undiagnosed for decades, as did this patient.

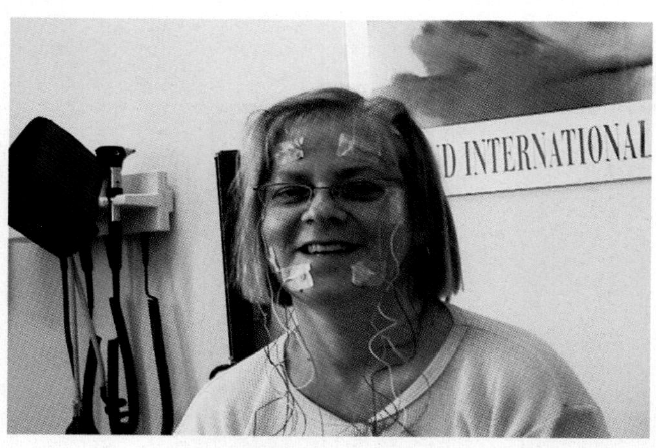

HALLUCINATIONS IN A MALE NARCOLEPSY PATIENT (VIDEO 11)

Vivid hypnagogic hallucinations and dream imagery are common in narcolepsy. Some patients may have the perception that they are floating out of their body. This patient had almost all of the symptoms of narcolepsy.

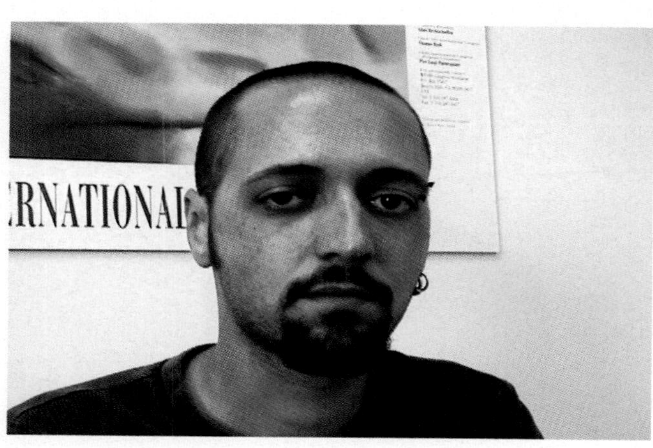

NARCOLEPSY PATIENT WITH SLEEP APNEA (VIDEO 12)

This patient was referred for evaluation because of suspected OSA. The history revealed some classic narcolepsy symptoms.

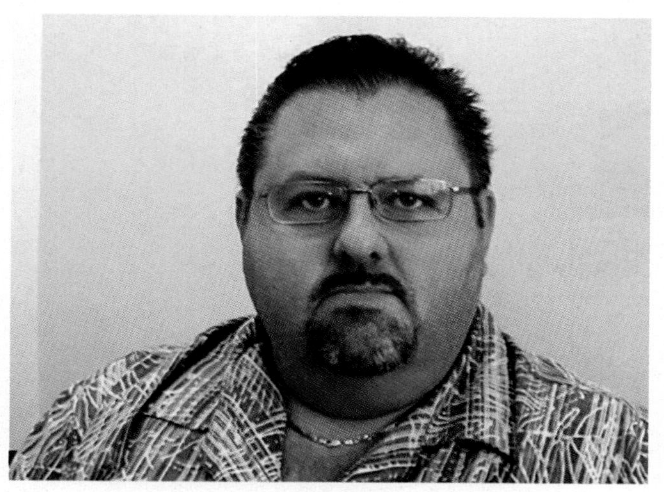

RESTLESS LEGS SYNDROME IN A MALE (VIDEO 13)

Restless legs syndrome is common and is found in all age groups, as in this young adult male. He is French Canadian and the disorder is common in that population.

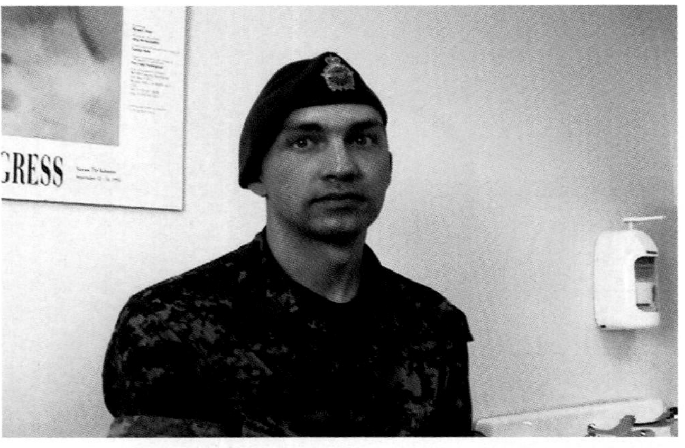

MIDDLE-AGED WOMAN WITH RESTLESS LEGS SYNDROME (VIDEO 14)

Different people use different terms to discuss the sensation of restless legs. This patient said it felt like insects crawling under her skin.

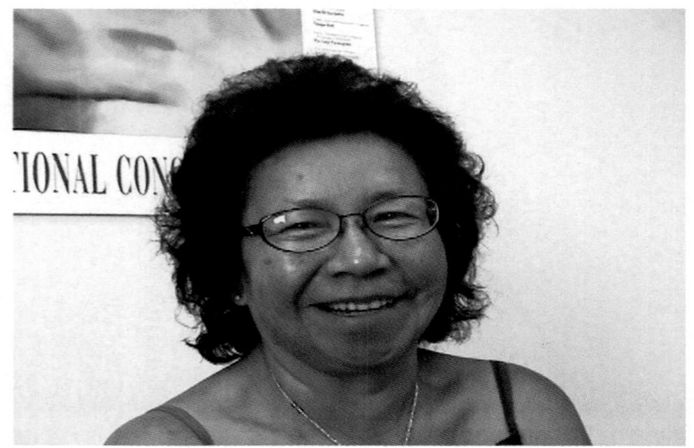

REM SLEEP BEHAVIOR DISORDER (VIDEO 15)

REM sleep behavior disorder can be terrifying. It is a sleep disorder in which the reaction to a dream can result in harm to the patient's bed partner.

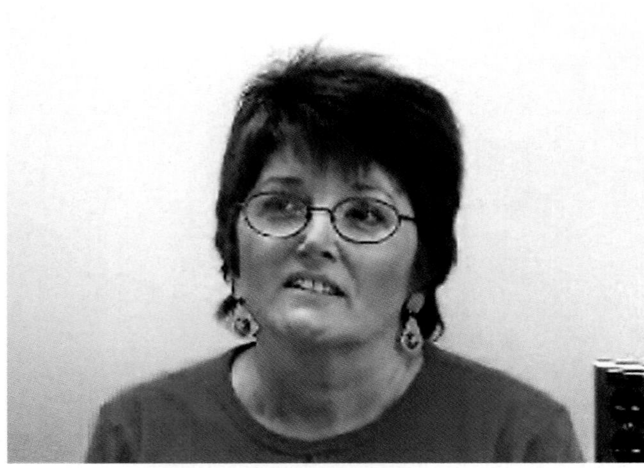

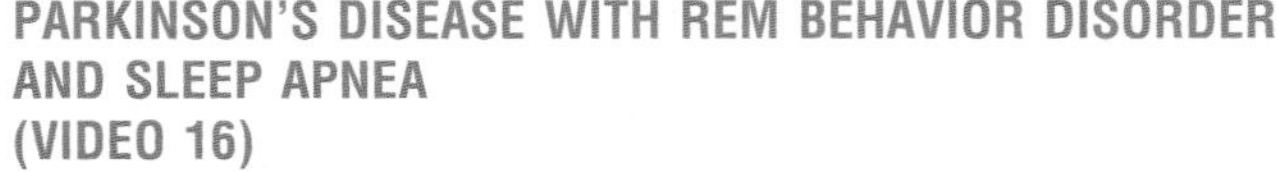

PARKINSON'S DISEASE WITH REM BEHAVIOR DISORDER AND SLEEP APNEA (VIDEO 16)

This patient with Parkinson's disease had several common sleep complications including REM sleep behavior disorder and sleep apnea.

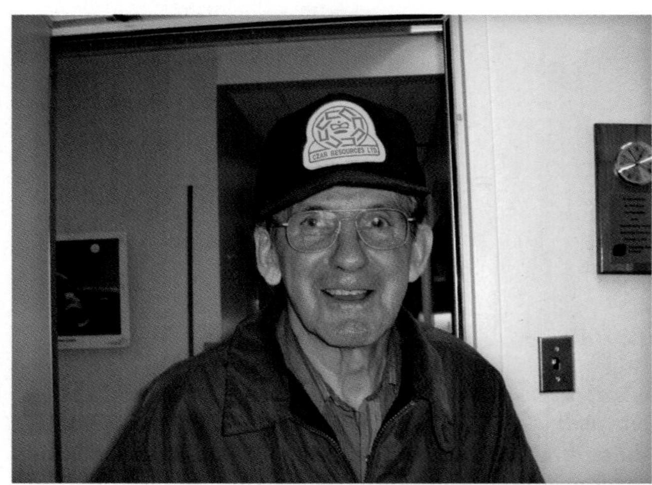

MULTIPLE SCLEROSIS, SLEEP APNEA, AND HYPNAGOGIC HALLUCINATIONS (VIDEO 17)

This patient had multiple sclerosis and developed central apnea that required treatment. He also had the features of narcolepsy.

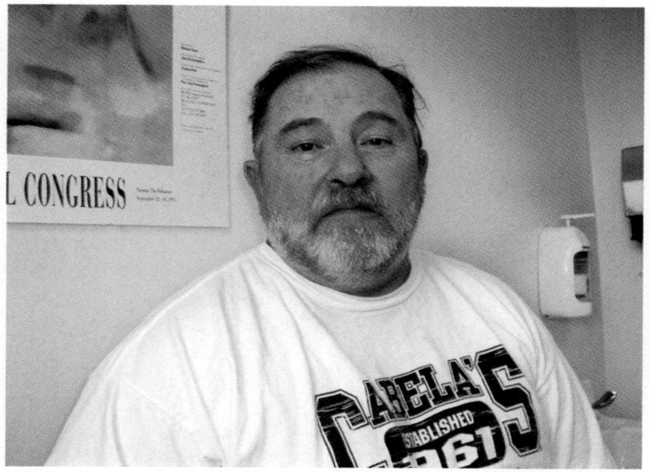

ARNOLD-CHIARI MALFORMATION (VIDEO 18)

Patients with Arnold-Chiari malformation may have abnormal control of breathing and develop sleep apnea.

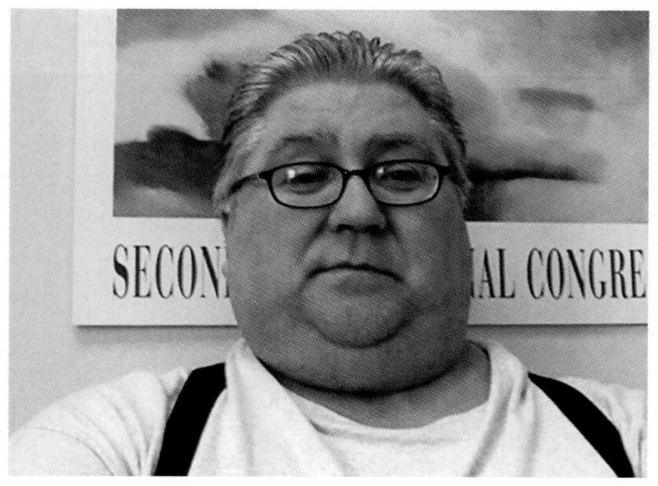

SYRINGOMYELIA (VIDEO 19)

In this patient, the syrinx affected the brain stem. This had an effect not only on the structures that control breathing and the centers involved in REM sleep, but also on the motor pathways that control the legs.

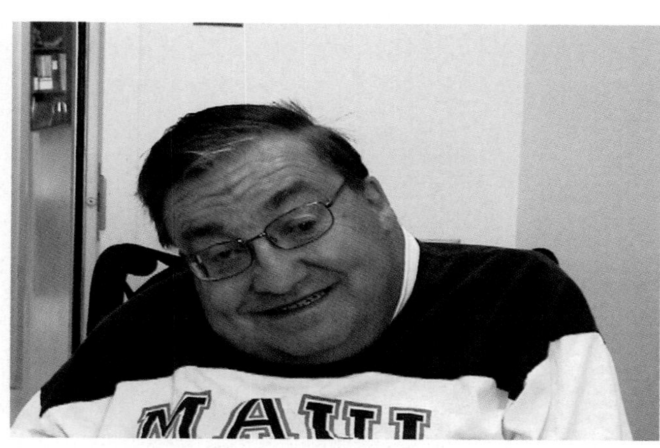

BECKER'S MUSCULAR DYSTROPHY (VIDEO 20)

The muscular dystrophies may be associated with sleep apnea as in this patient with Becker's muscular dystrophy.

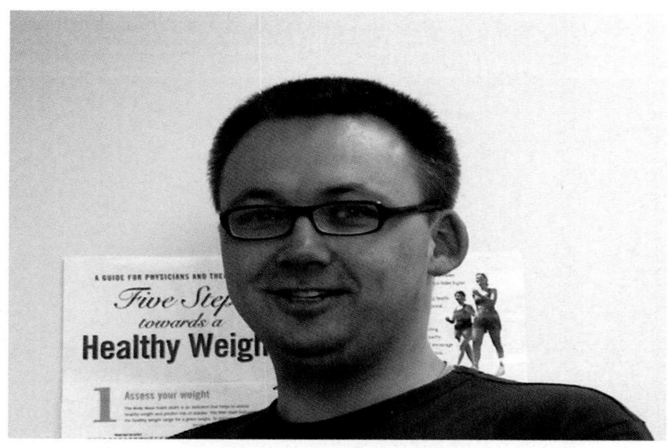

PSYCHIATRIC DISORDERS (VIDEO 21)

Psychiatric disorders and their treatment may result in sleep problems. Hypnagogic hallucinations (in this patient associated with sleep apnea) differ from psychotic hallucinations, and both may be found in the same patient.

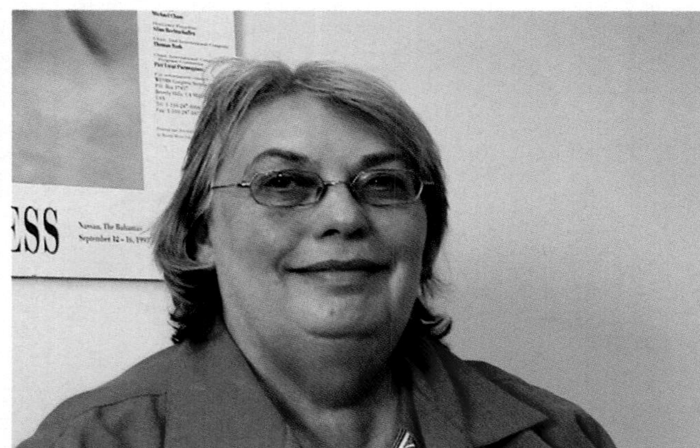

GALLERY OF SLEEP LABORATORY VIDEO FINDINGS

CHAPTER 20

Meir Kryger

This chapter contains examples of video findings obtained in a typical sleep medicine clinic polysomnography lab. They are grouped into categories. Most modern sleep lab acquisition systems allow the collection of synchronized digital videos. The videos can be played back in real time or can be sped up. Video clips referred to here are of patients with sleep disorders obtained during sleep studies and can be seen on the Web at www.expertconsult.com.

Obstructive Sleep Apnea

APNEA, RESTLESSNESS IN CHILD

This 12-year-old boy presented with restless sleep. This is a common presentation of sleep apnea in children of all ages. The restlessness is often present the entire night (Video 22).

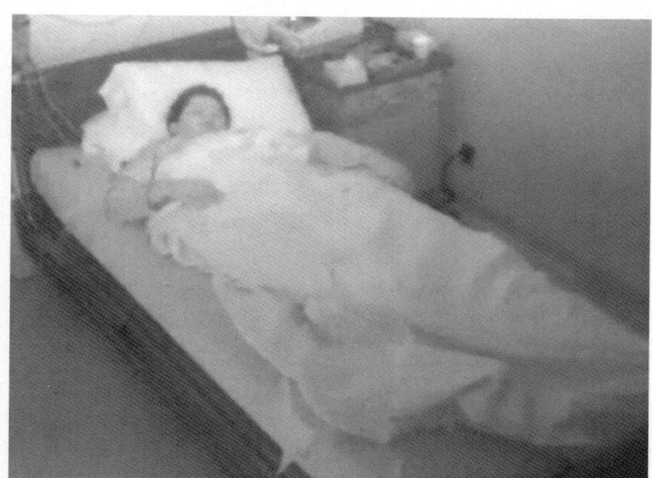

NASAL OBSTRUCTION AND APNEA

This patient had been a boxer, had his nose fractured several times, and could not breathe via his nasal airway. He demonstrated periods of silence, noisy breathing, and restlessness (Video 23).

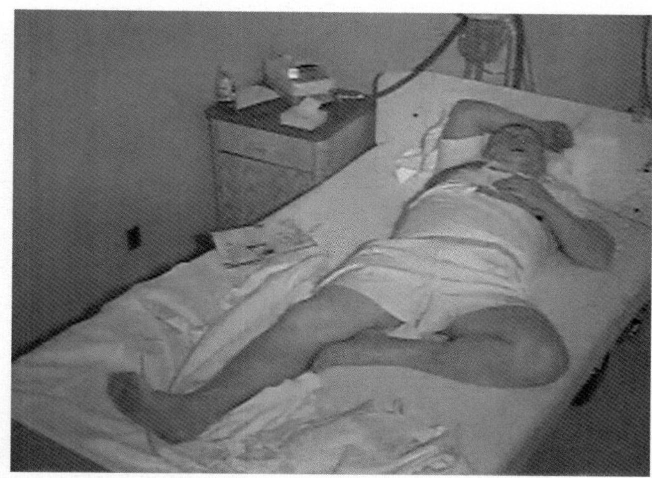

AROUSAL THRESHOLD TO NOISE IN OSA

This patient with sleep apnea is snoring loudly and sleeping on his side when a fire alarm goes off. The patient does not arouse and awaken in response to the noise (Video 24).

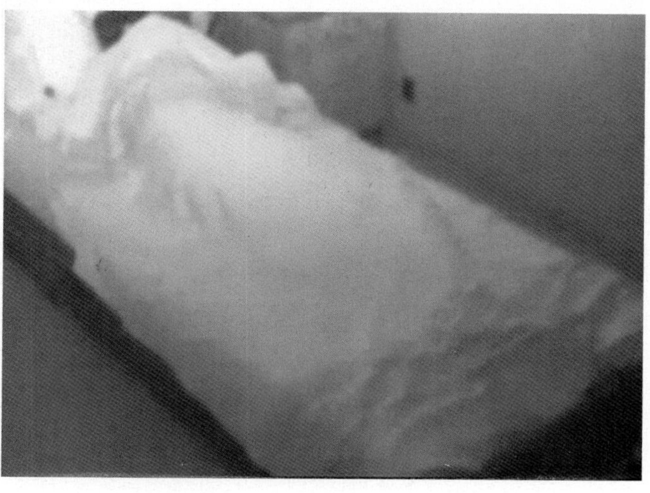

OSA, VIOLENT BODY MOVEMENTS

Excessive body movements linked to the episodes of apnea are evident in this patient with obstructive sleep apnea (OSA) (Video 25).

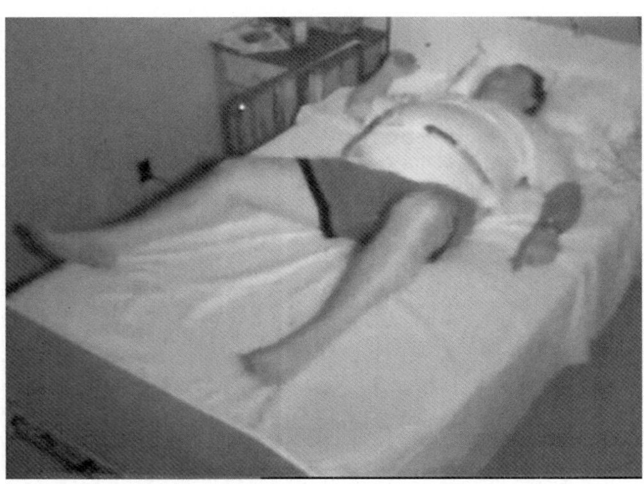

ATYPICAL SNORING POST-UPPP

This patient had uvulopalatopharyngoplasty, which removed part of the soft palate. The patient continued to have sleep apnea, but the snoring noises were atypical and quite different than preoperatively (Video 27).

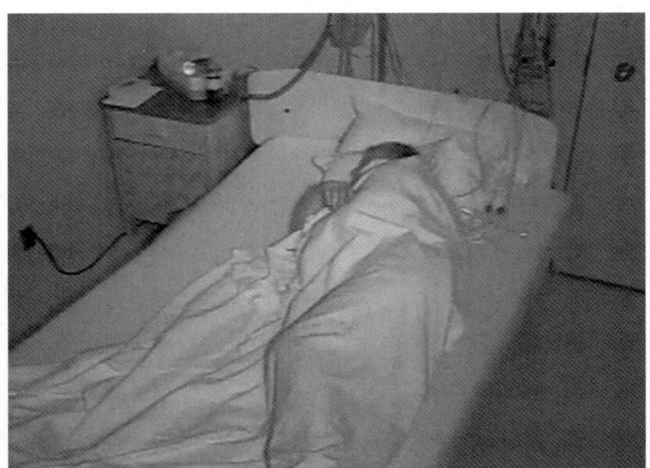

OSA, VIOLENT BODY MOVEMENTS × 10

In this same patient with OSA, this video is sped up by a factor of 10 to better show the frequency and vigor of the movements (Video 26).

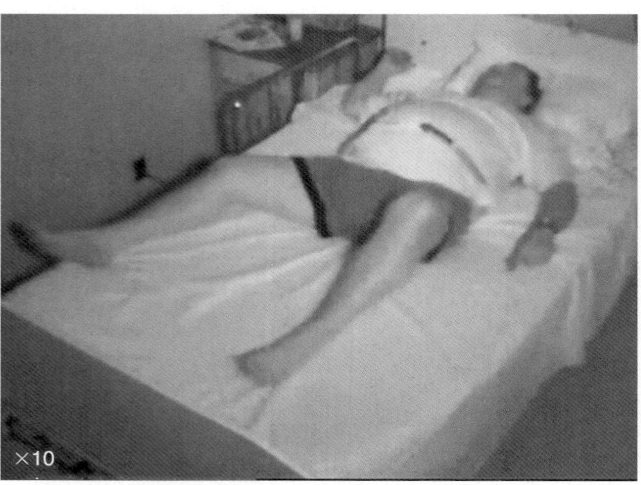

VIGOROUS MOVEMENTS IN OSA × 10

In many patients with sleep apnea, there are vigorous movements often associated with the apnea. These sometimes result in the patient being diagnosed as having periodic limb movements disorder. These movements often resolve with treatment. This clip has been sped up by a factor of 10 (Video 28).

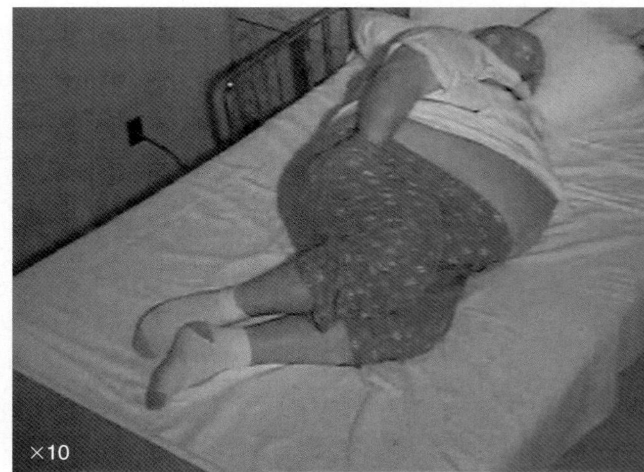

Obstructive Sleep Apnea in Special Populations

OBESITY HYPOVENTILATION

This patient had obesity hypoventilation syndrome and evidence of both obstructive apnea and hypoventilation (Video 29).

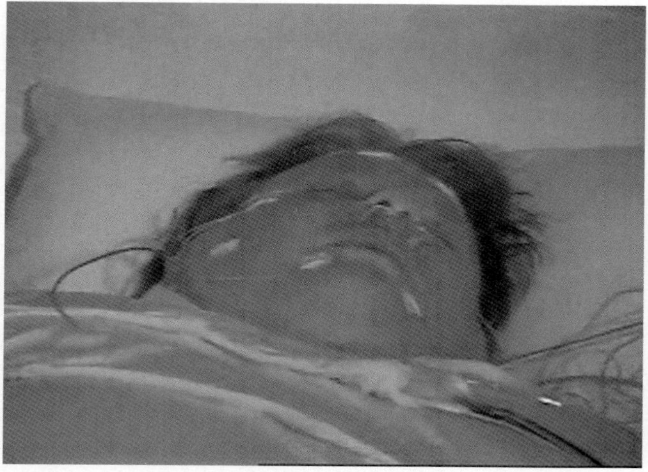

OBESITY HYPOVENTILATION, TREATED

The same patient was treated with bilevel pressure with an excellent response (Video 31).

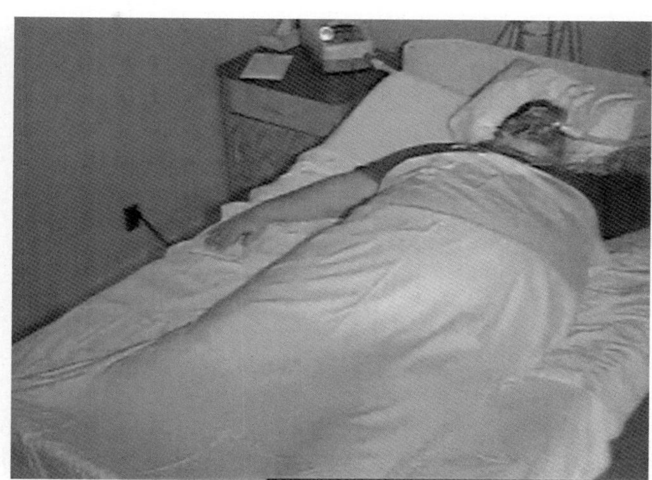

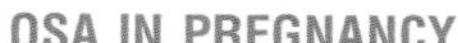

OBESITY HYPOVENTILATION, HEART FAILURE

The same patient as above had the features of severe right-sided heart failure with massive peripheral edema. During times when he hypoventilates, he is relatively quiet. When obstructed, he demonstrates chest wall abdominal paradox and then loud snoring (Video 30).

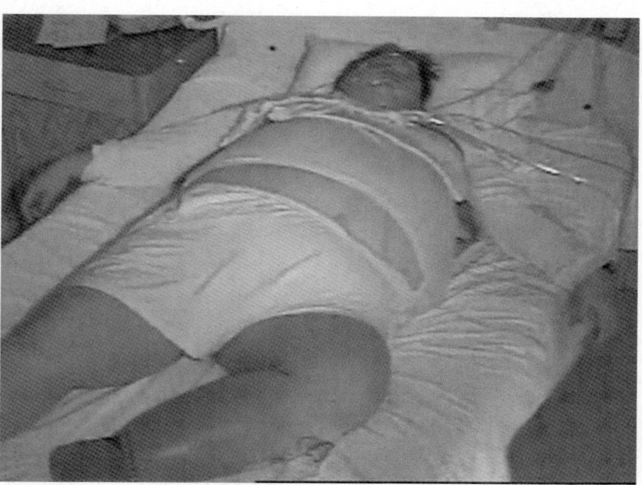

OSA IN PREGNANCY

This pregnant woman had severe obstructive apnea related to obesity. She had a very high breathing frequency that was especially noticeable during unobstructed breathing (Video 32).

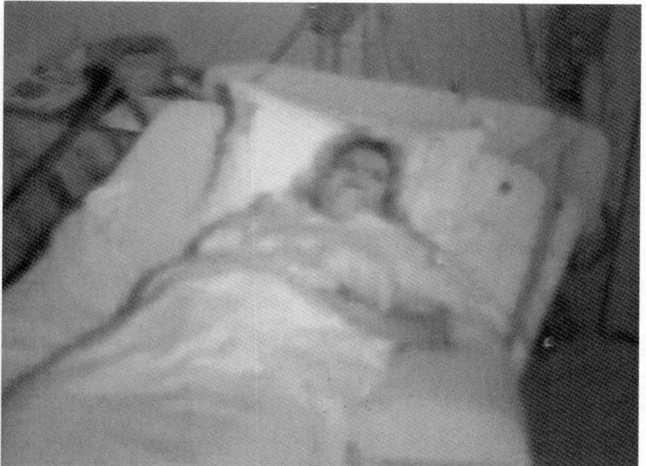

OSA POSTPARTUM

This woman was 4 months' postpartum and had difficulty caring for her new baby. She had had undiagnosed apnea for years. A previous pregnancy ended with a miscarriage (Video 33).

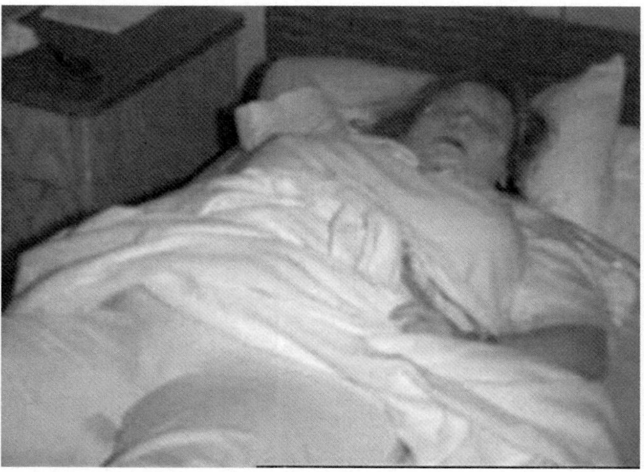

OSA POSTPARTUM ON TREATMENT

The same patient as above is on continuous positive airway pressure (CPAP) and sleeps with her mouth closed. The CPAP is much quieter than her snoring (Video 34).

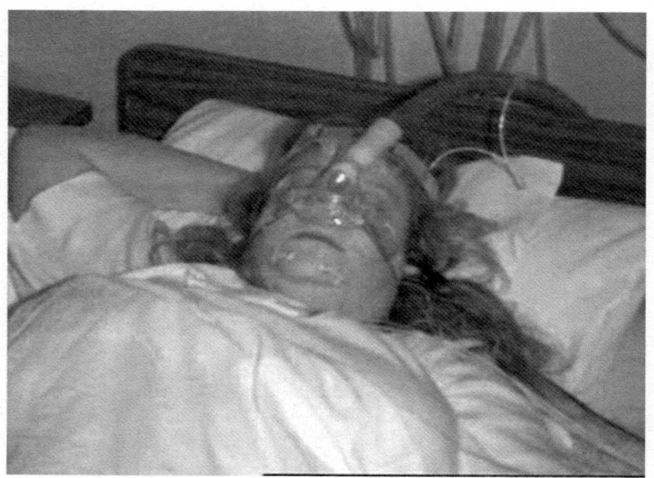

APNEA IN ACROMEGALY

This 71-year-old woman had acromegaly with abnormalities in her jaw structure and an enlarged tongue. She had stridor noted (Video 35).

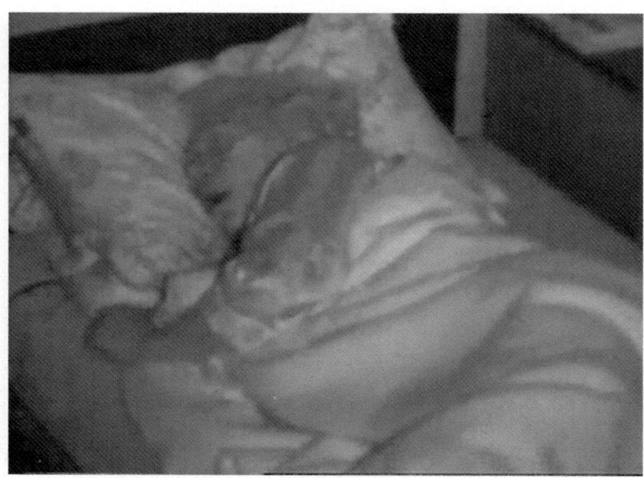

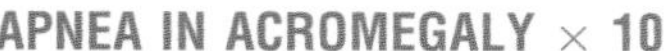

APNEA IN ACROMEGALY × 10

In the same patient with acromegaly, the video has been sped up by a factor of 10 to show the marked movements of the jaw during sleep (Video 36).

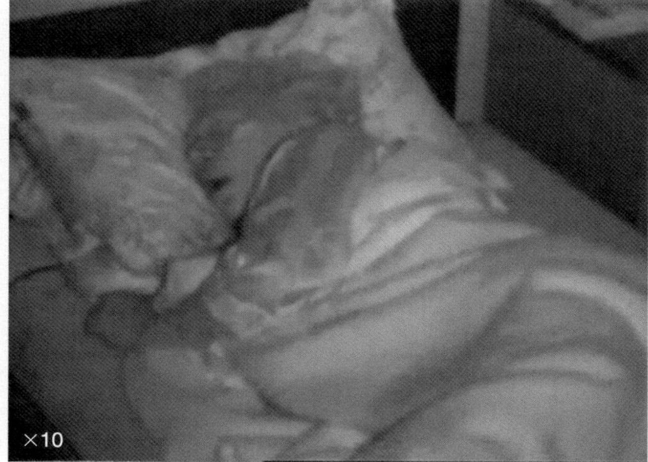

APNEA AND DOWN SYNDROME

Sleep apnea is common in children and adults with Down syndrome (Video 37).

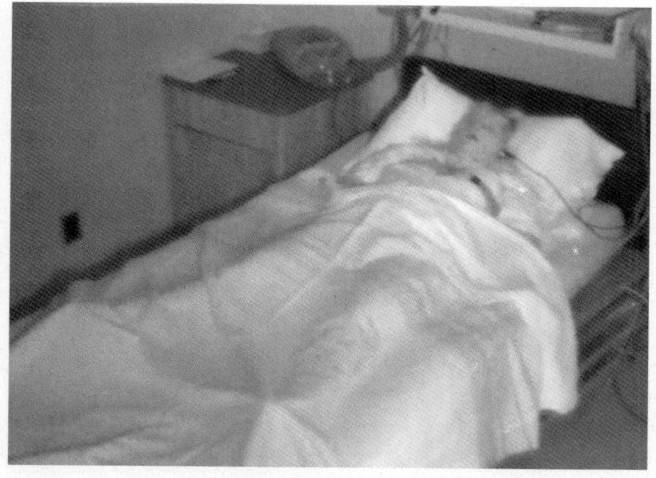

UARS, QUIET SNORING × 7

This is the same patient with UARS with the clip sped up by a factor of 7. Note the movements of the jaw at the beginning and the end of the clip and that she closes her mouth to reestablish breathing (Video 39).

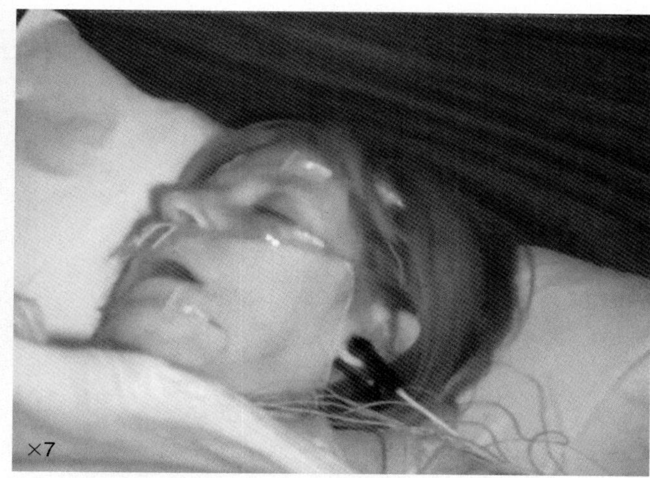

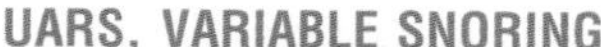

Upper Airway Resistance Syndrome

UARS, QUIET SNORING

This woman has upper airway resistance syndrome (UARS). Notice the initially quiet and high-pitched snoring noises. Notice at 1 minute 10 seconds she closes her mouth and moves her head to reestablish breathing. When the patient breathes via her mouth, the nasal sensor will not detect the breaths (Video 38).

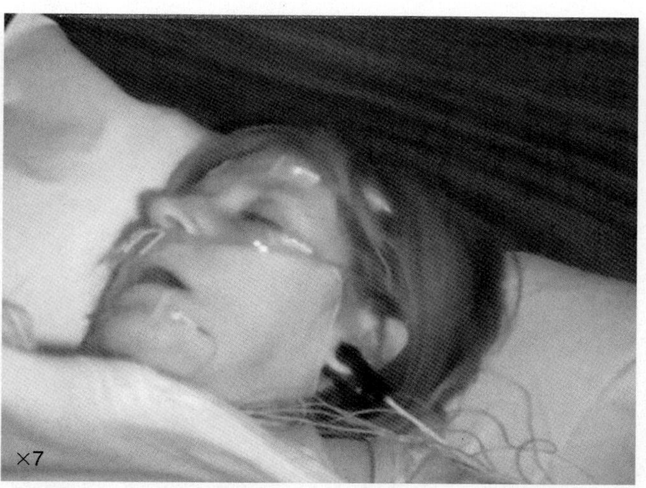

UARS, VARIABLE SNORING

This patient had UARS and snoring with different sounds. Note that the sensor over the mouth is likely to miss when he breathes via his mouth. Notice that at the end of the clip he reestablishes unobstructed breathing (Video 40).

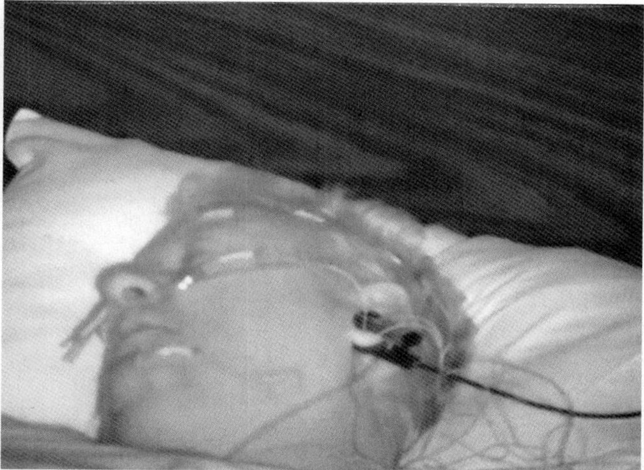

UARS, VARIABLE SNORING × 5

The same patient with UARS with the clip sped up by a factor of 5. At such high speed, the movements of the mouth and jaw become apparent in this patient with upper airway resistance syndrome (Video 41).

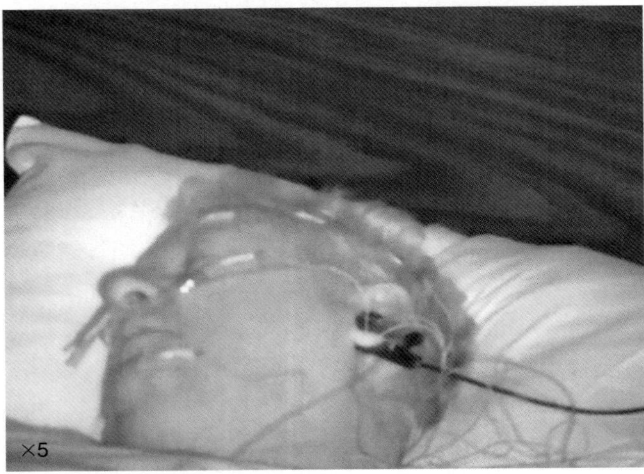

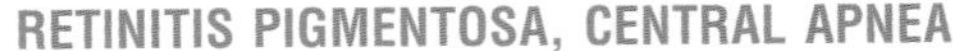

RETINITIS PIGMENTOSA, CENTRAL APNEA

An older male with retinitis pigmentosa had severe central apnea. There is little effort to breathe during the episodes (Video 43).

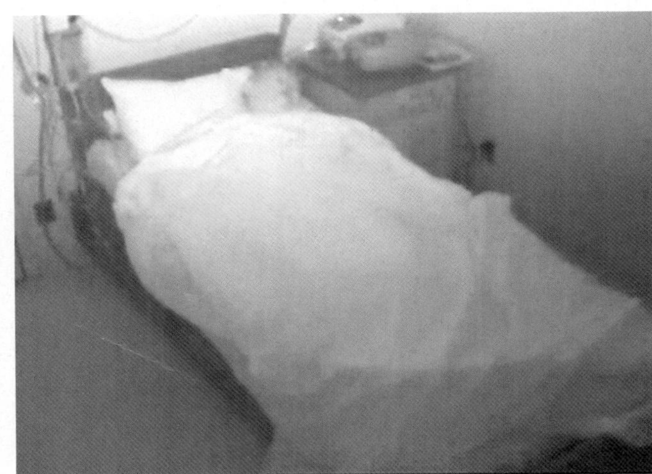

Central Sleep Apnea and Cheyne Stokes Respiration

IDIOPATHIC CENTRAL APNEA

This young adult male had idiopathic central apnea. During apnea there is virtually no effort to breathe. At apnea termination there is sometimes a snort (Video 42).

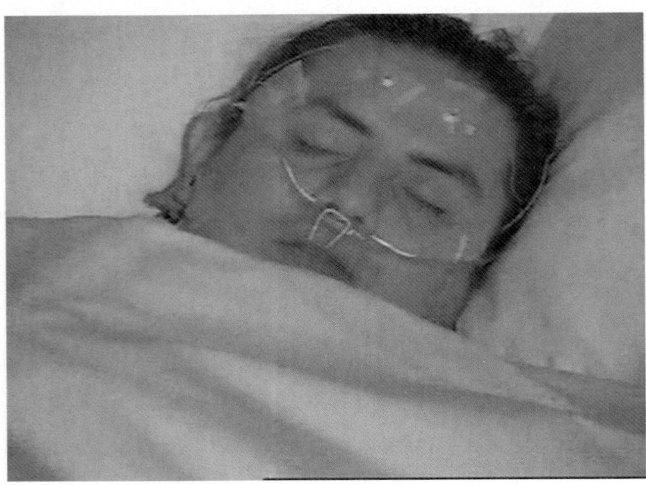

CENTRAL APNEA, OBESITY

An obese male with symptoms of obstructive apnea was found to have primarily central apnea. Note the deep unobstructed breaths after apnea termination (Video 44).

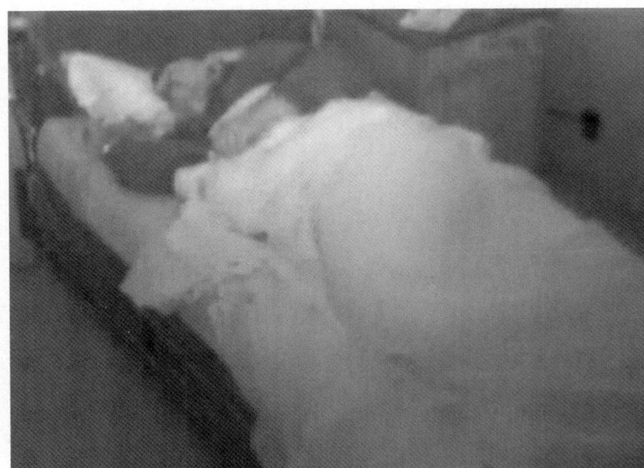

OSA AND CHEYNE STOKES BREATHING

This patient with obstructive apnea developed heart failure, which led to Cheyne Stokes breathing. Thus the patient had evidence of two types of abnormal breathing patterns and pathology (Video 45).

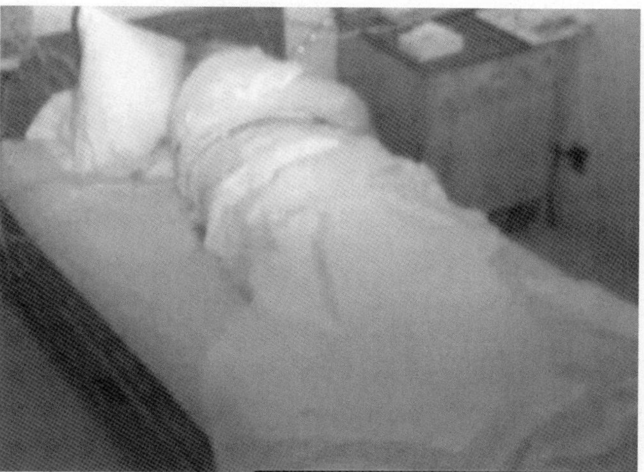

Respiratory Diseases

ASTHMA

Patients with asthma wheeze on expiration. This obese patient with asthma makes loud inspiratory snoring noises and higher-pitched expiratory wheezing sounds (Video 47).

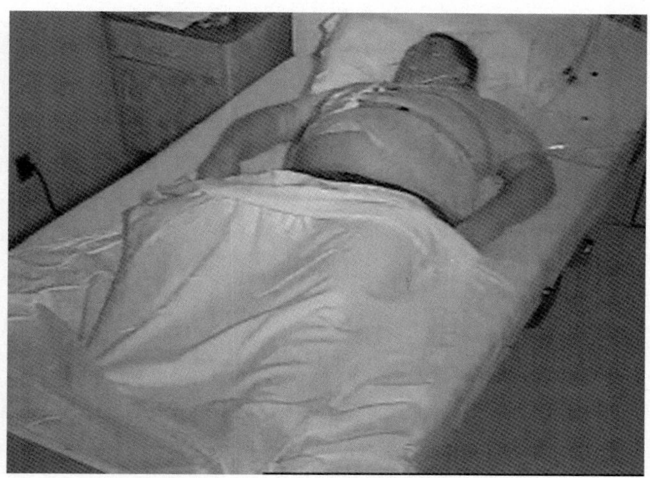

PULMONARY EDEMA

This patient has obstructive sleep apnea and pulmonary edema caused by left heart failure. He had Cheyne Stokes breathing while awake and asleep. The loud gurgling noises are made by the edema fluid (Video 46).

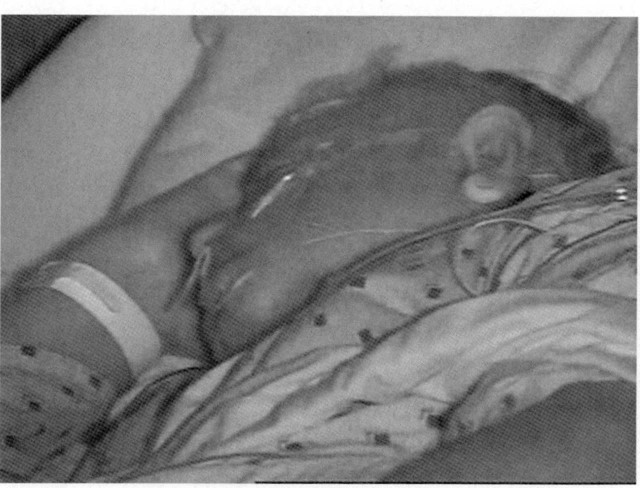

COPD

This chronic obstructive pulmonary disease (COPD) patient made loud sounds on expiration (from his lung disease) that could be confused with inspiratory snoring (Video 48).

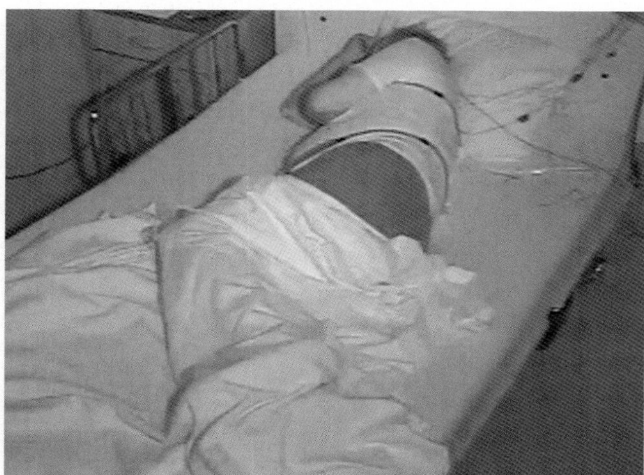

COPD, UPPER AIRWAY OBSTRUCTION

This is the same COPD patient as above. Here the sounds are inspiratory due to upper airway obstruction (Video 49).

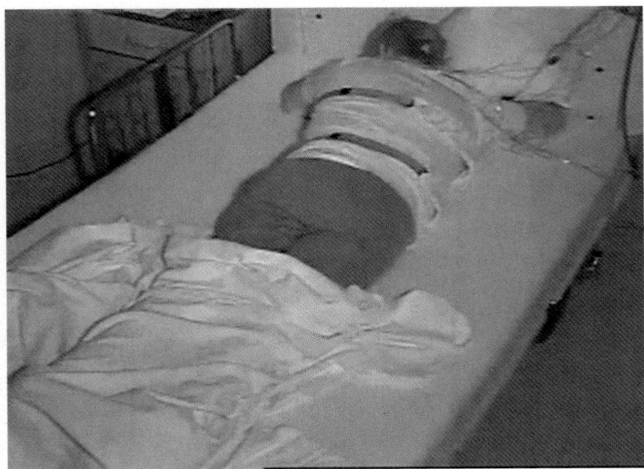

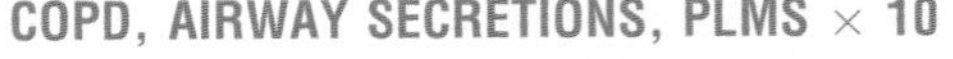

COPD, AIRWAY SECRETIONS, PLMS × 10

This is the same COPD patient as above. The video has been sped up by a factor of 10 to make the periodic movements more apparent. Look at the patient's feet beneath the cover (Video 51).

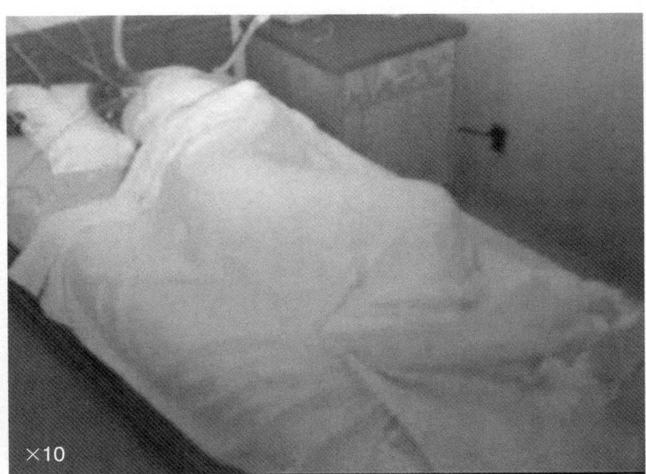

COPD, AIRWAY SECRETIONS, PLMS

This COPD patient has poor-quality sleep because of secretions in her airways that make her breathing noisy. She also has periodic limb movements disorder (Video 50).

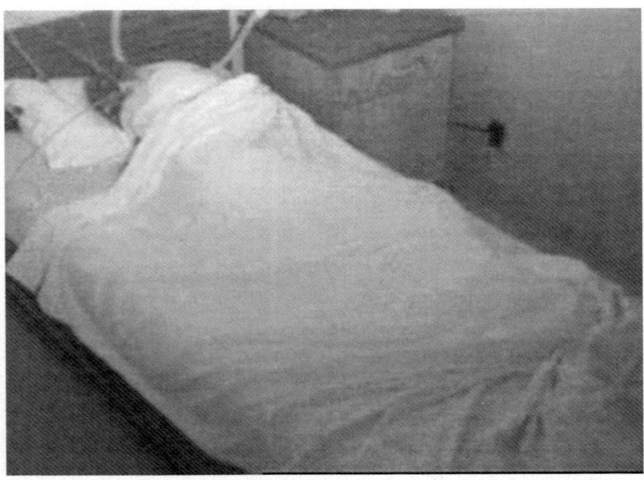

OVERLAP SYNDROME

This patient has the overlap syndrome, the combination of COPD and obstructive sleep apnea. This clip in REM sleep shows the patient hypoventilating. Toward the end of the clip the upper airway obstruction becomes more apparent (Video 52).

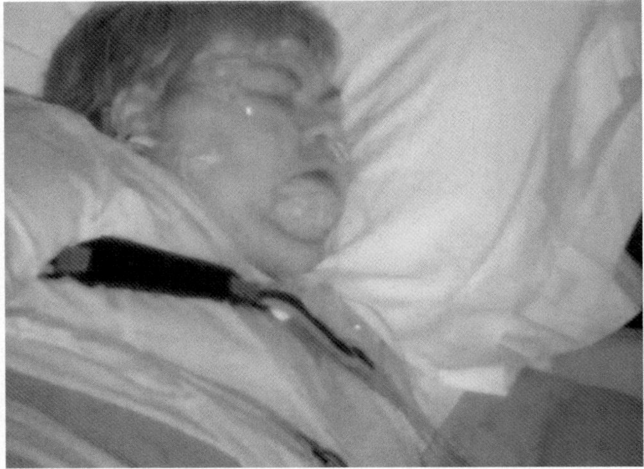

OVERLAP SYNDROME ON TREATMENT

The same patient with overlap syndrome is being treated with bilevel positive airway pressure and oxygen. One can hear the machine generating the pressure changes (Video 53).

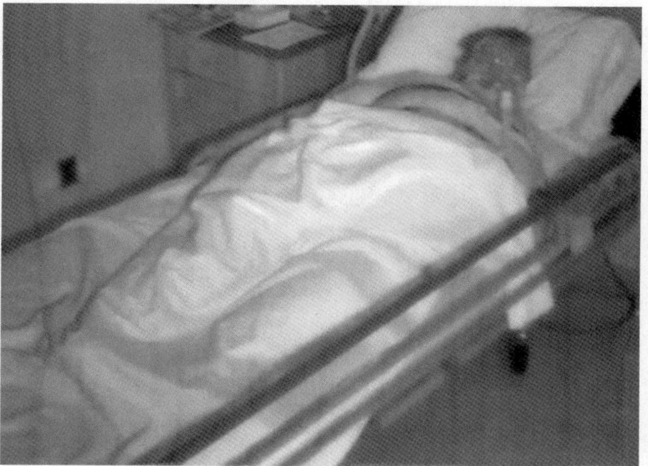

PULMONARY FIBROSIS

This patient has severe interstitial pulmonary fibrosis caused by rheumatoid lung disease. This shows severe dyspnea, and the patient had difficulty achieving persistent sleep (Video 54).

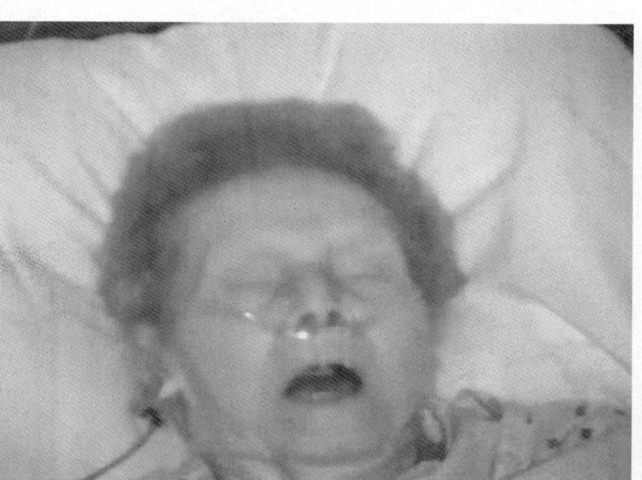

Neurologic and Other Disorders

RLS, INSOMNIA

This patient had sleepiness and obesity, which were thought to be caused by sleep apnea. Her main problem was severe restless legs syndrome (RLS), which led to her being awake for much of the night (Video 55).

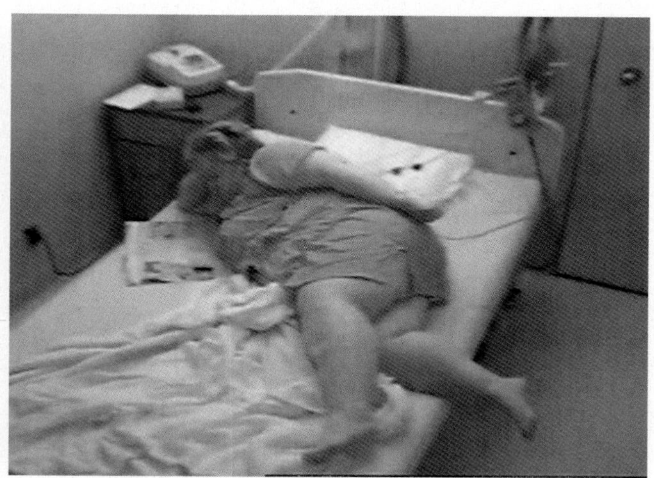

RLS AND PLM × 25

This patient with restless legs syndrome was originally referred for sleep apnea. Her problem ended up being a movement disorder caused by iron deficiency (ferritin level was 12). Note that she keeps her feet exposed in this video, sped up 25 times to show the periodic limb movements (PLM) in sleep (Video 56).

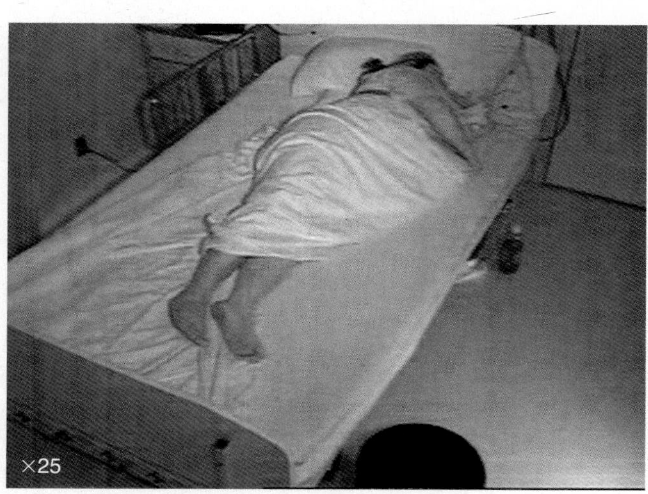

RLS, SLEEP APNEA

Restless legs syndrome in a patient with sleep apnea. The irresistible urge to move the legs and the onset of obstructed breathing cause sleep-onset insomnia in this patient (Video 57).

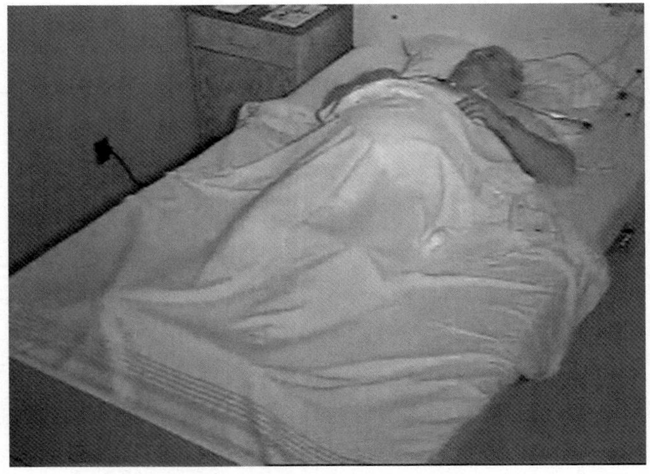

PLMD, APNEA × 10

Periodic limb movements disorder masquerading as sleep apnea. The patient had frequent movements and movements that resulted in overbreathing followed by apnea. Video sped up by a factor of 10 (Video 59).

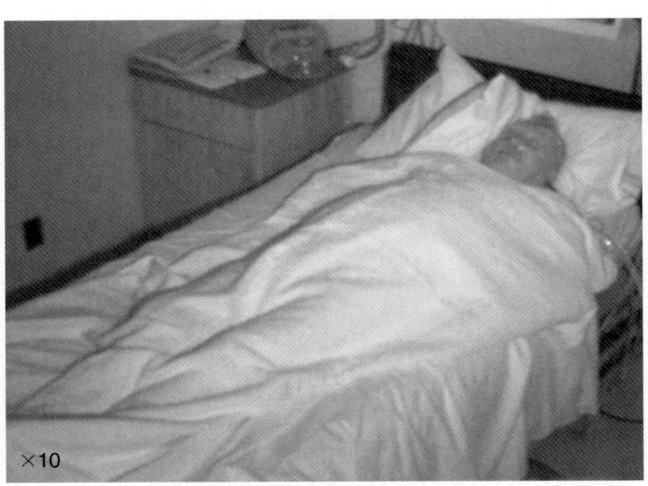

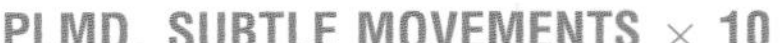

RLS, SLEEP APNEA × 10

Same patient as above. The video has been sped up to emphasize the frequency and severity of the movements (Video 58).

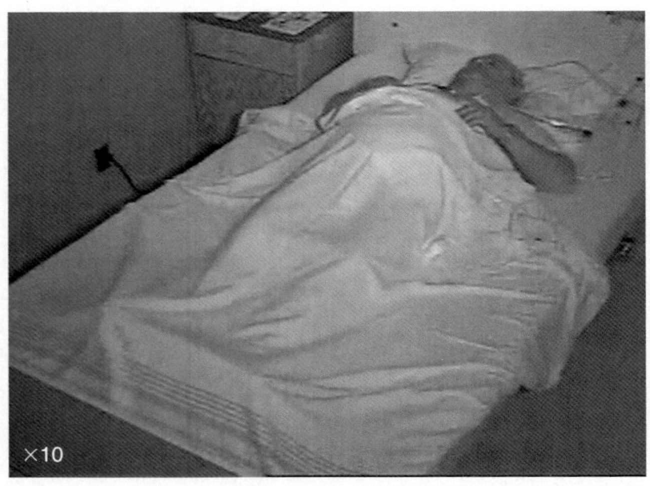

PLMD, SUBTLE MOVEMENTS × 10

In the same patient as above, this video sped up by a factor of 10 shows more subtle movements in the legs (Video 60).

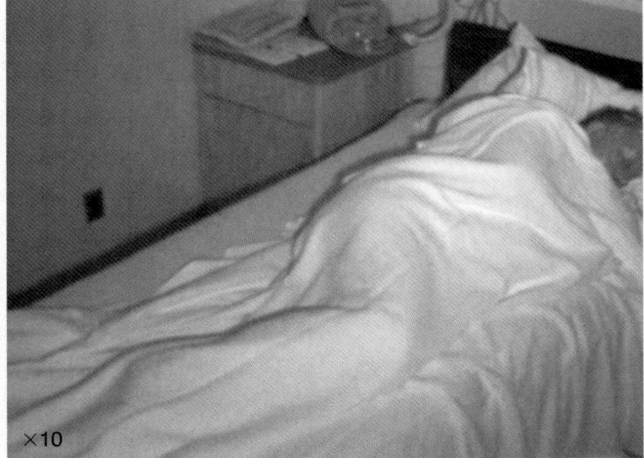

REM SLEEP BEHAVIOR DISORDER

This patient had REM behavior disorder. At times the movements during REM can be subtle, as in this study. This is REM sleep. Notice the movement of the right hand toward the end of the clip (Video 61).

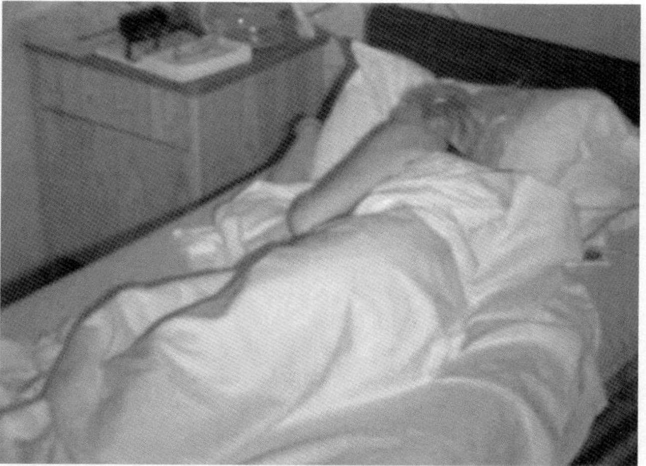

SLEEP PARALYSIS

Sleep paralysis in a patient without narcolepsy. The patient recalled trying to call the technician but was heard only to moan. REMs were present throughout this segment (Video 63).

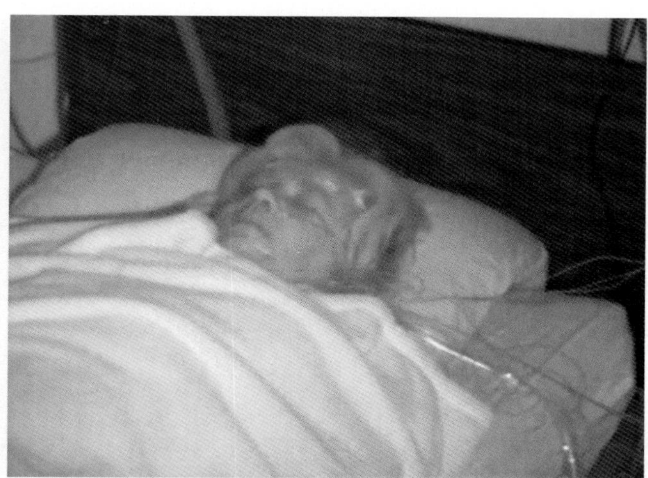

REM SLEEP BEHAVIOR DISORDER, OSA

This patient had OSA and was being treated with CPAP. This treatment, which restores more normal sleep and amounts of stages R and N3 sleep, may unmask parasomnia. This patient developed REM sleep behavior disorder on CPAP (Video 62).

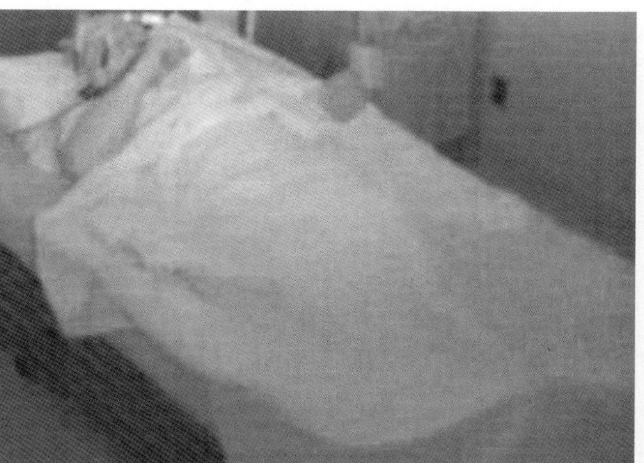

DELAYED SLEEP PHASE SYNDROME

Delayed sleep phase. This is a time-lapse clip of the entire night of a patient referred for severe sleep-onset insomnia. Notice the activities during the night, including watching a movie on a laptop. Once asleep, all findings were normal (Video 64).

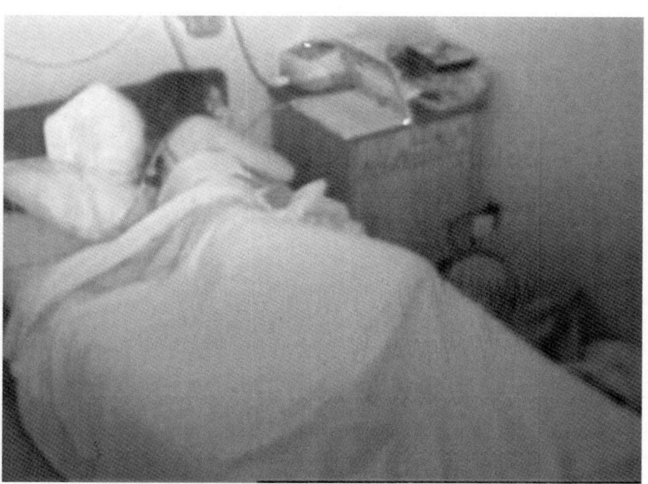

EPILEPSY

This patient had two seizures during the night. One was at about 12:29 A.M. and another at about 2:15 A.M. (Video 65).

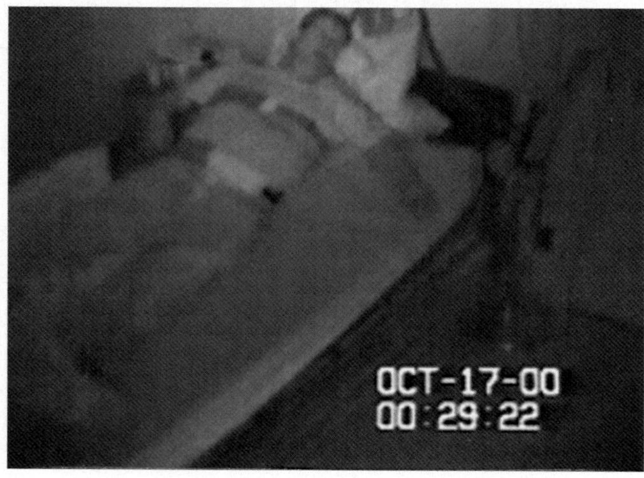

PSYCHOGENIC "SEIZURES"

This patient presented with "seizures" during sleep. This video clip is sped up to emphasize the movements. This patient had psychiatric problems, and it was concluded that she was "simulating" seizures. She was awake during this clip (Video 67).

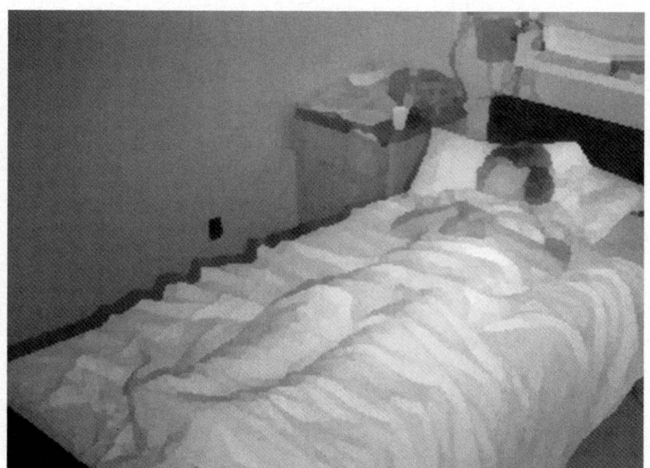

SEIZURE INVOLVING LEG

This patient had a history of seizures. During a multiple sleep latency test, she had a seizure that resulted in movement only of her right leg (Video 66).

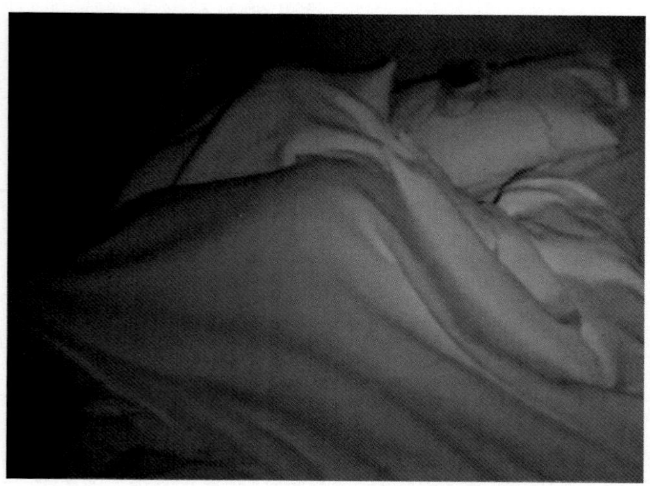

PSYCHOGENIC "SEIZURES," EDGE ENHANCED

The same patient and video clip as above modified to show additional detail. Note that during the seizure, she at times straightens her hair (Video 68).

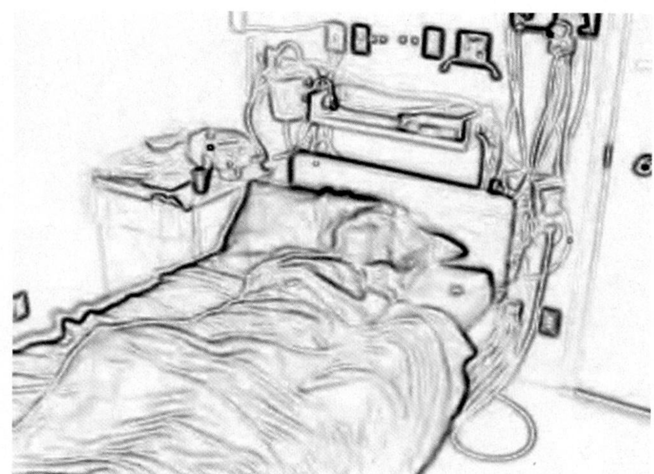

Index

Page numbers followed by *f* indicate figures; those followed by *t* indicate tables; those followed by *b* indicate boxes.